HANDBOOK OF PHARMACY HEALTH-CARE
Diseases and Patient Advice

HANDBOOK OF PHARMACY HEALTH-CARE

Diseases and Patient Advice

Editor
Robin J. Harman

Editorial Staff
Gail C. Neathercoat *and* Prakash Gotecha

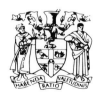

London
THE PHARMACEUTICAL PRESS
1990

Copies of this book may be obtained through any good bookseller or, in any case of difficulty, direct from the publisher or the publisher's agents:

The Pharmaceutical Press
(publications division of the Royal Pharmaceutical Society of Great Britain)
1 Lambeth High Street, London SE1 7JN, England

Australia
The Australian Pharmaceutical Publishing Co. Ltd
40 Burwood Road, Hawthorn, Victoria 3122;

and

Pharmaceutical Society of Australia
Pharmacy House, PO Box 21, Curtin, ACT 2605

Japan
Maruzen Co. Ltd
3–10 Nihonbashi 2-chome, Chuo-ku, Tokyo 103

New Zealand
The Pharmaceutical Society of New Zealand
124 Dixon Street, PO Box 11–640, Wellington

U.S.A.
Rittenhouse Book Distributors, Inc.
511 Feheley Drive, King of Prussia, Pennsylvania 19406

CONTENTS

PREFACE

The *Handbook of Pharmacy Health-care: Diseases and Patient Advice* is produced by direction of the Council of the Royal Pharmaceutical Society of Great Britain, and is one of a new series of books to replace the *Pharmaceutical Handbook* (19th Edition, 1980) and *The Pharmaceutical Codex* (11th Edition, 1979). This new '*Handbook*' comprises completely new material, and covers the fundamentals of disease, the provision of patient advice, symptoms and disease identification, and a comprehensive glossary of medical terms.

Historically, the *Pharmaceutical Handbook* evolved from the *Pharmacy Students' Pocket Note-book* (first published in 1906) through *The Pharmacy Students' Guide* and *The Pharmaceutical Pocket Book*. The 19th Edition of the *Pharmaceutical Handbook* was primarily intended as a companion volume to *Martindale: The Extra Pharmacopoeia*. The '*Handbook*' provided a tremendous variety of information for practising pharmacists, including background and easily accessible tabulated information on chemical nomenclature, pharmaceutics, disease names, and drug absorption. The preparation and supply of medicines and the types of medicinal products were also covered in considerable detail. Chapters on sterilisation, immunology, and microbiology complemented the discussions of fundamental topics, and understanding was further encouraged by a range of glossaries (including synonyms, and medical and pharmaceutical terms).

The Pharmaceutical Codex has had an equally distinguished history. From its origins in 1907 as *The British Pharmaceutical Codex (BPC)*, editions containing standards for a wide range of preparations that could be made extemporaneously in the pharmacy were published at regular intervals under the same title until the 1973 edition. The change in name and content at that time was a consequence of the request of the Medicines Commission (formed as a result of the Medicines Act 1968) that all official standards for drugs should be published in a single volume rather than distributed between the *British Pharmacopoeia* and the *BPC*. The Council of the Society agreed to the change of status of the *BPC*, and for the 11th edition it was retitled *The Pharmaceutical Codex*. The prime function of the new (1979) edition was as a compendium of drug information. However, it significantly diversified its scope by also including the causes, signs, symptoms, and treatment of many common diseases; various aspects of clinical pharmacy (e.g. advice to patients and drug metabolism); details of chromatographic and spectrophotometric analyses of drugs and their metabolites; and information on bioavailability and pharmacokinetics.

The content of both the '*Handbook*' and '*The Codex*' had evolved arbitrarily in response to need, and the opportunity has now been taken to rationalise the content of the replacement volumes. At the time of planning further editions of each of these two volumes, it was recognised that considerable changes had taken place in the practice of pharmacy since the publication of the most recent editions of the '*Handbook*' and '*The Codex*'. Whilst remaining an important function in manufacturing units within hospital pharmacy, and of occasional importance in community pharmacy, the traditional expertise required by pharmacists in the production of extemporaneous medicines has been almost completely replaced by the supply of products from the pharmaceutical industry. It is likely that, with the advent of increased legislation to ensure that producers are liable for defective products (e.g. the Consumer Protection Act 1987 in the UK) and the consequent trend towards original pack dispensing, such basic skills will inevitably be in less demand.

Whereas many pharmacists may view the demise of their traditional role with regret, the opportunities that it also creates cannot be underestimated. At the time at which compounding of medicines was at its zenith (possibly around the time of the birth of the NHS in 1948), almost all available drugs were generic and required full use of pharmacists' skills in preparation. Since that time, the numbers and range of therapeutic products available have grown dramatically until, in 1989, the *British National Formulary (BNF)* contains monographs for over 1000 drugs. The vast majority of these drugs are contained in products manufactured by the industry. Over the same period, the number of prescriptions dispensed in the UK has risen from 225 million in 1949 to 397 million in 1987. The corresponding number of pharmacies decreased from 12 883 in 1949 to 11 621 in 1987, indicating a rise over 40 years in prescriptions per pharmacy from 17 465 to 33 000.

What are the opportunities that all these facts and figures represent? One of the most important factors in pharmacy today is that considerably less time is now spent dispensing each prescription (estimates range from 5 to 7 minutes, but clearly this calculated average is subject to wide variation). With the introduction of original pack dispensing, it is likely that this 'average' time will be further reduced, releasing pharmacists from the workbench and allowing them to adopt a more positive and pro-active (as opposed to reactive) approach in, for example, talking to patients. What is possibly a more important measure than time spent on each prescription is the overall amount of time that pharmacists can allocate to a particular patient who presents a prescription or seeks advice. Pharmacists should be prepared to discuss all matters of concern that patients may raise about their illnesses and their treatment, and to advise patients on general health matters when such opportunities arise.

However, in order to communicate confidently and effectively with patients, pharmacists must possess knowledge not only of the medicines that patients are receiving but also of the diseases for which those medicines are prescribed. The primary aim of **Part A** of the *Handbook of Pharmacy Health-care: Diseases and Patient Advice* is to provide a comprehensive but concise account of a wide range of diseases for which medicines are prescribed, or for which non-prescription medicines are purchased. Because the range is intended to be comprehensive, many of the diseases included are unlikely to be encountered on a regular basis. However, their inclusion is justified on the grounds of completeness and because incidents can occur in which a particular disease may achieve prominence. Examples of less common diseases that have gained ephemeral, but prominent, publicity in the last 12 months include outbreaks of legionellosis and of listeriosis. There will no doubt be many more examples in the future. By using the '*Handbook*', pharmacists can obtain a concise summary of the causes, symptoms, and treatment, and provide information to members of the public to help put into perspective the frequently emotive reports in the media.

The role that the media play in highlighting health issues is complex[1]. Because of their personal, and sometimes dramatic, appeal, health matters are attractive to the media. On the one hand, promotion of the positive aspects of health, and creation of an open and frank discussion on emotive health topics (e.g. heart, lung, and liver transplants, and abortion), can make a positive contribution to health. On the other hand, however, sensationalised and unbalanced reports on health matters

have considerable potential for harm. People's expectations (e.g. of a particular form of treatment) are unwarrantably raised, and the ready availability of pharmacists to the general public makes them an early target for enquiries. Many pharmacists will be only too familiar with the image of the patient entering the pharmacy carrying a newspaper cutting which suggests some new form of treatment, or 'explains' aspects of life-style relating to health. In order to be able to respond constructively and effectively in such situations, pharmacists must obviously possess a sound and broad scientific and medical knowledge-base.

One of the significant purposes in producing a book orientated towards 'patient' aspects of pharmacy, rather than the more commonly produced 'drug-related' aspects, is to encourage pharmacists to remember the basic concept that all those receiving drugs and medicines are people, and not solely patients. As such, each individual brings to the pharmacy a complete range of unique experiences and characteristics. In the provision of medicines, pharmacists must remember the likely circumstances that have brought that person (who has now become classed as a patient) to the pharmacy. Patients may be unwell themselves, or a person may be concerned about a friend or relative who is unwell. At such times of stress, people can become confused and can act irrationally and sometimes unreasonably.

In recognition of this awareness of individuality and personality, the aim of **Part B** of the book is to direct pharmacists towards the most effective ways in which they can apply the knowledge outlined in **Part A**. The emphasis is on particular groups (i.e. the very young and the elderly) who provide a range of specific management problems. In coping with these and other problems in the pharmacy, pharmacists and all health-care professionals must be able to communicate effectively with patients, and at the same time impart the information that patients require in a professional manner. Equally importantly, pharmacists must be able to **listen**, and be aware of questions that patients may ask which can have a more fundamental meaning than the spoken words suggest. Enquiries from patients about use of medicines can, on occasion, mask the unspoken desire to know more about the illness that confronts them, and which is perhaps the most important factor in their life at that time. Obviously, pharmacists must approach such requests for further information with sensitivity, but the great satisfaction that pharmacists as individuals can derive from the knowledge that they have been of assistance to another person is one of the foundation stones of good professional practice.

One of the most significant recent events in pharmacy, which has acted as a focus and impetus for the development of pharmacy practice in the UK, has been the Nuffield Report of 1986[2]. Throughout production of this book, many of the recommendations and conclusions of the report have been consistently borne in mind. Recommendations concerning community and hospital pharmacy, and educational recommendations, have significant implications for the future of pharmacy. Those recommendations which have been considered in this book include greater collaboration with other health-care professionals, greater personal involvement with the public in giving advice on taking of medicines, involvement in the treatment of individual patients that does not conflict with the responsibilities of the clinician, development of communication skills, and inclusion of training in pathology.

Although it is obvious that pharmacists do not normally enter the minefield of diagnosis (primarily because they are not trained for that role), an awareness of the range of possible diseases that may cause a particular symptom can be a useful tool when supplying medicines and talking to patients. In responding to symptoms (*see* Section 20.3), pharmacists must be able to distinguish between those signs which are symptomatic of potentially serious diseases, and those which reflect 'trivial' illness. As a quick reference guide, and using the information covered in Chapters 1 to 13, **Part C** lists all symptoms mentioned in the disease monographs and the diseases in which these symptoms can occur.

Although pharmacists are correctly seen as specialists in drug knowledge, the future development of the profession and its usefulness within the overall framework of the health-care team requires that this specialist knowledge should be supplemented by a knowledge of the language of other professions. An understanding of medical terminology is therefore vital to be able to communicate with medical practitioners and other clinicians on equal terms, and this subject is addressed in **Part D** of the book.

1. A. Karpf, *Doctoring the Media: The Reporting of Health and Medicine*, London, Routledge, 1988

2. *Pharmacy: The Report of a Committee of Inquiry appointed by the Nuffield Foundation*, London, The Nuffield Foundation, 1986

Acknowledgements

Certain Chapters of the *Handbook* were written by external authors, and the invaluable contribution of the following experts is gratefully acknowledged:

Clive Edwards, BPharm, PhD, MRPharmS
Responding to Symptoms

Roger Hicks,
MPharm, PhD, MRPharmS, FRCPath
General Pathology *and* Pathophysiology

Michael H. Jepson, BPharm, MSc, FRPharmS
Communication, Counselling, and Compliance

To confirm the accuracy of the medical information, the content of each of the disease monographs in Chapters 1 to 13 was reviewed by Dr B.J. Whitby-Smith, MBBS, MRCS, LRCP, MRCGP, DRCOG, a general practitioner in Ash Vale, Aldershot, Hampshire. I am grateful to Dr Whitby-Smith for carrying out this task efficiently and for making many useful suggestions.

All diagrams are reproduced from the *Sourcebook of Medical Illustration*, Parthenon Publishing, 1989; the co-operation of the editor, Peter Cull, is acknowledged.

Photographs were supplied by St Bartholomew's Hospital, London.

It is a pleasure to acknowledge the commitment and enthusiasm of the editorial staff, Gail Neathercoat, BSc, MRPharmS and Prakash Gotecha, BSc, MRPharmS. I am also delighted to acknowledge the contribution made by John Martin, BPharm, PhD, MRPharmS, who was temporarily seconded to the project. The contribution of Irvine J.C. MacKenzie, BSc, MRPharmS and Janet M. Batson, BSc, CChem, MRSC in the earlier stages of production is also gratefully acknowledged. The secretarial assistance provided by Miss Thelma M. Roberts has been greatly appreciated.

Especial thanks are due to the Director, W.G. Thomas, MSc, PhD, FRPharmS and other staff of the Department of Pharmaceutical Sciences, including Ainley Wade, BPharm, MPhil, FRPharmS, General Editor of Scientific Publications. The support given by Pamela North, BPharm, MRPharmS, MIInfSc and all the staff of the library has been a much valued asset.

Robin J. Harman, BPharm, PhD, MRPharmS

January 1990

PART A
FUNDAMENTALS OF DISEASE

INTRODUCTION

Pharmacists have traditionally been involved almost exclusively with the therapeutic use of drugs, and their expertise in this field is well recognised. However, this role cannot be considered in isolation from an awareness of the diseases for which drugs are administered. To provide this essential foundation for the use of drugs, **Part A** of the *Handbook of Pharmacy Health-care: Diseases and Patient Advice* details the fundamentals of disease.

A knowledge of the causes and symptoms of disease is an essential prerequisite for an understanding of the rationale for, and mechanisms of, drug treatment, and this fact is used as the basis for therapeutics teaching in many undergraduate pharmacy courses. As part of the learning process it is also useful to be aware of the classification of disease, and recognition of this fact has been adopted as the starting point for the presentation of the disease monographs in **Chapters 1 to 13** inclusive. Diseases have been classified according to their occurrence in the body, using the same classification of body systems as that contained within the British National Formulary (BNF). The reasons for linking this book so closely with the BNF are twofold. Firstly, its frequent use means that many pharmacists are familiar with this classification. By following the same classification, it is hoped that readers will quickly gain familiarity with the '*Handbook*', and its effective use may be expedited. Secondly, a conscious decision was made at the outset of compilation of the '*Handbook*' to omit references to specific examples of drugs used to treat a particular disease. Instead, the reader is referred to the relevant Section in the BNF (usually in an analogous Chapter) where detailed information can be found. Duplication of information is therefore minimised and the clear distinction in emphasis of the two books between diseases and drugs is maintained.

The Chapters containing disease monographs have been subdivided into further classifications. These have been derived from detailed consideration of '*Martindale Thesaurus*' (*Martindale Online: Drug Information Thesaurus and User's Guide*, The Pharmaceutical Press, London, 1984), *The Merck Manual, 15th Edition* (Merck, Sharp, and Dohme, New Jersey, 1987), and the *World Health Organization Manual of the International Statistical Classification of Diseases, Injuries, and Causes of Death (ICD) Volumes 1 and 2* (WHO, Geneva, 1977 and 1978). Where more than one classification could be possible for a particular disease (based on its local manifestation or its occurrence as a complication, or on a generalised underlying disease process), the classification determined by the WHO as the underlying disease process has been selected for this book.

Disease monographs have been written concisely and provide a brief but detailed summary of the major aspects of each disease. Each monograph has been divided into three sections: definition and aetiology, symptoms, and treatment.

The **aetiology** of diseases can be influenced by a wide variety of factors. Infections can be contracted by personal contact with others; environmental causes are becoming increasingly recognised; and genetic predisposition (i.e. autosomal and recessive traits) can be a determining factor (e.g. cystic fibrosis and inborn errors of metabolism).

In recording the **symptoms** of each disease, no attempt has been made to define their relative occurrence, other than to specify whether one or more symptoms is predominant (e.g. diarrhoea in cholera; petechiae in thrombocytopenia). Equally, although non-specific symptoms (e.g. malaise, fatigue, and nausea) are mentioned, by definition their occurrence cannot be definitely correlated with that disease. What is more important is the sequence of development and the range of symptoms which, when considered together, provide a composite picture which is characteristic of a particular disease. Certain disease states benefit from illustration with black-and-white photographs.

To enable pharmacists to recognise the diverse range of diseases of which many common symptoms can be a component, and to assist them in assessing the possible causes of an individual symptom, symptoms recorded in the disease monographs have been collated into **Part C, Symptom and Disease Identification**. A detailed discussion of the criteria for selection of symptoms in this list can be found in the Introduction to Part C.

To emphasise the patient and disease aspects of the book, as opposed to therapeutic aspects, general classes rather than specific examples of drugs are detailed in the **treatment** section of disease monographs. The only exceptions to this general rule are instances where a specific drug is used. For further information, readers are referred to the appropriate Section within the BNF in which detailed data about drugs and their use may be found. **All cross-references specified within the treatment sections are to BNF No. 19 (March 1990).**

Pharmacists are often asked for advice about organisations that patients suffering from a particular condition can join, or from whom information may be sought. The tremendous importance and reassurance that patients can derive from contact with others in a similar predicament should not be underestimated. To help pharmacists readily identify those organisations which have an interest in a particular condition, many disease monographs are supplemented by the names of one or more relevant **self-help organisations**. Full details (including

UK address and telephone number, and a brief summary of aims and services) of all organisations are given in Part B, Chapter 21.

Each Chapter (except Chapters 5 and 8) includes an illustrated description of relevant anatomy and physiology. (An analogous, but more detailed, section designed to complement Chapter 5 can be found in Chapter 14; and morphological descriptions of terms used in Chapter 8 are explained in detail in Section 15.7.) Many pharmacists will have studied biology (including human biology) before entering undergraduate pharmacy, but it was deemed useful to include in each Chapter a brief resumé of those anatomical and physiological systems referred to within the disease monographs. It must be stressed, however, that these sections on anatomy and physiology are not intended to provide a comprehensive discussion of anatomy and physiology, for which there are innumerable excellent specialised textbooks (*see* Selected Bibliography and Reference Sources).

To complement the detailed description of infections covered in Chapter 5, the section in the former *Pharmaceutical Handbook* on 'Microbiology' has been rewritten as Chapter 14, **Medical Microbiology**. It provides background information on the causative agents of infections, stressing the importance of correct classification and nomenclature, and describing the means by which infections are transmitted to humans.

The importance of pathology and pathophysiology in understanding the therapeutic use of drugs has been recognised by the Council of the RPSGB by publication of a report on pathology and therapeutics in pharmacy practice (*Pharm. J.*, 1984, *233*, 240). The study of pathology was considered especially relevant because of the increasing clinical bias of pharmacy practice, and recommendations were made for its inclusion in the pharmacy undergraduate curriculum. It had been previously recognised that pharmacists required a more detailed knowledge of disease states and medical terminology, and that their lack could be an obstacle to the integration of pharmacists in the health-care team.

Chapters 15 and 16 address this problem by providing a detailed, and fully illustrated, discussion of pathology and pathophysiology. The fundamental concept in health is that the human body is continually undergoing adaptation, adjusting to changes in the internal and external environment. Pathology, in contrast, is the study of inappropriate or inadequate adaptation, when the host can turn against itself; in other words, it is the study of what goes wrong. The emphasis in each of these sections on a disturbance of homoeostasis is a necessary prerequisite to understanding the dual roles that many physiological systems and components can play (e.g. the protective role of antibodies on the one hand and their involvement in the aetiology of disease on the other). The activities are in essence the same, but their usefulness to the body has been drastically altered in disease.

Introduction to Anatomy and Physiology

Many of the terms used within the disease monographs refer to anatomical positions in relation to another organ or tissue within the body. Medically, these relationships may be given directional terms, some of which are described below. Organs within the body may also be described in terms of planes or sections, illustrating the direction in which an organ lies or in which vessels pass. All of these terms are based on a person in a standing position looking forward with the palms of the hands facing forward (frontal position), and are commonly grouped in pairs of opposites.

Directional terms

superior	– above or higher, situated nearer to the top of the head
inferior	– below or to the base of the body
anterior/ventral	– closer to or on the front surface of the body
posterior/dorsal	– closer to or on the rear surface of the body
midline	– an imaginary vertical line down the centre of the body
medial	– closer to the midline or the middle portion
lateral	– further away from the midline or towards the side
ipsilateral	– on the same side (of the body)
contralateral	– on the opposing side (of the body)
proximal	– nearer to the point of attachment (e.g. of a limb to the trunk)
distal	– further away from the point of attachment (e.g. the distal convoluted tubule in the kidney is further away from the glomerulus than the proximal convoluted tubule)
superficial	– on or toward the surface of the body or of an organ
deep	– further away from the surface of the body or of an organ

Planes   Medically, nomenclature also exists for the different planes of the body. These imaginary flat surfaces may be considered to dissect the body into regions and may be used to describe the predominant direction in which an organ lies (Fig. 1).

Vertical planes are described as sagittal, and may be midsagittal or parasagittal. A midsagittal plane passes

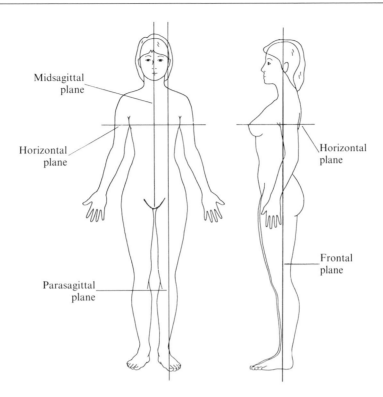

Fig. 1
Planes of the body.

through the midline and divides the body into two equal halves. A parasagittal plane is parallel to the sagittal plane but the division produces two unequal portions. A further vertical division may be considered with the body turned at a right angle to the frontal position. A vertical division down the side of the body produces the frontal plane which divides the body into anterior (front) and posterior (rear) portions.

A horizontal (transverse) plane is situated at right angles to the sagittal plane and divides the body into superior (upper) and inferior (lower) portions.

Common names and anatomical terms   Pharmacists act at the interface between the medical world and the general public. They have to be capable of communication with medical practitioners, nurses, and other medical personnel who may be familiar with a comprehensive medical vocabulary. They also have to be able to impart information to members of the public for whom an aura of mystique, and sometimes confusion, may exist around medical terminology. Pharmacists must therefore be able to readily interconvert medical and lay terminology, and the list below is intended to provide a guide to the most commonly used terms.

Common name	Anatomical term
Head	
head	cephalic
neck	cervical
skull	cranial
face	facial
eye	orbital or ocular
ear	otic
cheek	buccal
nose	nasal
mouth	oral
chin	mental
Trunk – front	
chest	thoracic
breast	mammary
navel	umbilical
hip	coxal
groin	inguinal
pubis	pubic
Trunk – rear	
shoulder	acromial
back	dorsal

Common name	Anatomical term
Trunk – rear (*contd*)	
loin	lumbar
buttock	gluteal
Limbs – upper	
arm pit	axillary
arm	brachial
front of elbow	antecubital
back of elbow	olecranal
forearm	antebrachial
wrist	carpal
palm	metacarpal
thumb	pollex
fingers	digital or phalangeal
anterior surface of hand	palmar or volar
posterior surface of hand	dorsal
Limbs – lower	
thigh	femoral
front of knee	patellar
hollow behind knee	popliteal
leg	crural
calf	sural
ankle	tarsal
toes	digital or phalangeal
great toe	hallux
sole of foot	plantar
heel of foot	calcaneal

Chapter 1

GASTRO-INTESTINAL AND RELATED DISORDERS

1.1 GENERAL DISORDERS

Appendicitis

Definition and aetiology
Appendicitis is acute inflammation of the vermiform appendix, which occurs most commonly in children and young adults. A carcinoid tumour may be the cause through obstruction of the lumen.

Symptoms
It usually starts with referred, colicky, central abdominal pain, which may be only moderately severe; anorexia, nausea and vomiting, and mild fever may develop within 1 to 2 hours of the onset of the pain. Classically, the central pain shifts to the right iliac fossa (Fig. 1.1) within 6 hours, becoming persistent, steady, and localised. The pain is accentuated on movement, deep breathing, and coughing.

Other symptoms include constipation, dysuria, and abdominal tenderness, although diarrhoea is relatively uncommon. Complications include perforation, which may lead to peritonitis, formation of an appendix mass palpable in the right iliac fossa, and abscess formation.

Treatment
Treatment is by appendicectomy.

Colic

Definition and aetiology
Colic consists of spasms of severe griping pain, which increase in intensity to a peak, remit for a short period, and then recur. The condition may arise in the stomach, intestines, kidneys, ureters (*see* Renal Calculi and Colic), or biliary tract (*see* Cholecystitis).

Intestinal colic may be due to relatively trivial causes

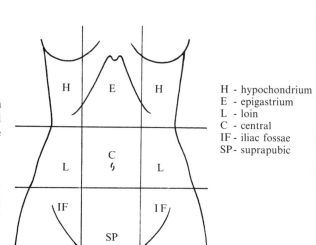

H - hypochondrium
E - epigastrium
L - loin
C - central
IF - iliac fossae
SP - suprapubic

Fig. 1.1
Abdominal regions.

(e.g. aerophagia), emotional upset, and over- or under-feeding. It may, however, also be associated with more serious complaints (e.g. food poisoning and intestinal obstruction).

Symptoms
Infants in the first months of life are commonly affected by intestinal colic. It is characterised by paroxysms of crying associated with pulling up of the knees and irritability in an otherwise thriving infant. Attacks commonly occur in the evening, but unlike crying caused by loneliness or a soiled napkin, are not usually relieved by picking up the child.

Treatment
Non-drug remedies include lying the infant on his abdomen or changing feeding equipment or technique. Persistent colic may be treated with anticholinergic antispasmodics (BNF 1.2), although dicyclomine is now contra-indicated in infants under six months of age and it is rare for colic to still be a problem at this age.

Constipation

Definition and aetiology
Constipation is defined as increased difficulty and reduced frequency of bowel evacuation, and may be chronic or acute. Normal frequency of defaecation varies from three times a day to once every three days. Failure to appreciate this normal variation has lead to widespread and unnecessary laxative abuse.

Simple (chronic) constipation is usually due to lack of dietary fibre or poor bowel training. Acute constipation implies a definite, sudden change in bowel habit. It may be due to organic causes (e.g. mechanical obstruction by impacted faeces, paralytic ileus, or confinement to bed). If a sudden change in bowel habit persists for some weeks, colorectal cancer or other causes of partial bowel obstruction may be responsible.

Further causes of constipation include anal fissures, haemorrhoids, proctitis, irritable bowel syndrome, diverticular disease, megacolon, pregnancy, pelvic masses, diminished muscle tone particularly in the elderly, hypothyroidism, parkinsonism, hypercalcaemia, spinal lesions, and depressive disorders. Constipation may be a side-effect of drug administration and laxative abuse.

Treatment
Most cases of constipation can be successfully treated by dietary measures alone. Long-term constipation should be treated by increasing the bulk of intestinal contents with the use of a high-fibre diet (e.g. bran) and increased fluid intake or, failing this, by artificial means using bulk-forming drugs (BNF 1.6.1). If these measures are unsuccessful stimulant laxatives (BNF 1.6.2), faecal softeners (BNF 1.6.3), or osmotic laxatives (BNF 1.6.4) may be used.

Diarrhoea

Definition and aetiology
Diarrhoea is caused by an increased frequency and fluidity of defaecation. The cause may be a disorder of the stomach, biliary system, small or large bowel, a systemic illness (e.g. hyperthyroidism or diabetes mellitus), or the ingestion of drugs, toxins, or poisons. Patients often overstress the severity of the condition.

In its acute form it may be caused by food poisoning, dietary indiscretion, by bowel infection (viral, bacterial, or parasitic), or ingestion of bacterial toxins. Traveller's diarrhoea is normally caused by bacterial toxins, in particular by pathogenic *Escherichia coli, Campylobacter,* or *Shigella* species.

Chronic diarrhoea may be due to malabsorption, Crohn's disease, diverticular disease, ulcerative colitis, malignant disease, protozoal or occasionally helminthic infections, disturbances of intestinal motility (e.g. irritable bowel syndrome), or to the effects of drugs. Pseudomembranous colitis may develop after antibacterial therapy and cause acute or chronic diarrhoea. Faecal impaction occurs mainly in the elderly and may give rise to spurious diarrhoea.

Treatment
Treatment is directed if possible to the underlying cause. Prophylaxis is not usually recommended. For symptomatic treatment in adults a fluid-only diet may be sufficient, although antidiarrhoeal adsorbent powders or mixtures (BNF 1.4.1) may be useful to treat mild diarrhoea. Antidiarrhoeal drugs which reduce motility (BNF 1.4.2) may be given in more severe cases. Bulk-forming drugs (BNF 1.6.1) may be used to remove excess fluid and to control faecal consistency in patients with an ileostomy or colostomy. The risk of dehydration in severe diarrhoea is especially high in the very young, the old, and choleraic patients, and rehydration should be carried out by means of oral (BNF 9.2.1) or, if necessary, intravenous administration of fluids (BNF 9.2.2). Spurious diarrhoea may be overcome through evacuation of the rectum by the administration of suppositories or enemas (BNF 1.6), or by manual removal.

Diverticular Disease

Definition and aetiology
Diverticular disease is the term which has now replaced the former terms diverticulosis and diverticulitis.

A diverticulum is a small saccular mucosal pouch, which distends outwards from the external muscle wall of the gastro-intestinal tract. Diverticula occur most commonly in the sigmoid colon, but may also develop in other regions of the gut (e.g. oesophagus, duodenum, and small intestine). Their incidence increases with age (over half occur in patients of over 50 years of age) and appears to be associated with diets low in fibre and with prolonged raised pressure within the colon. Inflammatory complications of diverticular disease are rare but potentially dangerous.

Symptoms
The occurrence of diverticula is frequently asymptomatic, and they are only detected on unrelated pelvic

investigation. Symptomatic diverticular disease is characterised by abdominal pain and altered bowel function (e.g. diarrhoea, constipation, or both). Pain, located usually in the left iliac fossa, may be relieved by defaecation.

Inflammation may be associated with abdominal tenderness, fever, and constipation; an inflammatory mass may be present. Symptoms may also arise from complications which include abscesses, fistulas (e.g. to the bladder or vagina), peritonitis, rectal bleeding, and intestinal obstruction.

Treatment
Symptomatic diverticular disease may be treated with a high-fibre diet, bran supplements, bulk-forming drugs (BNF 1.6.1), and antispasmodics and other drugs altering gut motility (BNF 1.2).

In the event of inflammation or associated complications, bed rest, fasting, intravenous nutrition (BNF 9.3), and intravenous antibacterial drugs (BNF 5.1) are indicated. Opioid analgesics (BNF 4.7.2) may be required for severe abdominal pain. Surgery may be necessary for complications, failure to respond to treatment, or recurrent attacks.

Gastritis

Definition
Gastritis is defined as inflammation of the gastric mucosa, which may be acute or chronic.

Acute Gastritis

Definition and aetiology
Acute gastritis may result from irritation due to drugs (e.g. salicylates and systemic chemotherapeutic agents), alcohol, corrosive agents, irradiation, bacterial toxins (e.g. staphylococcal), or can be associated with bacterial infection (e.g. salmonellal infections). Stressful events (e.g. trauma and surgery) may also precipitate symptoms.

Symptoms
Acute gastritis is usually asymptomatic, but anorexia, epigastric pain, and nausea and vomiting may occur. Gastritis is an important cause of upper gastro-intestinal haemorrhage, which is characterised by haematemesis or melaena. Acute gastritis due to the ingestion of corrosive materials is characterised by severe chest and epigastric pain; haemorrhage, vomiting, hypotension, shock, and perforation may occur.

Treatment
Conservative measures include removal of the causative agent (e.g. cessation of alcohol intake and avoidance of non-steroidal anti-inflammatory drugs). Antacids (BNF

1.1) may be required in symptomatic patients. Severe bleeding associated with acute gastritis is treated with intravenous administration of fluids (BNF 9.2.2), antacids (BNF 1.1), gastric aspiration, and lavage. Blood transfusion may be necessary. Surgery is associated with high morbidity and mortality and is avoided if possible.

Chronic Gastritis

Definition and aetiology
The causes of chronic gastritis are not clear but are thought to include auto-immune diseases (e.g. thyroid disease, Addison's disease, and diabetes mellitus) and prolonged gastric irritation. *Helicobacter pylori* (formerly called *Campylobacter pylori*) has been implicated as a cause of non-auto-immune disease. Chronic gastritis occurs commonly in association with peptic ulceration, cancer of the stomach, and following gastric surgery. The condition has also been reported in megaloblastic anaemia and iron-deficiency anaemia.

Symptoms
Chronic gastritis varies in severity. It may affect only superficial tissue or cause a variable degree of glandular atrophy. Metaplasia frequently occurs in atrophic gastritis. Uncomplicated forms are usually asymptomatic although anorexia, epigastric pain, nausea and vomiting, and hypochlorhydria or achlorhydria may occur.

Treatment
Treatment is not usually necessary for uncomplicated chronic gastritis. Dyspepsia may be relieved by antacids (BNF 1.1) even if hypochlorhydria is present. Iron-deficiency anaemia or megaloblastic anaemia should be treated with replacement therapy (BNF 9.1.1 and 9.1.2).

Gastro-enteritis

Definition and aetiology
Gastro-enteritis is a group of clinical syndromes characterised by acute inflammation of the stomach, intestine, or both. It may be due to food poisoning, and bacterial, viral, or protozoal infections.

In food poisoning, gastro-enteritis is due to ingestion of food contaminated by bacterial enterotoxins, and bacteria which invade the gut mucosa. Non-bacterial causes include ingestion of poisonous or chemically contaminated food (e.g. mushroom poisoning from *Amanita* toadstools and solanine poisoning from green potatoes).

Bacterial gut infections are varied in aetiology. Epidemics of infantile gastro-enteritis may be caused by enteropathogenic strains of *Escherichia coli*. Viral infections are a common cause of gastro-enteritis and are usually due to rotaviruses in young children.

Symptoms

Nausea, vomiting, and diarrhoea are classical symptoms. Abdominal pain and fever may also be present. In severe cases, dehydration, prostration, and shock may develop. Incubation periods and clinical features vary according to the causative toxin or bacteria. The incubation period for *E. coli* in infantile gastro-enteritis is 8 to 48 hours, and diarrhoea and vomiting may lead to dehydration and severe illness. Alternatively the illness may be mild, and vomiting and malaise absent. The incubation period for rotaviruses is 24 to 72 hours, and gastro-intestinal symptoms are frequently preceded or accompanied by upper respiratory symptoms (including otitis media). Diarrhoea, vomiting, or both often occur and the illness is usually self-limiting, lasting between 3 and 8 days.

Treatment

Gastro-enteritis is treated by the oral administration of fluids (BNF 9.2.1) to prevent or alleviate dehydration, and by avoidance of solids until symptoms have subsided. In severe cases, intravenous administration of fluids (BNF 9.2.2) may be required. Antidiarrhoeal drugs (BNF 1.4) may be given as an adjunct to fluid and electrolyte replacement, but in general should not be used in infants or children. Antibacterials are generally unnecessary in simple gastro-enteritis and may in fact prolong symptoms.

Ileus

Definition and aetiology

Ileus is a condition in which the transit of intestinal contents is arrested or severely impaired.

Paralytic (adynamic) ileus is due to functional failure of normal intestinal peristalsis. It commonly occurs postoperatively following abdominal surgery. It may also occur in patients with acute pancreatitis, ischaemic gastro-intestinal disease, choledocholithiasis, peritonitis, and external trauma, or may be induced by ganglion-blocking antihypertensive drugs.

Mechanical ileus is mechanical or organic obstruction of the small intestine or colon and may be complete or partial (subacute obstruction). It is commonly caused by fibrous bands and adhesions, hernias, malignant disease, impacted faeces, or inflammatory bowel disease.

Symptoms

The symptoms vary according to the site and extent of the obstruction, but include abdominal distension, colicky pain, anorexia, constipation, and nausea and vomiting; dehydration and shock may develop. Complications include strangulation or infarction, leading to gangrene, perforation, and peritonitis. Complete mechanical obstruction is fatal if untreated.

Treatment

Paralytic ileus is usually self-limiting and is initially treated conservatively. Recovery may be expedited with intravenous fluid replacement (BNF 9.2.2) and gastric aspiration. Mechanical ileus is treated similarly but surgery should be carried out as soon as the patient's condition allows.

Immediate surgery is required for strangulation or infarction. Parasympathomimetics (BNF 1.6.2) may be required for paralytic ileus, but should be avoided if organic obstruction is present. Opioid analgesics (BNF 4.7.2) may be required and antibacterial drugs (BNF 5.1) should be given if peritonitis is present.

Irritable Bowel Syndrome

Definition and aetiology

The irritable bowel syndrome (IBS) is a chronic motility disorder of the colon with no demonstrable organic cause.

Symptoms

It is characterised by recurrent episodes of abdominal discomfort, pain, and altered bowel habit. The pain may be colicky or a continuous dull ache and is commonly related to food intake. It may be relieved by defaecation or on the passage of flatus. There may be a history of diarrhoea or constipation, or alternating diarrhoea and constipation; the faeces may be described as 'marbles', 'pellets', or 'rabbit droppings' (scybala), and mucus may be present. Rectal bleeding does not occur unless haemorrhoids or other lesions are also present.

Other symptoms include abdominal distension and flatulence; non-intestinal symptoms (e.g. fatigue and headache) are thought to be psychosomatic. Symptoms may be aggravated by emotional stress, anxiety, or depressive disorders. Diagnosis is made by suspecting IBS to be the cause of the patient's symptoms and excluding other causes.

Treatment

Many patients may be reassured when the benign nature of the condition is explained to them. Treatment may consist of a high-fibre diet (e.g. bran). Drug therapy should be avoided if possible, but bulk-forming drugs (BNF 1.6.1) may be required for constipation and antidiarrhoeal drugs (BNF 1.4.2) may occasionally be necessary. Antispasmodic drugs and other drugs altering gut motility (BNF 1.2) may be required for abdominal colic. Underlying anxiety or depression should be treated.

Ischaemic Gastro-intestinal Disorders

Definition and aetiology

Ischaemic gastro-intestinal disorders may be acute or

chronic, and vary from mild ischaemia with superficial necrosis causing no permanent damage to massive ischaemia and infarction. Ischaemia may result from arterial occlusion due to atherosclerosis with or without thrombosis, embolism, or less commmonly aortic aneurysm or polyarteritis nodosa. Other causes include thrombosis of the mesenteric vein (e.g. as a complication of abdominal surgery or cirrhosis of the liver), and hypotension occurring as a complication of shock.

Acute Intestinal Ischaemia

Definition and aetiology
Acute intestinal ischaemia occurs primarily in older patients with degenerative cardiovascular disease.

Symptoms
The onset is usually abrupt, but may be insidious. It is characterised by colicky abdominal pain in the right iliac fossa, which later becomes constant, severe, and diffuse. Other early symptoms include diarrhoea which may be bloody, nausea and vomiting, anxiety, dyspnoea, pallor, and sweating. Later symptoms include anuria, cyanosis, and hypotension followed by necrosis leading to infarction, gangrene, peritonitis, shock, and death.

Treatment
Treatment consists of intravenous administration of fluids (BNF 9.2.2) to correct fluid and electrolyte imbalance and intravenous antibacterial drugs (BNF 5.1). Blood is also given if necessary. Surgery should be carried out as soon as possible; resection of the intestine is usually necessary but embolectomy or thrombectomy may reduce the length of intestine that has to be resected (e.g. in patients who are already compromised by cardiovascular disease). The mortality rate is high.

Chronic Intestinal Ischaemia

Definition and aetiology
Chronic intestinal ischaemia is usually associated with extensive atherosclerosis involving at least two of the visceral arteries and may progress to acute intestinal ischaemia.

Symptoms
It is characterised by chronic postprandial abdominal pain (usually occurring 20 to 60 minutes after eating), which is unrelieved by antacids. As the condition progresses, the patient becomes afraid to eat and marked weight loss occurs.

Treatment
Treatment consists of surgical reconstruction of the arteries.

Focal Ischaemia of the Small Intestine

Definition and aetiology
In focal ischaemia of the small intestine, only a segment of the small intestine is affected, causing local ulceration which on healing leads to stenosis. It may be caused by vascular disorders (*see above*) or may be due to a strangulated hernia, blunt trauma to the abdomen, or irradiation. Drug-induced ulceration (e.g. from ingestion of potassium salts) is another important cause. A rare cause is localised vasculitis secondary to infections or collagen disorders.

Symptoms
Focal ischaemia is characterised by colicky abdominal pain occurring 2 to 3 hours after eating, associated with nausea, abdominal distension, and occasional vomiting.

Treatment
Treatment consists of surgical resection of the obstructed segment.

Ischaemic Colitis

Definition and aetiology
Ischaemia of the colon may be widespread or segmented. It may be caused by vascular disorders (*see above*), by venous occlusion, or may be associated with colorectal cancer, colonic prolapse, or volvulus.

Symptoms
It is characterised by abdominal pain in the left iliac fossa and nausea and vomiting, followed by the passage of loose faeces darkly stained with blood.

Treatment
Treatment consists of intravenous administration of fluids (BNF 9.2.2) and intravenous antibacterial drugs (BNF 5.l). Surgical resection may be required if a stricture develops or if there is evidence of peritonitis, persistent bleeding, or an underlying colonic disorder (e.g. malignant disease). However, more than 90% of cases resolve spontaneously.

Megacolon

Definition
Megacolon (Fig. 1.2) is a condition in which there is acute or chronic dilatation of the colon.

Congenital Megacolon

Definition and aetiology
In congenital megacolon (Hirschprung's disease), the absence of neurones in a distal portion of the colon results in a narrowed segment. This 'bottleneck' effect produces dilatation of the colon proximal to the affected segment.

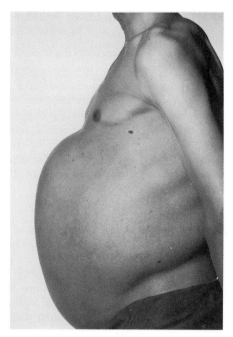

Fig. 1.2
The severe abdominal dilatation produced by megacolon.

Symptoms
The condition usually presents in the first few days of life and is characterised by severe constipation, abdominal distension, vomiting, and poor feeding. Presentation in the later weeks of life is associated with mild constipation, which dates back to the neonatal period; anorexia and failure to thrive may also be present. If only a very short section of bowel is involved, the presentation may be delayed into adult life.

Treatment
Congenital megacolon should be treated by resection of the affected portion of bowel, although temporary colostomy may be necessary to relieve acute obstructions.

Acquired Megacolon

Definition and aetiology
Acquired megacolon is dilatation that occurs as a result of chronic constipation. It usually occurs in mentally retarded or psychotic children and in infirm or elderly subjects.

Symptoms
Symptoms are similar to those of congenital megacolon, although faecal incontinence due to impacted faeces is also common.

Treatment
Acquired megacolon is treated with rectally administered laxatives (BNF 1.6) followed by retraining of bowel habits.

Peptic Ulceration

Definition and aetiology
Peptic ulcers develop through loss of tissue of the mucosa, submucosa, and muscularis mucosae in regions of the gastro-intestinal tract exposed to gastric secretions, which contain acid and pepsin. They may occur in the lower oesophagus, the stomach (gastric ulcers), and the duodenum (duodenal ulcers). Ulceration results from an imbalance between the damaging actions of acid and pepsin, and the mucosal defence mechanisms. Certain drugs (e.g. aspirin and other anti-inflammatory drugs) have been linked to the occurrence of peptic ulceration, but the evidence that they cause chronic ulceration is not convincing.

Gastric Ulceration

Definition and aetiology
Gastric ulcers may be benign or malignant. Benign gastric ulcers are usually single, circular, or semi-circular discrete breaks in the gastric mucosa, which frequently penetrate deeply into the muscularis mucosae. Acute or chronic ingestion of aspirin or other anti-inflammatory drugs may cause acute gastric ulceration.

Symptoms
They are characterised by localised epigastric pain, which may become worse after eating; unlike duodenal ulcers the pain is worse during the day, although differentiation on clinical grounds is unreliable. Other symptoms include anorexia, nausea and vomiting, excess salivation, and weight loss. Acute or occult haemorrhage or perforation are the commonest complications and are sometimes the presenting features. Relapses after healing occur less frequently than in duodenal ulceration.

Treatment
Treatment is as described below under duodenal ulceration. Surgery may also be required for persistent, bleeding, malignant ulcers, or ulcers which fail to heal.

Duodenal Ulceration

Definition and aetiology
Duodenal ulcers usually occur as benign, single, circular areas in the mucosa of the duodenal bulb. There is a possible association between duodenal ulceration and smoking, and genetic factors may be involved. They

are more common in people with blood group O. Duo-denal ulceration is a very common condition, with 10% to 15% of the population likely to suffer from duodenal ulceration some time during their lives.

Symptoms
Duodenal ulceration is typically characterised by epigastric pain, which is often localised. The pain may be described as gnawing, burning, boring, aching, or as a sensation of pressure, heaviness, or hunger, and may be mild or severe. The pain may be relieved by food, but commonly recurs 2 to 3 hours after eating and is worse at night. Nausea and vomiting are relatively uncommon unless there is severe pain or pyloric stenosis. Haemorrhage may occur, causing haematemesis, melaena, and iron-deficiency anaemia. Perforation will produce severe acute pain, collapse, and peritonitis. Haemorrhage, perforation, or both may occur in patients without previous symptoms. Duodenal ulceration is frequently associated with spontaneous remissions and relapses.

Treatment
Treatment consists of rest, avoidance of gastro-intestinal or mucosal irritants (e.g. smoking and alcohol), regular meals, and symptomatic treatment with antacids (BNF 1.1) and ulcer-healing drugs (BNF 1.3). Surgery still has a role in the treatment of acute complications (e.g. haemorrhage and perforation) and for unsuccessful medical treatment.

Acute Erosive Ulceration

Definition and aetiology
Multiple superficial ulcers may develop in the oesophagus, stomach, or duodenum of acutely stressed patients, particularly after major trauma, extensive burns, or during shock or hypoxia. These 'stress ulcers' can also develop in patients whose upper gastro-intestinal mucosa is damaged by alcohol or non-steroidal anti-inflammatory drugs.

Treatment
Antacids (BNF 1.1) and ulcer-healing drugs (BNF 1.3) may be used for the prophylaxis and treatment of stress ulceration.

Polyps

Definition and aetiology
A polyp is a growth which protrudes from a mucous membrane. Polyps found in the large intestine are usually adenomas with malignant potential. Their origin is uncertain, but their incidence has been linked to dietary factors which alter the flora of the colon and cause the production of carcinogens through bacterial action. Genetic factors may also be important (e.g. in familial adenomatous polyposis).

Symptoms
Polyps frequently occur asymptomatically and tend to be diagnosed on associated investigation. They vary considerably in size, and occur singly or in groups, with the greatest incidence in the rectum and sigmoid colon. The most common symptom is rectal bleeding which, if persistent, may cause mild anaemia. In familial adenomatous polyposis, there is a widespread covering of polyps over the lining of the colon and rectum.

Treatment
The polyps should be removed for assessment of the tissue type. Follow-up is necessary to monitor for the development of adenocarcinoma. The very poor prognosis of familial adenomatous polyposis may be improved by continuous monitoring. Total proctocolectomy with ileostomy formation or ileo-anal anastomosis may be necessary in severe cases which may progress to carcinoma.

Pyloric Stenosis

Definition and aetiology
Pyloric stenosis is the obstruction of the pyloric outlet (pylorus) of the stomach. It may arise congenitally, through a complex multifactorial inheritance, due to thickening of the pyloric muscle. It may also be acquired through inflammation or fibrosis of the pylorus as a late complication of chronic peptic ulceration or malignant disease.

Symptoms
Congenital hypertrophic pyloric stenosis, which most commonly arises in first-born males, usually produces symptoms within the first weeks of life. It is characterised by vomit (without bile) projected up to a metre, constipation, dehydration, weight loss, and hunger. Rarer and less severe forms may not be detected until early adult life. Acquired pyloric stenosis occurs in adults, and produces vomiting (several hours after eating) and weight loss, both of which may be associated with a long history of ulceration and its symptoms.

Treatment
Treatment consists of intravenous nutrition (BNF 9.3) and fluid and electrolytes (BNF 9.2), followed by surgery. Hypertrophied muscle may be divided surgically in the congenital condition or the obstruction bypassed in the acquired form.

1.2 OESOPHAGEAL DISORDERS

Achalasia

Definition and aetiology
Achalasia (cardiospasm) is a rare idiopathic condition in which there is a failure of peristalsis in the oesophagus combined with a failure of relaxation of the cardiac sphincter. It may be caused by local nerve cell degeneration.

Symptoms
Achalasia is characterised by dysphagia; chest pain may also occur. Nocturnal regurgitation of undigested food, which occurs in about 30% of patients, may produce pulmonary aspiration leading to lung abscess, bronchiectasis, or pneumonia. Distal oesophageal cancer is a late complication in 5% to 10% of cases regardless of treatment.

Treatment
Achalasia may be treated by dilatation of the cardiac sphincter, but surgery (cardiomyotomy) may be necessary.

Dyspepsia

Definition and aetiology
Dyspepsia (indigestion) is a collection of symptoms which may occur shortly after eating or drinking. Acute episodes may be due to overindulgence in food or alcohol. Chronic dyspepsia may occur in peptic ulceration, hiatus hernia, reflux oesophagitis, chronic gastritis, cholecystitis, or ischaemic heart disease, or it may occur independently of any pathological change (non-ulcer dyspepsia). Dyspepsia is aggravated by heavy smoking, stress, and anxiety and may be psychosomatic.

Symptoms
The major symptoms are epigastric discomfort, chest pain, or both. It may be accompanied by a feeling of fullness after eating, heartburn, abdominal distension, flatulence, eructation, anorexia, and nausea and vomiting; a change in bowel habit may also be reported. Eructation may occur in anxious patients due to aerophagia.

Treatment
Dyspepsia may be treated with antacids (BNF 1.1); antispasmodics and other drugs altering gut motility (BNF 1.2) may also be useful in non-ulcer dyspepsia. It is recommended (BNF 1.3) that the use of cimetidine in undiagnosed dyspepsia is restricted to younger patients. All patients should be advised to stop smoking, moderate their alcohol intake, and to eat regularly, avoiding foods which aggravate the problem.

Dysphagia

Definition and aetiology
Dysphagia is an awareness of difficulty in swallowing, due to solids or liquids sticking in the oesophagus. It should be differentiated from neurotic dysphagia (globus hystericus) in which there is a feeling of a lump in the throat, which is not associated with swallowing.

Dysphagia may be due to lesions of the mouth or tongue. Neuromuscular disorders of the pharynx (e.g. myasthenia gravis and bulbar palsy) or of the oesophagus (e.g. achalasia, systemic sclerosis, and diabetes mellitus) may be aetiological factors. Other causes include extrinsic pressure (e.g. mediastinal glands and thyroid enlargement) or intrinsic lesions (e.g. foreign body, benign or malignant strictures, and pharyngeal pouch).

Treatment
Treatment may involve dilatation or surgery.

Hiatus Hernia

Definition and aetiology
Hiatus hernia is the protrusion of a portion of the stomach into the thorax through the oesophageal hiatus of the diaphragm.

In 'sliding' hiatus hernia, the gastro-oesophageal junction is displaced upwards into the chest. In 'rolling' hiatus hernia, the gastro-oesophageal junction remains in its normal position, but a portion of the stomach herniates into the chest by rolling up alongside the oesophagus. Hiatus hernia is common in obese subjects and during pregnancy; rolling hernias occur more frequently in women than in men and the incidence increases with age.

Symptoms
Most patients with hiatus hernia are asymptomatic. If symptoms are present, they are usually related to reflux oesophagitis and include heartburn, chest pain, and regurgitation; chest pain without reflux oesophagitis may also occur and cause confusion with cardiac pain. Haemorrhage may occur with both types of hiatus hernia, leading to iron-deficiency anaemia. Rolling hernias may produce vague chest discomfort and occasionally become incarcerated or strangulated.

Treatment
Patients with hiatus hernia presenting with symptoms of reflux oesophagitis are treated for this latter condition. Surgery may be required if symptoms persist and for rolling hernias to avoid the risk of incarceration or strangulation.

Reflux Oesophagitis

Definition and aetiology
Reflux oesophagitis is a condition in which reflux of gastric and duodenal contents into the oesophagus, caused by incompetence of the lower oesophageal sphincter, produces inflammation. It is commonly associated with hiatus hernia, but may occur independently of any anatomical abnormality, particularly in the obese and during pregnancy.

Symptoms
It is characterised by heartburn or chest pain (which may be confused with cardiac pain) and is aggravated by stooping or lying down. Pain may occur whilst eating or drinking. Other symptoms include regurgitation of gastric contents into the mouth, and dysphagia of solids. Hoarseness and nocturnal cough or wheeze are signs of pulmonary aspiration. Complications of reflux oesophagitis are few, but may include oesophageal erosions and shallow ulcers. Resultant blood loss may produce iron-deficiency anaemia; rarely, deep oesophageal ulcers may develop, producing severe pain radiating to the back or neck. Oesophageal strictures are a further complication.

Treatment
Treatment consists of elevation of the head of the bed, avoidance of stooping and tight clothing, and administration of antacids (BNF 1.1). Ulcer-healing drugs (BNF 1.3) and metoclopramide (BNF 1.2) may also be used. Patients should be advised to lose weight and avoid alcohol, caffeine, smoking, and any foods (e.g. chocolate, fatty foods, and onions) which aggravate symptoms. Food and drink should also be avoided late at night, before retiring. Dilatation may be required if strictures are present and surgery indicated for resistant cases.

1.3   NON-SPECIFIC INFLAMMATORY BOWEL DISORDERS

Crohn's Disease

Definition and aetiology
Crohn's disease is a chronic granulomatous and inflammatory disease of unknown cause affecting any part of the gastro-intestinal tract, particularly the terminal ileum. The disease most commonly begins in young adults, and remissions and relapses occur during its course. Some cases may not be distinguishable from ulcerative colitis.

Symptoms
It is characterised by abdominal pain, chronic diarrhoea, mild fever, and weight loss. In some cases, the symptoms may mimic those of appendicitis. Rectal bleeding occasionally occurs in colonic forms of the disease. Fistulas and abscesses commonly occur and may penetrate the intestine in the abdomen or perianal region. Non-intestinal complications include anaemia, aphthous stomatitis, arthritis, erythema nodosum, growth retardation in children, and nutritional deficiencies. Eye, hepatic, and renal complications may also occur. In children, and more rarely in adults, non-intestinal symptoms may predominate in the absence of abdominal pain and diarrhoea.

Treatment
No specific treatment is available for Crohn's disease. Diarrhoea and anaemia may be treated symptomatically. Rest and treatment with corticosteroids (BNF 6.3.4) may be of value. Antibacterial drugs (BNF 5.1) may be required in the presence of overwhelming infection or abscess. Sulphasalazine may be helpful in suppressing colonic disease and azathioprine has been used for maintenance (BNF 1.5). Intravenous nutrition (BNF 9.3) or elemental diets may produce remission or be required during acute relapses. Surgery may be required, but is often complicated by fistula and abscess formation. Relapses often occur.

Self-help organisation
National Association for Colitis and Crohn's Disease

Toxic Megacolon

Definition and aetiology
Toxic megacolon is an acute dilatation of the colon (principally affecting the transverse and ascending colon), which may occur as a complication of ulcerative colitis or, more rarely, of Crohn's disease.

Symptoms
It is characterised by abdominal distension and tenderness, dehydration, diarrhoea, fever, malaise, and tachycardia, and may lead to perforation, peritonitis, and septicaemia.

Treatment
It is treated by intravenous administration of fluids (BNF 9.2.2), 'nil by mouth', discontinuation of antidiarrhoeal drugs, gastric aspiration, intravenous antibacterial drugs (BNF 5.1), and intravenous corticosteroids (BNF 6.3.4). Surgery (colectomy) should be carried out if there is no response to medical treatment within 24 to 48 hours and can considerably reduce the overall mortality.

Ulcerative Colitis

Definition and aetiology
Ulcerative colitis is a chronic condition of unknown cause in which there are changes in the structure of the mucosa and submucosa of the wall of the colon, with widespread inflammation and superficial ulceration. The inflammatory process appears to begin in the rectum (or rectosigmoid area) and usually spreads proximally to a variable extent. The disease most commonly begins in late adolescence or in young adults, although it may occur at any age.

There is an overlap between ulcerative colitis and Crohn's disease, and 10% of cases are unable to be differentiated. Ulcerative colitis is twice as common as Crohn's disease.

Symptoms
Symptoms vary from diarrhoea in mild disease to septicaemia, dehydration, and malnutrition in severe forms. Diarrhoea, with blood and mucus in the faeces, is a common sign, although if the disease is confined to the rectum there may paradoxically be constipation. Tenesmus and pain frequently precede defaecation; abdominal cramp may be due to colonic spasm. Other common symptoms are anaemia, anorexia, fatigue, fever, and weight loss. Remissions and relapses occur in most patients, although a small number have chronic disease. Gastro-intestinal complications include toxic megacolon, perforation, severe haemorrhage, pseudopolyposis, fibrous strictures, and colorectal cancer. Rectal complications may occur (e.g. abscesses and fistulas), though they are less common than in Crohn's disease. Non-intestinal complications include erythema nodosum, pyoderma gangrenosum, rashes, arthritis, aphthous stomatitis, and eye disorders. Ankylosing spondylitis, liver and biliary diseases, and growth retardation in children have also been associated with ulcerative colitis.

Treatment
Symptomatic treatment may be required, with intravenous administration if necessary, to correct deficiency of electrolytes (BNF 9.2), vitamins (BNF 9.6), minerals (BNF 9.5), and other nutrients. Blood transfusion may be necessary for anaemic patients and antibacterial drugs (BNF 5.1) may be required for treatment of infections. Corticosteroids, sulphasalazine, and azathioprine are used in the treatment of ulcerative colitis (BNF 1.5). Symptoms of mild ulcerative colitis may be relieved with antidiarrhoeal drugs (BNF 1.4), but these should be used with caution in moderate or severe disease because of the risk of precipitating ileus or toxic megacolon. Regular follow-up examinations (sigmoidoscopy and colonoscopy) should be made to detect the possible development of colorectal cancer, which has a much greater incidence in patients with a long history (more than 10 years) of extensive ulcerative colitis. Surgery is required for cases unresponsive to medical therapy.

Self-help organisations
Ileostomy Association of Great Britain
National Association of Colitis and Crohn's Disease

1.4 MALABSORPTION SYNDROMES

Coeliac Disease

Definition and aetiology
Coeliac disease (idiopathic steatorrhoea or gluten-sensitive enteropathy) is a chronic disorder of the small intestine in which there is an unusual sensitivity to gluten, sometimes associated with secondary lactose intolerance. It is a common disorder with a UK incidence of approximately 1 in 2000. Coeliac disease may occur in children or adults and is sometimes familial, with 10% to 15% of siblings being affected. Dermatitis herpetiformis is a related condition.

Symptoms
It is characterised by abnormalities of the jejunal mucosa, which cause malabsorption and steatorrhoea. The malabsorption leads to weight loss and deficiency of minerals and vitamins. Other non-specific symptoms include fatigue, malaise, abdominal distension, anaemia, aphthous stomatitis, bone pain, and oedema.

Treatment
In most cases, avoidance of foods containing gluten (e.g. those prepared from wheat, rye, barley, and oats) results in normal intestinal function, but the disease returns if gluten is again ingested. A range of gluten-free foods is available (BNF 9.4.1). Some medicines (e.g. tablets) may be prepared with gluten-containing ingredients and should be avoided. Administration of nutritional supplements (BNF 9.1, 9.5, and 9.6) may be necessary if deficiencies occur.

Self-help organisation
Coeliac Society of the United Kingdom

Short-bowel Syndrome

Definition and aetiology
The short-bowel syndrome is a term used to describe the effects which may occur after extensive surgical resection of the small intestine. Up to 60% of the small intestine may be resected without causing the syndrome.

Symptoms

Symptoms depend upon the length of residual small intestine, the site of resection, and the presence or absence of residual disease. It is characterised by malabsorption with associated nutritional deficiencies. Resection of the ileum allows the passage of bile salts and fatty acids into the colon. The resultant interference with water and electrolyte absorption may lead to diarrhoea, steatorrhoea, and gallstone formation. Megaloblastic anaemia may follow ileal resection. There may be an increased risk of renal calculi, due to increased oxalate absorption. Jejunal resection may cause gastric hypersecretion, which may lead to peptic ulceration.

Treatment

Treatment consists of intravenous administration of fluids (BNF 9.2.2) in the early postoperative period, intravenous nutrition (BNF 9.3) if severe diarrhoea is prolonged postoperatively, and antidiarrhoeal drugs which reduce motility (BNF 1.4.2). Oral feeding should be introduced gradually and elemental diets (BNF 9.4.2) may be useful. Patients should be encouraged to take frequent small meals, and a relatively high calorie intake may be necessary to avoid the effects of malabsorption. Minerals (BNF 9.5) and vitamins (BNF 9.6) may be required for deficiencies and pancreatin supplements (BNF 1.9.4) for pancreatic insufficiency.

Tropical Sprue

Definition and aetiology

Tropical sprue is a chronic malabsorption syndrome which occurs in patients who live in or have visited the tropics. The condition may be caused by an infection.

Symptoms

It is characterised by diarrhoea or steatorrhoea, abdominal discomfort and distension, anorexia, malabsorption, and weight loss. Glossitis and stomatitis are common, and pigmentation of the skin and oedema may occur. The condition may have an acute onset with severe diarrhoea, fever, and blood and mucus in the faeces; remission may occur on leaving the tropics. Malabsorption may lead to vitamin deficiencies and megaloblastic anaemia.

Treatment

Treatment consists of administration of a tetracycline (BNF 5.1.3), folic acid, and hydroxocobalamin (BNF 9.1.2). Treatment should be continued for at least 6 months and relapses may occur. Antidiarrhoeal drugs (BNF 1.4.2) may be necessary and intravenous administration of fluids (BNF 9.2.2) may be required in acute illness. Mineral (BNF 9.5) or vitamin (BNF 9.6) supplements may be required for other nutritional deficiencies.

Whipple's Disease

Definition and aetiology

Whipple's disease is a rare malabsorption syndrome, which usually occurs in middle-aged and elderly men. There is a diffuse infiltration of the mucosa of the small intestine by unidentified bacilli.

Symptoms

It is characterised by arthritis, steatorrhoea, and weight loss. Other common symptoms include abdominal pain, clubbing of the fingers, fever, lymphadenopathy, nutritional deficiencies, skin pigmentation, and weakness. Anaemia may develop.

Treatment

Treatment consists of prolonged administration of antibacterial drugs (BNF 5.1) and correction of nutritional deficiencies (BNF 9.3 and 9.4).

1.5   LIVER DISORDERS

Cirrhosis of the Liver

Definition and aetiology

Cirrhosis of the liver is a group of chronic diseases of multiple aetiology. It is characterised by destruction of parenchymal cells, loss of their normal lobular structure with widespread fibrosis, and regeneration of the remaining cells to form nodules. Alcoholism and hepatitis B (*see* Acute Viral Hepatitis) are common causes of cirrhosis in the western world. Congenital causes include hereditary haemorrhagic telangiectasia and inborn errors of metabolism (e.g. hepatolenticular degeneration and haemochromatosis, which are both inherited and treatable causes of cirrhosis). Up to 30% of cases in the UK are of unknown origin (cryptogenic cirrhosis). Prolonged cholestasis may lead to biliary cirrhosis. Cirrhosis can also result from adverse reactions to drugs (e.g. isoniazid, methotrexate, and methyldopa).

Symptoms

The disease may have a long latent period and be far advanced before symptoms appear. The disturbance of liver architecture may produce a blockage of venous flow causing portal hypertension. This gives rise to ascites, with abdominal distension and pain, oesophageal varices resulting in haematemesis, and splenomegaly. The disturbed liver structure may also lead to biliary obstruction, with associated jaundice and pruritus.

The loss of liver cells and an inefficient blood supply to the regenerated cells results in liver-cell failure, primarily affecting the metabolism of ingested substances.

Toxic products of protein metabolism may cause hepatic encephalopathy leading to coma, and the toxic effects of drugs are increased and prolonged.

Other metabolic consequences of liver-cell failure include oedema, impaired synthesis of albumin and various clotting factors, and delayed breakdown of hormones (e.g. hydrocortisone and oestrogens). Excess quantities of these hormones can lead to the formation of spider telangiectasia, erythema of palms and soles and, in the male, gynaecomastia and atrophy of the testes. Other clinical features include whitened nails (having a pink area at the tip), finger clubbing, glossitis, paraesthesia, parotid-gland enlargement, pyrexia, muscle wasting, and weight loss. In some patients, the regenerative activity in the hepatic nodule becomes neoplastic, resulting in hepatoma.

Treatment
Since the disease process cannot be reversed, treatment is designed to prevent further fibrosis and limit the development of fluid retention and encephalopathy. A diet rich in energy and protein should be given unless encephalopathy is present, when protein intake should be limited. In general, alcohol should be avoided.

Hepatic coma due to encephalopathy is prevented or treated by reducing the absorption of toxic nitrogenous substances from the intestine. This is achieved by reducing protein intake and reducing the bacterial population of the gut by administration of antibacterials (e.g. neomycin, BNF 5.1.4). Salt intake should be restricted when ascites or oedema are present, and potassium-sparing diuretics (BNF 2.2.3) administered if required. In severe ascites, abdominal paracentesis may be required.

Surgery may be required when cirrhosis is due to obstruction of the bile ducts. Pruritus, which is most commonly associated with cirrhosis caused by biliary obstruction, may be relieved by the use of antihistamines (BNF 3.4.1) and cholestyramine (BNF 1.5). Cortico-steroids (BNF 6.3.4) may relieve symptoms and prolong life when used in the active phases of the disease, particularly if there is evidence of progressive active hepatitis.

Hepatitis

Definition and aetiology
Hepatitis is an inflammatory condition of the liver characterised by diffuse or patchy hepatocellular necrosis, and may be acute or chronic (Fig. 1.3). Acute forms may be due to viral infections, alcohol, drugs, or toxins and if they persist can develop into chronic episodes.

Acute Viral Hepatitis

Definition and aetiology
Acute viral hepatitis may be caused by hepatitis A, hepatitis B, or by non-A, non-B hepatitis viruses. More rarely yellow fever and infectious mononucleosis together with cytomegalovirus, herpes simplex virus, or rubella virus infections may lead to an acute hepatitis syndrome.

Hepatitis A (infectious hepatitis) is usually spread by faecal-oral contamination (e.g. of food), although transmission by blood transfusion is also theoretically possible. Outbreaks occur sporadically, but small epidemics may develop in institutions. More significant outbreaks can accompany large movements of population (e.g. in war) and there appears to be an increased incidence among promiscuous homosexuals. The incubation period is from 2 to 6 weeks. There is no carrier state.

Hepatitis B (serum hepatitis or post-transfusion hepatitis) is usually transmitted in transfused blood or plasma, by the use of non-sterile needles and syringes, by sexual intercourse, oro-genital contact, or by contact with infected secretions. High-risk groups include haemophiliacs, homosexuals, drug addicts, haemodialysis patients, and health-care and laboratory

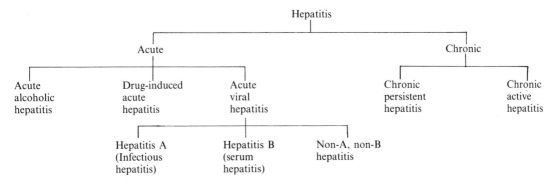

Fig. 1.3
Classification of hepatitis.

personnel. The incubation period is from 1 to 6 months. Some patients may become asymptomatic carriers.

Non-A, non-B hepatitis is caused by one or more viruses. It is the major cause of post-transfusion hepatitis and is common in drug addicts and other needle-users. It accounts for more than 20% of sporadic cases (i.e. of unknown aetiology) and is diagnosed by exclusion of hepatitis A or B. The incubation period is 2 to 20 weeks. Many patients become carriers.

Symptoms
The first (prodromal) phase of hepatitis A is usually rapid in onset and characterised by mild fever, malaise, anorexia, nausea and vomiting, abdominal distension, rashes, and arthralgia. Classically, the patient may describe a loss of taste for coffee or tobacco. After 3 to 10 days jaundice may rapidly develop, the fever subsides, and the patient feels better. The stools are pale, the urine is dark, and hepatomegaly occurs, accompanied by mild splenomegaly, in about 20% of cases. In elderly patients there may be disorientation and confusion. Jaundice usually subsides after 2 to 4 weeks. However, in many patients, especially children, jaundice does not develop and the illness is perceived as a nonspecific influenza. The prognosis is usually good, but complications (e.g. acute hepatic necrosis, hepatic cirrhosis, and aplastic anaemia) may occur.

Clinically, hepatitis B follows a similar pattern to hepatitis A, but tends to be more prolonged and have a greater mortality. Up to 90% of patients with hepatitis B recover completely. About 1% may develop acute hepatic failure (fulminant hepatitis), characterised by progressive mental changes, deepening jaundice, and the development of encephalopathy. Some patients will become chronic carriers of the infection, or develop chronic persistent hepatitis or chronic active hepatitis. Hepatitis B virus has also been associated with the development of primary hepatocellular carcinoma.

Clinically, non-A, non-B hepatitis is similar to hepatitis B. There is a similar incidence of acute hepatic failure and non-A, non-B hepatitis is also associated with an apparent carrier state. The incidence of chronic hepatitis after non-A, non-B hepatitis is greater than 25%, but in many of these cases the disease is mild and may spontaneously remit after about one year.

Treatment
In most cases of acute viral hepatitis, no special treatment is required. Patients should be advised to rest, but strict confinement to bed is not necessary. A diet low in fat but high in protein and carbohydrate should be instituted. Corticosteroids should not be given unless there is prolonged jaundice. Alcohol should be avoided throughout the course of the acute illness. The condition

is infectious during the prodromal phase, and strict personal hygiene is important in preventing the spread of infection. Contacts may be given normal immunoglobulin (BNF 14.5) for prophylaxis following which protection lasts for about 3 to 6 months, depending on dosage.

Hepatitis B vaccine (BNF 14.4) is used for prophylaxis in individuals at high risk of contracting the infection. Accidental contamination with hepatitis B virus-infected blood may be treated by passive immunisation with specific anti-hepatitis B virus immunoglobulin (BNF l4.5).

General measures for the treatment of non-A, non-B hepatitis are the same as for hepatitis A.

Acute Alcoholic Hepatitis

Definition and aetiology
Acute alcoholic hepatitis is characterised by diffuse hepatic inflammation (fatty and hyaline) and necrosis, and is a precursor of cirrhosis.

Symptoms
Patients may present with symptoms similar to those of acute viral hepatitis, although unlike acute viral hepatitis, cholestasis may be a dominant early feature.

Treatment
There is no specific treatment, but patients should be advised to abstain from alcohol and adopt a well-balanced diet. About 10% of cases will proceed to cirrhosis in spite of abstention from alcohol.

Drug-induced Acute Hepatitis

Definition and aetiology
Certain drugs and chemicals can cause an idiosyncratic acute hepatitis, which may mimic the broad clinical spectrum associated with acute viral hepatitis. Examples of offending agents include halothane, isoniazid, methyldopa, gold, rifampicin, paracetamol, and sulphonamides.

Treatment
Most patients will make a complete recovery provided the responsible agent is identified and withdrawn.

Chronic Persistent Hepatitis

Definition and aetiology
Chronic persistent hepatitis is defined as a sustained, non-progressive, inflammatory condition of the liver lasting for more than 6 to 12 months, which is largely confined to the portal areas. It usually follows acute viral hepatitis.

Symptoms

It may be entirely asymptomatic or associated with non-specific symptoms (e.g. fatigue, anorexia, abdominal discomfort, or pain). There may be mildly tender hepatomegaly, but extrahepatic manifestations are uncommon.

Treatment

There is no specific treatment, although exposure to potential hepatotoxins should be avoided. Provided alcohol has been excluded as the cause, small amounts are permissible if there is no worsening of symptoms or laboratory tests. The prognosis is excellent.

Chronic Active Hepatitis

Definition and aetiology

Chronic active hepatitis is a progressive inflammatory condition involving portal and periportal areas of the liver. About 20% of cases are caused by hepatitis B viral infection, but it may also follow non-A, non-B hepatitis. Other causes include drugs (e.g. isoniazid and methyldopa), alcohol, hepatolenticular degeneration, and auto-immune reactions. The disease occurs primarily in young women.

Symptoms

Clinical features include malaise, fatigue, variable jaundice, spider telangiectasia, variable hepatosplenomegaly, and anorexia. Cellular damage is characterised by piecemeal necrosis, fibrosis, and bridging necrosis and may progress to cirrhosis of the liver or acute hepatic failure. Occasionally chronic active hepatitis may be discovered incidentally in asymptomatic patients. Evidence of an auto-immune mechanism is indicated by the occurrence of rashes, arthralgia, amenorrhoea, and other extrahepatic features.

Treatment

Treatment consists of removal of any causative factors (e.g. drugs and alcohol) and immunosuppression using corticosteroids (BNF 6.3.4), with or without low-dose azathioprine (BNF 8.2.1).

Self-help organisations

Alcoholics Anonymous
Health Education Authority

Jaundice

Definition

Jaundice (icterus) is a yellow discoloration of the skin, sclera, and mucous membranes caused by the accumulation of bilirubin. Depending on the cause of the jaundice, the bilirubin may be conjugated (in the liver cell), water-soluble, and excreted in the urine (conjugated hyperbilirubinaemia). This occurs in cholestatic jaundice. In other forms of jaundice (e.g. haemolytic), the bilirubin is unconjugated, water-insoluble, and not excreted in the urine (unconjugated hyperbilirubinaemia). In all types, tissues and fluids throughout the body (except mucous secretions) accumulate bilirubin.

Cholestatic Jaundice

Definition and aetiology

Cholestatic (obstructive) jaundice is caused by obstruction in the bile ducts (extrahepatic) or between the liver cells and bile ducts (intrahepatic), and results in conjugated hyperbilirubinaemia. Numerous drugs and chemicals may cause intrahepatic cholestatic jaundice (e.g. phenothiazines, anabolic steroids and, more rarely, oral contraceptives). Intrahepatic jaundice may also occur in primary biliary cirrhosis, in pregnancy, and in rare inherited disorders. Extrahepatic cholestatic jaundice may be due to gallstones, strictures, pancreatitis, or malignant disease.

Symptoms

The condition is usually insidious in onset, of variable intensity, and characterised by pruritus and anorexia. The faeces are pale or clay-coloured and contain excessive amounts of fat, and the urine is dark.

Treatment

Treatment is related to the cause, and in extrahepatic obstruction, surgery may be necessary.

Haemolytic Jaundice

Definition and aetiology

In haemolytic (acholuric) jaundice, excessive destruction of erythrocytes results in the release of more bilirubin than the liver can metabolise. It may be due to excessive fragility of the erythrocytes, as in certain congenital diseases (e.g. sickle-cell anaemia and beta thalassaemia), or it may be caused by toxin-producing micro-organisms, haemolytic poisons, megaloblastic anaemia, or circulating erythrocyte antibodies. Jaundice is likely to be particularly severe in neonates with haemolytic anaemia, and if the plasma-bilirubin concentration is not controlled, kernicterus may develop. Haemolytic jaundice may develop as a result of the administration of drugs (e.g. methyldopa). Mild unconjugated hyperbilirubinaemia may also occur in the absence of liver disease or overt haemolysis (Gilbert's syndrome, an hereditary disorder affecting approximately 2% of the population).

Symptoms

The faeces may be darker than normal and there may be splenomegaly.

Treatment

Treatment depends on the cause of the disease, but surgery and the administration of corticosteroids (BNF 6.3.4) may be required.

Hepatocellular Jaundice

Definition and aetiology

Damage to the parenchymal cells of the liver may occur due to acute viral hepatitis, acute alcoholic hepatitis, or drug-induced hepatitis. As a result, the cells fail to take up bilirubin, conjugate it, and pass the complex to the bile ducts. Congenital abnormalities and deficient enzyme systems are also causative factors.

Symptoms

Intrahepatic cholestasis may develop. The onset of jaundice is usually rapid and the disease varies from mild to severe.

Treatment

Treatment depends on the underlying cause, but generally surgery is of no value and should be avoided.

Physiological Jaundice

Definition and aetiology

Physiological (neonatal) jaundice due to hepatic immaturity is a common condition, particularly in premature neonates. It usually appears after the first 24 hours in full-term neonates and after 48 hours in premature neonates.

Treatment

It may be treated by phototherapy.

Kernicterus

Definition and aetiology

Kernicterus is degeneration of brain tissue in neonates. It is caused by bilirubin crossing the blood-brain barrier as a result of high plasma concentrations of unconjugated bilirubin (unconjugated hyperbilirubinaemia), and is usually associated with haemolytic disease of the newborn. This is now rare due to careful monitoring during pregnancy and the use of anti-D (Rh$_o$) immunoglobulin in rhesus-negative women who have previously carried a rhesus-positive baby.

Symptoms

The development of kernicterus in full-term jaundiced neonates may be characterised by drowsiness, anorexia, vomiting, and convulsions. In premature neonates there are usually no clinical symptoms other than jaundice. It may be fatal or result in permanent brain damage.

Treatment

Plasma-bilirubin concentrations should be monitored in jaundiced neonates. Phototherapy may be effective in alleviating hyperbilirubinaemia and is used in the prevention of kernicterus, but exchange blood transfusion may also be required.

1.6   BILIARY-TRACT DISORDERS

Cholangitis

Definition and aetiology

Cholangitis is inflammation of the bile ducts (Fig. 1.4), usually due to bacterial infection. It is commonly associated with gallstones partially obstructing the common bile duct or benign biliary strictures. It may be mild and intermittent or severe (suppurative cholangitis).

Symptoms

Cholangitis is characterised by malaise, fever, and chills, followed by pain (which may be colicky and severe) in the right upper quadrant of the abdomen. Vomiting, cholestatic jaundice, and pruritus may also ensue; the urine becomes dark and the faeces are pale. Recurrent attacks may result in the formation of an hepatic abscess. Suppurative cholangitis may lead to septicaemia and shock.

Treatment

Treatment consists of parenteral antibacterial drugs (BNF 5.1) and intravenous administration of fluids (BNF 9.2.2) to correct fluid and electrolyte imbalance. Surgery may be required to remove bile-duct stones (choledochotomy) and the gall bladder (cholecystectomy), or for surgical repair of a biliary stricture.

Cholecystitis

Definition

Cholecystitis is an inflammatory condition of the gall bladder, which may be acute or chronic.

Acute Cholecystitis

Definition and aetiology

Acute cholecystitis occurs at the same time as gallstones in nearly all patients. It results from the toxic effects of retained bile on the gall bladder wall, following the obstruction of the outlet (cystic duct) of the gall bladder by a gallstone. Secondary bacterial infection frequently occurs.

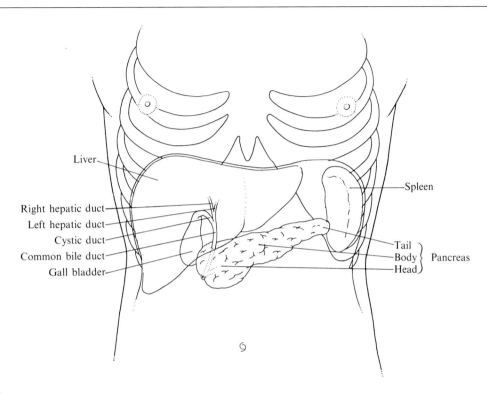

Fig. 1.4
Accessory digestive organs.

Symptoms

Acute cholecystitis is characterised by severe pain of relatively sudden onset localised in the right hypo-chondrium or in the epigastrium. The pain is continuous and often radiates to the back. In uncomplicated cases it gradually subsides over a period of 12 to 18 hours. Flatulence and nausea are common and mild fever may occur. Persistent vomiting and jaundice may be present, but are more likely in obstruction of the common bile duct. Complications include empyema of the gall bladder, cholangitis, gangrene, and perforation, which may lead to abscess formation, fistulas, or peritonitis.

Treatment

Treatment consists of parenteral opioid analgesics (BNF 4.7.2), intravenous administration of fluids (BNF 9.2.2), and for all except mild cases, treatment with antibac-terial drugs (BNF 5.1). Surgery may be required urgently if complications develop; otherwise cholecystectomy is performed after the acute symptoms have resolved, either within 2 to 3 days or after an interval of 2 to 3 months.

Chronic Cholecystitis

Definition and aetiology
Chronic cholecystitis is the most common form of gall bladder disease resulting from gallstones. It usually develops insidiously, but may follow an attack of acute cholecystitis.

Symptoms
It may be characterised by recurrent attacks of biliary colic or by recurrent episodes of constant right hypo-chondrial or epigastric pain. The pain may radiate to the right shoulder or the back and lasts for periods ranging from about 15 minutes to several hours. It commonly occurs after a meal or wakes the patient at night, and symptoms are frequently related to the ingestion of fatty foods. However, in a significant number of patients the symptoms are vague and ill-defined and include ab-dominal discomfort and distension, nausea, flatulence, and intolerance of fatty foods. Complications include acute cholecystitis, passage of stones into the common bile duct (choledocholithiasis), pancreatitis, formation of fistulas, gallstone ileus, and rarely cancer of the gall bladder. Occasionally the accumulation of mucus and

gallstones produces hydrops, which is characterised by constant right hypochondrial discomfort and a tender mass, without the occurrence of acute cholecystitis.

Treatment
Treatment consists of surgical removal of the gall bladder (cholecystectomy) for established cases of chronic cholecystitis. If the diagnosis is in doubt (e.g. vague symptoms associated with a well-functioning gall bladder containing stones), conservative treatment may be tried (e.g. weight reduction and a low-fat diet). Drugs acting on the gall bladder (BNF 1.9.1) may also be used.

Gallstones

Definition and aetiology
Gallstones (cholelithiasis) are stones formed in the gall bladder. Gallstone disease is common and the incidence increases progressively with age. The stones may be classified as cholesterol stones, bile-pigment stones, or mixed stones.

Cholesterol stones are usually solitary, large, and faceted. They occur more commonly in women and obese subjects and are thought to be associated with raised biliary-cholesterol secretion and diminished bile-acid synthesis. Racial differences, diet, drugs (e.g. oral contraceptives), and gastro-intestinal disease (e.g. Crohn's disease) also influence the development of cholesterol stones. Bile-pigment stones are either composed purely of bile pigment or of bile pigment and calcium. Pure pigment stones are black, hard, and brittle; they are commonly found in patients with haemolytic anaemia, cirrhosis of the liver, chronic bile-duct obstruction, and malaria. Stones formed of bile pigment and calcium are brown, soft, and pliable and have been associated with infections of the biliary tract. Mixed stones, composed of cholesterol, bile pigment, and calcium are usually multiple and faceted.

Symptoms
The majority of gallstones remain in the gall bladder and may be asymptomatic (silent gallstones). If the neck of the gall bladder becomes obstructed by a gallstone, biliary colic will occur and acute or chronic cholecystitis may develop. Multiple small stones may cause intermittent episodes of biliary colic when a small stone passes into the common bile duct (*see below*). If the bile duct becomes obstructed cholestatic jaundice may develop. Other complications of gallstones include cholangitis, biliary cirrhosis, and development of an internal biliary fistula. Acute pancreatitis and cancer of the gall bladder have been associated with gallstone disease. Patients with uncomplicated gallstones may complain of abdominal discomfort and distension,

flatulence, and intolerance to fatty foods, but it is uncertain whether these symptoms are directly related to the gallstones.

Treatment
Gallstones may be treated surgically by removal of the gall bladder (cholecystectomy). Certain patients with cholesterol stones may be treated with chenodeoxycholic or ursodeoxycholic acid (BNF 1.9.1).

Choledocholithiasis

Definition
Choledocholithiasis is the occurrence of gallstones in the common bile duct.

Symptoms
Classically, it is characterised by biliary colic, cholestatic jaundice, and fever. It is commonly associated with cholangitis, in which case fever and chills are present. Nausea and vomiting occur frequently and pruritus may be severe. Choledocholithiasis may, however, be asymptomatic or present with only one of the classical symptoms. Prolonged choledocholithiasis may eventually lead to obstructive biliary cirrhosis.

Treatment
Treatment consists of surgical removal of the gallstones (choledochotomy) and cholecystectomy if the gall bladder is present. In some cases, the stone may be removed from the bile duct using an endoscope. Parenteral antibacterial drugs (BNF 5.1) may be required if cholangitis is present, and intravenous fluids (BNF 9.2.2) may be required for fluid and electrolyte imbalance.

1.7   PERITONEAL DISORDERS

Ascites

Definition and aetiology
Ascites is the accumulation of fluid within the peritoneal cavity. It is most commonly caused by cirrhosis of the liver, malignant disease, advanced congestive heart failure, or tuberculosis. Other causes include hepatic-vein obstruction, hypothyroidism, hypoalbuminaemia (e.g. as a result of nephrotic syndrome), ovarian disease, pancreatitis, and inflammatory diseases of the peritoneum.

Symptoms
Symptoms may include abdominal pain and distension (Fig. 1.5), dehydration, dyspnoea, and muscle wasting. Minor occurrences of ascites may be asymptomatic.

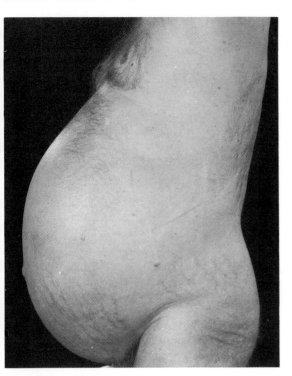

Fig. 1.5
Ascites in a male adult.

Treatment
Treatment consists of bed rest, adoption of a low-sodium diet (BNF 9.4.1), and restricting fluid intake if required. If the condition does not improve, potassium-sparing diuretics (BNF 2.2.3 and 2.2.4) may be given. Drainage of fluid may relieve severe discomfort and shorten the period of hospitalisation.

Peritonitis

Definition and aetiology
Peritonitis is the acute inflammation of the peritoneum. It is usually caused by bacterial infection secondary to gastro-intestinal perforation, and may be localised or diffuse.

Common causes of localised peritonitis are appendicitis, Crohn's disease, diverticular disease, peptic ulceration, salpingitis, and chemical irritation (e.g. in severe acute pancreatitis).

Diffuse (generalised) peritonitis may result from a ruptured appendix, perforated peptic ulcer, or perforation of the colon (e.g. due to infarction, obstruction, or ulcerative colitis).

Tuberculous peritonitis may accompany pulmonary tuberculosis, while rarer causes are fungal or parasitic infections.

Granulomatous peritonitis may develop postoperatively from the presence of starch and magnesium oxide used to reduce the stickiness of surgical rubber gloves.

Symptoms
Bacterial peritonitis is usually characterised by acute abdominal pain and tenderness, dehydration, fever, hypotension, ileus, nausea and vomiting, and tachycardia. These symptoms are not always present, however, particularly in elderly patients and in patients undergoing corticosteroid therapy. Complications include abscess formation, oliguria (occasionally leading to acute renal failure), and shock. In tuberculous peritonitis, the development of symptoms is often insidious, but may include anorexia, fever, malaise, and weight loss. Abdominal distension and ascites are present in about 70% of cases. Fungal peritonitis usually occurs only in immunosuppressed patients.

Treatment
Peritonitis should be treated with antibacterial drugs (BNF 5.1), intravenous administration of fluids (BNF 9.2.2), gastric aspiration, and opioid analgesics (BNF 4.7.2). Blood transfusion may be required. Surgery should be carried out as soon as possible to correct the underlying cause.

Self-help organisation
British Kidney Patients Association

1.8   ANORECTAL DISORDERS

Anal Fissure

Definition and aetiology
An anal fissure is an acute lengthways tear or a chronic circular ulcer in the epithelial lining of the anal canal. Acute tears are usually caused by large hard faeces or are idiopathic. They may also arise through childbirth and diarrhoea (e.g. in Crohn's disease). Young children may also develop acute tears. Chronic fissures comprise circular or elliptic ulcers, which are secondary to fibrosis due to chronic infection.

Symptoms
Patients with a chronic anal fissure may report an external skin tag (sentinel pile). Painful symptoms are produced by all fissures, particularly during defaecation. Marked spasm of the anal sphincter and slight bleeding may also occur.

Treatment
Adoption of a high-fibre diet (e.g. bran), administration of faecal softeners (BNF 1.6.3), and application of topi-

cal soothing agents (BNF 1.7.1) are all beneficial and are used in conjunction with rectal dilators. Bathing in warm salt water may also provide relief. Surgery may be necessary for chronic fissures.

Anorectal Fistula

Definition and aetiology
An anorectal fistula (fistula in ano) is a hollow fibrous tract, usually connecting the anal canal or rectum to an opening in the perianal skin. It may result from the rupture or surgical drainage of an anorectal abscess, or be due to Crohn's disease, diverticular disease, tuberculosis, sexually-transmitted disease, malignant disease, or anal fissure. In neonates, fistulas are congenital and are more common in boys. Rectovaginal fistulas may also occur, arising congenitally or following radiotherapy, pelvic surgery, childbirth, or malignant disease.

Symptoms
Continual discharge of pus, blood, mucus, and occasionally faeces through the perianal opening results in discomfort, irritation, and pruritus ani. Pain from an underlying abscess may also be present.

Treatment
Soothing preparations (BNF 1.7.1) may be applied topically, but surgery (fistulotomy) is the only effective treatment.

Haemorrhoids

Definition and aetiology
Haemorrhoids (piles) are varicosities of the network of veins which line the anus and rectum (haemorrhoidal plexus). They are commonly caused by straining as a result of constipation, low-fibre diets, and pregnancy.

Haemorrhoids may be classified as internal or external. Internal haemorrhoids, which do not prolapse, are termed primary (or first-degree); those which prolapse on defaecation but withdraw again are termed secondary (second-degree); and permanently prolapsed haemorrhoids are referred to as tertiary (third-degree) haemorrhoids. External haemorrhoids (a subcutaneous haematoma at the anal verge) often leave a permanent protruding fold or skin-tag.

Symptoms
The principal symptom is the discharge of bright red blood from the rectum, which at first occurs only on defaecation but later may occur independently of bowel action. Persistent blood loss may lead to a secondary anaemia. Soreness, pruritus ani, discharge of mucus, and pain on defaecation may occur. Haemorrhoids which have prolapsed and thrombosed are painful and may become infected or gangrenous.

Treatment
Treatment consists of the adoption of a high-fibre diet, the use of faecal softeners (BNF 1.6.3), and the application of soothing preparations (BNF 1.7.1). Warm salt baths may give symptomatic relief. Patients should be instructed in hygienic measures and to replace protruding piles after defaecation. Uncomplicated internal haemorrhoids which bleed may be treated by injection of a rectal sclerosant (BNF 1.7.3). Rubber-band ligation and cryosurgery are also used. In the presence of complications (e.g. prolapse), haemorrhoids require surgical treatment (haemorrhoidectomy).

Proctitis

Definition and aetiology
Proctitis is an inflammation of the rectal mucosa. Infectious proctitis may be caused by *Shigella* spp. or sexually-transmitted diseases (especially in male homosexuals). Non-infectious causes include radiation injury, trauma, ischaemia, or chronic inflammatory disease (e.g. Crohn's disease). Ulcerative proctitis (haemorrhagic proctitis) is a form of ulcerative colitis in which inflammation is limited to the rectum.

Symptoms
It is characterised by rectal bleeding, discharge of mucus, tenesmus, and anal or perianal soreness. The frequency of defaecation may be increased, but the faeces are often normal or hard and dry. Anaemia may occur, but other systemic symptoms are rare. Remissions and relapses are common.

Treatment
Treatment of proctitis depends on the underlying cause. In infectious proctitis the infecting micro-organism should be identified and treatment directed accordingly. Ulcerative proctitis may be treated with corticosteroid suppositories or enemas or with sulphasalazine (BNF 1.5). Treatment may be supplemented by adopting a high-fibre diet to avoid hard faeces, and soothing preparations (BNF 1.7.1).

1.9   PANCREATIC EXOCRINE DISORDERS

Cystic Fibrosis

Definition and aetiology
Cystic fibrosis is an inherited disease affecting infants, children, and young adults. It is characterised by the widespread secretion of abnormally viscid mucus and by

sweat containing high electrolyte concentrations. It is transmitted by an autosomal recessive gene. Approximately 1 in 20 people carry the gene and 1 in 2000 Caucasian births are affected. Detection of the carrier state may be possible in the near future.

Symptoms

Respiratory-tract disorders and pancreatic insufficiency are the most important manifestations, but symptoms vary in severity. Bronchial obstruction, recurring respiratory-tract infection, bronchiectasis, emphysema, and pulmonary insufficiency leading to cor pulmonale are respiratory complications. Pancreatic insufficiency may be asymptomatic, although the pancreatic ducts become blocked. Diabetes mellitus and hepatic changes may also occur. Meconium ileus may be the presenting symptom in the newborn, indicating intestinal obstruction. Vitamin deficiency is likely due to malabsorption. Other common symptoms include diarrhoea, steatorrhoea, failure to thrive despite hyperphagia, and rectal prolapse. The prognosis beyond early adulthood is poor due to progressive pulmonary and pancreatic degeneration, although the outlook has steadily improved over recent years.

Treatment

Drug treatment comprises the administration of pancreatin supplements (BNF 1.9.4), parenteral fat-soluble vitamins (BNF 9.6), and appropriate high-dose antibacterial drugs (BNF 5.1). Bronchodilators (BNF 3.1) may also be necessary. Mucolytics (BNF 3.7) have been used, and drug treatment for diabetes mellitus may be required. Bronchodilators, mucolytics, and antibacterial drugs delivered via a nebuliser in the home are gaining in popularity. Foods for special diets are available (BNF 9.4.1 and BNF Appendix 3), and surgery may be needed for intestinal obstruction. Physiotherapy with postural drainage is beneficial for pulmonary symptoms and needs to be a daily routine.

Self-help organisation

Cystic Fibrosis Research Trust

Pancreatitis

Definition

Pancreatitis is inflammation of the pancreas and may be acute or chronic.

Acute Pancreatitis

Definition and aetiology

Acute pancreatitis is an inflammatory and sometimes haemorrhagic process in the pancreas. Ischaemia and activation of proteolytic enzymes result in damage to the pancreas and surrounding tissues. Its aetiology is unknown, but it may be associated with biliary-tract disease, abdominal surgery, or a bout of excessive alcoholic drinking. Recurrent acute pancreatic disease is almost always associated with biliary-tract disease. Other diseases associated with the development of acute pancreatitis include hyperparathyroidism, hyperlipidaemia, and mumps. It may also arise following drug therapy (e.g. thiazide diuretics, azathioprine, and overdosage with paracetamol).

Symptoms

The primary symptoms are extreme epigastric pain often radiating to the back, abdominal tenderness, and, in severe cases, hypovolaemic shock. The abdominal wall may be rigid and there are signs of peritoneal irritation. Nausea and vomiting are common and fever, jaundice, and ileus may develop. In severe cases ascites, pleural effusions, hypoxia, and adult respiratory distress syndrome may occur. Complications include pseudocysts and abscesses.

Treatment

Treatment should be conservative, with laparotomy performed only if there is diagnostic difficulty or underlying biliary-tract disease. No fluids or solids should be given by mouth and any shock should be treated. Opioid analgesics (BNF 4.7.2) may be required for pain relief. In severe cases, the stomach should be aspirated. A range of treatments has been tested in acute pancreatitis. Aprotinin, a proteolytic enzyme inhibitor (BNF 1.9.3), may reduce the effects of released pancreatic enzymes; and glucagon (BNF 6.1.4) has also been used. The value of any of these treatments is currently unsubstantiated.

Chronic Pancreatitis

Definition and aetiology

Chronic pancreatitis is characterised by the progressive destruction and fibrosis of pancreatic glandular tissue, resulting in the failure of endocrine and exocrine pancreatic function. It may arise through chronic alcoholism, chronic protein malnutrition, hyperparathyroidism, or hyperlipidaemia.

Symptoms

Recurrent episodes of severe epigastric pain lasting about 24 to 48 hours commonly occur and these may be aggravated by a heavy meal or by alcohol. Alternatively, the pain may be relatively constant, but aggravated by food. Pain may be accompanied by nausea and vomiting and is not relieved by antacids. Jaundice may occur and pseudocysts are common. Chronic pancreatitis results in a reduction in pancreatic size and a dilatation of the pancreatic ducts. Lack of pancreatic enzyme secretion gives rise to malabsorption from the intestine, characterised by steatorrhoea. Initially the endocrine function of the pancreas may continue, but eventually mild diabetes mellitus may occur.

Treatment
Chronic pancreatitis is treated symptomatically. Acute attacks are treated with analgesics (BNF 4.7). A low-fat high-protein diet should be given, alcohol forbidden, and replacement therapy with pancreatin supplements (BNF 1.9.4) provided when required. Insulin (BNF 6.1.1) may be needed for the treatment of diabetes, as oral hypoglycaemic agents are unlikely to be effective. Surgical treatment may be necessary.

1.10 ANATOMY AND PHYSIOLOGY OF THE DIGESTIVE SYSTEM

The digestive system (Fig. 1.6) comprises the gastro-intestinal tract and associated organs. Its structure is modified along its length to allow the sequential processes of intake, digestion, absorption, and excretion. (For a description of the anatomy and physiology of the oropharynx, *see* Section 12.4.)

The oesophagus channels food and liquids downward from the mouth to the stomach, aided by mucus and peristalsis. The contents of the stomach are prevented from regurgitating into the oesophagus by the muscular cardiac sphincter.

The stomach is a muscular reservoir whose convoluted inner surface secretes gastric juice (which includes hydrochloric acid, and the proteolytic enzyme precursor, pepsinogen) in response to the release of the hormone gastrin from the stomach mucosa. Rennin is also secreted in young children. The internal surface of the stomach is protected from the potentially harmful effects of these secretions by the continual regeneration of epithelial cells, the regulation of output so that food is always present when secretion occurs, and the presence of the glycoprotein, mucin, which provides a physical and chemical barrier, particularly to the effects of gastric acid. Retention of ingested material occurs mainly in the fundus, but also to a lesser extent in the body of the stomach. Mixing and homogenisation of ingested material into a suspension (chyme) occurs in the body and distal antrum. When the lower portion of the stomach contracts, small quantities of acidic chyme are propelled through the pyloric sphincter into the small intestine.

The small intestine consists sequentially of the duo-denum, jejunum, and the ileum. When food enters the duodenum, it is modified by secretions from the intestine wall, the liver, and the pancreas. Intestinal mucosal and submucosal cells secrete an alkaline mucus which neutralises the acidic character of the chyme.

The liver (*see also below*) secretes bile which is stored in the gall bladder. In the presence of food in the duodenum, the release of bile is stimulated by the action of pancreozymin. Bile contains steroidal bile salts (e.g. sodium glycocholate) which emulsify fats and lipids; bile pigments (containing the breakdown products of haemoglobin), which colour the faeces; and cholesterol, lecithin, water, and electrolytes.

The release of exocrine pancreatic secretions is also controlled by pancreozymin. These secretions include amylase, which digests polysaccharides to disaccharides; lipase, which converts lipids to fatty acids and glycerol; and the enzyme precursors trypsinogen and chymotrypsinogen, which are converted to active proteolytic enzymes.

The small intestine is the primary site of absorption of the initial products of digestion. The presence of gently oscillating villi (Fig. 1.7), tightly packed in the duodenum and jejunum, but more sparsely populating the ileum, greatly enhances the absorptive capacity. These finger-like projections comprise cells which constantly migrate upwards from the base, to be shed within 2 to 3 days of formation. As the relatively alkaline luminal emulsion (chyle) is absorbed by the villi, digestion continues within the lining cells. Proteases break down peptides to amino acids; lactase, maltase, and sucrase break down disaccharides to (mainly) glucose; lipase breaks down the macrostructure of fat droplets to form simple fatty acids and glycerol; and long-chain fatty acids and glycerol, together with phospholipids and proteins, recombine to produce chylomicrons. Water-soluble vitamins including vitamin B_{12}, iron, and folic acid are also absorbed.

The intestinal liquid chyle enters the ascending colon through the ileocaecal valve. The colon acts as the final site of water and electrolyte reabsorption, causing the intestinal mass to become firmer as it passes towards the rectum. The presence of a bulky mass produces stimulation of the stretch receptors in the colon and rectum, inducing peristalsis and initiating the evacuation of the faeces.

The liver lies in the upper portion of the peritoneal cavity, immediately beneath the diaphragm. It is composed of lobules (Fig. 1.8) formed of sheets of radiating cells orientated around a central branch of the hepatic vein. The hepatic arteries bring oxygenated blood from the general circulation, and the hepatic portal veins collect nutrients from along the lower gastro-

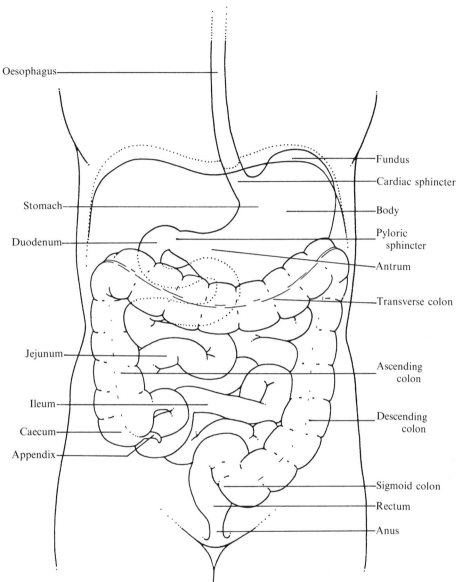

Oesophagus

Fundus

Cardiac sphincter

Stomach

Body

Duodenum

Pyloric sphincter

Antrum

Transverse colon

Jejunum

Ascending colon

Ileum

Caecum

Descending colon

Appendix

Sigmoid colon

Rectum

Anus

Figure 1.6
Anatomy of the digestive system.

intestinal tract. Both supplies drain into sinusoids between the liver cells.

The liver has many diverse functions. It secretes bile into canaliculi between the sheets of liver cells, from where the bile drains into the bile ducts. Excess glucose is removed from the hepatic-portal system and stored as glycogen or fat. In hypoglycaemia, glycogen is reconverted into glucose and released into the circulation. The iver also stores vitamins A, D, and B$_{12}$, and iron and deaminates amino acids. One fragment of the amino acid is converted into glucose and utilised as energy. The second fragment is converted into ammonia in the liver and excreted via the urea cycle (*see* Section 15.2). The synthesis of non-essential amino acids is also carried out by the liver through transamination reactions. It produces plasma proteins and blood coagulation factors. The liver also has an important protective role. Bacteria are removed by phagocytosis, drugs and chemicals are detoxified, and aged erythrocytes and leucocytes are destroyed. Homoeostatic regulation is also achieved through the controlled inactivation of endocrine hormones.

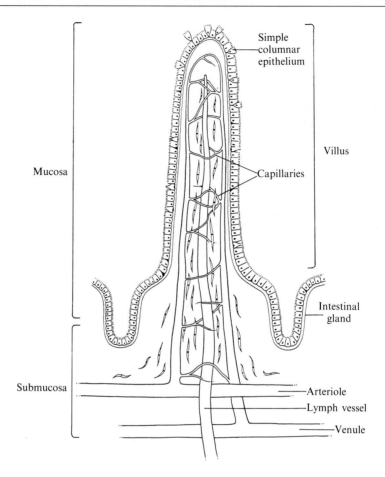

Fig. 1.7
Cross-section of a villus.

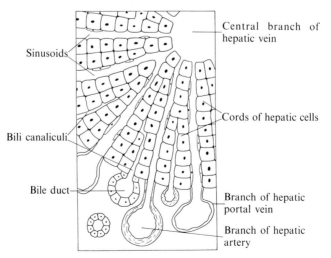

Fig. 1.8
Schematic diagram of a portion of a liver lobule.

Chapter 2

CARDIOVASCULAR SYSTEM DISORDERS

2.1 GENERAL DISORDERS

Aneurysm

Definition and aetiology

An aneurysm is a localised dilatation of an artery. Saccular aneurysms usually occur at arterial junctions (e.g. cerebral aneurysm). Longitudinal aneurysms occur along the complete length of a vessel (e.g. aortic aneurysm) due to replacement of the vessel wall with fibrous tissue. If blood penetrates the vessel wall and separates its layers it is termed a dissecting aneurysm. Aneurysms are commonly caused by atherosclerosis, but may also arise due to congenital abnormalities, injury, or inflammation.

Aortic Aneurysm

Definition and aetiology

Abdominal aortic aneurysms are more common than thoracic aortic aneurysms. Both types are usually caused by atherosclerosis, although injury and syphilis are other causes.

Symptoms

Abdominal aortic aneurysm is characterised by severe abdominal tenderness and pain which may radiate to the back. Equally, however, it may arise asymptomatically and be detected only on rupture, resulting in acute circulatory failure and shock.

Thoracic aortic aneurysm is often asymptomatic, but chest pain radiating to the back may occur. Pressure on adjacent organs may produce dysphagia and cough. Rupture may result in sudden death.

Dissecting aneurysm of the thoracic aorta (Fig. 2.1) is usually associated with atherosclerosis and hypertension. It produces chest and back pain, which may radiate to the neck or arms and can be difficult to differentiate from the pain of myocardial infarction.

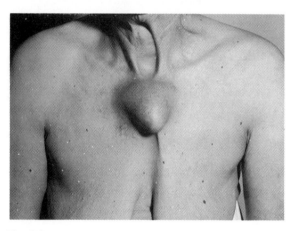

Fig. 2.1
A dissecting aortic aneurysm in which blood has penetrated the vessel walls, producing dilatation.

Treatment

Treatment is by surgery. Antihypertensive therapy (BNF 2.5) may be useful in dissecting aneurysms.

Cerebral Aneurysm

Definition and aetiology

Cerebral (berry) aneurysms occur in intracranial arteries. They may be caused by congenital abnormalities or may develop as a result of atherosclerosis or hypertension.

Symptoms

Cerebral aneurysms are often multiple and may be asymptomatic. They can rupture resulting in subarachnoid haemorrhage, which is characterised by severe headache and often results in death.

Treatment

Treatment consists of hospitalisation and the administration of beta-adrenoceptor blocking drugs (BNF 2.4) or antihypertensive therapy (BNF 2.5). Antifibrinolytic drugs (BNF 2.11) have also been used. Surgery may be indicated, but is hazardous.

Arteriosclerosis

Definition and aetiology

Arteriosclerosis is the term applied to a group of blood vessel diseases in which loss of elasticity and increased thickening occur, caused by the replacement of muscle and elastic tissue by fibrous tissue.

The most common form of arteriosclerosis is atherosclerosis, although arteriolosclerosis (affecting the arterioles) may also occur, usually as a consequence of hypertension.

Atherosclerosis

Definition and aetiology

Atherosclerosis is characterised by the development of yellowish-fatty plaques (atheromas), containing cholesterol and other lipids. The plaques subsequently haemorrhage, calcify, and become ulcerated. They are formed within the endothelial lining of the walls of large and medium-sized arteries. They most commonly cause problems when they arise in coronary and cerebral arteries, and peripheral arteries of the lower limbs. Their development is part of a natural ageing process, and the disease is progressive. Factors which predispose to the development of atherosclerosis include hyperlipidaemia, diabetes mellitus, obesity, lack of exercise, genetic factors, smoking, and possibly emotional disturbances.

Symptoms

Atheromas cause narrowing and ultimately occlusion of the arteries, resulting in chronic ischaemia of the structures supplied by the arteries. Atheromas also provide a surface on which thrombosis can occur, producing acute ischaemia and infarction.

The symptoms of ischaemia depend upon the organ supplied by the artery and upon whether occlusion is acute or chronic, as the latter may be offset by the development of a collateral circulation. Atherosclerosis occurring in coronary vessels can give rise to angina pectoris, myocardial infarction, and arrhythmias. Its occurrence in cerebral arteries can cause forgetfulness, confusion, personality changes, or a stroke. In the arteries of the leg, intermittent claudication of calves and gangrene of toes may develop.

Atherosclerosis may cause hypertension through increased peripheral resistance of the narrowed arteries or because of stenosis of the renal artery. A long-standing atheroma may extend into the wall, with weakening of the artery. Aneurysms are formed when rupture of the lining of the artery wall allows blood to collect beneath the outer fibrous coat, which becomes grossly distended. They produce symptoms by pressing on the surrounding structures or by rupturing.

Treatment
Control of predisposing factors is the most important element of prevention and control of atherosclerosis. Plasma-lipid concentrations may be lowered by dietary control and by the administration of lipid-lowering drugs (BNF 2.12). The patency of severely narrowed arteries may sometimes be restored by surgery and by transluminal angioplasty using balloon catheters.

Cardiac Arrest

Definition and aetiology
Cardiac arrest is the sudden arrest of cardiac function and often occurs in conjunction with respiratory failure. Cardiac contraction is absent or inadequate, resulting in the termination of an effective cardiac output. It is a common cause of death. It usually occurs as a result of ventricular fibrillation, heart block, or acute circulatory failure.

Symptoms
It is characterised by absent pulse, heart sounds, and blood pressure. Apnoea, dilated pupils, and unconsciousness also occur.

Treatment
Immediate treatment is essential and initially consists of artificial respiration and external cardiac massage. Normal heart function may be restored by cardioversion. Drug treatment appropriate to the underlying cause may be necessary.

Circulatory Failure, Acute

Definition and aetiology
Acute circulatory failure, or lack of an adequate blood supply to the tissues and organs, results from arterial hypotension caused by a substantial uncompensated reduction in cardiac output. In transient form this gives rise to syncope, and in more prolonged form to shock.

Syncope

Definition and aetiology
Syncope (faint) is a transient reversible loss of consciousness caused by an acute reduction in blood supply to the brain (cerebral ischaemia), resulting from acute circulatory failure. Reduction in cardiac output may be the consequence of insufficient venous return to the heart caused by peripheral vasodilatation (e.g. in hot weather) or by venous pooling below the heart (e.g. after prolonged standing). It may also be caused by instability of vasomotor control (e.g. orthostatic hypotension caused by ganglion-blocking agents or bilateral sympathectomy). Cardiogenic syncope, caused by transient failure of the diseased heart to provide sufficient cardiac output (e.g. in myocardial infarction), may be followed by shock. Psychogenic factors may also precipitate syncope through vagal overactivity.

Symptoms
Syncope is usually preceded by feelings of lightheadedness, nausea, pallor, sweating, and tachypnoea. The hypotensive episode may be accompanied by bradycardia, particularly if due to vagal overactivity.

Treatment
Unconsciousness is brief and recovery may be hastened by laying the patient flat and raising the legs. Further treatment is usually unnecessary.

Shock

Definition and aetiology
Shock is caused by derangement of circulatory control or loss of circulating fluid, resulting in severe reduction in cardiac output. Intense sympathetic vasoconstriction initially maintains the arterial pressure and blood flow to the brain and other vital organs, although at inadequate levels.

Hypovolaemic shock may be caused by massive loss of body fluids arising from haemorrhage, fractures, extensive muscle trauma, burns, vomiting, or diarrhoea. It may also be caused by release into the circulation of endotoxins (septic shock) or tissue breakdown products which cause vasodilatation and increased capillary permeability (e.g. in peritonitis, septicaemia, and pancreatitis).

Cardiogenic shock results from a marked decrease in cardiac output and may be caused by heart disease (e.g. myocardial infarction and serious arrhythmia) or pulmonary embolism (*see also* Cardiac Arrest).

Anaphylactic shock occurs as a result of a specific antigen-antibody reaction, which results in the release of histamine and other chemical mediators. In addition to cardiovascular symptoms, respiratory and skin reactions are common.

Symptoms
All vital activities are depressed, causing weakness, subnormal temperature, sweating, and apathy. Con-

sciousness is generally maintained, although syncope (*see above*) may occur if the patient stands up. The skin is pale, cold, and cyanotic and the pulse is weak and rapid. There is hypotension, tachypnoea, hypoxia, and a reduction in renal blood flow which results in decreased urinary output and fluid and electrolyte retention. Metabolic disturbances result in a metabolic acidosis.

Treatment
The incidence and severity of shock may be minimised by gentle handling of injuries, protection from cold, and prevention of further losses of blood and electrolytes. Treatment should be instituted as soon as possible and consists of the administration of opioid analgesics (BNF 4.7.2), fluid and electrolytes (BNF 9.2), correction of blood loss, oxygen therapy (BNF 3.6), and the correction of metabolic acidosis (BNF 9.2.2). In addition, antiarrhythmic drugs (BNF 2.3) or sympathomimetics with inotropic activity (BNF 2.7.1) may be of value in cardiogenic shock and adrenaline, followed by corticosteroids (BNF 6.3.4), may be given in anaphylactic shock.

Cor Pulmonale

Definition and aetiology
Cor pulmonale is pulmonary hypertension complicated by right ventricular hypertrophy and right heart failure, developing as a result of lung diseases (e.g. asthma, chronic bronchitis and emphysema, pulmonary fibrosis, or pulmonary embolism).

Symptoms
All symptoms of cor pulmonale are associated with pulmonary hypertension, right ventricular hypertrophy, and right heart failure and include arrhythmias, hepatomegaly, increased venous pressure, oedema, and hypercapnia. In severe disease, the nephrotic syndrome may develop.

Treatment
Treatment involves identification and treatment of the underlying lung disorder. Oxygen therapy (BNF 3.6) and respiratory stimulants (BNF 3.5) may be necessary in some patients. Diuretics with potassium salts (BNF 2.2) are used to control heart failure, and venesection may be indicated.

Heart Failure

Definition and aetiology
Heart failure is an acute or chronic condition in which the heart fails to maintain an adequate blood supply to the tissues despite normal ventricular filling. It may occur in the left heart (left ventricular failure), the right heart (right ventricular failure), or both sides (congestive

heart failure). Since coronary arteriosclerosis, hypertension, and rheumatic heart disease (arising from rheumatic fever) affect mainly the left heart, left ventricular failure is more common than right. Left ventricular failure, however, is the most common cause of right heart failure.

Causes of heart failure include myocardial disorders and valvular heart disease, anaemia, hyperthyroidism, hypertension, and arrhythmias. Right heart failure may be secondary to lung disease (e.g. pulmonary embolism and chronic bronchitis and emphysema), and under such circumstances it is termed cor pulmonale.

Symptoms
Failure of one side of the heart leads to congestion and oedema in the tissues from which the venous supply is drained. Thus left heart failure produces pulmonary oedema, pulmonary hypertension, and breathlessness (dyspnoea, orthopnoea, and paroxysmal nocturnal dyspnoea) caused by pulmonary congestion. Other symptoms are cyanosis, fatigue, haemoptysis, and tachycardia. Right heart failure produces peripheral oedema (e.g. of ankles), cyanosis, fatigue, hepatic enlargement and tenderness, and sometimes ascites. In addition, the inadequate cardiac output leads to a disproportionate reduction in renal blood-flow, resulting in sodium and water retention. In congestive heart failure the symptoms are a combination of those described above and result in marked physical incapacity, breathlessness, and peripheral oedema.

Treatment
Treatment should be directed at the underlying cause and patients advised to rest in order to reduce cardiac work. Positive inotropic drugs (BNF 2.1), diuretics with potassium supplements (BNF 2.2), angiotensin-converting enzyme inhibitors (BNF 2.5.5), or vasodilators (BNF 2.6) are used in the treatment of heart failure.

Self-help organisations
British Heart Foundation
Chest Heart and Stroke Association

Hypertension

Definition and aetiology
Hypertension is abnormally high arterial blood pressure. The blood pressure of healthy individuals may extend over a wide range of values which tend to increase with age. The pressure at which blood pressure is described as abnormal is at present controversial. In the young or middle-aged, a resting systolic pressure in excess of 150 mmHg or a diastolic pressure greater than 100 mmHg would warrant treatment by most

authorities, although these pressures apparently have no ill effects in some subjects.

Essential (primary) hypertension is idiopathic and is the most common form of the disease. Age, arteriosclerosis, diet, family history, and obesity may be factors in its development.

Secondary hypertension occurs as a result of other underlying disorders. Possible causes include renal disease (e.g. renal artery stenosis and pyelonephritis), endocrine disorders (e.g. Cushing's syndrome, primary aldosteronism, and phaeochromocytoma), and drug administration (e.g. oral contraceptives and corticosteroids). Other causes are coarctation of the aorta and eclampsia.

Malignant (accelerated) hypertension is usually characterised by a diastolic pressure greater than 140 mmHg. It is most common in patients over 40 years of age and in those with chronic renal disorders.

Symptoms
Hypertension is usually asymptomatic, although blurred vision, dizziness, dyspnoea, and nocturia may occur. Although headaches are commonly thought to be associated with hypertension, they are usually only a symptom of severe hypertension. The main complications of hypertension, which may be fatal, are heart failure, myocardial infarction, renal failure, ruptured aneurysm, and stroke. These complications are often the presenting features of hypertension.

Treatment
The initial approach to the treatment of hypertension is the identification and treatment of any underlying cause. If no cause can be found, patients should be encouraged to alter their life-style, lose excess weight, stop smoking, and reduce alcohol consumption. Low-salt diets and stress reduction may also be beneficial. Drug treatment may be necessary and includes the use of thiazide and related diuretics (BNF 2.2.1), beta-adrenoceptor blocking drugs (BNF 2.4), calcium-channel blockers (BNF 2.6.2), or other antihypertensive therapy (BNF 2.5). Periodic examination of heart size and of the retina, and testing urine for proteins, are desirable in such subjects to assess deterioration of cardiovascular and renal function.

Malignant hypertension is a medical emergency and requires immediate hospitalisation.

Self-help organisations
British Heart Foundation
Chest Heart and Stroke Association

Orthostatic Hypotension

Definition and aetiology
Orthostatic (postural) hypotension is a fall in blood pressure which occurs upon rising abruptly from the supine to the erect position. It may also occur when standing motionless in a fixed position. It is often caused by drug therapy (e.g. benzodiazepines, levodopa, phenothiazines, thiazides, and tricyclic and related antidepressants). It may also occur after prolonged bed rest and as a result of autonomic nervous system disorders (e.g. Shy-Drager syndrome), and is common in the elderly.

Symptoms
Orthostatic hypotension is often asymptomatic. It may, however, result in blurred vision, dizziness, and syncope caused by impairment of the cerebral circulation.

Treatment
Treatment consists of withdrawal or dosage reduction of the offending drug. Patients should be advised to stand up slowly and to wear graduated compression hosiery. Fludrocortisone (BNF 6.3.1) may have a role in the treatment of severe orthostatic hypotension.

Pericarditis

Definition and aetiology
Pericarditis is inflammation of the membranous sac (the pericardium) surrounding the heart. It may be caused by viral, bacterial (including tuberculous), or fungal infection, and can also follow myocardial infarction or heart surgery. Other causes include rheumatic fever, connective tissue disorders, hypothyroidism, and malignant disease. It may also arise as a result of irradiation, trauma, or the administration of drugs (e.g. hydralazine and procainamide).

Symptoms
Pericarditis is characterised by arrhythmias and a sharp continuous chest pain which is relieved by sitting up. Symptoms may be preceded by a general influenza-like malaise. Breathing may also be painful, resulting in dyspnoea. Pericarditis may result in accumulation of fluid within the pericardium (pericardial effusion), causing cardiac tamponade in which the pressure of accumulated fluid interferes with ventricular filling. Ventricular filling may also be restricted by thickening of the pericardium.

Treatment
Pericarditis may be self-limiting and require only symptomatic treatment. The underlying cause should, however, be treated. Indomethacin (BNF 10.1.1) may be given to reduce pain and inflammation, and corticosteroids (BNF 6.3.4) may be indicated. Emergency treatment of cardiac tamponade by pericardial aspiration

may be necessary. Surgery may be required in cases of pericardial constriction caused by thickening of the pericardium.

Pulmonary Hypertension

Definition and aetiology
Pulmonary hypertension is abnormally high blood pressure in the pulmonary circulation in which the systolic pressure rises above 30 mmHg or the diastolic pressure rises above 15 mmHg. Lung disease (e.g. chronic bronchitis and emphysema, or pulmonary embolism) produces an increase in pulmonary vascular resistance due to chronic hypoxia. The ensuing pulmonary hypertension is followed by right ventricular hypertrophy and subsequent right heart failure (cor pulmonale).

Other causes of pulmonary hypertension include congenital heart disease and mitral stenosis. Increased pulmonary blood pressure of unknown cause is termed primary pulmonary hypertension.

Symptoms
Severe pulmonary hypertension is characterised by fatigue and dyspnoea on effort together with chest pain, haemoptysis, peripheral cyanosis, and syncope.

Treatment
Treatment of pulmonary hypertension is directed toward the underlying heart or lung disease. The use of anticoagulants (BNF 2.8.2) has been proposed. The course is relentlessly downhill for most patients, and heart-lung transplantation offers the only hope of prolonged survival.

Pulmonary Oedema

Definition and aetiology
Pulmonary oedema is the abnormal accumulation of fluid in pulmonary tissue and the alveoli. It is often due to left ventricular failure, but may also occur as a result of mitral stenosis, pneumonia, or the accidental inhalation of gastric contents.

Symptoms
Pulmonary oedema is characterised by acute worsening dyspnoea. Anxiety and a sensation of suffocation are common symptoms, and a cough together with the production of pink frothy sputum may occur. Cyanosis may develop and the condition can be fatal.

Treatment
Early treatment is essential and comprises sitting the patient up and administering oxygen (BNF 3.6), diuretics (BNF 2.2), bronchodilators (BNF 3.1), vasodilators

(BNF 2.5.1 and 2.6.1), and an opioid analgesic (BNF 4.7.2). The underlying disorder must be identified and treated.

Valvular Heart Disease

Definition
Valvular heart disease is characterised by inadequate functioning of the mitral, aortic, and tricuspid valves of the heart. Pulmonary valve disease also occurs but is uncommon.

Mitral Stenosis

Definition and aetiology
Mitral stenosis is a narrowing of the orifice of the left atrioventricular (mitral) valve. It is usually caused by rheumatic heart disease (arising from rheumatic fever), and it may also develop as a result of congenital abnormalities, infective endocarditis, and systemic lupus erythematosus. Disease of rheumatic origin is much more common in women.

Symptoms
Mitral stenosis usually develops insidiously over several years, but may occur abruptly. The most common symptoms are reduced exercise tolerance, followed later in the disease by paroxysmal nocturnal dyspnoea caused by pulmonary oedema. Palpitations may arise through atrial fibrillation. Haemoptysis may be a consequence of bronchial vein rupture, left heart failure, and pulmonary embolism. Angina may occasionally occur. Severe cases may be complicated by pulmonary hypertension, which leads to right heart failure.

Treatment
Treatment of atrial fibrillation with anti-arrhythmic drugs (BNF 2.3), fluid retention with diuretics (BNF 2.2), chest infections with antibacterial drugs (BNF 5.1), and anticoagulants (BNF 2.8) for atrial fibrillation and pulmonary embolism should be undertaken. Surgical treatment may be necessary, and mitral valve dilatation (valvotomy) or replacement may be performed. Antibacterial prophylaxis (BNF 5.1, Table 2) is necessary in patients requiring minor surgery (e.g. dental surgery).

Mitral Regurgitation

Definition and aetiology
Mitral regurgitation is the backflow of blood from the left ventricle to left atrium, caused by a defective mitral valve. It may be due to rheumatic heart disease, and other causes include a floppy mitral valve, infective

endocarditis, ischaemic heart disease, cardiomyopathy, and valve calcification. 50% of cases are associated with mitral stenosis (*see above*).

Symptoms

Symptoms are variable, developing gradually or suddenly, and include fatigue, dyspnoea, pulmonary oedema and embolism, congestive heart failure, heart murmurs, and conduction defects.

Treatment

Mild mitral regurgitation often requires no treatment, apart from antibacterial prophylaxis (BNF 5.1, Table 2) as appropriate, although treatment of the underlying disease may be necessary. In severe disease, surgical repair or replacement of the mitral valve may be indicated.

Aortic Stenosis

Definition and aetiology

Aortic stenosis is characterised by a narrowing of the aortic orifice of the heart. It may be caused by congenital abnormalities (e.g. an abnormal bicuspid valve) or may result from rheumatic heart disease, valve calcification, or infective endocarditis.

Symptoms

Symptoms tend to occur late in the course of the disease and include anginal pain, dyspnoea, and syncope. Sudden death may occur.

Treatment

Most asymptomatic patients require little treatment, apart from appropriate antibacterial prophylaxis (BNF 5.1, Table 2). The symptomatic patient may, however, benefit from bed rest, diuretics (BNF 2.2), and surgical aortic valve replacement. Angina should be treated with beta-adrenoceptor blocking drugs (BNF 2.4) as vasodilators may aggravate symptoms.

Aortic Regurgitation

Definition and aetiology

Aortic regurgitation is the backflow of blood from the aorta into the left ventricle caused by a defective aortic valve. It may develop as a result of rheumatic heart disease, rheumatoid arthritis, ankylosing spondylitis, infective endocarditis, trauma, dissecting aneurysm, syphilis, ulcerative colitis, or congenital conditions (e.g. Marfan's syndrome or abnormal bicuspid valves).

Symptoms

It may be asymptomatic for many years. Dyspnoea, however, is a common symptom, particularly on exercising, and chest pain and heart murmurs may also occur.

Treatment

Antibacterial prophylaxis (BNF 5.1, Table 2) is appropriate and surgical valve replacement may be necessary in severe cases.

Tricuspid Stenosis

Definition and aetiology

Tricuspid stenosis is a narrowing of the tricuspid orifice of the heart, which is almost always caused by rheumatic heart disease.

Symptoms

Symptoms are similar to those of mitral and aortic valve disease (*see above*), but ascites and peripheral oedema may be prominent in severe stenosis.

Treatment

Treatment includes the administration of diuretics (BNF 2.2). Although valve replacement should be avoided, dilatation (valvotomy) or repair may be necessary.

Tricuspid Regurgitation

Definition and aetiology

Tricuspid regurgitation is the backflow of blood from the right ventricle to the right atrium caused by a defective tricuspid valve. It may arise as a result of rheumatic heart disease, infective endocarditis, carcinoid syndrome, pulmonary hypertension, or congenital abnormalities.

Symptoms

Symptoms include raised venous blood pressure, oedema, ascites, and hepatomegaly with nausea and epigastric pain. Mild jaundice may occur.

Treatment

Treatment comprises bed rest and the administration of diuretics (BNF 2.2) and vasodilators (BNF 2.6). Surgical valve replacement may be beneficial.

Self-help organisations

British Heart Foundation
Chest Heart and Stroke Association

2.2   MYOCARDIAL DISEASE

Cardiomyopathy

Definition and aetiology

A cardiomyopathy is a disorder of the myocardium. Most cases are of unknown aetiology and cardiomyopathy is a frequent cause of sudden death.

Dilated (congestive) cardiomyopathy is the dilatation

of left or right ventricles, or both. It is thought to be due to inflammation of the myocardium, alcohol abuse, or hypertension.

Hypertrophic cardiomyopathy, which may be familial, consists of hypertrophy of the left, and occasionally right, ventricle.

Restrictive cardiomyopathy is due to fibrosis or scarring of the endomyocardium, which becomes rigid.

Symptoms
Dyspnoea is common to each cardiomyopathy. Oedema and embolism may occur in dilated and restrictive cardiomyopathies, whereas angina pectoris and syncope are characteristic of hypertrophic cardiomyopathy. Tachycardia may develop in dilated and hypertrophic forms of the disease, although both may be asymptomatic.

Treatment
The treatment of cardiomyopathies varies according to symptoms and may include the use of anticoagulants (BNF 2.8), diuretics (BNF 2.2), vasodilators (BNF 2.6.1), beta-adrenoceptor blocking drugs (BNF 2.4), and anti-arrhythmic drugs (BNF 2.3). Bed rest, weight loss, and avoidance of alcohol are useful measures in the management of dilated cardiomyopathy. Surgery may be carried out in all forms of cardiomyopathy, and heart transplantation may be necessary in severe cases of dilated and restrictive cardiomyopathy.

Myocarditis

Definition and aetiology
Myocarditis is inflammation of the myocardium. It is usually caused by viral, bacterial, fungal, or parasitic infections, or may be secondary to an underlying systemic disease process (e.g. connective tissue disorders). It may also occur as a side-effect of drug administration (e.g. cytotoxic drugs and chloroquine) and lead poisoning.

Symptoms
Myocarditis may be asymptomatic, or may present with the symptoms of myocardial infarction or angina pectoris. Symptoms include arrhythmias, tachycardia, chest pain, dyspnoea, fatigue, fever, oedema, and heart failure. Sudden death may occur.

Treatment
Treatment is directed towards the underlying cause. Heart failure and arrhythmias may also require treatment.

2.3   ISCHAEMIC HEART DISEASE

Angina Pectoris

Definition and aetiology
Stable angina pectoris arises through cardiac muscle ischaemia, resulting from coronary artery insufficiency and hypertension or, rarely, anaemia and valvular heart disease. Attacks may be precipitated by exertion or emotional disturbances, are relieved by rest, and are most likely in patients whose coronary arteries are partially occluded by arteriosclerotic lesions. In unstable angina pectoris, symptoms may occur at rest and be caused by coronary vasospasm.

Symptoms
Angina pectoris is characterised by paroxysmal pain (or tightness) in the chest which may extend to the shoulder, arms, throat, back, and jaw. Other symptoms are dyspnoea, dizziness, nausea, and sweating.

Treatment
Patients should regulate the amount of exercise taken to minimise the occurrence of attacks. Emotional disturbances, temperature extremes, and overwork should be avoided. Losing excess weight and abstention from smoking should be encouraged. Beta-adrenoceptor blocking drugs (BNF 2.4), nitrates (BNF 2.6.1), or calcium-channel blockers (BNF 2.6.2) may be employed to prevent or relieve attacks. Coronary bypass surgery or angioplasty may be required for failure of medical management and in younger patients with extensive coronary artery disease.

Self-help organisations
British Heart Foundation
Chest Heart and Stroke Association

Myocardial Infarction

Definition and aetiology
Myocardial infarction (coronary thrombosis) is occlusion of a coronary vessel which leads to ischaemia and subsequently destruction (necrosis) of heart muscle. The occlusion is usually caused by coronary-artery thrombosis, resulting from coronary atherosclerosis. Occlusion may also be due to coronary-artery spasm or stenosis. An increased risk of myocardial infarction has been associated with hypertension, hypercholesterolaemia, smoking, emotional disturbances, and lack of exercise.

Symptoms
If the affected area is localised, the unaffected remainder of the myocardium continues to function, although often

with a decreased cardiac ouput which can cause hypotension. This may be accompanied by severe prolonged chest pain, which resembles the pain of angina pectoris. However, it cannot be relieved by rest or the administration of vasodilators. Other symptoms include anxiety, dyspnoea, sweating, and nausea and vomiting. Acute myocardial infarction may lead to arrhythmias, heart block, and cardiogenic shock.

Treatment

Treatment, which is commonly undertaken in a coronary-care unit, consists initially of complete bed rest. The value of fibrinolytic drugs (BNF 2.10) has been demonstrated. A wide range of other drugs may be administered, which include oxygen (BNF 3.6), opioid analgesics (BNF 4.7.2), anti-emetics (BNF 4.6), anxiolytics (BNF 4.1.2), parenteral anticoagulants (BNF 2.8.1), beta-adrenoceptor blocking drugs (BNF 2.4), nitrates (BNF 2.6.1), and calcium-channel blockers (BNF 2.6.2). For the treatment of complications, *see* Arrhythmias, Heart Failure, *and* Shock.

Patients may be maintained on beta-adrenoceptor blocking drugs, oral anticoagulants (BNF 2.8.2), or antiplatelet drugs (BNF 2.9). They must be encouraged to avoid risk factors and return to a full and active life.

Self-help organisations

British Heart Foundation
Chest Heart and Stroke Association

2.4   ARRHYTHMIAS

Bradycardia

Definition and aetiology

Bradycardia is an unusually slow heart-rate (less than 60 beats per minute), resulting from increased vagal or diminished sympathetic tone. It may occur normally during sleep and in healthy young adults and athletes. Bradycardia also occurs after myocardial infarction and certain infections, and in raised intracranial pressure, hypothyroidism, and jaundice. Cardiac glycosides, beta-adrenoceptor blocking drugs, opioid analgesics, and some centrally acting antihypertensive drugs also slow the heart-rate, leading to bradycardia.

Treatment

Although bradycardia does not normally require treatment, the administration of atropine (BNF 2.3.2) or surgical placement of a pacemaker may be necessary.

Ectopic Beats

Definition and aetiology

Ectopic beats (extrasystoles) are cardiac contractions which arise earlier than expected in the cardiac cycle.

They are caused by impulse formation at an abnormal focus of electrical activity in the atria or ventricles. Most ectopic beats are followed by a diastolic pause, as the arrhythmia renders the cardiac muscle refractory to the effects of the next normal impulse. This results in coupling of heart beats, followed by a long pause. Ectopic beats may be associated with rheumatic heart disease (arising as a consequence of rheumatic fever), ischaemic heart disease, and acute myocardial infarction. They may occasionally occur in the absence of cardiac disease. Large quantities of alcohol, caffeine, or tobacco, and overdosage with cardiac glycosides may also cause ectopic beats.

Treatment

Ectopic beats may be asymptomatic. If palpitations occur in the absence of heart disease, patients should be advised to avoid fatigue, emotional disturbances, and excessive consumption of alcohol, caffeine, or tobacco. Anti-arrhythmic drugs (BNF 2.3) may be needed to prevent the development of more serious arrhythmias.

Fibrillations

Definition

A fibrillation is a small rapid series of unco-ordinated contractions of muscle which, in cardiac tissue, produces irregular and ineffective emptying of the heart chambers.

A flutter is a less disturbed, more regular, form of a fibrillation.

Atrial Fibrillation

Definition and aetiology

Atrial fibrillation is a common and important arrhythmia. Integrated atrial contractions disappear and are replaced by rapid fibrillary twitching of the atria. This leads to random rapid ventricular contractions, and the pulse is irregular in rhythm and force. Atrial fibrillation is usually associated with rheumatic heart disease (arising as a consequence of rheumatic fever), mitral stenosis, ischaemic heart disease, hyperthyroidism, and hypertension. Less commonly, lung cancer, other malignant diseases, congenital heart disease, infective endocarditis, and pericarditis may be involved. In the presence of other serious heart disease, the onset of atrial fibrillation may lead to congestive heart failure. Systemic embolism is a common complication when atrial fibrillation is caused by valvular heart disease. Onset of atrial fibrillation may be precipitated by alcohol and mental or physical stress.

Symptoms

Some patients may be unaware of the arrhythmia, although many experience palpitations. Attacks of atrial fibrillation may be accompanied by dizziness, syncope, and chest pain.

Treatment
Any underlying cause should be treated. When there is tachycardia (*see below*) or any evidence of congestive heart failure, positive inotropic drugs (BNF 2.1) are used to reduce the rapid ventricular rate. If there is no evidence of serious organic disease, atrial fibrillation may be converted to normal (sinus) rhythm by cardioversion (direct-current shock). Anti-arrhythmic drugs (BNF 2.3) may be used to maintain normal rhythm and oral anticoagulants (BNF 2.8.2) to prevent embolism.

Atrial Flutter

Definition and aetiology
Atrial flutter is similar to atrial fibrillation. There is co-ordinated, but rapid, atrial muscle action, slower than in atrial fibrillation, but more rapid than in paroxysmal atrial tachycardia (*see below*). Atrial flutter is almost always associated with organic heart disease, and rapidly progresses to the more commonly encountered atrial fibrillation.

Symptoms and treatment are similar to those of atrial fibrillation.

Ventricular Fibrillation

Definition and aetiology
Ventricular fibrillation is a serious condition in which the ventricles fail to contract effectively and cardiac output falls, so that perfusion of vital organs (e.g. the brain) ceases. Death rapidly follows if the condition is not reversed. The causes are the same as those of ventricular tachycardia (*see below*).

Treatment
Treatment comprises cardioversion or the administration of anti-arrhythmic drugs (BNF 2.3).

Heart Block

Definition and aetiology
In heart block (atrioventricular block), there is a defective conduction of the impulse which arises in the sino-atrial (SA) node in the right atrium and passes to the ventricles. This may be due to a defect in the atrioventricular (AV) node or the bundle of His. In partial heart block, the atrial impulse may be delayed in its conduction from the atria to the ventricles (first degree block). Intermittent failure of atrioventricular conduction may cause beats to be missed (second degree block). In complete heart block, there may be atrioventricular dissociation, causing the ventricles to beat at their intrinsic rate of about 30 to 40 beats per minute (third degree block). This rate is completely dissociated from and unaffected by external stimuli. However, because of the slow rate, there is increased ventricular filling which may maintain a normal cardiac output. Heart block is usually due to idiopathic fibrosis or congenital lesions of the conducting system, myocardial infarction, or cardiac glycoside toxicity.

Symptoms
First degree block is asymptomatic. Second degree block may be asymptomatic, although it may suddenly become a complete block. In complete heart block, sudden attacks of syncope commonly occur (Stokes-Adams syndrome). The loss of consciousness is abrupt, with little or no preceding aura, and is associated with extreme bradycardia. Consciousness returns when the ventricular rate increases.

Treatment
Sympathomimetics with inotropic activity (BNF 2.7.1) may be given to increase the heart-rate and prevent the Stokes-Adams syndrome, although intolerable palpitations or ventricular ectopic beats may prevent their continued use. In established heart block, artificial pacemaking of the heart is indicated.

Tachycardias

Definition and aetiology
In tachycardia, the heart-rate is abnormally rapid (more than 100 beats per minute), usually because of increased sympathetic or decreased vagal tone. It often occurs in congestive heart failure and as a result of anaemia, anxiety, exercise, haemorrhage, hyperthyroidism, hypotension, or infections. It may be caused by excessive consumption of caffeine or tobacco, or by anticholinergic drugs.

Paroxysmal Atrial Tachycardia

Definition and aetiology
Paroxysmal atrial (supraventricular) tachycardia is characterised by sudden onset and termination of periods of tachycardia. It may be associated with various forms of heart disease.

Treatment
Attacks of paroxysmal atrial tachycardia may be terminated by massage of the carotid sinus. Beta-adrenoceptor blocking drugs (BNF 2.4), anti-arrhythmic drugs (BNF 2.3), or positive inotropic drugs (BNF 2.1) may also be used.

Ventricular Tachycardia

Definition and aetiology
In ventricular tachycardia, the rapid beating of the ventricles (120 to 250 beats per minute) is caused by an abnormal focus of excitation within the ventricles themselves. It is usually caused by ischaemic heart disease, myocardial infarction, mitral valve disease, cardiomyopathy, or to overdosage with cardiac glycosides or

sympathomimetics. Acute heart failure, ventricular fibrillation, and death may follow if the condition is not treated.

Treatment
Treatment comprises cardioversion or administration of anti-arrhythmic drugs (BNF 2.3).

2.5 PERIPHERAL VASCULAR DISEASE

Acrocyanosis

Definition and aetiology
Acrocyanosis is characterised by a persistent symmetrical blue discoloration (cyanosis) of the hands and, less commonly, feet. It is thought to arise from excessive vasoconstriction of the arterioles and occurs almost exclusively in women.

Symptoms
The affected extremities are blue, cold, sweat profusely, and may become swollen, although the condition is painless. The condition is more severe in cold weather.

Treatment
Treatment is usually unnecessary although cold should be avoided.

Chilblains

Definition and aetiology
Chilblains are local inflammatory lesions, bluish-red in colour, which occur as an abnormal reaction to cold damp weather. They are less common in cold dry conditions.

Their aetiology is unclear, but a possible mechanism involves vasoconstriction of subcutaneous arteries and arterioles and vasodilatation of surface capillaries produced by low temperatures. Arteriolar constriction is less persistent than venule constriction, and re-warming therefore leads to an accumulation of fluid in the tissues.

Symptoms
Chilblains appear on dorsal surfaces of fingers, hands, or feet, or on the ears or nose. They may also appear on lower parts of the leg. They are often accompanied by tenderness and intense pruritus; more severe cases may blister, ulcerate, and blacken due to tissue necrosis. Chronic ulcers may occur on repeated exposure to cold and these can cause atrophy and scarring of the tissue.

Treatment
Treatment is usually unnecessary, as chilblains may be prevented by wearing warm clothing in cold weather and by adequate indoor heating. Peripheral vasodilators

(BNF 2.6.3) have been used, and topical preparations for circulatory disorders (BNF 13.14) are also available, but are of debatable value.

Raynaud's Syndrome

Definition and aetiology
Raynaud's syndrome is vasospasm of arterioles or arteries in the distal areas of limbs, and may be triggered by cold or emotional disturbances. Idiopathic disease occurs mainly in young women. Secondary causes include occlusive artery disease, connective tissue disorders, trauma, or administration of drugs (e.g. beta-adrenoceptor blocking drugs). When the condition is secondary to underlying disease, it is termed Raynaud's phenomenon.

Symptoms
Symptoms include blanching, cyanosis, and numbness, followed by reactive hyperaemia which causes redness and throbbing pain. Ischaemia may lead to atrophy of the skin or small painful ulcers on the digital tips. Attacks may last for minutes or hours.

Treatment
Patients should be advised to avoid extreme cold and factors which may produce occlusive artery disease (e.g. smoking). Treatment with nifedipine (BNF 2.6.2) or by surgery (regional sympathectomy) may be necessary.

Varices

Definition
Varices are abnormally dilated tortuous veins, arteries, or lymphatic vessels. They commonly occur in veins of the gastro-intestinal tract (e.g. oesophageal varices) and of the legs (varicose veins).

Oesophageal Varices

Definition and aetiology
Oesophageal varices often arise as a consequence of portal hypertension (e.g. in cirrhosis of the liver).

Symptoms
Bleeding may occur, resulting in haematemesis or melaena. However, massive haemorrhage may occur, leading to shock. Symptoms of the underlying liver disease (e.g. ascites, hepatic encephalopathy, hepatomegaly, and jaundice) may be present.

Bleeding varices may also occur in the veins of the stomach.

Treatment
Treatment is by transfusion, and administration of vitamin K (BNF 9.6.6) and certain posterior pituitary hormones (BNF 6.5.2). Sclerotherapy may be used and,

if bleeding persists, emergency surgery may be necessary. Treatment of the underlying liver disease may be required.

Varicose Veins

Definition and aetiology

Varicose veins (Fig. 2.2) are varices which usually involve the superficial (saphenous) veins of the leg. They are associated with defective valves, particularly between the superficial and deep veins of the leg. They may be due to congenital valve defects, thrombophlebitis, deep vein thrombosis, pregnancy, ascites, malignant disease, and excessive body-weight.

Symptoms

The affected superficial veins are often visible and symptoms may include local pain and oedema, which may be exacerbated by prolonged standing, but disappear on resting. The calf muscles often become easily fatigued. Varices of the deep veins may result in chronic venous insufficiency, and are characterised by oedema and fibrosis. Local brown pigmentation may develop together with a pruritic eczematous rash. Ulceration of the skin may occur.

Treatment

Treatment consists of support with graduated compression hosiery or bandages, and elevation of the legs. Local sclerosants (BNF 2.13) may be useful and surgical ligation or stripping may be necessary.

2.6 ANATOMY AND PHYSIOLOGY OF THE CARDIOVASCULAR SYSTEM

The cardiovascular system comprises a pump, the heart, and the circulatory system, which may be divided into the systemic (peripheral) and pulmonary branches.

The heart lies behind the sternum and costal cartilages in the mediastinum, and ventral to the oesophagus. The heart and great vessels are enclosed within a sac, the pericardium, which consists of an outer fibrous layer and an inner membranous layer, the epicardium. The epicardium is continuous with the outermost surface of the heart muscle, while the pericardium acts to limit the movement of the heart as it contracts.

The heart is composed of cardiac muscle, the myocardium, which has an inner lining, the endocardium.

Internally, the heart (Fig. 2.3) consists of two pairs of chambers, the right pair being separated from the left by a continuous septum. Deoxygenated blood enters the heart at the right atrium via the inferior vena cava (bring-

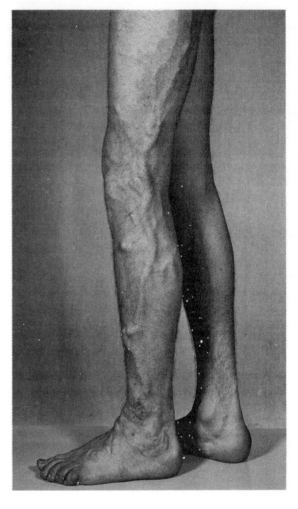

Fig. 2.2
Varicose veins. Note the area of pigmentation at the top rear of the thigh, and the early signs of ulceration of the ankle.

ing blood from all lower parts of the body) and the superior vena cava (carrying blood from the brain and tissues lying above the plane of the heart). On contraction of the atrium, blood passes through the right atrioventricular (tricuspid) valve into the right ventricle. The valve, as the name implies, consists of three cusps formed from a fold of the endocardium. All valves of the heart open and close passively (i.e. when the forward or backward pressure is sufficient to force them to do so). The tricuspid valve closes on ventricular systole to prevent the backflow of blood into the atrium. Blood leaves the right ventricle through the semi-lunar (pulmonary) valve.

Once the blood has been oxygenated in its passage through the lungs, it returns to the heart via two pul-

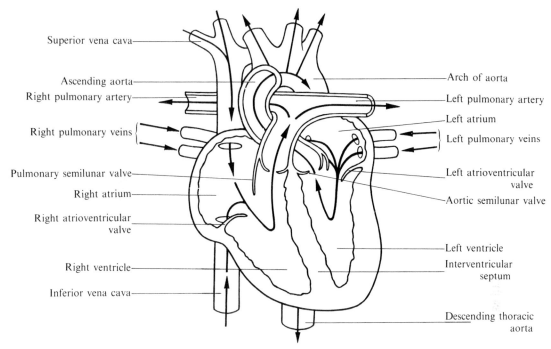

Superior vena cava

Ascending aorta

Right pulmonary artery

Right pulmonary veins

Pulmonary semilunar valve

Right atrium

Right atrioventricular valve

Right ventricle

Inferior vena cava

Arch of aorta

Left pulmonary artery

Left atrium

Left pulmonary veins

Left atrioventricular valve

Aortic semilunar valve

Left ventricle

Interventricular septum

Descending thoracic aorta

Fig. 2.3
Anterior view of the heart.

monary veins from each lung, to re-enter the left atrium. From there, it passes through the left atrioventricular (mitral) valve into the thick-walled left ventricle, from which it is pumped through the semi-lunar (aortic) valve via the aorta to all parts of the body.

The cardiac cycle is the period between two successive heart contractions. The cycle is initiated by the spontaneous generation of an action potential in the sinoatrial node (the pacemaker), which is located in the right atrium near the point of entry of the superior vena cava. The action potential travels rapidly through both atria to depolarise the atrioventricular node. From here it passes via the atrioventricular bundle (bundle of His) to the furthermost point of the ventricles. Contraction of the atria occurs fractionally ahead of the ventricles, allowing the blood to enter the ventricles from the atria before it is pumped around the body.

The action potential of heart activity may be monitored using an electrocardiogram (ECG). This technique also provides a powerful means of assessing defects in cardiac contractility. The P wave is produced by depolarisation of the atria immediately before contraction. The characteristic QRS complex is caused by depolarisation of the ventricles prior to contraction, and the T wave indicates the period of repolarisation of the ventricles (the repolarisation of the atria is not recorded as it

is swamped by the considerably greater QRS complex). The PR interval is about 0.16 seconds and the total duration of the cardiac cycle is about 0.8 seconds.

Heart sounds may also be an important indicator of cardiac disease, particularly disease affecting the valves. Sounds are produced by the closure of the valves, and are commonly described as 'lub' and 'dup'. The resonant 'lub' sound is produced during ventricular systole when the left and right atrioventricular valves close to prevent the backflow of blood into the atria. The more abrupt 'dup' sound indicates the closure of the semi-lunar valves as the ventricles enter a diastolic phase. 'Murmurs' may be produced by diseased valves.

The heart is a thick-walled muscle. The presence of a supply of blood continually bathing its internal surfaces is not sufficient to satisfy the muscle's energy requirements. To allow for this, coronary vessels supply the external layers of the cardiac muscle with oxygenated blood. Two coronary arteries branch off from the aorta almost immediately after its emergence from the left ventricle. These arteries divide rapidly to produce a fine capillary network visible over the heart's external surface. The competence of this network is essential to the viability of cardiac function.

The systemic circulation consists of all blood vessels, except the pulmonary vessels. The arteries transport

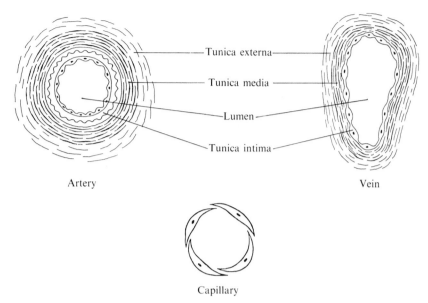

Artery   Vein

Capillary

Fig. 2.4
Cross-section of blood vessels.

blood under high pressure to tissues and modulate the beating impulse of blood flow by their inherent elasticity. The wall of an artery consists of three layers (Fig. 2.4):

- the outermost layer, the tunica externa (composed of connective tissue)
- the tunica media (a mixture of smooth muscle and elastic tissue)
- the innermost layer, the tunica intima (elastic tissue lined by a smooth endothelium).

The arterioles contain a higher proportion of muscle tissue than other vessels, and provide the greatest resistance to the flow of blood. This bottle-neck effect is reflected by a drop in pressure from a mean of 90 mmHg in the smaller arteries to 30 mmHg in the arterioles. The arterioles act as 'control valves', through which blood is released to the capillaries. The return of blood in the venous system occurs via the venules, veins, and the venae cavae. The blood is at negligible pressure within these vessels, and from many parts of the body it has to flow against gravity. The return is encouraged by the muscular pump (particularly within the legs); by negative intrathoracic pressure, which effectively draws blood from the lower vessels in the abdomen into thoracic vessels; and by the presence of valves within the veins, which help prevent the backflow of blood.

The pressure within the cardiovascular system is produced by the pumping action of the heart, the elasticity of the blood vessels, and blood viscosity. It is homoeostatically maintained by the stimulation of baroreceptors, which lie in the aorta and carotid arteries. Increased pressure within the system increases the stimulation of the baroreceptors, which transmit an inhibitory response affecting the activity of the sympathetic neurones in the cardiovascular centre in the medulla. As a result, sympathetic tone in the arterioles is decreased and peripheral resistance is reduced.

Average figures are often quoted for blood pressure (e.g. 120 mmHg systole and 80 mmHg diastole). However, these figures do not reflect the wide range of values which may be recorded in a representative cross-section of the healthy population. The residual diastolic resistance is generally taken as the most useful indicator of cardiovascular integrity and health, as it indicates the minimum pressure within the system at all times.

The pulmonary circulation consists only of the blood supply to and from the lungs. Despite receiving a volume of blood equivalent to the aortic output, the blood flow to the lungs is considerably less regulated than that to other parts of the body. Pulmonary vessels offer little resistance to flow and the pressure within the system is consequently much lower (average values of 24 mmHg systole and 9 mmHg diastole).

Chapter 3

DISORDERS OF THE RESPIRATORY SYSTEM

3.1 GENERAL DISORDERS

Alveolitis

Definition
Alveolitis is inflammation of the alveoli.

Fibrosing Alveolitis

Definition and aetiology
Fibrosing alveolitis is a syndrome characterised by inflammation and fibrosis of the alveoli, and production of exudate. It is idiopathic, although it may be associated with a concurrent connective tissue disorder or exposure to ionising radiation (e.g. X-rays).

Symptoms
Common symptoms include dyspnoea on exertion, dry cough, arthralgia, weight loss, and malaise. Bacterial infection is a common complication.

Treatment
See Extrinsic Allergic Alveolitis below.

Extrinsic Allergic Alveolitis

Definition and aetiology
Extrinsic allergic alveolitis is alveolar inflammation caused by vasculitis and leading to fibrosis. It occurs as a result of a hypersensitivity reaction to prolonged exposure to high concentrations of an allergen (e.g. avian protein causing bird-fancier's lung and organic dust causing farmer's lung), which may be encountered in the course of work or leisure pursuits.

Symptoms
Symptoms usually occur 4 to 8 hours after exposure and subside within 24 to 48 hours. They include dry cough (which may become productive if the disease becomes chronic), dyspnoea, tightness in the chest, fever with

rigors, and general malaise. The disease may become chronic on continued allergen exposure and such exposure should be avoided.

Treatment

Treatment of fibrosing and extrinsic allergic alveolitis includes the administration of corticosteroids (BNF 6.3.4) and oxygen therapy (BNF 3.6).

Bronchiectasis

Definition and aetiology

Bronchiectasis is chronic dilatation of the bronchi. It may develop as a result of infection (e.g. pneumonia, tuberculosis, measles, or pertussis), but this has become considerably less common with the advent of antimicrobials. It may also occur as a result of bronchial obstruction, cystic fibrosis, or the inhalation of toxins (e.g. from smoking), or it can be congenital (e.g. Kartagener's syndrome).

Symptoms

Repeated respiratory-tract infections, cough, and purulent sputum production are the most common symptoms. Other symptoms include dyspnoea, haemoptysis, wheezing, and malaise.

Treatment

Treatment consists of the systemic and nebulised administration of appropriate antibacterial drugs (BNF 5.1), often in high doses. Postural drainage is a vital daily routine. Surgery may occasionally be useful in localised disease. Bronchodilators (BNF 3.1) may be beneficial in patients with demonstrable reversible airways obstruction. Patients should be advised to stop smoking.

Cough

Definition and aetiology

Coughing arises through a defensive reflex mechanism caused by the stimulation of receptors in the upper respiratory tract by irritant substances (e.g. dust, foreign bodies, mucus, or smoke). It is characterised by forced expiration against a closed glottis, which suddenly opens to expel air and unwanted substances from the lungs. It is symptomatic of a wide range of underlying disorders (e.g. asthma, bronchiectasis, bronchitis, lung cancer, heart failure, pneumonia, pulmonary fibrosis, and tuberculosis). Its most common cause is a minor self-limiting upper respiratory-tract infection.

Symptoms

A dry cough, characterised by the absence of sputum, may be irritating, hacking, short, and repetitive; or harsh, hoarse, and painful (croup) when associated with laryngitis.

The appearance of sputum (which may be clear to white, or yellowish-green and offensive in the presence of infection) is indicative of a 'productive' cough. If coughing is rapidly repetitive, the pressure build-up behind the glottis may impede venous filling of the heart and cough syncope may result from the decreased cardiac output.

Treatment

Treatment involves the administration of cough suppressants (BNF 3.9.1) to control a dry cough, demulcents (BNF 3.9.2) for their soothing action on the pharyngeal mucosa, and expectorants (BNF 3.9.2), which may increase bronchial secretions and facilitate expulsion of tenacious mucus. Water is of value in treating dry and productive coughs, taken orally or as inspired humidified air. In the presence of a prolonged cough, the possibility of an underlying disorder should be considered.

Croup

Definition and aetiology

Croup (acute laryngotracheobronchitis) occurs in young children (usually between 6 months and 3 years of age) and arises as a result of narrowing of the airway in the region of the larynx. The most common cause is a viral infection (particularly parainfluenza viruses), although bacteria may also be responsible (*see also* Epiglottitis). The partial obstruction is due to inflammation and oedema. Other causes include allergic responses or the presence of foreign bodies.

Symptoms

Croup is characterised by a paroxysmal 'barking' cough and inspiratory stridor, which may be accompanied by fever, wheezing, and tachypnoea. The symptoms often occur at night and, if severe, may cause respiratory distress, leading to cyanosis and exhaustion. Respiratory failure and pneumonia are potentially fatal complications.

Mild cases are self-limiting and symptoms resolve within 3 to 4 days. In severe cases, complete obstruction of the airway may occur.

Treatment

There is no specific antiviral therapy, but antibacterials (BNF 5.1) may be indicated in the presence of bacterial infection. Mild cases may be treated at home. Bed rest and adequate fluid intake are essential and home humidifiers or vaporisers may prove beneficial. Severe cases should be treated in hospital and may require oxygen therapy (BNF 3.6), intubation, or assisted ventilation.

Pneumoconioses

Definition and aetiology
Pneumoconioses are a group of chronic pulmonary conditions resulting from prolonged inhalation of dust. The dust is usually of occupational or environmental origin (e.g. coal dust causing coal-miner's pneumoconiosis, silicon dioxide causing silicosis, and asbestos fibres causing asbestosis). Inhalation results in fibrosis of the lung.

Symptoms
Symptoms include cough, dyspnoea, and obstructive airways disease (e.g. emphysema). Respiratory failure may occur in severe cases and death may follow. Silicosis is associated with an increased risk of tuberculosis, and asbestosis with an increased incidence of malignant disease.

Treatment
Patients should be advised to avoid further exposure to the offending dust, and aggravating factors (e.g. cigarette smoke).

Respiratory Distress Syndrome

Definition
Respiratory distress syndrome is an acute respiratory insufficiency, which may arise in adults with previously normal function or in neonates.

Neonatal Respiratory Distress Syndrome

Definition and aetiology
Neonatal respiratory distress syndrome is one of the most frequent life-threatening disorders in neonates. It occurs most commonly in premature infants, but also occasionally develops in those born to diabetic mothers or by caesarean section. It is thought to be due to hyaline membrane disease in which alveolar surfactant is deficient.

Symptoms
Symptoms develop soon after birth and include dyspnoea and tachypnoea, expiratory grunting, and cyanosis. The syndrome may be fatal, although the large majority of infants survive with appropriate treatment.

Treatment
Urgent supportive treatment is essential and consists of assisted ventilation with oxygen (BNF 3.6). The probability of premature infants developing the syndrome may be predicted by amniocentesis.

Adult Respiratory Distress Syndrome

Definition and aetiology
Adult respiratory distress syndrome (ARDS) is a non-specific reaction of the lungs, which commonly follows a clinical crisis (e.g. major trauma, hypovolaemic or septic shock, aspiration pneumonia, burns, smoke inhalation, drug overdose, embolism, or surgery). Its development is characterised by pulmonary oedema and fibrosis, and it can be fatal.

Symptoms
The symptoms of the syndrome occur in a recognised pattern of four stages. The initial stage is characterised by hyperventilation with alkalosis, soon after the precipitating event. Mild tachypnoea may develop within 24 to 72 hours, although the patient may appear stable. Pulmonary oedema follows, together with dyspnoea, cyanosis, and worsening hypoxaemia. Finally, hypoxaemia, hypercapnia, and acidosis develop and lead to coma and heart failure.

Treatment
Treatment is directed at preventing the last two stages of the syndrome and comprises assisted ventilation and careful fluid management. Corticosteroids (BNF 6.3.4) have been used. The administration of diuretics (BNF 2.2) and sympathomimetics with inotropic activity (BNF 2.7.1) may be necessary. Antibacterial therapy (BNF 5.1) is indicated for any underlying infection.

Respiratory Failure

Definition and aetiology
Respiratory failure arises as a result of impaired pulmonary gas exchange. It is characterised by abnormally low arterial oxygen tension (PaO_2) or high arterial carbon dioxide tension ($PaCO_2$). It usually occurs when a chronic illness (e.g. chronic bronchitis and emphysema, myasthenia gravis, pleural effusion, or poliomyelitis) undergoes an exacerbation as a result of an acute precipitating illness (e.g. infection, asthma, heart failure, or pneumothorax). It may also be precipitated by sedative drugs or following surgery.

Treatment
Treatment consists of controlled oxygen therapy (BNF 3.6) with assisted ventilation, if necessary. The administration of a respiratory stimulant (BNF 3.5) may be helpful. Appropriate antibacterial therapy may be necessary and bronchodilators (BNF 3.1), diuretics (BNF 2.2), and corticosteroids (BNF 6.3.4) may be indicated.

Sudden Infant Death Syndrome

Definition and aetiology
The sudden infant death syndrome (SIDS) or 'cot death' is the unexplained and unexpected death of an otherwise previously healthy baby. It is the most common cause of death in babies under one year of age, with the incidence reaching a peak in the third and fourth month of life. A greater prevalence has been associated with prematurity, social poverty, and bottle-feeding.

Almost all deaths occur during sleep between the hours of midnight and 0900 hrs. As its definition implies, the aetiology of sudden infant death syndrome is unclear, although various factors appear to culminate in a final disorder of respiratory mechanism.

Chronic hypoxia may occur immediately before death, due to prolonged periods of apnoea. Laryngospasm or nasal obstruction have been implicated in the development of apnoea.

Cardiovascular abnormalities (e.g. arrhythmias, conduction disturbances, or an electrolyte imbalance) have been proposed as possible causative factors. Other general aetiological mechanisms suggested include overheating, nitrous fumes from domestic gas burning, or the use of drugs such as phenothiazines. The evidence to support these suggestions, however, is limited.

Prevention
Some health authorities have adopted a multifactorial approach to accumulate data from patients in obstetric units and following delivery in an effort to identify those infants thought to be at risk. Certain common factors emerging (e.g. age of parents, similar sibling death, parity, antenatal care, obstetric complications, and environmental factors) may allow identified infants to be closely monitored during the high-risk period. Parents should be educated about nutrition (stressing the importance of breast-feeding) and the general care of the infant.

Self-help organisation
Foundation for the Study of Infant Deaths

3.2 OBSTRUCTIVE AIRWAYS DISEASE

Asthma

Definition and aetiology
Asthma is a reversible obstructive airways disease of varying severity. The symptoms are caused by constriction of bronchial smooth muscle (bronchospasm), oedema of bronchial mucous membranes, and blockage of the smaller bronchi with plugs of mucus. Asthma may occur, particularly in children, as a result of identifiable trigger factors or allergens (extrinsic asthma). Immunological mechanisms involving specific allergens (e.g. house-dust mite, pollens, and animal danders) may be responsible. Non-specific trigger factors include viral infection, exercise, dust and irritants (e.g. cigarette smoke), beta-adrenoceptor blocking drugs, emotional disturbances, and non-steroidal anti-inflammatory drugs (e.g. aspirin and indomethacin).

Asthma may arise, however, in the absence of trigger factors (intrinsic asthma), and this commonly occurs in middle-aged patients. As many as 10% to 15% of the population may suffer from asthma at some stage of life.

Symptoms
Symptoms of asthma range from mild to severe and life-threatening. The main symptoms are dyspnoea, wheezing, and tightness of the chest. Cough, with or without the production of sputum, is common and is often the presenting symptom. Other symptoms include tachycardia, tachypnoea, fatigue, and drowsiness.

Treatment
Reassurance and education are important components of treatment. Patients should be advised to avoid known trigger factors and encouraged to maintain an active life. Smoking should be discouraged. Drug treatment includes the use of bronchodilators (BNF 3.1). Prophylaxis with inhaled corticosteroids (BNF 3.2), or other agents such as sodium cromoglycate and nedocromil (BNF 3.3), is recommended. Oxygen therapy (BNF 3.6) may be necessary and hyposensitisation (BNF 3.4.2) may be considered.

Treatment of severe asthma comprises the administration of adrenoceptor stimulants (BNF 3.1.1), most commonly via a nebuliser, assisted ventilation, and parenteral corticosteroids (BNF 3.1.1). Oxygen therapy (BNF 3.6) may be necessary.

Self-help organisations
Action Against Allergy
Asthma Society and Friends of the Asthma Research
  Council

Bronchitis

Definition and aetiology
Bronchitis is characterised by inflammation of the trachea and bronchi and may be acute or chronic (*see* Chronic Bronchitis and Emphysema).

Acute Bronchitis

Definition and aetiology
Acute bronchitis is usually self-limiting and is commonly due to viral infection. It often follows a cold or

influenza; the causative micro-organisms of secondary bacterial infection are commonly *Streptococcus pneumoniae* and *Haemophilus influenzae*.

Symptoms
Common symptoms include cough, which may be dry or productive, tracheitis, and expiratory wheezing, which can be cleared by coughing.

Treatment
In otherwise healthy patients, treatment is not usually necessary, although antibacterials (BNF 5.1) are often given due to the probability of bacterial infection. A cough suppressant (BNF 3.9.1) may be indicated in the presence of a troublesome dry cough.

Chronic Bronchitis and Emphysema

Definition and aetiology
Chronic bronchitis is an irreversible obstructive airways disease, which usually results from smoking or prolonged exposure to environmental irritants. It is defined as cough with the production of sputum for at least three months of the year and for more than one year. Repeated respiratory-tract infections may contribute to its development.

Emphysema is an irreversible chronic obstructive airways disease, which is characterised by dilatation of the air spaces distal to the terminal bronchioles and destruction of the alveolar walls. The outstanding feature is loss of the elastic tissue of the lungs. It usually develops in association with chronic bronchitis, and is invariably due to smoking. Rarely, it may be caused by an enzyme (alpha-1-antitrypsin) deficiency.

Symptoms
Chronic bronchitis and emphysema are characterised by a chronic or recurrent cough and the production of excess sputum, which may be clear, or purulent in the presence of concurrent infection. Symptoms tend to be more marked on waking and during the winter months. Other symptoms include dyspnoea and tachypnoea on exercise, and wheezing. In severe disease, drowsiness, headache, weight gain, and peripheral oedema may occur.

Treatment
Patients should be advised to stop smoking and avoid exposure to other irritants, and attempts made to increase exercise tolerance. Drug treatment comprises the administration of bronchodilators (BNF 3.1). Antibacterial therapy (BNF 5.1, Table 1) is indicated in the presence of respiratory-tract infection. Oxygen administration (BNF 3.6) may be necessary. Mucolytics (BNF 3.7) and cough suppressants (BNF 3.9.1) are sometimes used, and physiotherapy may be beneficial.

Self-help organisation
Chest Heart and Stroke Association

3.3 PLEURAL DISORDERS

Pleurisy and Pleural Effusion

Definition and aetiology
Pleurisy is inflammation of the pleura. It may be accompanied by pleural effusion, which is characterised by the presence of fluid (exudate or transudate) in the pleural space. The accumulated fluid may be purulent (empyema) or contain blood (haemothorax). Common causes include heart failure, hepatic or renal impairment, infection (e.g. pneumonia and tuberculosis), malignant disease, pancreatitis, pulmonary infarction or oedema, and physical trauma.

Symptoms
Pleurisy is characterised by sudden sharp chest pain, which is exacerbated by movement and inspiration. This pain may disappear on the development of pleural effusion, which may be asymptomatic. Dyspnoea and dull chest pain may occur as the volume of accumulated fluid increases, and there may be poor expansion of the affected side of the chest.

Treatment
Treatment is directed at the underlying cause. In pleural effusion, surgical aspiration may be necessary and continuous drainage indicated.

Pneumothorax

Definition and aetiology
Pneumothorax is the accumulation of air in the pleural space. It often occurs spontaneously, usually in thin young men. It may also arise as a result of physical trauma, underlying pulmonary disease (e.g. asthma, bronchitis, cystic fibrosis, emphysema, and tuberculosis), or malignant disease.

Symptoms
Pneumothorax may be asymptomatic, with only a vague discomfort in the chest, but severe chest pain, dyspnoea, and cyanosis may occur.

Treatment
Pneumothorax may resolve without treatment, but underwater seal drainage may be required and thoracic surgery is indicated in resistant or recurring cases.

3.4 ANATOMY AND PHYSIOLOGY OF THE RESPIRATORY SYSTEM

The respiratory system in man is responsible for the processes of gas exchange between the atmosphere, the circulation, and the cells of the body; the homoeostatic maintenance of blood pH; and for the provision of vocal expression (i.e. speaking and singing).

Air enters the respiratory tree through the nasal passages and the mouth, and is warmed, humidified, and partially filtered as it passes over the mucosal membranes and cilia. From the nasal passages, the air passes through the pharynx (Fig. 3.1). The upper portion of the pharynx (above the level of the soft palate) is called the nasopharynx, from which the Eustachian tubes branch off. These link the middle ear with the nasopharynx, and assist in the maintenance of atmospheric pressure within the tympanic cavity (*see* Section 12.4). The lower reaches of the pharynx may be subdivided at the upper edge of the epiglottis into the oropharynx and the hypopharynx (laryngopharynx). The entry to the trachea is guarded by the larynx, situated immediately below the pharynx. The larynx also produces vocal sounds through the action of the vocal cords in the glottis. Food and liquids are prevented from entering the larynx by a flap of cartilage, the epiglottis, which closes over the entrance to the larynx on swallowing.

The trachea links the larynx to the right and left bronchi and is prevented from collapsing by the presence of approximately 20 horseshoe-shaped rings of cartilage. The incomplete sections of cartilage are located adjacent to the oesophagus.

On passing through the trachea, air enters the lungs via the bronchi, bronchioles, and alveoli (Fig. 3.2). The bronchi walls contain rings of cartilage interspersed throughout smooth muscle, and their inner surface is lined by cilia whose roots are in the mucous membrane. The rings of cartilage prevent the collapse of the bronchi when the internal pressure changes, and the beating cilia assist in the upward and outward movement of unwanted fine particles.

The bronchioles are narrower versions of the bronchi, usually of less than 1 mm diameter. However, unlike the bronchi, their walls are not reinforced with cartilage, and they may open and narrow to modify the resistance to the passage of air. Deeper within the lung, the bronchioles repeatedly branch, giving rise to terminal bronchioles. The terminal bronchioles divide further into respiratory bronchioles, which possess end outgrowths, the alveoli (Fig. 3.3). The walls of the respiratory bronchioles and alveoli are thin, covered in a network of fine capillaries, and are the sites of gaseous exchange.

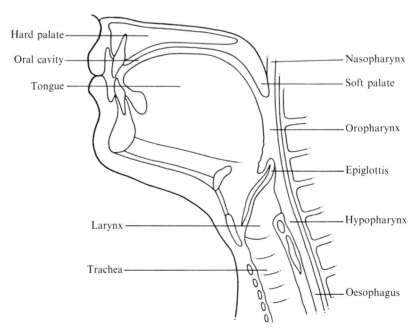

Hard palate
Oral cavity
Tongue
Larynx
Trachea

Nasopharynx
Soft palate
Oropharynx
Epiglottis
Hypopharynx
Oesophagus

Fig. 3.1
Upper respiratory tract.

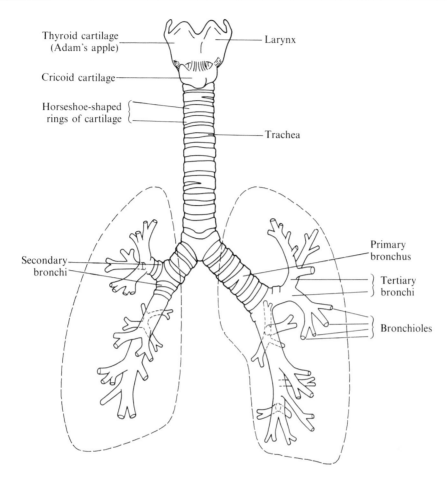

Thyroid cartilage (Adam's apple)

Larynx

Cricoid cartilage

Horseshoe-shaped rings of cartilage

Trachea

Secondary bronchi

Primary bronchus

Tertiary bronchi

Bronchioles

Fig. 3.2
Anterior view of bronchial tree.

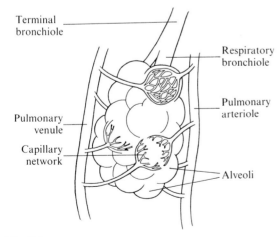

Terminal bronchiole

Respiratory bronchiole

Pulmonary arteriole

Pulmonary venule

Capillary network

Alveoli

Fig. 3.3
Areas of gaseous exchange.

An alveolar surfactant is present in the fluid lining the surface of the air sacs. This surfactant, which consists of phospholipids and is secreted by the alveolar cells, reduces surface tension and hence the energy required to keep the alveoli inflated.

The lungs are located in the thoracic cavity, and the two non-identical lobes are separated by the heart in the mediastinum. The right lung consists of an upper, middle, and lower lobe, while the left lung comprises only an upper and lower lobe. Internally, each lobe is further subdivided into 2 to 5 segments, which may provide the localised sites of many pulmonary disorders.

Each lung is surrounded by two closely associated membranes, the pleura. The space between the two membranes (the pleural cavity) is filled with fluid (cf. two plates of glass separated by a thin film of water). The outer parietal membrane lines the inner wall of the thoracic cavity, and the inner visceral pleural membrane follows the contours of the outer surfaces of the lungs. The pleura of each lung are not linked.

Chapter 4

DISORDERS OF THE NERVOUS SYSTEM

4.1 GENERAL DISORDERS

Cerebral Oedema

Definition and aetiology
Cerebral oedema is the excessive accumulation of fluid in the brain and is accompanied by an increase in intracranial pressure (*see also* Papilloedema). It is often due to physical trauma or malignant disease, but may also result from hypoxia at high altitude (high-altitude cerebral oedema), poisoning (e.g. with CNS depressants, carbon monoxide, or lead), or meningitis.

Symptoms
It is characterised by altered consciousness followed by coma. Other symptoms include slow respiration leading to apnoea, pupillary dilatation, and a decerebrate posture. Death may follow.

Treatment
Early treatment is essential, and neurosurgical decompression or assisted ventilation may be necessary. Drug treatment consists of the administration of intravenous osmotic diuretics (BNF 2.2.5); corticosteroids (BNF 6.3.4) are used to treat cerebral oedema due to trauma.

Cerebral Palsy

Definition and aetiology
Cerebral palsy constitutes a group of non-progressive neurological disorders, resulting from faulty development of the brain or damage sustained in the uterus or in early infancy. Causes include foetal disorders, birth trauma, birth asphyxia, neonatal jaundice, cerebral haemorrhage or infarction, or severe systemic disease (e.g. meningitis) in early infancy. It is more common in premature infants.

Symptoms
The characteristics and symptoms of cerebral palsy depend on the cause, extent, and location of the brain damage. Spastic syndromes (e.g. hemiplegia, paraplegia, quadriplegia, and diplegia) occur most commonly, and are characterised by muscular hypertonicity, weakness, and contractures. There may also be auditory and visual impairment, athetosis, ataxia, dysarthria, dysphagia, persistent dribbling, epilepsy, and temper tantrums. Mental retardation may occur on its own or in conjunction with any of the above problems.

Treatment
Treatment depends on the severity of physical and mental disability, and is likely to be long-term. Physiotherapy, occupational and speech therapy, and educational and social support may be necessary. Ortho-paedic surgery may be beneficial in selected cases. Antiepileptics (BNF 4.8) may be required to control seizures.

Self-help organisations
Leonard Cheshire Foundation Spastics Society

Headache

Definition and aetiology
Headache may be idiopathic or a symptom of a disease process, with its frequency, duration, nature, and location depending on the disease. It may arise from systemic infection (e.g. syphilis and tuberculosis), meningitis, osteitis deformans, trigeminal neuralgia (*see below*), vascular disturbances, head injuries, severe hypertension, and giant cell arteritis. It may also be caused by disease of the nose, sinuses, eyes, ears, or teeth. Headaches are commonly due to muscle tension, which may be associated with anxiety, emotional disturbances, and fatigue.

Migraine

Definition and aetiology
Migraine is of unknown aetiology. Disturbances of cranial-blood circulation have been demonstrated and it may be familial. Migraine usually begins between 10 and 30 years of age and is more common in women. It may be triggered by agents (e.g. chocolate, tyramine-containing foods, combined oral contraceptives, and alcohol) or by hunger, smoking, or emotional disturbances.

Symptoms
Migraine without an aura has been defined as a succession of five unilateral pulsating headaches lasting 4 to 72 hours. Their severity restricts normal daily activities and they may be accompanied by nausea or vomiting, or both, and sensitivity to light or noise.

In migraine with an aura, visual disturbances (e.g. flashing lights and blurred vision) occur between 5 and 20 minutes before the headache, but last less than an hour. Paraesthesia in the face, hands, and feet can also develop.

Treatment
Treatment of migraine consists of the administration of non-opioid analgesics (BNF 4.7.1) for mild attacks and ergotamine preparations (BNF 4.7.4.1) for more severe attacks. Anti-emetics (BNF 4.6) and anxiolytics (BNF 4.1.2) may also be useful. Prophylactic treatment may be given by pizotifen, clonidine, and methysergide (BNF 4.7.4.2), antidepressant drugs (BNF 4.3.1), and selected beta-adrenoceptor blocking drugs (BNF 2.4). Patients should be advised to avoid known trigger factors.

Cluster Headache

Definition and aetiology
Cluster headache (migrainous neuralgia or histamine headache) consists of paroxysmal acute pain centred around one eye, which may last for 20 to 60 minutes. Cluster headache is more common in men and appears to be due to an abnormality of the autonomic nervous system.

Symptoms
The attacks tend to occur 3 to 4 times daily in clusters over a period of several weeks, followed by a prolonged attack-free period. The affected eye may appear bloodshot, with swelling of the eyelids. Pupillary constriction, enophthalmos, ptosis, and loss of sweating on the same side of the face may accompany the headache. Vasodilatation and nasal congestion on the same side of the face are common.

Treatment
Non-opioid analgesics (BNF 4.7.1) and certain anti-migraine drugs (BNF 4.7.4) may be of value. Antimanic drugs (BNF 4.2.3) have also been used.

Tension Headache

Definition and aetiology
Tension headache is due to sustained contraction of skeletal muscle of the scalp, jaw, and neck. It is often associated with anxiety and emotional disturbances and is the most common form of chronic and recurrent headache. Tension headache may be differentiated from migraine as the pain is continuous, not pulsatile, giving the impression of pressure on both sides of the head.

Symptoms
It is characterised by a steady nonpulsatile ache, which may be unilateral or bilateral in the temporal, occipital, parietal, or frontal regions. It may last for hours or occur intermittently for years.

Treatment
Treatment consists of the administration of non-opioid analgesics (BNF 4.7.1) or the removal of any underlying stress.

Trigeminal Neuralgia

Definition and aetiology
Trigeminal neuralgia (tic douloureux) is a syndrome characterised by brief attacks of severe pain over an area of the face innervated by one or more branches of the trigeminal nerve. The pain may be triggered by touching hypersensitive areas on the skin, by face and jaw movements, or exposure to cold draughts on the face. It is generally of unknown aetiology and encountered in people over 50 years of age. In younger patients, it may be due to multiple sclerosis.

Treatment
Treatment consists of the administration of carbamazepine, phenytoin, or both (BNF 4.7.3).

Self-help organisations
Action Against Allergy
British Migraine Association
Migraine Trust

Definition and aetiology
Hydrocephalus is an increase in the volume of cerebrospinal fluid (CSF) within the skull. It is caused by increased secretion of CSF or by interference with the flow of CSF within the ventricles of the brain. In infants (infantile hydrocephalus), it may be due to congenital brain abnormalities which interfere with CSF circulation. It can also be caused by meningitis, subarachnoid haemorrhage arising from birth trauma, or in association with spina bifida. Hydrocephalus may also occur in adults as a result of malignant disease, meningitis, or subarachnoid haemorrhage.

Symptoms
Symptoms are due to increased intracranial pressure. In infants, they include head enlargement, bulging of the forehead, and prominent scalp veins. In severe cases, mental retardation may occur, with limb spasticity and visual disturbances. Other symptoms are headache and convulsions.

Treatment
Treatment is by the surgical insertion of a valve or shunt.

Self-help organisation
Association for Spina Bifida and Hydrocephalus

Insomnia

Definition and aetiology
Insomnia is the disturbance of normal sleep patterns, which may be manifested by difficulty in falling asleep, early waking, intermittent waking, or fitful sleep.

Transient insomnia may occur due to extraneous factors (e.g. noise, room-temperature changes, or shift work). Short-term insomnia may be caused by emotional disturbances or medical illness. It usually lasts a few weeks, but can recur. Chronic insomnia may be associated with psychiatric disorders (e.g. depressive disorders and anxiety), daytime sleeping, abuse of drugs and alcohol, pain, cough, pruritus, or dyspnoea.

Some patients who complain of insomnia may be found on enquiry to have adequate sleep, and others may sleep better if they avoid excitement or stimulants (e.g. coffee or tea).

Treatment
Patients, especially the elderly, should be advised to avoid alcohol, daytime sleeping, and to take some form of physical exercise (e.g. walking). Any underlying disorder should be treated and any causative factor remedied.

Drug treatment consists of the judicious administration of hypnotics (BNF 4.1.1), whose choice depends on the type of insomnia.

Malignant Hyperthermia

Definition and aetiology
Malignant hyperthermia (malignant hyperpyrexia) is a rare, but potentially fatal, disorder characterised by a sudden and dramatic increase in body metabolism and temperature. It occurs in susceptible patients on exposure to anaesthetics (e.g. succinylcholine and halothane), and is due to an hereditary disorder of muscle metabolism.

Symptoms
The chief symptoms are high fever, acidosis, and widespread muscular rigidity. Death may ensue.

Treatment
Treatment consists of the administration of dantrolene sodium (BNF 15.1.8). Offending anaesthetics should be avoided in susceptible patients and their families.

Motion Sickness

Definition and aetiology
Motion sickness is caused by repetitive movement (e.g. that experienced when travelling by air, rail, road, and sea). Its exact mechanism is unknown, but it is thought to be due to excessive stimulation of the vestibular system.

Symptoms
It is characterised by dizziness and nausea and vomiting. Increased salivation, pallor, and cold sweating of the face and hands may also occur. If prolonged, motion sickness can lead to anorexia, apathy, dehydration, and depression, and it may have a marked adverse effect on performance.

Treatment
Prevention is more successful than treatment and comprises the administration of hyoscine or an antihistamine (BNF 4.6) before travelling. Visual mechanisms are thought to be significant and, when travelling, subjects should be advised to focus on distant objects or to keep their eyes closed with the head in a fixed position.

Myasthenia Gravis

Definition and aetiology
Myasthenia gravis is a neuromuscular disorder characterised by muscle weakness and arising from defective neuromuscular transmission. It is thought to be caused by an auto-immune mechanism involving the production of antibodies to the acetylcholine receptors present in the neuromuscular junction.

Symptoms
Symptoms may be episodic, with patients experiencing permanent or temporary remissions. Relapses may occur, however, after months or years.

The primary symptom is muscle weakness affecting most commonly the muscles of the eyes, lips, tongue, throat, neck, and shoulders. This results in diplopia and ptosis, chewing and swallowing difficulties, speech disorders, and drooping of the head. Limb muscles may also be affected and movement may become restricted. Dyspnoea and respiratory paralysis may arise from involvement of the respiratory muscles and the consequences may be fatal. Symptoms are exacerbated by strenuous exercise, emotional disturbances, fatigue, pregnancy, and by the administration of certain drugs (e.g. aminoglycosides). Myasthenia gravis may be accompanied by thymic enlargement, which may be caused by a thymoma.

Treatment
Treatment is by the administration of an anticholinesterase (BNF 10.2.1). Corticosteroids (BNF 10.2.1) can also be given in unresponsive cases. Thymectomy may be beneficial in some patients and plasmapheresis may be indicated in severe cases.

Nausea and Vomiting

Definition and aetiology
Nausea and vomiting are common symptoms. Examples of disturbances which can cause nausea and vomiting include gastric irritation, irradiation (radiation sickness), or travel (motion sickness) or in pregnancy (morning sickness). Nausea and vomiting may also be due to psychogenic factors, occur postoperatively, or following the administration of certain drugs. Haematemesis or 'coffee-ground vomitus' are indications of serious organic disease. Projectile vomiting is the forceful ejection of vomit without prior retching, and is characteristic of pyloric stenosis.

Treatment

Nausea and vomiting may be prevented or treated by the administration of anticholinergic drugs, phenothiazines, or other anti-emetics (BNF 4.6). The most powerful of these drugs may also be effective in the treatment of post-operative vomiting and radiation sickness. Drug treatment for 'morning sickness' should be avoided if possible because of teratogenic risk. Persistent nausea and vomiting may be an indication of serious gastro-intestinal, neurological, or metabolic disorders, and if this is suspected it may be desirable to withhold treatment until a diagnosis has been made. Complications of persistent vomiting include dehydration, hypokalaemia, and alkalosis, for which fluid and electrolyte replacement (BNF 9.2) may be necessary.

Pain

Definition and aetiology

Pain may be caused by physical or psychological disturbances, or a combination of both. It may be characteristic of a disease and is sometimes the only presenting symptom. The nature of a particular pain may help in the diagnosis of the underlying condition. The location of a pain may indicate the part of the body affected, although pain felt in one position may sometimes be referred from pathology in another part of the body (e.g. shoulder-tip pain occurs with gall bladder disease). This occurs when pain cannot be felt in the affected area (e.g. the viscera) or when it causes pressure on a nerve. Some forms of pain do not remain localised in one area, but move from one place to another. The pain may radiate to a characteristic region where discomfort is felt (e.g. cardiac pain is usually felt as central chest pain, but often radiates to the shoulders and left arm).

Symptoms

Pain varies in severity from mild to severe. It may only appear at certain times of the day or night, or be continuous for many hours. Varied descriptions may be given by the patient (e.g. stabbing, crushing, gnawing, burning, or throbbing), and pain may be acute, chronic, or intractable.

Treatment

Treatment, which is symptomatic, is usually directed towards the underlying cause. Pain may resolve with re-assurance in the absence of treatment, or relief may be obtained by rest, warming, cooling, or changing position. Patients should be advised to avoid any aggravating factors. Drug treatment for the relief of pain consists of the administration of analgesics (BNF 4.7). Local anaesthesia (BNF 15.2) may be used for certain types of localised pain. Antidepressant drugs (BNF 4.3),

anxiolytics (BNF 4.1), and corticosteroids (BNF 10.1.2) may be used in the treatment of certain types of pain. In various cases of intractable pain, relief may be obtained from surgical section of the afferent sensory pathways.

Self-help organisations

Back Pain Association
Intractable Pain Society of Great Britain and Northern Ireland

Restless Leg Syndrome

Definition and aetiology

Restless leg syndrome (Ekbom's syndrome) is characterised by unpleasant sensations in the legs, which only develop at rest. The cause is unknown, although iron-deficiency anaemia, pregnancy, and uraemia may be contributory factors.

Symptoms

The symptoms, which may be intolerable, only occur when the legs are at rest and include 'pins and needles', burning sensations, twitching, and, sometimes, pain. These sensations, which usually occur between the ankle and knee, may be relieved by movement, but return when movement ceases. Insomnia frequently occurs as a consequence.

Treatment

Many patients do not require drug treatment. Should drug treatment be considered, oral iron (BNF 9.1.1), clonazepam (BNF 4.8), carbamazepine (BNF 4.7.3), and orphenadrine (BNF 4.9.2) have been used, although only clonazepam and carbamazepine have been proven clinically effective.

Spina Bifida

Definition and aetiology

Spina bifida is an idiopathic congenital neural tube disorder characterised by defective closure of the spinal column. The defect occurs most commonly in the lower thoracic, lumbar, and sacral regions. In spina bifida occulta, there is no outward sign of a spinal defect. In spina bifida cystica, the meninges and cerebrospinal fluid (CSF), and more commonly also the nerves and part of the spinal cord, protrude in a sac through the vertebral defect (Fig. 4.1). It is the most common defect present at birth in the UK.

Symptoms

The severity of the disorder varies according to the type and location of the defect. Varying degrees of paralysis and sensory loss may occur. The lower limbs may be affected, and incontinence may be caused by paralysis of the rectal and bladder sphincters. In spina bifida cystica,

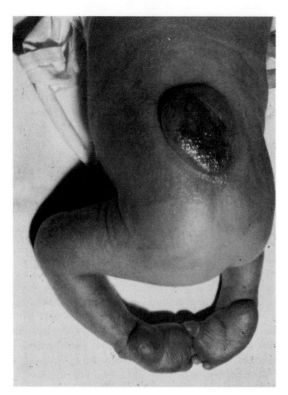

Fig. 4.1
Spina bifida cystica in a neonate.

the sac containing the protruding cord and meninges may rupture, resulting in leakage of CSF and an increased risk of meningitis. Hydrocephalus and multiple congenital defects may accompany spina bifida at birth.

Treatment
Treatment consists of surgical closure of the defect, although the patient will often remain paraplegic and incontinent. Surgery may also be necessary if hydrocephalus is present, and appropriate antibacterial therapy (BNF 5.1) is indicated if meningitis develops. In many cases, long-term medical and nursing care is necessary.

Self-help organisations
Association for Spina Bifida and Hydrocephalus
Urostomy Association

Vertigo

Definition and aetiology
Vertigo is the sensation of movement, particularly of rotation. It may occur normally in response to certain stimuli (e.g. motion sickness), but may be the symptom of labyrinthine disorders (e.g. Ménière's disease or vestibular neuronitis). Vertigo may also arise as a result of central disorders (e.g. epilepsy, migraine, and multiple sclerosis) or as a side-effect of administration of drugs (e.g. aminoglycosides).

Symptoms
Vertigo, which is often described as dizziness, is frequently accompanied by nausea and vomiting, and nystagmus.

Treatment
Treatment varies according to the underlying disorder, but may include the administration of antihistamines or phenothiazines (BNF 4.6).

Vestibular Neuronitis

Definition and aetiology
Vestibular neuronitis is a labyrinthine disorder in which vestibular function is disturbed in the absence of deafness. It usually occurs between 30 and 50 years of age. It often follows a febrile illness and, although its cause is unknown, it may be associated with viral infection.

Symptoms
It is characterised by severe vertigo, which may be precipitated by the adoption of certain positions of the head, but may also be exacerbated by movement. The vertigo decreases in severity over a period of days, although occasional attacks may occur for weeks or even months.

Treatment
Treatment is symptomatic, and antihistamines and phenothiazines (BNF 4.6) may be helpful.

4.2 CEREBROVASCULAR DISORDERS

Stroke

Definition and aetiology
A stroke (cerebrovascular accident) is caused by an acute vascular lesion in the brain and is characterised by an area of ischaemic infarction. It is usually due to cerebral embolism or thrombosis, and less commonly due to cerebral haemorrhage. These in turn may be caused by aneurysm, atherosclerosis, heart disease, hypertension, diabetes mellitus, alcohol, and smoking. Stroke may follow a transient ischaemic attack.

Symptoms
Symptoms vary according to the area and site of brain tissue affected. The onset of symptoms may be sudden,

particularly if stroke is due to cerebral embolism or haemorrhage. Alternatively, there may be a short prodromal or warning phase prior to actual onset, particularly when cerebral thrombosis is the cause. Symptoms are usually limited to the side of the body opposite to the half of the brain in which the stroke occurs (i.e. stroke in the left half of the brain produces right-sided symptoms).

Common symptoms, which by definition last more than 24 hours (*see also* Transient Ischaemic Attacks), include hemiplegia, hemiparesis, sensory loss, speech disorders, and visual disturbances. A sudden loss of consciousness may occur which, although often regained, can deepen and lead to death. Surviving patients may suffer permanent neurological damage, resulting in marked suffering and loss of dignity through disability (e.g. incontinence, amnesia, paralysis, and speech disorders). Some patients become 'locked-in' and, although conscious, are unable to move, speak, or swallow. Cerebral oedema is an important local complication of stroke, and other general complications associated with paralysis are decubitus ulcers, pneumonia, and urinary-tract infections.

Treatment
Treatment depends on the severity of the symptoms and aims to overcome any resultant disability. Any underlying cause should be treated to prevent further attack. The use of dipyridamole and low-dose aspirin (BNF 2.9) has been advocated in all stroke victims. Long-term nursing care and physiotherapy are often necessary.

Self-help organisations
Action for Dysphasic Adults
Chest Heart and Stroke Association

Subarachnoid Haemorrhage

Definition and aetiology
Subarachnoid haemorrhage is bleeding into the subarachnoid space (i.e. between the arachnoid membrane and the pia mater). It is commonly due to a ruptured cerebral aneurysm, but may also be a consequence of congenital vascular abnormalities, cerebral haemorrhage, head injury, or a blood clotting disorder.

Symptoms
The onset of symptoms is usually very sudden and is characterised by severe headache, which may spread into the neck and back by the passage of blood down the spinal cord. Vomiting is common, and confusion, drowsiness, hemiplegia, neck stiffness, and occasionally convulsions, may occur. Patients may subsequently become irritable, drowsy, and confused. Consciousness is often impaired and coma may develop. Prolonged coma usually results in death.

Treatment
A small number of patients may benefit from surgery. Antifibrinolytic drugs (BNF 2.11) and dexamethasone have been used, but their benefits are not proven. Vascular spasm may be reduced by the administration of beta-adrenoceptor blocking drugs (BNF 2.4).

Subdural and Extradural Haemorrhage

Definition and aetiology
Subdural haemorrhage is bleeding into the subdural space (i.e. between the dura mater and arachnoid membrane). It is usually due to trauma, and elderly, alcoholic, or epileptic patients are particularly at risk.

Extradural haemorrhage is a consequence of a tear in a middle meningeal artery. It is commonly caused by a skull fracture, which can follow a direct blow to the temple.

Symptoms
The onset of symptoms in subdural epidsodes is usually insidious, and they may not develop until several weeks after the trauma. Symptoms often mimic those of a slowly developing stroke and include a changing level of consciousness, headache, muscle weakness, personality changes, spasticity, and unequal-sized pupils.

In extradural haemorrhage, the patient may report a minor head injury which resulted in brief unconsciousness. Subsequently, a full recovery appears to take place, but within a few hours there is a rapid deterioration into confusion, hemiparesis, and unequal-sized pupils.

Treatment
Treatment consists of prompt surgery (craniotomy), following which complete recovery is likely.

Transient Ischaemic Attacks

Definition and aetiology
Transient ischaemic attacks are brief cerebral disturbances of vascular origin whose effects, by definition, last less than 24 hours (*see also* Stroke). They have the same causes as stroke, but are often associated with occlusion of the carotid artery. They may also be due to anaemia, epilepsy, hypotension, hypoglycaemia, or migraine. Smoking and hypertension are particularly high-risk factors in patients who have had a stroke.

Symptoms
Attacks may be single or multiple. The onset is usually abrupt, and common symptoms include hemiparesis, sensory loss, speech disorders, and visual disturbances. Ataxia, deafness, dysphagia, nausea and vomiting, and

vertigo may also occur. Each attack usually lasts only a few minutes, and never longer than 24 hours. Unlike stroke, there is no permanent neurological damage, but an attack may warn of an impending stroke.

Treatment

Treatment comprises the administration of oral anti-coagulants (BNF 2.8.2). Aspirin (BNF 2.9) and dipyridamole may be of value in some patients. Corrective surgery of the carotid artery (carotid endarterectomy) may be beneficial. Patients should be advised to avoid smoking following an attack.

4.3 DISORDERS OF HIGHER FUNCTION

Amnesia

Definition and aetiology

Amnesia is characterised by an inability to remember information, and is a common sign of many CNS pathologies (e.g. Alzheimer's disease). If the lesions in brain tissue are localised, memory impairment may be limited. Severe amnesia involves much more generalised pathology and may be due to thiamine deficiency, tumours around the third ventricles, meningitis, Alzheimer's disease, and severe head injuries which produce prolonged unconsciousness.

Symptoms

Impairment of short-term memory involves difficulty in remembering recent conversation, names, messages, and recently read material. Severe amnesia produces extreme problems in retaining material for more than a few seconds, and even this may be lost if the patient is distracted. Severe cases commonly produce retrograde amnesia, in which memory loss of events prior to the cerebral pathology may also occur.

Treatment

Treatment consists of the management of the underlying condition. Although amnesia may resolve spontaneously, there is no recognised treatment.

Anxiety

Definition and aetiology

Anxiety is a normal response to stress or anticipated danger, and is characterised by feelings of apprehension and fear. It is considered abnormal when it is excessive, inappropriate, or without obvious cause. If anxiety occurs in response to everyday problems, it tends to become chronic with acute exacerbations. Acute anxiety

to specific stimuli (e.g. spiders) is classed as a phobic state.

Anxiety is more common in women and typically occurs in early adulthood. Family history and current environmental circumstances are possible contributory factors. It is often a symptom of depressive or other psychiatric disorders (e.g. delirium, dementia, and schizophrenia).

Panic attacks are acute bouts of anxiety with marked physical symptoms, usually associated with chronic anxiety. The precipitating factor can be an emotional stress (e.g. bereavement), but it may be a more trivial distressing event in the presence of chronic anxiety. The attacks can occur irregularly and unpredictably, each lasting up to several hours.

Symptoms

Central symptoms include irritability, poor memory, loss of concentration, insomnia, and nightmares. These are accompanied by physical symptoms, which include tension headache, tremor, chest pain, dizziness, dyspnoea, palpitations, gastro-intestinal disturbances, urinary frequency, back pain, and a general feeling of weakness. The prognosis is good, provided the precipitating factor is self-limiting.

Treatment

Reassurance and explanation may be sufficient for many patients, and relaxation techniques may be beneficial. Anxiolytics (BNF 4.1.2), beta-adrenoceptor blocking drugs (BNF 4.1.2), and antidepressant drugs (BNF 4.3) have been used with varying degrees of success. Short-term treatment with antipsychotic drugs (BNF 4.2.1) may be used in severe anxiety.

Autism

Definition

Autism is a syndrome which usually occurs in infancy.

Symptoms

It is characterised by the failure to develop social relationships (e.g. lack of attachment to parents and avoidance of eye gaze), by resistance to change (e.g. rituals, attachment to familiar objects, and repetitive acts), and by language and speech disorders (e.g. delayed onset of speech, total muteness, and idiosyncratic use of language). In addition, there is usually mental retardation.

Treatment

Treatment consists of behaviour therapy for very severe cases and psychotherapy and special schooling for less severe cases.

Self-help organisation

National Autistic Society

Dementia

Definition and aetiology

Dementia is an acquired general impairment of intellect, memory, and personality, which occurs in the absence of drowsiness or agitation. It is usually chronic and progressive, and the majority of cases are irreversible. Dementia is primarily a disease of the elderly, with up to 10% of the over-65's suffering from mild or severe forms.

It often accompanies irreversible degenerative processes in the brain (e.g. Alzheimer's disease, arteriosclerosis, Pick's disease, multiple sclerosis, or Huntington's chorea). Reversible causes include megaloblastic anaemia, hypothyroidism, heart block, alcohol, and normal pressure hydrocephalus.

Senile dementia usually occurs in patients over 70 years of age, is more common in women, and consists of a gradual (though sometimes rapid) and progressive decline.

Pre-senile dementia is a syndrome with a slowly progressive decline, usually occurring under 60 years of age. It occurs without apparent cause, although a family history may exist. Alzheimer's disease is the most common cause of pre-senile dementia, but other causes include Pick's disease and Huntington's chorea.

Alzheimer's disease is the commonest cause of the progressive dementias and affects both men and women. Rarely, it may begin as early as the late teens or 20s. The frequency increases progressively with age, affecting about 5% of people over 65 years of age and 20% of people over 80 years of age. Formerly, patients under 65 years of age were classified as having pre-senile dementia and older patients as having senile dementia, as they were thought to be different illnesses. Clinically and pathologically, however, Alzheimer's disease and senile dementia are identical. The disease may, however, progress more rapidly in older patients, and the onset may be abrupt and associated with minor illnesses or operations.

Arteriosclerotic dementia usually occurs in the middle-aged or elderly. It is more common in men, and consists of repeated episodes of cerebral function impairment leading to a fluctuating decline. There may be evidence of arterial disease, hypertension, or a history of cerebrovascular disease.

Symptoms

The onset of dementia is insidious, and initial symptoms include a decreasing ability to concentrate, memory impairment, and an inability to cope with intellectual demands. This may progress to further memory loss, with thoughts becoming few and disconnected. The personality may deteriorate, leading to self-neglect, rigidity, depressive disorders, and unpredictable behaviour. Emotions may become blunted, shallow, or labile, and incontinence may occur. There may also be symptoms of brain damage (e.g. aphasia, apraxia, agnosia, or convulsions).

Treatment

Treatment consists of the management of underlying or associated conditions (e.g. depressive disorders), together with psychological and social support. Patients with potentially reversible causes of dementia require prompt treatment if permanent damage is to be avoided. Social contact with friends and relatives should be encouraged, and occupational therapy may be beneficial. In severe cases, hospitalisation may be necessary. Cerebral vasodilators (BNF 2.6.4) have been used in the treatment of dementia.

Self-help organisation

Alzheimer's Disease Society

Depressive Disorders

Definition and aetiology

Depressive disorders are affective conditions characterised by an abnormal experience of sadness and misery, accompanied by loss of interest, a decreased capacity for enjoyment or productive work, and a feeling of dejection and unworthiness. They should be distinguished from a normal response to unhappy events, physical illness, or environmental stresses, which lessen with the passage of time.

Previously, depressive disorders were classified as reactive or endogenous, but this classification has now been superseded by reference to the severity of symptoms (i.e. mild, moderate, or severe).

Aetiological factors in depressive disorders are varied, and include genetic predisposition, adverse childhood experiences, personality, and persistent socio-economic difficulties (e.g. single-parent mothers). These factors may operate through abnormal biochemistry in brain tissue, which affects neurotransmitters (e.g. serotonin and noradrenaline).

Symptoms

Mild depressive disorders are characterised by apathy, low mood, lack of interest, and irritability. Sleep disruption may occur through early waking or difficulty in falling asleep. Mild disorders may be characterised by anxiety, phobic states, and obsession, which are commonly classified as neurotic symptoms.

Moderate depressive disorders have similar, but worsened, symptoms of lack of energy, disinterest, and irritability. Speech is drone-like and slowed. The patient becomes withdrawn, and feels that everyday tasks are major obstacles. Somatic features include loss of appetite and weight, malaise, reduced libido, and, in women, amenorrhoea. These symptoms may antagonise the depressive state, as patients worry that they have a serious illness.

Depressive disorders of a severe nature present with all the above symptoms, but to a greater degree. Additionally, delusions and hallucinations may occur (commonly classified as psychotic symptoms) in which guilt and persecution may be prominent. Such patients present a high risk of suicide.

Treatment
Mild cases of depressive disorders usually require only supportive treatment and behaviour therapy. Moderate to severe manifestations may require additional anti-depressant drugs (BNF 4.3). Anxiolytics (BNF 4.1.2) may be used with caution in depressive states associated with agitation. Hospitalisation can be helpful in moderate cases and is often essential in severe conditions. In severe cases, electroconvulsive therapy may be indicated.

Drug Dependence

Definition and aetiology
Drug dependence is a psychic, and sometimes physical, state characterised by behavioural and other responses. It always includes a compulsion to take a drug on a continuous or periodic basis in order to experience its psychic effects, and sometimes to avoid the discomfort of its absence (i.e. withdrawal symptoms).

Psychic dependence is characterised by an intense craving and compulsive need to take a drug in order to produce its pleasurable psychic effects or to avoid withdrawal symptoms. Physical dependence is an adaptive state, characterised by intense physical trauma on withdrawal of the drug, which can only be relieved by the administration of the same drug or another with similar pharmacological action. Tolerance, which may or may not be present, is the requirement to increase the dose to maintain the desired effect. Cross-tolerance between drugs may also occur, and dependence is often not restricted to one drug.

Symptoms
The psychic and physical characteristics of drug dependence vary with the type of drug, amount used, frequency of use, and the route of administration.

Treatment
General measures used in the treatment of drug dependence are described below.

Alcohol-type Drug Dependence

Definition
Drug dependence of the alcohol-type is characterised by mild to marked psychic and physical dependence, with some tolerance to its effects. There is mutual, but incomplete, cross-tolerance between alcohol and barbiturates.

Symptoms
Alcohol-dependent patients may experience impairment of judgement, thought, and psychomotor co-ordination, which may result in deterioration of work performance and in accidents, exhibitionism, aggressive behaviour, and violence. Patients may be predisposed to physical illness, which may also arise through personal neglect. The intensity of the withdrawal symptoms, which include delirium tremens and convulsions, vary with the duration and amount of alcohol taken. They may be mild, but life-threatening symptoms may occur.

Amphetamine-type Drug Dependence

Definition
Dependence of the amphetamine-type occurs with the amphetamines and other central nervous stimulants. It is characterised by mild to marked psychic dependence, little (if any) physical dependence, and by marked tolerance.

Symptoms
Persons dependent on these drugs may be prone to accidents, aggressive behaviour, and, particularly after intravenous use, to psychotic episodes involving hallucinations and delusions. There are no characteristic withdrawal symptoms, but mental and physical depression may occur.

Barbiturate-type Drug Dependence

Definition
Dependence of the barbiturate-type occurs with barbiturates and other sedative drugs (e.g. chloral hydrate, meprobamate, and the benzodiazepines). It is characterised by mild to marked psychic and physical dependence, and substantial tolerance. There is mutual, but incomplete, cross-tolerance between these drugs and alcohol.

Symptoms
Persons dependent on these drugs may show impaired mental function, confusion, increased emotional instability, and a distorted perception of time. They may also be accident-prone and violent. There may be a risk of sudden overdosage, and relatively limited tolerance to the lethal dose. The intensity of the withdrawal symptoms, which include anxiety, headache, vomiting, insom-

nia, and tachycardia, varies with the type of drug, dose, duration, and method of use. They may only be mild but life-threatening symptoms (e.g. convulsions) may develop.

Cannabis-type Drug Dependence

Definition
Dependence of the cannabis-type is characterised by mild to moderate psychic dependence, with little (if any) physical dependence. There may be some tolerance at higher doses and acute psychotic episodes may occur.

Symptoms
On long-term regular use, persons dependent on cannabis may show impaired psychomotor co-ordination and perception. There are no characteristic withdrawal symptoms.

Cocaine-type Drug Dependence

Definition
Cocaine-type dependence is characterised by mild to marked psychic dependence (with a strong tendency to continue administration), and no physical dependence or tolerance.

Symptoms
On long-term use, persons dependent on cocaine may show personality deterioration, unreliability, and loss of self-control. High doses may precipitate a psychotic state with hallucinations and delusions, which may result in aggressive and violent behaviour. There are no characteristic withdrawal symptoms, but depressive disorders and delusions may occur.

Hallucinogen-type Drug Dependence

Definition
Dependence of the hallucinogen-type occurs with lysergide (LSD) and other hallucinogens (e.g. dimethyltryptamine, mescaline, and psilocybin). It is characterised by mild to moderate psychic dependence and no physical dependence. The degree of tolerance (which may be marked) varies according to the drug used, and cross-tolerance occurs within the group.

Symptoms
Persons dependent on hallucinogens may suffer from serious impairment of judgement. Reactions, including panic reactions to the hallucinations and delusions, may lead to accidents. There are no characteristic withdrawal symptoms, but agitation or psychotic episodes may occur.

Opiate-type Drug Dependence

Definition
Dependence of the opiate-type occurs with opium, morphine, diamorphine, codeine, and synthetic opioid drugs (e.g. methadone and pethidine). It is characterised by moderate to marked psychic dependence and marked physical dependence and tolerance, each of which develop readily with low doses, and produce cross-tolerance within the group.

Symptoms
Persons dependent on these drugs may be prone to physical neglect, malnutrition, and infection. There may also be apathy, lethargy, and a disruption of interpersonal relationships. These drugs produce characteristic withdrawal symptoms, which include yawning, lachrymation, rhinorrhoea, sneezing, muscle tremor, agitation, and diarrhoea. The intensity of withdrawal symptoms depends on the drug, dose, and method of use.

Volatile Solvent-type Drug Dependence

Definition
Dependence of the volatile solvent-type (inhalant-type) occurs with volatile solvents (e.g. acetone or toluene as found in some types of glue, and petrol) and anaesthetic agents (e.g. ether and chloroform). It is characterised by mild to moderate psychic dependence with little, if any, physical dependence. Tolerance may develop with some agents (e.g. toluene), and there is cross-tolerance between alcohol and some anaesthetic agents.

Symptoms
Persons dependent on these agents may show aggressive and violent behaviour, impaired psychomotor co-ordination, and may be prone to physical illness. Reactions to the hallucinations caused by the agents may lead to accidents. There are no characteristic withdrawal symptoms, but acute psychotic episodes may occur.

Treatment of Drug Dependence
Treatment, which is usually long-term, depends on the type of dependence and includes identification of predisposing factors, drug or agent withdrawal and, in some cases, substitution. If withdrawal symptoms occur, symptomatic drug treatment may be necessary. Psychotherapy and supportive counselling may be helpful.

Self-help organisations
Alcoholics Anonymous
Institute for the Study of Drug Dependence
National Campaign against Solvent Abuse
Standing Conference on Drug Abuse

Epilepsy

Definition and aetiology

Epilepsy is characterised by seizures caused by recurrent paroxysmal disturbances in the electrical activity of the brain. An epileptic seizure may be defined as a transitory disorder of cerebral function, usually associated with a disturbance of consciousness and accompanied by sudden excessive electrical changes in the cerebral neurones. It may be idiopathic or precipitated by an underlying disease (e.g. infection, metabolic disorders, or an intracranial tumour). It may also be due to head injury or the administration of some drugs (e.g. phenothiazines) or abrupt withdrawal of antiepileptics or benzodiazepines.

Treatment

Measures used in the treatment of the various forms of epilepsy are described below.

Generalised Seizures

Definition and aetiology

Generalised seizures are usually characterised by a loss of, or alteration to, consciousness. This accompanies generalised symmetrical electrical changes, which spread rapidly to all parts of the brain.

Tonic-clonic (grand mal) seizures, absence (petit mal) seizures, and myoclonic seizures are examples of generalised attacks. Other types of seizure, which are generalised at the outset, include tonic seizures, clonic seizures, atonic or akinetic seizures, atypical absence seizures, and infantile spasms.

Symptoms

Tonic-clonic seizures are characterised by a loss of consciousness, followed by a tonic phase in which the muscles become rigid. A characteristic cry may be heard, and there may be tongue biting and incontinence. Cyanosis may develop due to interrupted respiration. The tonic phase is followed by a clonic phase, which produces rhythmic contraction and relaxation of the limbs and trunk. A period of deep stupor and confusion precedes regaining consciousness. Headache and muscle soreness are common post-seizure symptoms. The seizures may last several minutes, and can occur at any age.

Absence seizures usually begin in childhood, but rarely persist into adult life. They are characterised by very brief lapses of consciousness, which begin and end abruptly and may go unnoticed. Occasionally, there is clonic jerking of the arms, although a blank expression or fluttering of the eyelids may be the only signs.

Myoclonic seizures occur as random involuntary movements, usually involving the limbs, and are frequently provoked by noise or other sensory stimuli. They may be associated with tonic-clonic or absence seizures.

Partial Seizures

Definition and aetiology

Partial (focal) seizures are usually caused by a disturbance in electrical activity in a localised area (the focus) of the brain, and which does not spread. Partial seizures can become generalised, and the symptoms of the partial seizure appear as an aura prior to rapid generalisation. Types of partial seizures include psychomotor (temporal lobe) epilepsy, jacksonian epilepsy, and sensory epilepsy.

Psychomotor seizures may develop at any age, and are usually associated with structural lesions, often in the temporal lobe of the brain.

Symptoms

Partial seizures are characterised by a dream-like state and amnesia. Consciousness is not usually lost, and the location of the focus determines the symptoms.

Symptoms of psychomotor seizures depend on the site of the lesion. A very common initial symptom is a vague feeling of discomfort in the upper abdomen and a sense of fullness in the head. These symptoms constitute the aura, which may be experienced if the seizure becomes secondarily generalised. Other symptoms may include memory loss, disorientation, feeling of re-experiencing the environment (*déjà-vu*), and a sense of unreality. Initially motor activity ceases, to be replaced by simple movements (e.g. swallowing and chewing). Fear, dizziness, and hallucinations may occur.

Status Epilepticus

Definition and aetiology

Status epilepticus can occur with tonic-clonic seizures (tonic-clonic status), absence seizures (absence status), and psychomotor seizures (psychomotor status). It is characterised by a rapid succession of seizures without a recovery period, and may consequently be fatal unless rapidly controlled. It may be precipitated by alcohol or abrupt withdrawal of antiepileptic drugs.

Treatment of Epilepsy

Treatment of all types of epilepsy consists of the administration of antiepileptics (BNF 4.8). The choice of drug is governed by the type of seizure, which is usually confirmed by reference to an electroencephalogram. Drug combinations may be needed where different types of seizure co-exist, although the use of more than two antiepileptics is rarely justified.

Patients should be advised to avoid any causative

factors, and underlying disorders (e.g. metabolic disorders) should be treated. Children with seizures unresponsive to antiepileptics may benefit from a ketogenic diet (BNF 9.4), and some types of seizure and refractory cases may benefit from surgery.

Status epilepticus requires immediate control with parenteral antiepileptics (BNF 4.8.2), and steps may be necessary to maintain the airway.

Self-help organisations
British Epilepsy Association
National Society for Epilepsy

Mania and Manic-depressive Illness

Definition and aetiology
Mania is an uncommon affective disorder, which is characterised by elation, hyperactivity, hyperirritability, and delusions. It may occur as an uncomplicated disorder, but may also exist in combination with depressive disorders as a bipolar manic-depressive illness. The exact cause of mania and manic-depressive illness is unclear, but several theories exist as to their aetiology. They may arise as a result of disordered brain biochemistry, or electrolyte or endocrine disturbances. Childhood experiences or life events may also have some bearing.

Symptoms
The onset of mania is often gradual with only mild symptoms (hypomania), which may include early waking, excitement and restlessness, and loss of concentration. The patient may indulge in irrational behaviour and become sexually promiscuous. This may be followed by more severe symptoms characteristic of true mania. These include hyperactivity and hyperirritability, wild illogical speech, marked elation, and delusions of grandeur. The patient may lose weight as a result of a failure to eat, and may become exhausted.

In manic-depressive illness, a period of depression follows the manic phase, and this is characterised by the gradual onset of depressive symptoms.

Treatment
Antipsychotic drugs (BNF 4.2.1) may be administered for the short-term treatment of acute mania, and antimanic drugs (BNF 4.2.3) may also be useful. Antimanic drugs are also given as prophylaxis for manic-depressive illness, and electroconvulsive therapy may be beneficial. In severe cases of mania and manic-depressive illness, hospitalisation may be necessary, and psychotherapy and occupational therapy are often employed.

Mental Retardation

Definition and aetiology
Mental retardation is a state of permanent impaired intelligence, which may be present at birth or appear during the first two years of life. As a consequence of the abnormality, special care and training is required, which in severe cases must be continuous.

Prenatal causes of mental retardation include chromosome disorders (e.g. phenylketonuria), congenital infections (e.g. rubella), drugs and alcohol, maternal illness, and radiation. Children born to very young mothers present a high risk of cerebral palsy, whereas children produced late in the mother's reproductive life are particularly prone to Down's syndrome.

Complications that arise at birth may also cause mental retardation. Premature and underweight babies have an increased risk, and trauma during birth (e.g. breech or high-forceps delivery) increases the likelihood of impaired mental development.

After birth, encephalitis and meningitis, lead poisoning, and physical injury or asphyxiation are possible causes of mental retardation.

Symptoms
The outward signs of mental retardation may vary significantly according to the cause of the condition. Stature and unusual head growth may be indicative of certain types of prenatal lesions. Metabolic disorders may present as a failure to thrive, lethargy, vomiting, convulsions, and external manifestations (e.g. coarse facial features).

Developmental tests are used to assess children who produce no outward signs of illness, but who are apparently slow to develop. Developmental milestones (*see* Section 17.4) may be missed, and this may be the only outward indication of retardation.

Educational assessment in older children is based on intelligence quotient (IQ) tests. Moderately subnormal and severely subnormal children possess an IQ of 50-69 and below 50 respectively. Profound retardation is indicated by an IQ of less than 30.

Treatment
Most cases of mental retardation are not treatable, although the causes may be treatable to prevent their worsening. Those that are amenable to treatment often have fluctuating symptoms, and include phenylketonuria, galactosaemia, hydrocephalus, and some epileptic syndromes.

Self-help organisations
Downs Syndrome Association
MENCAP
Leonard Cheshire Foundation
National Autistic Society
Spastics Society

Phobic States

Definition

A phobic state is characterised by the emergence of inappropriate anxiety or panic attacks, and morbid fear of certain objects or situations. It is usually a chronic condition, which may begin in early adulthood, with various degrees of remission and relapse. It results in the avoidance of the phobic stimulus, and anticipatory anxiety may be present before subsequent exposure to the stimulus. The condition can become disabling if the stimulus cannot be easily avoided.

Agoraphobia is a phobic state due to open and public places or crowds. Claustrophobia is due to confined or enclosed spaces. Other types of phobia include those of objects (e.g. spiders) or social phobias (e.g. the presence of other people or eating in public places).

Treatment

Treatment consists of behaviour therapy to condition the patient to the phobic stimulus, and hypnotherapy. Drug treatment with anxiolytics (BNF 4.1.2) may be used to alleviate anticipatory anxiety, and antidepressant drugs (BNF 4.3) to prevent panic attacks.

Schizophrenia

Definition and aetiology

Schizophrenia is a psychotic state with disturbance of mind and personality, but without impairment of consciousness. It may be caused by a combination of environmental and genetic factors.

Symptoms

Schizophrenia is usually insidious in onset, tends to be chronic, and remissions and relapses commonly occur. It is characterised by disturbance of mental processes, thought, and mood.

The diagnostic symptoms of schizophrenia are termed first-rank symptoms. The occurrence of any one of these symptoms in the absence of other physical disease is strongly suggestive of schizophrenia. First-rank symptoms include auditory hallucinations (in which patients hear their own thoughts spoken aloud or others talking about them), disordered thoughts, delusions, and control of emotions by others. Other symptoms include behaviour disorders, hallucinations, and, in chronic schizophrenia, social withdrawal.

Treatment

Treatment consists of the long-term administration of antipsychotic drugs (BNF 4.2.1 and 4.2.2). In certain cases electroconvulsive therapy may be useful. Psychotherapy, counselling, occupational therapy, and social rehabilitation and support may also be necessary.

Self-help organisation

Schizophrenia Association of Great Britain

Speech Disorders

Definition and aetiology

Disorders of speech indicate a derangement of higher nervous function caused by lesions at specific sites within the cerebral cortex.

Aphasia

Definition and aetiology

Aphasia (dysphasia) is the disturbance of language function caused by damage to the language centres, which are located primarily in the left cerebral hemisphere of most people, whether right- or left-handed. It is due to transient ischaemic attacks or to intracranial tumours, and may occur in children or adults.

Symptoms

Disturbances to the delivery of speech may range from complete loss to speech which is non-fluent, ungrammatical, and difficult to comprehend. The presence of aphasia is frequently accompanied by writing disorders of a similar degree.

Treatment

Spontaneous recovery from aphasia may occur over a period of months, although this happens less frequently in affected adults than children.

Dysarthria

Definition and aetiology

Dysarthria is a disorder of speech which arises through disruption of the mechanical production of speech. The muscles which generate speech may themselves be damaged, or they may malfunction secondary to cerebral cortex damage.

Symptoms

Speech in dysarthria often contains the correct words, but they may not be understandable.

Stuttering

Definition and aetiology

Speech production may be impaired due to the disturbance of the normal sequence of muscular function in the larynx. It may be of psychogenic origin, and occurs occasionally in conjunction with aphasic symptoms.

Symptoms

Stuttering is characterised by hesitation and repetition in speech delivery, which produces disjointed conversation in which words or syllables may be missing altogether.

Self-help organisations
Action for Dysphasic Adults
Association for Stammerers
Chest Heart and Stroke Association
Dyslexia Institute
Motor Neurone Disease Association

4.4   DEGENERATIVE DISORDERS

Bell's Palsy

Definition and aetiology
Bell's palsy is facial paralysis due to a lesion of the seventh cranial nerve within the facial canal. It is of unknown aetiology, of rapid onset, and usually occurs unilaterally. The nerve is inflamed, and compression within the facial canal may contribute to axonal damage. Mild cases are due to a local conduction block within the facial canal, which may be due to demyelination without axonal degeneration. In more severe cases, there may be total paralysis and axonal degeneration.

Symptoms
Paralysis usually reaches its maximum in 1 to 2 days, and may be accompanied by transient pain below the ear or in the mastoid region. Other symptoms may include dysarthria, difficulty in eating, dribbling, impairment of taste, intolerance of noise, and sagging of the face. Voluntary eye closure is usually impossible, and the eye may water or be dry. Ectropion may also be present, especially in the elderly. Patients with no axonal degeneration usually recover within a few weeks. If axonal degeneration is present, recovery usually begins after about three months with regeneration, but may be incomplete or fail to occur.

Treatment
In the early stages of the condition, treatment is directed towards preventing axonal damage, and corticosteroids (BNF 6.3.4) may be administered. Preparations for tear deficiency (BNF 11.8.1) should be used if the eye is dry, and patients advised to protect the eye from light.

Carpal Tunnel Syndrome

Definition and aetiology
Carpal tunnel syndrome is compression of the median nerve within the wrist. It most commonly occurs in middle-aged women and is usually idiopathic. It may, however, be due to tenosynovitis of the flexor tendons after excessive or unaccustomed use of the hand, to rheumatoid arthritis, or osteoarthritis. Other predisposing factors include hypothyroidism, acromegaly, pregnancy, the menopause, oral contraceptive use, and diabetic neuropathy.

Symptoms
Numbness and tingling (paraesthesia), and a burning pain in the hand, thumb, fingers, and occasionally the forearm, commonly occur at night. The hand may feel useless on waking. There may also be weakness and wasting of the muscles involved, and sensory loss over the tips of the affected fingers (acroparaesthesia).

Treatment
Treatment depends on the severity of the symptoms. If acroparaesthesia is the only symptom, reduced use of the hand may be all that is required. Splinting of the wrist and local corticosteroid injections (BNF 10.1.2.2) may help. If symptoms persist, or if muscle weakness and wasting are present, surgical decompression of the nerve may be indicated.

Diabetic Neuropathy

Definition and aetiology
Diabetic neuropathy is a peripheral neuropathy, which occurs as a complication of diabetes mellitus. Contributory factors include the age of the diabetic and the duration of his diabetes, poor diabetic control, and nerve damage due to ischaemia or compression. It affects the legs and feet predominantly, but the arms and hands may also be affected.

Symptoms
Symmetrical polyneuropathy may occur, ranging from numbness to total loss of sensation, together with loss of joint-position sense, muscular pain, and weakness. Dysaesthesia may occur and include feelings of numbness, compression, warm or cold, tingling, pricking, or diffuse irritation. Motor neuropathy may occur, causing sudden knee and hip weakness with pain and wasting of the thigh muscles. Autonomic neuropathy, involving the sympathetic ganglia, may occur and result in orthostatic hypotension, diarrhoea, impotence, urinary retention, and sweating at the start of a meal (gustatory sweating). Mononeuropathy may also occur (e.g. carpal tunnel syndrome).

Treatment
Drug treatment of diabetic neuropathy (BNF 6.1.5) is symptomatic. Close diabetic control may be beneficial. Patients with sensory loss should be advised about their vulnerability to injury, which may predispose the patient to infection, ulceration, and gangrene.

Encephalopathy

Definition
Encephalopathy is any degenerative disease of the brain.

Dialysis Encephalopathy

Definition and aetiology
Dialysis encephalopathy may occur after prolonged repeated haemodialysis, possibly as a result of high aluminium concentrations in haemodialysis solutions.

Symptoms
Symptoms include amnesia, convulsions, dementia, somnolence, and speech disorders.

Treatment
Treatment consists of reducing the aluminium concentration of haemodialysis solutions, withdrawing oral aluminium preparations, or both.

Hepatic Encephalopathy

Definition and aetiology
Hepatic encephalopathy is a neurological syndrome which occurs as a result of advanced liver disease. It may be due to the toxic effects of substances (e.g. ammonia) normally metabolised by the liver.

Symptoms
It is characterised by altered consciousness and may result in coma (hepatic coma). Other symptoms include anxiety, ataxia, mania, speech disorders, somnolence, tremor, and rigidity.

Treatment
Treatment comprises the withdrawal of dietary protein, and the administration of lactulose (BNF 1.6.4) and neomycin (BNF 5.1.4).

Hypertensive Encephalopathy

Definition and aetiology
Hypertensive encephalopathy consists of a group of neurological symptoms associated with severe hypertension.

Symptoms
It is characterised by severe headache, convulsions, and nausea and vomiting. Stupor and coma may follow.

Treatment
Urgent treatment is essential, and involves the reduction of blood pressure. Antiepileptic drugs (BNF 4.8) may be required.

Guillain-Barré Syndrome

Definition and aetiology
Guillain-Barré syndrome is characterised by proximal, distal, or generalised polyneuropathy, with inflammation, oedema, and demyelination of the affected nerves. It is idiopathic, but many cases follow viral infection or surgery.

Symptoms
Motor nerves are predominantly affected, usually starting distally and slowly ascending, resulting in paralysis of all limbs and loss of tendon reflexes. In severe cases facial, trunk, and respiratory muscles may be involved. Sensory nerve involvement may result in touch, vibratory, and postural sensory loss. There may also be autonomic involvement.

Treatment
Treatment is supportive and may include assisted ventilation. Patients usually recover within weeks or months, but recovery may be prolonged in severe cases and muscle weakness may remain.

Motor Neurone Disease

Definition and aetiology
Motor neurone disease is a rare, progressive, degenerative disorder of the motor neurones, which occurs most commonly in middle-age. Its cause is unknown.

Symptoms
Symptoms include muscle wasting and weakness in the hands and arms, and spasticity of the legs. Muscle cramps, occasionally with pain, may occur. Dysphagia and speech disorders are also common. There is no sensory loss. The disease is always fatal and death usually occurs within 3 to 5 years of the onset.

Treatment
No treatment is known.

Self-help organisation
Motor Neurone Disease Association

Multiple Sclerosis

Definition and aetiology
Multiple sclerosis (disseminated sclerosis) is characterised by patches of demyelination of nerves within the central nervous system, including the optic nerves. The axons are initially unaffected, but in later stages axonal degeneration occurs. The peripheral nervous system is not affected. It is of unknown aetiology, has a peak onset around 30 years of age, and is usually chronic.

Its course is highly variable and unpredictable, and

remissions and relapses are common. After an initial attack there may be complete recovery, but subsequent relapses may lead to a progressive decline. It may also be chronically progressive from onset, especially in older patients.

Symptoms

The presence and severity of symptoms is variable and depends on the sites of the lesions. Initial symptoms may include weakness in one or both legs, dysarthria, loss of co-ordination, and sensory loss, visual disturbances due to retrobulbar neuritis, and vertigo. Other symptoms include nystagmus, ataxia, tremor, facial twitching, dementia, muscle spasms of the limbs, urgency of micturition, incontinence, and impotence. Trigeminal neuralgia may occur in younger patients. Symptoms tend to worsen with small increases in body temperature (e.g. during fever and hot baths), fatigue, or exertion. In advanced stages, and in conjunction with a variety of other disabilities, patients may become confined to a wheelchair or require full nursing care, or both. Complications (e.g. urinary-tract infection, decubitus ulcers, and coma) may be fatal.

Treatment

No special treatment exists. Corticosteroids (BNF 6.3.4), corticotrophin (BNF 6.5.1), and immunosuppressants (BNF 8.2.1 and 8.2.2) have been used to treat acute relapses and delay progression. Skeletal muscle relaxants (BNF 10.2.2) are used to treat muscular spasm. Patients should be advised to avoid fatigue, and physiotherapy may be beneficial early in the course of the disease. Incontinence aids may benefit some patients.

Self-help organisations

Action Research into Multiple Sclerosis
Leonard Cheshire Foundation
Multiple Sclerosis Society of Great Britain and Northern Ireland

Reye's Syndrome

Definition and aetiology

Reye's syndrome is an acute encephalopathy, which affects children between 2 and 16 years of age. The syndrome is also characterised by fatty droplets present in the liver, and with impaired liver function. It tends to follow an acute viral infection (e.g. upper respiratory-tract infection, chickenpox, or influenza), although the link between the precipitating illness and Reye's syndrome is not known.

Recent studies have indicated that the use of aspirin, but not paracetamol, in the preceding viral illness may be associated with the development of Reye's syndrome.

Symptoms

Symptoms develop in a child recovering from a viral infection. Intractable vomiting develops suddenly, followed by lethargy, disorientation, and irritability. Without medical intervention, convulsions, coma, and death occur within 3 to 5 days. Hepatomegaly may also occur in up to half the cases, but jaundice is absent. Irreversible brain damage may occur in 50% of the surviving children.

Treatment

There is no specific treatment for Reye's syndrome, although improved survival may result from symptomatic therapy. Fluid and electrolyte disturbances may be treated by intravenous administration of fluids (BNF 9.2.2) containing glucose. Cerebral oedema may be treated by osmotic diuretics (BNF 2.2.5) and corticosteroids (BNF 6.3.4).

Syringomyelia and Syringobulbia

Definition and aetiology

Syringomyelia is the occurrence of a tubular fluid-filled cavity (the syrinx) in the spinal cord, often in the cervical region. It is termed syringobulbia when the brain stem is involved. It is thought to be a congenital disorder, although symptoms do not usually develop until early adulthood.

Symptoms

Symptoms of syringomyelia include sensory loss in the hands, which also become wasted, and lower limb spasticity. Syringobulbia is characterised by atrophy of the tongue, dysphagia, speech disorders, deafness, vertigo, nystagmus, and sensory loss over the face.

Sensory loss may become widespread. Symptoms may be mild and stable, but may become progressive and rapidly deteriorate.

Treatment

Treatment is by surgical decompression.

4.5 EXTRAPYRAMIDAL DISORDERS

Chorea

Definition and aetiology

Chorea is characterised by brief involuntary muscle contractions. It results in a continuous series of irregular jerky movements, which move rapidly from one part of the body to another at random. It may be due to an underlying disorder or to certain drugs (e.g. antipsychotic drugs and phenytoin). Hemichorea affects only one side of the body.

Huntington's Chorea

Definition and aetiology

Huntington's chorea is a rare, dominantly inherited, progressive disease characterised by chorea and dementia.

Symptoms

There is general brain damage and atrophy, with extensive neuronal loss. Onset is insidious and usually occurs between 30 and 50 years of age. Initial symptoms include personality disorders (e.g. loss of drive and irritability), followed by progressive dementia and chorea. Severe depression is common. In advanced stages, the chorea may be slowed due to the development of rigidity and akinesia. The patient finally becomes bedridden, and death eventually follows.

Treatment

No specific treatment exists. Tetrabenazine (BNF 4.9.3) may be necessary to control the movement disorder. Permanent hospitalisation is almost inevitable, and family support may be required.

Sydenham's Chorea

Definition and aetiology

Sydenham's chorea (St. Vitus' dance) is a rare disease characterised by chorea and psychological disturbances and accompanied by inflammatory encephalitis. It commonly occurs up to six months after rheumatic fever.

Symptoms

Onset is frequently insidious and usually occurs between 7 and 12 years of age. It may recur in later life, especially in pregnant women and in those taking oral contraceptives. Initial symptoms include psychological disturbances (e.g. irritability, agitation, and inattentiveness), followed by a generalised chorea resulting in difficulty in walking and handling objects, and impaired speech. In severe cases, flaccidity and weakness may also be present.

Treatment

The condition is self-limiting, but drug treatment for chorea may be necessary (BNF 4.9.3), in conjunction with bed rest. Antibacterial prophylaxis (BNF 5.1, Table 2) may be necessary to prevent recurrence of rheumatic fever.

Parkinsonism

Definition and aetiology

Parkinsonism is a syndrome commonly caused by Parkinson's disease (paralysis agitans), a progressive disorder of insidious onset which usually begins between 50 and 65 years of age. In the majority of cases, there is no definable cause (idiopathic parkinsonism), although it may be due to poisoning with carbon monoxide, manganese or other metals, brain tumours in the basal ganglia, cerebral trauma, degenerative diseases, or following encephalitis (post-encephalitic parkinsonism). Drug-induced parkinsonism may also occur (e.g. following administration of antipsychotic drugs).

In Parkinson's disease, there are degenerative changes with loss of cells in the substantia nigra and basal ganglia. There may also be degenerative changes in the brain stem or cranial nerve nuclei, or atrophy of the cerebral cortex. Depletion of the neurotransmitter, dopamine, results in an imbalance between the cholinergic and dopaminergic neurones in the extrapyramidal system.

Symptoms

Parkinsonism is characterised by tremor, muscular rigidity, loss of postural reflexes, and akinesia (with hypokinesia and bradykinesia). The patient has a mask-like expression and a monotonous voice, and may experience fatigue, drooling of saliva, dysphagia, constipation, and excessive sweating. Speech disorders and depressive disorders are common.

Treatment

Treatment consists of the administration of dopaminergic drugs (BNF 4.9.1), anticholinergic drugs (BNF 4.9.2), or both. Drug-induced parkinsonism, however, may only be treated with anticholinergic drugs, and remission often occurs on withdrawal of the causative drug. Physical therapy and aids may also be useful.

A high level of physical activity is recommended to prevent the worsening of rigidity and akinesia.

Self-help organisations

Age Concern England
Leonard Cheshire Foundation
Parkinson's Disease Society

Tardive Dyskinesia

Definition and aetiology

Tardive dyskinesia is a chronic movement disorder usually associated with antipsychotic drug treatment. It is characterised by repetitive uncontrollable movements, occurring most noticeably on the face and upper trunk.

It occurs most commonly in women, the elderly, and in those with brain injury. Although it is usually precipitated by antipsychotic therapy, symptoms may persist after treatment has stopped. It is thought to be associated with increased sensitivity of dopaminergic receptors as a consequence of their constant blockade by antipsychotics.

Symptoms

Symptoms appear usually after at least six months dosage with antipsychotics, and their onset may be associated with a reduction or cessation of dosage. The most apparent signs are continuous chewing movements, lip smacking, and continual darting of the tongue from the mouth. Body-rocking and incessant movement of the fingers and toes also occur. 'Marching in place' may appear as a result of repetitive movement of the legs. The most distressing symptom described is the feeling that the person is about to jump out of his skin. Anticholinergic drug administration aggravates the symptoms.

Treatment

Reintroduction of the antipsychotic drug (BNF 4.2.1) may ameliorate symptoms, although in some cases paradoxical worsening of the condition may occur. Reserpine and clonazepam have been found useful in some patients.

Tics

Definition and aetiology

Tics are rapid, involuntary, twitching movements which are repetitive and occur at the same site, usually the face or shoulders. They commonly occur in childhood and are usually self-limiting, but may persist into adult life. Tics are rarely considered abnormal, but may become severe and be associated with a psychological disorder.

Gilles de la Tourette Syndrome

Definition and aetiology

Gilles de la Tourette syndrome is a chronic disorder characterised by multiple tics and involuntary verbal manifestations. It is idiopathic, but may be due to organic disease of the central nervous system.

Symptoms

Typical onset is before 15 years of age. Initial symptoms include blinking, nodding, sniffing, or stuttering, but other tics may appear. Involuntary noises (e.g. grunting or barking) subsequently develop and are commonly transformed into swear-words (coprolalia). Patients may also repeat words spoken to them (echolalia), words spoken by them (palilalia), and may indulge in obscene gesturing (copropraxia) or imitation of the movement of others (echopraxia).

Treatment

Treatment consists of the administration of haloperidol (BNF 4.9.3) to control the symptoms.

4.6 ANATOMY AND PHYSIOLOGY OF THE NERVOUS SYSTEM

Introduction

The nervous system is the medium through which the body experiences changes in the internal and external environments, and co-ordinates the responses made to these changes. It may be classified anatomically into two major components. The central nervous system (CNS) comprises the brain and spinal cord, and the peripheral nervous system is made up of the nerves and ganglia throughout the rest of the body.

Functionally, the nervous system may also be classified as the somatic (voluntary) nervous system, which receives impulses from skeletal muscles, ligaments, bone, eye, ear, and skin and returns impulses to skeletal muscles; and the autonomic (involuntary) nervous system (ANS), which co-ordinates the activities of heart muscle, smooth muscle, and glands and therefore the major organs of the body. The autonomic nervous system comprises the sympathetic and parasympathetic divisions. Most visceral organs are innervated by both components. In general, stimulation of the sympathetic division produces responses that prepare the body for an emergency (e.g. increased cardiac output, increased blood pressure, and bronchodilatation), while stimulation of the parasympathetic division produces opposing actions. Autonomic nervous system function is regulated by the relative activity of the two divisions.

The brain is the highly developed outgrowth of the spinal cord, which is contained within and protected by the cranium. The brain stem connects the spinal cord to the two cerebral hemispheres, and is divided into the medulla, midbrain, and pons. The cerebellum is closely linked anatomically to the brain stem. It consists of two hemispheres connected by a central mass, the vermis.

The Cerebral Hemispheres

The two cerebral hemispheres develop as the enlarged outgrowths of the brain stem. On continued evolutionary development, the outermost surfaces of the two hemispheres have become highly convoluted, and this distinguishes gross human brain structure from that in other animals. The folds (gyri) in the outer surface of the cerebral hemispheres produce deep fissures and more shallow sulci. In the hemispheres, the grey matter containing cell bodies overlies white matter formed of tracts of nervous tissue, whereas in the brain stem and spinal cord, the reverse is true. The two cerebral hemispheres are connected by a tract of white matter, the corpus callosum.

The cortical surfaces of the cerebral hemispheres are divided into four main regions, and each region has distinct sensory or motor functions. The sensory cortex comprises the parietal lobe (e.g. concerned with sensations of touch) and the occipital lobe (which contains the visual cortex). The temporal lobe is also largely concerned with sensory input, converting and interpreting the information received. The frontal lobe of the cerebral cortex is the main site of motor control (e.g. affecting the movements of the hands and facial muscles) (Fig. 4.2).

The Cranial Nerves

Information is transmitted to and from the brain via the spinal cord and the 12 pairs of cranial nerves. Ten pairs of cranial nerves originate in the underside of the brain stem, and innervate primarily the head and neck. They are numbered with Roman numerals according to the order in which they arise from brain tissue. The nerves may be sensory (e.g. the optic (II) nerve); exhibit a mixture of sensory and motor functions (e.g. the vagus (X) nerve and the trigeminal (V) nerve); or mixed, but primarily motor (e.g. the oculomotor (III) nerve).

Cerebrospinal Fluid

Brain tissue is very soft and easily traumatised. In order to reduce potential damage, it floats in cerebrospinal fluid (CSF) located between two of the three membranes (the meninges), which encase the brain and spinal cord. CSF is also found in the spaces, the ventricles, within the brain. The outermost meningeal membrane (the dura mater) lies immediately inside the cranium and acts as the main buffer against movement of the brain within the skull. It also protects the delicate brain tissue from the comparatively rough inner surface of the skullbone. Immediately inside the dura mater is the arachnoid membrane. The space between the arachnoid membrane and the third membrane (the pia mater) is termed the subarachnoid space, and contains CSF. The pia mater is a thin highly vascularised membrane, which closely follows all the contours of the convoluted brain surface.

CSF is produced by projections of the pia mater (the choroid plexuses) within the hemispheres, which are located on the ventricles (Fig. 4.3). From here, it passes sequentially to the third and fourth ventricles. The CSF reaches the subarachnoid space through small holes in the roof of the fourth ventricle, and is distributed around the brain and spinal cord.

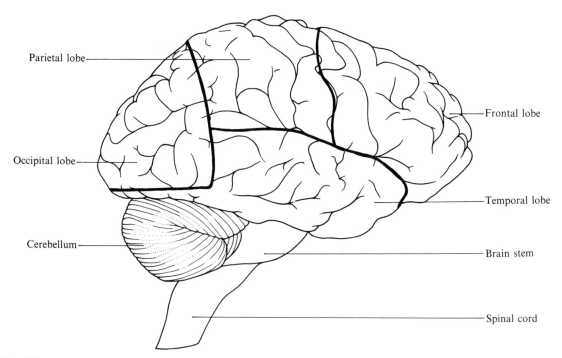

Parietal lobe

Occipital lobe

Cerebellum

Frontal lobe

Temporal lobe

Brain stem

Spinal cord

Fig. 4.2
Brain (lateral view).

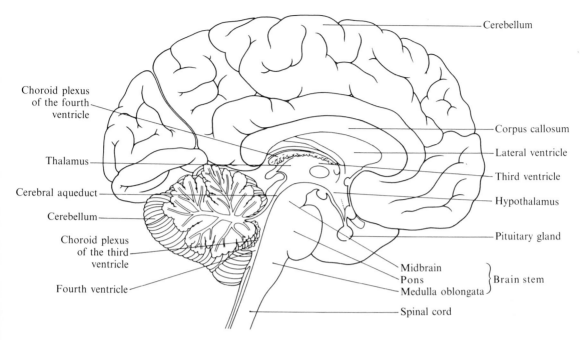

Cerebellum

Choroid plexus of the fourth ventricle

Corpus callosum

Lateral ventricle

Thalamus

Third ventricle

Cerebral aqueduct

Hypothalamus

Cerebellum

Choroid plexus of the third ventricle

Pituitary gland

Fourth ventricle

Midbrain
Pons
Medulla oblongata } Brain stem

Spinal cord

Fig. 4.3
Brain (sagittal section).

The Extrapyramidal System

The extrapyramidal system is one of the functional components involved in the control of movement in the body initiated by the motor cortex. The system comprises the basal ganglia, which lie deep within the cerebral hemispheres, and the upper portion of the brain stem. These interconnected masses of grey matter include the substantia nigra, the putamen, globus pallidus, and the caudate nucleus. Information received by these centres is passed to the extrapyramidal tract, from where it proceeds down the spinal cord to the effector muscle.

The Blood Supply to the Brain

The brain is a prolific metabolic organ, which uses a disproportionate amount of oxygen and glucose in rela-

tion to its size. The maintenance of an adequate blood supply to the brain to provide these nutrients is vital. Deficiencies for periods of as short as 1 or 2 minutes may result in unconsciousness, and permanent brain damage may result from an interruption of four minutes or longer.

Blood reaches the brain from the aorta via the brachiocephalic artery and the carotid artery. On the underside of the brain surface, the left and right carotid arteries join the basilar artery to form a circular arterial network called the circle of Willis, from which the arteries supplying the brain arise. The circle of Willis also equalises the pressure of blood supplied to the brain from different arteries, and enables alternative blood supply pathways to be adopted in the event of arterial damage.

Chapter 5

INFECTIONS

5.1 INFECTIONS OF NON-SPECIFIC ORIGIN

(For information on relevant medical microbiology, *see* Chapter 14.)

Dysentery

Definition and aetiology
Dysentery is a serious form of diarrhoea accompanied by the passage of blood and mucus. It is due to infection and inflammation of the colonic mucous membranes, resulting in ulceration. It is commonly caused by amoebiasis (amoebic dysentery) or shigellosis (bacillary dysentery).

Symptoms
Common symptoms include abdominal pain, colic, tenesmus, and the frequent passage of soft or watery stools containing blood and mucus. Vomiting may occur, and there may be a slight fever. In severe prolonged cases, patients may become emaciated and debilitated. Dehydration may be life-threatening, particularly in infants, the elderly, and malnourished individuals, and perforation and peritonitis may occasionally occur.

Treatment
Dehydration should be prevented or treated by admin-
istration of oral (BNF 9.2.1) or intravenous (BNF 9.2.2) fluids. All patients with amoebiasis should be treated by administration of amoebicides (BNF 5.4.2), but only severe cases of shigellosis require specific antibacterial therapy (BNF 5.1, Table 1).

Infective Arthritis

Definition and aetiology
Infective arthritis (septic arthritis) is arthritis which occurs as a result of infection of a joint and associated tissues. It may occur in a previously healthy or already diseased joint. Only one or a limited number of joints may be involved, which points to an infective cause, particularly if only one joint is affected. Patients with existing rheumatoid arthritis, especially those receiving corticosteroid therapy, are particularly at risk. Infective arthritis is often transmitted via the circulation from some primary infection, but it may also occur following joint surgery or an intra-articular injection. The infection is commonly staphylococcal, but other micro-organisms (e.g. *Haemophilus influenzae*) may be responsible.

Symptoms
The onset is usually marked by an acutely painful joint, which becomes hot, stiff, and swollen. Fever and rigors

frequently develop and, in the absence of treatment, joint destruction may occur.

Treatment

Treatment consists of the prompt administration of an appropriate antibacterial drug (BNF 5.1, Table 1). Aspiration or surgical drainage of the joint may be indicated, and immobilisation (i.e. splinting) may be necessary. Physiotherapy is often beneficial in restoring joint function after recovery.

Infective Endocarditis

Definition and aetiology

Infective endocarditis is an infection of the endocardium, which results in vegetation and inflammation of the heart chambers or, more commonly, the heart valves. It may be acute or subacute. It usually occurs as a result of bacterial infection, with streptococci or staphylococci the most common infecting micro-organisms. Streptococcal infection commonly derives from dental procedures (e.g. extraction and de-scaling). Fungi may also be responsible. It may arise in the presence of existing cardiac lesions (e.g. rheumatic or congenital heart disease) or of prosthetic heart valves, or it may occur in the absence of underlying heart disease. It may also develop as a consequence of the intravenous abuse of drugs.

Symptoms

The symptoms of acute infective endocarditis are severe and rapid in onset. The subacute form commonly develops insidiously, usually in patients with acquired or congenital heart disease. Such patients may suffer non-specific chronic ill-health. The symptoms are, however, similar for both forms of the disease and both may be fatal if untreated. The condition commonly occurs in the elderly. Characteristic symptoms are fever, embolisms, and heart murmurs. Other symptoms may include malaise, arthralgia, congestive heart failure, petechial and ophthalmic haemorrhages, renal impairment with haematuria, and splenomegaly. Meningitis is a possible complication. Confusion and memory loss may occur, particularly in the elderly.

Treatment

Treatment comprises the intravenous administration of antibacterial drugs (BNF 5.1, Table 1). Surgery may be necessary in unresponsive cases. Antibacterial prophylaxis (BNF 5.1, Table 2) is indicated in susceptible patients undergoing dental, gastro-intestinal, or genito-urinary procedures.

Meningitis

Definition and aetiology

Meningitis is inflammation of the meninges, which comprise the dura mater, pia mater, and arachnoid membranes. It may be caused by bacterial, fungal, or viral infection, cerebral abscess, demyelinating disorders, and malignant diseases.

Pyogenic Meningitis

Definition and aetiology

Pyogenic meningitis is due to infection by pyogenic micro-organisms and usually results from bacterial infection of the upper respiratory tract, lungs, middle ear, or nasopharynx. Micro-organisms commonly involved include *Streptococcus pneumoniae* (pneumococcus), *Neisseria meningitidis* (meningococcus, *see* Meningococcal Infections), and *Haemophilus influenzae* type B.

Symptoms

Onset is usually rapid and characterised by fever, headache, vomiting, neck stiffness, rigors, and delirium. Other symptoms may include sensorineural deafness, facial palsy, and loss of consciousness. In meningococcal infections, there is usually an associated rash.

Treatment

Treatment consists of the identification of the infecting micro-organism and appropriate parenteral antibacterial therapy (BNF 5.1, Table 1). Fluid and electrolytes (BNF 9.2) may be necessary. Symptomatic treatment may be necessary for headache, restlessness, or convulsions.

Tuberculous Meningitis

Definition and aetiology

Tuberculous meningitis is a secondary infection of the meninges resulting from infection elsewhere, usually the chest, by *Mycobacterium tuberculosis* (*see also* Tuberculosis).

Symptoms

It is usually insidious in onset with a prodrome of mild fever, general malaise, and loss of appetite. This is followed by headache and vomiting, and more severe symptoms which may include ocular and facial palsy, deafness, stupor, and coma. Convulsions may occur in later stages.

Treatment

Antituberculous drugs (BNF 5.1.9), fluid and electrolytes (BNF 9.2), and symptomatic treatment of convulsions is necessary.

Viral Meningitis

Definition and aetiology

Viral meningitis is commonly due to enteroviruses or mumps virus.

Symptoms

It may be characterised by headache and neck stiffness. Other symptoms may include back pain, myalgia, retro-orbital pain, pain on lateral movement of the eyes, fever, vomiting, anorexia, lassitude, and photophobia.

Treatment

There is no specific treatment, but symptomatic treatment for headache, pain, and fever may be required. Viral meningitis is self-limiting and usually results in complete recovery. Lumbar puncture is required to differentiate viral from bacterial infection.

Paronychia

Definition and aetiology

Paronychia is an infection of the nail fold and may be acute or chronic. *Staphylococcus aureus*, usually the offending micro-organism in the acute form, penetrates the skin at a site of local trauma. The chronic condition is generally of fungal origin, most often due to *Candida albicans*. Chronic infection occurs in people whose hands are frequently immersed in water, as the micro-organism gains entry through the macerated and damaged cuticle. Absent or poor nail manicuring, and nail-biting are also frequent causes.

Symptoms

The symptoms of acute paronychia are usually more severe than in the chronic form. It is characterised by a painful red swelling of the nail fold, and in some cases a purulent exudate. A similar, although less painful, lesion occurs in chronic paronychia, and may spread to other fingers with loss of the cuticle. If the condition persists untreated, the nail matrix may become infected, resulting in a deformed and discoloured nail body. Occasionally, the micro-organism may directly attack the nail body. The condition may be complicated by acute attacks due to secondary bacterial infection.

Treatment

The hands should be kept dry for as long as is possible. Treatment consists of the local application of an appropriate anti-infective skin preparation (BNF 13.10), or a skin disinfecting and cleansing agent (BNF 13.11). A systemic antibacterial drug (BNF 5.1) or antifungal drug (BNF 5.2) may be indicated. Surgical removal of the nail body is occasionally necessary in chronic cases where it has become directly infected.

Pneumonia

Definition and aetiology

Pneumonia is inflammation of the lungs with the production of exudate, which enters the alveoli causing con-solidation. The lesions may be localised and confined to a complete lobe (lobar) or lobule (segmented or lobular). Diffuse lesions affect the bronchi and bronchioles (bronchopneumonia) causing consolidation in adjacent lobules. The distribution may be unilateral or bilateral. Most cases of pneumonia are due to infection with bacteria. Some bacteria are capable of invading normal lung, whereas others can only invade the lung when resistance to infection is lowered (opportunistic infection). Common micro-organisms which cause pneumonia include *Streptococcus pneumoniae* (the pneumococcus), *Staphylococcus pyogenes*, and *Klebsiella pneumoniae*. Infections due to *Mycoplasma* and *Chlamydia* species and *Legionella pneumophila* are less common. Pneumonia may also be caused by viruses, fungi, protozoa (e.g. *Pneumocystis carinii*), chemical or physical irritants, or allergic reactions in the lung.

Symptoms

Common symptoms include cough, dyspnoea with tachypnoea, chest pain, purulent sputum production (initially scanty), haemoptysis, and diminished chest movements on the affected side. There is fever with rigors, and other symptoms of systemic infection (e.g. insomnia, headache, delirium, and weakness). Complications of pneumonia include pleural effusion, empyema, lung abscess, spontaneous pneumothorax, pericarditis, and meningitis.

Treatment

Treatment consists of bed rest, and the administration of oral (BNF 9.2.1) or intravenous (BNF 9.2.2) fluids and appropriate antibacterial drugs (BNF 5.1, Table 1). Oxygen therapy (BNF 3.6) and regular physiotherapy may be necessary. A vaccine is available (BNF 14.4) to provide protection against pneumococcal pneumonia.

Salpingitis

Definition and aetiology

Salpingitis is infection of the Fallopian tubes. It is usually bilateral and occurs predominantly in young sexually-active women. It may be gonococcal, or due to infection with a non-gonococcal micro-organism (e.g. *Chlamydia trachomatis* and *Mycoplasma hominis*), enteric anaerobic micro-organisms, or viruses. Rarely, salpingitis may result from tuberculosis. Non-gonococcal salpingitis may be associated with minor gynaecological procedures, abortion, childbirth, previous pelvic inflammatory disease, or intra-uterine contraceptive devices, but frequently no factors are found.

Symptoms

Salpingitis is characterised by constant lower abdominal pain and tenderness. Vomiting, low back pain, and profuse vaginal discharge may also be present. Symptoms are usually more severe and abrupt when the infection is gonococcal and fever is often present. Complications include generalised pelvic inflammatory disease (e.g. peritonitis), pyosalpinx, tubal abscess, hydrosalpinx, pelvic abscess, infertility or reduced fertility, increased incidence of ectopic pregnancy, dyspareunia, and peri-hepatitis. Recurrent cases may also occur. These complications are more common in patients with non-gonococcal salpingitis.

Treatment
Treatment consists of bed rest, hospitalisation in severe cases, and administration of high doses of penicillins (BNF 5.1.1) for gonococcal infections or oral tetracyclines (BNF 5.1.3) for non-gonococcal salpingitis. Fluid and electrolytes (BNF 9.2) may be necessary.

Septicaemia

Definition and aetiology
Septicaemia (blood poisoning) is an acute and serious clinical condition arising as a result of the presence in the bloodstream of pathogenic micro-organisms or their toxins. Any micro-organism may be responsible, either singly or in conjunction with others, and originates from an existing focus of infection (e.g. appendicitis, cellulitis, cholecystitis, infections of the gastro-intestinal or genito-urinary tracts, pelvic inflammatory disease, pneumonia, or decubitus ulceration). Indwelling urinary catheters, intravenous lines, and surgical wounds may also provide points of entry in hospitalised patients.

Individuals most at risk of developing septicaemia are the elderly, malnourished, alcoholics, and those suffering from severe burns and with debilitating diseases (e.g. cirrhosis of the liver or diabetes mellitus).

Symptoms
The onset is abrupt (particularly if due to Gram-negative micro-organisms) and is marked by chills, fever, diarrhoea, and nausea and vomiting. There may be prior warning signs, which include apprehension, diminished consciousness, lethargy, and tachypnoea; further symptoms are hypotension and prostration. Secondary infections may arise in any organ and hypotension may cause heart failure, jaundice, or renal complications due to inadequate perfusion of vital organs. Death due to septic shock (*see below*) may be the final outcome.

Treatment
The prognosis is dependent on the virulence of the infecting micro-organism, the age of the patient, other predisposing factors, and the speed with which treatment is started.

The source of sepsis should be removed or drained where possible, and high-dose, intravenous, 'blind' antibacterial therapy (BNF 5.1, Table 1) initiated until the causative micro-organism has been identified. Large volume intravenous infusions may be required to restore normal blood pressure. Additional supportive measures may be necessary to manage underlying disorders and organ failure.

Septicaemia may be prevented in hospitals by strictly adhering to the rules for aseptic procedure at all times and closely monitoring those most at risk.

Septic Shock

Definition and aetiology
Septic shock is acute circulatory failure arising as a result of septicaemia (*see above*). It is most often caused by endotoxin-releasing Gram-negative bacteria, although Gram-positive infections are more likely to produce complications at sites distant from the causative infection.

It occurs most frequently in hospitalised patients, particularly in the newborn, elderly, or those with an underlying debilitating disorder. Patients receiving antimicrobials, corticosteroids, or cytotoxic drugs are also at risk.

Symptoms
The initial symptoms are as for septicaemia, with progression to shock as toxins in the blood activate a series of reactions, which include the complement and blood clotting systems. Disseminated intravascular coagulation, metabolic acidosis, and poor perfusion may all contribute to end organ damage. Complications (e.g. adult respiratory distress syndrome, heart failure, and renal failure) may occur.

Treatment
The prognosis is poor once shock has developed, and mortality may be as high as 50% to 90% if early therapy is not available. Antimicrobial therapy and preventive measures are as for septicaemia, and supportive measures are described under shock.

Tonsillitis

Definition and aetiology
Tonsillitis is inflammation of the tonsils, which may be due to streptococcal or viral infection. It is most common in children and young adults and is usually transmitted by droplets or dust, especially in crowded or poorly ventilated conditions. It may be acute or chronic.

Symptoms
Acute tonsillitis, which is sudden in onset, is characterised by marked soreness of the throat, with pain and

difficulty on swallowing. It may also be accompanied by pharyngitis. The tonsils become red and swollen and a purulent tonsillar exudate may be present. Fever, headache, and malaise are common and arthralgia and myalgia may develop. Rare complications include acute glomerulonephritis and rheumatic fever. A peritonsillar abscess (quinsy) may develop and is characterised by a marked increase in pain and fever. Repeated acute attacks may result in the development of chronic tonsillitis.

Treatment
Treatment includes bed rest and the administration of plenty of fluids. If a virus is responsible, treatment is symptomatic. A penicillin (BNF 5.1.1) may be beneficial in the presence of streptococcal infection. If an abscess forms, surgical drainage is essential. In chronic cases, tonsillectomy may be necessary.

Urinary-tract Infections

Definition and aetiology
Urinary-tract infection may be present at any level of the urinary tract, i.e. urethra (urethritis), bladder (cystitis), ureters, or the kidney (pyelonephritis). The infection is usually characterised by bacteriuria with symptoms of urinary-tract inflammation, although these symptoms are not a reliable guide to the exact location of the infection. It may be acute, chronic, or recurrent. Most urinary-tract infections are caused by Gram-negative bacteria, and common infecting micro-organisms include *Escherichia coli*, and species of *Proteus* and *Pseudomonas*. Occasionally *Klebsiella* spp. are involved. Gram-positive micro-organisms include *Staphylococcus* and *Streptococcus* spp.

Symptoms
Urinary-tract infection is common in women, and in both sexes on urinary catheterisation. Symptoms, which are usually confined to the lower urinary tract, include urinary frequency and urgency, dysuria, and occasionally haematuria. Asymptomatic infection may also occur, especially in pregnancy.

Urethritis

Definition and aetiology
Urethritis is an inflammation of the urethra, and can be gonococcal or non-specific (non-gonococcal). In both cases, transmission is by sexual intercourse. Although no infecting micro-organism can be detected, it is commonly attributed to species of *Chlamydia, Trichomonas, Corynebacterium*, and rarely *Mycobacterium*. Herpes simplex virus may also be responsible.

An attack of non-specific urethritis may be precipitated by a large intake of alcohol.

Symptoms
Urethritis is characterised by dysuria and frequency, and accompanied by a mucopurulent urethral or vaginal discharge, or both. Inflammation of the urinary meatus may occur in men, and cervicitis or vaginitis in women.

Complications include cystitis, epididymitis, prostatitis, salpingitis, and urethral stricture. Reiter's disease, in which urethritis is accompanied by arthritis and conjunctivitis, may develop in a few patients.

Treatment
Treatment is by the avoidance of sexual intercourse and alcohol, and the administration of a tetracycline (BNF 5.1.3) or other appropriate antimicrobial.

Cystitis

Definition and aetiology
Cystitis is inflammation of the bladder and may be acute or chronic. Acute attacks may occur in isolation with no indication of the underlying cause, or they may be the precursors of chronic infection.

Symptoms
Symptoms include dysuria and frequency, fever, haematuria, malaise, and suprapubic pain.

Treatment
Treatment is similar to that described under pyelonephritis.

Pyelonephritis

Acute pyelonephritis is an acute, sometimes pyogenic, infection resulting in inflammation of the pelvis and parenchyma of one or both kidneys. It may be associated with urinary-tract obstruction.

Symptoms
The onset of symptoms may be rapid with dysuria, fever and rigors, and loin pain and tenderness. It may, however, be insidious with anorexia and lethargy. Repeated attacks may result in chronic pyelonephritis, which is characterised by persistent inflammation and may eventually culminate in renal failure.

Treatment
Treatment consists of bed rest and the administration of appropriate antibacterial drugs (BNF 5.1, Table 1). Drugs to increase urinary pH (BNF 7.4.3) may relieve some symptoms, but will not eliminate the underlying infection. Patients should be encouraged to increase fluid intake. Sexual intercourse should be avoided for the duration of the infection. Surgery may be required for urinary-tract obstruction.

Vincent's Infection

Definition and aetiology

Vincent's infection (acute ulcerative gingivitis, acute necrotising ulcerative gingivitis, trench mouth, or Vincent's disease) is an acute or chronic infection of the gums, which usually begins in the gingival papillae between the teeth, but may extend throughout the gums. The micro-organisms responsible are often fusiform bacilli and spirochaetes. The most common cause is the presence of dental plaque arising from poor oral hygiene. Other precipitating factors include emotional disturbances, systemic disease, and smoking.

Symptoms

The onset is usually abrupt and is characterised by general malaise, marked gingival bleeding, inflammation, and swelling. Fever is generally absent, but pain may be so severe as to render eating and talking impossible. Halitosis and excessive salivation are also common. Characteristic 'punched-out' gingival ulcers often develop. These ulcers, which bleed readily, may develop a membranous covering.

Treatment

Patients should be advised to avoid precipitating factors. Proper oral hygiene and regular dental treatment should be encouraged. A non-opioid analgesic (BNF 4.7.1) may be necessary and an appropriate systemic oropharyngeal anti-infective drug (BNF 12.3.2) may be indicated. Minor surgery (i.e. gingivectomy) may be beneficial.

5.2 BACTERIAL INFECTIONS

(Background information on bacteria can be found in Section 14.2.)

Actinomycosis

Definition and aetiology

Actinomycosis is a chronic infection caused by *Actinomyces* spp., particularly *A. israelii*, which are Gram-positive, anaerobic or microaerophilic, filamentous bacteria.

   Actinomyces are present as part of the normal oral and gastro-intestinal flora, and actinomycosis usually arises endogenously. It is rarely transmitted from person-to-person. The micro-organism invades through breaks in mucous membranes and multiplies in anaerobic conditions (e.g. created by poor vascular supply or the presence of necrotic tissue).

   About 60% of cases are in the cervicofacial region (lumpy jaw), often associated with dental caries or gingivitis. Abdominal actinomycosis accounts for approximately 20% of cases and may be associated with appendicitis, gastrectomy, or other trauma. Pulmonary actinomycosis is usually associated with an underlying lung disorder. It results from inhalation of the micro-organism into the lungs, or contiguous spread from cervicofacial or abdominal actinomycosis. Pelvic actinomycosis is most commonly due to colonisation of intra-uterine contraceptive devices, but may also spread from an abdominal ulcer.

Symptoms

Actinomycosis is characterised by granulomatous suppurative lesions, draining sinuses, and fibrosis. Common systemic symptoms may include anorexia, fever, wasting, and leucocytosis. In addition, there are specific symptoms related to the site of the abscesses. Cervicofacial actinomycosis may involve the salivary glands, tongue, pharynx, and larynx. It occurs more commonly in males and symptoms include painful swellings, trismus, and a purulent discharge containing yellowish-white granules. Abdominal actinomycosis is characterised by an inflammatory mass on the abdominal wall, and may result in anaemia. Symptoms of pulmonary actinomycosis may be productive cough and haemoptysis. Pelvic actinomycosis may cause cervicitis, endometritis, or salpingitis, and common symptoms include vaginal discharge, irregular bleeding, abdominal pain, and, in severe cases, vomiting.

Treatment

Actinomycosis is a progressive disease and may be fatal. With prompt treatment, however, the prognosis is good.

   Treatment comprises prolonged administration of an antimicrobial, usually benzylpenicillin (BNF 5.1.1.1), and surgical drainage or excision of abscesses.

Anthrax

Definition and aetiology

Anthrax is a zoonotic infection caused by *Bacillus anthracis*, a Gram-positive, aerobic, rod-shaped sporeformer. It occurs worldwide, although it is no longer endemic in developed countries.

   Spores, which may remain viable for years under the right conditions, are formed from bacilli excreted into the external environment in faeces, urine, saliva, and other discharges from infected animals (particularly cattle, goats, and sheep). Alternatively, spores may form when an animal dies from anthrax, and they can contaminate animal products (e.g. bones, hair, hide, wool, and meat). Animals contract the infection by ingestion or inhalation of spores present in their immediate environment. Transmission of infection to humans is mainly by inoculation of spores into wounds or abraded skin (cutaneous anthrax), although inhalation (pulmonary anthrax) and ingestion (gastro-intestinal anthrax) may also occur.

It is primarily a disease of workers engaged in the processing of animal-derived products, particularly those imported from endemic areas. Shepherds and cattle rearers in underdeveloped countries are also at risk. Human-to-human transmission has not been known to occur.

Symptoms
The incubation period of cutaneous anthrax is 5 to 7 days, of pulmonary anthrax (which is less common) 3 to 4 days, and of gastro-intestinal anthrax (the least common and occurring mainly in endemic areas) 2 to 5 days.

Cutaneous anthrax is marked by a small pruritic papule at the inoculation site, which develops into a vesicle surrounded by a ring of erythema and, in some cases, further vesicles. The central area ulcerates and finally develops into a dry, black, adherent scab. This characteristic anthrax sore is called a 'malignant pustule', although it is neither malignant nor does it contain pus. Oedema may spread out from the sore into surrounding tissues, and local lymph nodes may become enlarged. General symptoms include anorexia, chills, headache, nausea, and, in some cases, fever. Mild cases may recover without treatment, but in severe cases septicaemia may occur and result in collapse and death within 3 to 5 days. Healing of the sore in surviving patients is slow and may leave a scar.

The onset of pulmonary anthrax is abrupt and common symptoms include non-productive cough, mild fever, malaise, and myalgia. Severe respiratory distress may follow an apparent improvement and can be rapidly fatal if untreated.

Gastro-intestinal anthrax initially resembles an acute case of gastro-enteritis, with rapid progression to toxaemia, shock, and death.

Anthrax meningitis may occur as a secondary complication of all types of anthrax as a result of bacteraemia. Death is usually inevitable.

Treatment
Anthrax responds readily to treatment, which comprises administration of benzylpenicillin (BNF 5.1.1.1), and antimicrobial resistance is rare. Anthrax sores may be covered with clean dressings, but require no further attention. Intensive supportive measures may be necessary in severe cases, particularly for pulmonary and gastro-intestinal anthrax, and when complicated by septicaemia.

Anthrax may be prevented in endemic areas by improvements in animal husbandry. Dead infected animals should be burned or buried deeply, their stalls disinfected, and bedding and straw burned. Stringent precautions are necessary in factories to prevent infection of workers. These include decontaminating raw materials by autoclaving, gamma irradiation, and using oxidising agents, and providing protective clothing and respirators where necessary. Anthrax vaccine (BNF 14.4) is also available for active immunisation of humans at risk.

Botulism

Definition and aetiology
Botulism is a severe disease caused by various highly potent exotoxins produced by *Clostridium botulinum*, a Gram-positive, spore-forming, anaerobic bacillus.

In most cases, the disease is caused by the ingestion of preformed toxin in poorly prepared canned, fermented, or smoked food, rather than by ingestion of spores, which are regularly consumed without causing illness. Spores, which are widely distributed in the environment, are highly resistant and able to withstand prolonged boiling at 100°C. They are able to germinate, multiply, and produce toxin in the anaerobic environment created by some methods of food preservation. Infants under 9 months of age can, however, develop botulism on ingestion of spores, which germinate and produce toxin in the gastro-intestinal tract. One source of infant botulism has been traced to spore-contaminated honey. Wound botulism is a rare form of the disease caused by bacilli producing toxin within a wound.

Symptoms
The incubation period varies from 2 hours to 8 days, although in most cases it is within 12 to 72 hours.

The toxin is absorbed through the mucous membrane and disseminated by the bloodstream. It irreversibly binds to receptors at cholinergic neuromuscular junctions blocking release of acetylcholine. Symptoms vary in severity from mild illness to severe, flaccid, and often bilateral paralysis, commencing with the cranial nerves and progressively descending. Initial neurological symptoms include dry mouth, dysphagia, diplopia, diminished acuity, loss of accommodation, speech difficulties, and dizziness. They may be preceded in some cases by symptoms of gastro-intestinal disturbance (e.g. nausea and vomiting, diarrhoea, and abdominal pain). As the disease progresses, there may be constipation, urinary hesitancy, hypotension, difficulty in holding up the head, and finally paralysis of respiratory muscles.

Very severe cases usually have a short incubation period and can progress to death within a day. Surviving patients generally show a complete recovery, as new nerve terminals may form from axons.

Wound botulism has a longer incubation period (ranging from 4 to 17 days) and shows fewer gastro-intestinal symptoms.

Treatment

The prognosis is good, with less than 10% mortality if there is adequate intensive respiratory support, which may be necessary for several weeks. Gastric lavage, enemas, or purgatives may be of value early in the course to eliminate toxin from the gastro-intestinal tract. Botulism antitoxin (BNF 14.4) may be administered at any time to neutralise toxin present in the bloodstream. It prevents further progress of the disease, but is unable to dislodge toxin already bound to receptor sites and is of little value in infant botulism. Guanidine has been used to increase acetylcholine release, although its efficacy remains unproven.

Botulism may be prevented by ensuring high standards of food preservation. Irradiation or exposure to moist heat for 30 minutes at 120°C will kill spores, while toxin already formed may be destroyed by heating food for 30 minutes at 80°C. Germination of spores may be prevented by a low pH, drying, refrigeration, freezing, or use of salt, sugar, and sodium nitrite as preservatives. Honey should not be given to infants under one year of age.

Brucellosis

Definition and aetiology

Brucellosis (Malta fever, Mediterranean fever, or undulant fever) is an infection of animals caused by species of the genus *Brucella*, which are Gram-negative, aerobic, non-sporing, pleomorphic coccobacilli. *Brucella abortus* affects mainly cattle and the disease occurs worldwide, although it has almost been eradicated in developed countries. *Br. melitensis* causes disease primarily in goats and sheep, particularly in the Mediterranean basin, Asia, Africa, and Central and South America, while *Br. suis* infects pigs, caribou, and reindeer in the Americas, South East Asia, and arctic Russia.

The disease in humans is contracted from infected animals by ingestion of untreated milk products or close contact with blood or secretions. Invasion occurs through the gastro-intestinal mucosa, conjunctiva, and skin abrasions. It is an occupational disease of abattoir workers, farmers, and veterinary surgeons.

Symptoms

Brucellosis may be acute with an incubation period of 2 weeks (range 1 to 3 weeks) or several months may elapse before symptoms present.

In acute cases, initial symptoms include headache, low back pain, and myalgia accompanied by fluctuating (undulant) fever, drenching sweats, rigors, and prostration. There may also be hepatosplenomegaly, palpitations, gastro-intestinal disturbances, and weight loss. The symptoms of chronic disease, which may be insidious in onset or follow an untreated acute attack, are similar, although the patient's temperature is very often normal.

Granulomatous nodules arising from phagocytosed micro-organisms may deposit in the bone marrow, liver, and spleen. They may suppurate in untreated cases, resulting in bacteraemia and spread to other organs. Complications include arthritis, pneumonia, cholecystitis, endocarditis, epididymo-orchitis, meningo-encephalitis, and sciatica. Abortion, which is the most common symptom in infected animals, does not appear to occur in humans.

The course is variable and many cases resolve spontaneously, although relapses may occur for up to two years, especially if untreated. Infections with *Br. suis* and *Br. melitensis* are generally more serious than *Br. abortus*. One attack of brucellosis usually confers lifelong immunity.

Treatment

All cases of brucellosis must be treated to prevent relapses and possible complications. Appropriate antibacterials include tetracyclines (BNF 5.1.3) and co-trimoxazole (BNF 5.1.8).

Brucellosis may be prevented by heat-treating all milk and milk products, and ensuring adequate protection for those in high-risk occupations. The micro-organism may be eradicated in farm stock by active immunisation of calves, destruction of infected animals, and effective controls over the sale of livestock.

Cellulitis

Definition and aetiology

Cellulitis is a diffuse inflammatory condition affecting subcutaneous tissues (*see also* Erysipelas). It is most commonly caused by Group A β-haemolytic streptococci or occasionally by *Staphylococcus aureus*. It may arise at a site of existing trauma or infection, or can develop in previously healthy skin.

Symptoms

Cellulitis most commonly affects the arms and legs and is characterised by red, hot, oedematous areas with ill-defined margins. Vesicles and bullae may be present. In severe cases, other symptoms may include fever, malaise, and headache. The condition frequently results in lymphangitis and lymphadenopathy.

Treatment

Treatment consists of bed rest and the oral, or if necessary intravenous, administration of an appropriate antibacterial drug (BNF 5.1). Elevation of the affected area may facilitate drainage.

Cholera

Definition and aetiology

Cholera is an acute infection of the bowel caused by *Vibrio cholerae*, a Gram-negative, aerobic rod. It is endemic in the Ganges delta and Bangladesh, and is responsible for epidemics throughout India. Pandemics also occur periodically, and the latest one, which commenced in 1961, has spread throughout Asia, Africa, Mediterranean Europe, and the Gulf coast of the USA. The causative strain is the El Tor biotype.

The only known reservoir of infection is man, and transmission occurs via faecal-contaminated drinking water. Occasionally, food washed with contaminated water, or shellfish harvested from contaminated sea water, may be the source. It is also possible that flies transfer bacteria from faeces to food.

Achlorhydria, antacid therapy, and gastric surgery render individuals particularly susceptible to developing cholera, as vibrios are very sensitive to gastric acid. Children and adults are equally at risk, except in endemic areas where repeated ingestion of vibrios confers some degree of immunity in adults. One attack does not, however, always produce immunity.

Symptoms

The number of micro-organisms necessary to produce clinical symptoms in previously healthy individuals is very large, and the degree of severity varies from an asymptomatic carrier state to severe, fulminating, and fatal disease. The incubation period is usually 12 to 72 hours (range 12 hours to 6 days).

Symptoms are caused by an enterotoxin, which disrupts intracellular transport mechanisms responsible for maintaining the optimum fluid and electrolyte balance. The onset is rapid, and characterised by large volumes of white, mucoid, odourless, isotonic stools ('rice-water' stools), which may be followed by vomiting and muscle cramps (especially in the calf muscles). Mild cases may start to resolve after 3 to 12 hours, but in severe cases, further symptoms may include intense thirst, cyanosis, exhaustion, hypothermia, hypotension, tachycardia, and reduced skin turgor. Children also develop hypoglycaemia, a consequence of which may be CNS complications (e.g. stupor, convulsions, or coma). Progressive fluid losses (exceeding one litre per hour in some cases) result in severe dehydration, hypovolaemia, and metabolic acidosis, and may prove rapidly fatal in

about 50% of untreated cases. Convalescent patients continue to excrete vibrios in their faeces for 1 to 3 weeks.

Treatment

There is complete recovery in almost all patients receiving adequate oral (BNF 9.2.1) or intravenous (BNF 9.2.2) electrolyte and water replacement therapy. The use of tetracycline may be indicated as an adjunct in severe cases to reduce the volume of diarrhoea, duration of illness, and carrier state. Emergence of resistant strains, however, precludes indiscriminate use.

Cholera may be prevented in endemic areas by improving sanitation and providing a clean water supply. Where this is not available, drinking water should be boiled and consumption of raw unpeeled fruit and vegetables avoided. A vaccine (BNF 14.4) is available, which confers immunity for 3 to 6 months in about 50% of individuals. It does not, however, prevent excretion of vibrios and is thus of no value in curbing the spread during an outbreak.

Diphtheria

Definition and aetiology

Diphtheria is an infection caused by *Corynebacterium diphtheriae*, a Gram-positive, aerobic, non-sporing bacillus. It occurs worldwide, particularly in temperate and cold climates in early winter, although active immunisation programmes in recent years have reduced the incidence and mortality.

It is directly transmitted from person-to-person by droplets. The reservoir of infection is maintained by asymptomatic nasal carriers and individuals suffering from chronic cutaneous diphtheria (a condition existing mainly in the tropics).

Children between 1 and 5 years of age are most susceptible to developing clinical illness, although non-immune adults are also at risk.

Symptoms

Diphtheria may be asymptomatic or symptoms may vary in severity from mild, to fulminating and life-threatening. The incubation period is short, usually two days, extending in some cases to five days.

The bacilli colonise the fauces, nose, larynx, pharynx, tonsils, and skin, and produce an exotoxin which can disseminate via the circulation to other organs and cause serious complications. A characteristic greyish-white membrane, composed of dead epithelial cells, fibrin, leucocytes, and red blood cells is produced in most forms of diphtheria as a response to the inflammatory process induced by the multiplying bacteria. It changes colour as the disease progresses and eventually sloughs off during recovery.

Anterior nasal diphtheria is a mild condition with few, if any, constitutional symptoms as the toxin is not absorbed from this site. It is characterised by the production of a nasal discharge, which becomes progressively thick, purulent, and blood-stained. A thin membrane develops in the nose, and there may be irritation of the nares and upper lips.

Tonsillar (faucial) diphtheria has a slow onset and is marked by a membrane which grows to cover the tonsils. Other symptoms caused by mild toxaemia may include fever, headache, malaise, fatigue, dysphagia, and nausea and vomiting. Local lymph nodes may become enlarged. The membrane may spread to the uvula, palate, pharynx, and nasal mucosa (nasopharyngeal diphtheria), becoming severe and life-threatening due to extreme toxaemia. Oedema and enlarged lymph nodes may result in a characteristic 'bull-neck', and breathing difficulties due to obstruction.

Symptoms of laryngeal diphtheria, which usually occur in conjunction with tonsillar diphtheria, are due to the presence of a membrane involving the larynx and extending in some cases to the trachea and bronchi. Symptoms include hoarseness, non-productive cough or croup, stridor, dyspnoea, and cyanosis. The condition may be fatal if breathing is obstructed, but there are generally no toxaemic complications.

Cutaneous diphtheria is usually a chronic condition marked by painless slow-growing ulcers, often on the legs. Constitutional symptoms are usually absent because little toxin is absorbed from the skin.

Common complications of toxaemia are myocarditis and neuritis, which may be fatal, but usually resolve completely in adequately treated patients.

Treatment

Treatment of cases and carriers comprises administration of an appropriate antibacterial preparation such as benzylpenicillin (BNF 5.1.1.1) or erythromycin (BNF 5.1.5) to destroy the bacteria. Symptomatic patients additionally require diphtheria antitoxin (BNF 14.4) to neutralise the toxin. Bed rest is also necessary. Intensive care, assisted ventilation, or tracheostomy may be necessary in the management of complications.

Diphtheria may be prevented by active immunisation (BNF 14.4) of all infants (*see also* Section 17.5). Spread of infection during an outbreak may be curbed by isolating patients and carriers until three consecutive negative nose and throat swabs have been obtained. Contacts may be protected by administration of diphtheria antitoxin (BNF 14.4), but should be closely observed for signs of developing infection.

Epididymitis

Definition and aetiology

Epididymitis is inflammation of the epididymis and is usually due to bacterial infection, which often results from a primary urinary-tract infection. The infection may be gonococcal, but other micro-organisms (e.g. *Escherichia coli* and *Pseudomonas* spp.) may be responsible.

Symptoms

The onset of symptoms may be sudden or insidious. The infection is usually unilateral and is characterised by acute pain, swelling, and scrotal redness. It is often accompanied by malaise and mild fever. Fibrosis may persist after recovery.

Treatment

Treatment comprises bed rest and the administration of an appropriate antimicrobial drug, usually a tetracycline (BNF 5.1.3). A non-opioid analgesic (BNF 4.7) may be required and the patient may find it helpful to wear a scrotal support. If the condition becomes chronic, surgery (epididymectomy) may be necessary.

Epiglottitis

Definition and aetiology

Epiglottitis is characterised by inflammation and oedema of the epiglottis. It is due to a *Haemophilus influenzae* infection, and is most common in children between 2 and 4 years of age.

Symptoms

It is usually preceded by an upper respiratory-tract infection, which suddenly worsens. The child becomes severely ill due to septicaemia and acute dyspnoea with stridor. Other symptoms include pain on swallowing with excessive drooling, muffling of the voice, and swelling of the neck. Epiglottitis may be fatal due to airway obstruction. The condition should be distinguished from the milder condition, croup.

Treatment

Immediate hospital treatment is essential. An adequate airway must be maintained and it may be necessary to insert an endotracheal tube or perform a tracheostomy. Appropriate antibacterial therapy (BNF 5.1) is indicated.

Erysipelas

Definition and aetiology

Erysipelas is an infection of the dermis (*see also* Cellulitis), most frequently caused by Group A β-haemolytic streptococci, which are Gram-positive facultative anaerobes. It may arise at a site of existing trauma or skin infection (e.g. impetigo), although in many cases, there is no obvious point of entry, and the offending micro-organism may be present in the eye, nose, or throat.

Symptoms

Erysipelas has an abrupt onset after an incubation period of 2 to 5 days. It most commonly affects the face, arms, and legs, and is characterised by a tender, red, oedematous area with well-defined borders. Vesicles and bullae are often present. The skin lesions are frequently preceded by headache, fever, malaise, and vomiting. The condition, if untreated, may result in nephritis and septicaemia, especially in infants and the elderly, and may even prove fatal. Recurrent attacks may cause lymphoedema.

Treatment

Treatment consists of the oral administration of an appropriate penicillin (BNF 5.1.1) or erythromycin (BNF 5.1.4). A non-opioid analgesic (BNF 4.7) may provide pain relief.

Furunculosis

Definition and aetiology

Furunculosis is the recurrence of furuncles over weeks or months, or the coincidental occurrence of several furuncles.

Furuncles

Definition and aetiology

Furuncles (boils) are acute inflammatory nodules arising from infection of the hair follicles. The micro-organism responsible is usually *Staphylococcus aureus*, a Gram-positive, facultatively anaerobic coccus, which is carried as part of the normal skin flora of many individuals. The nares and perineum are the most common reservoirs of the micro-organism. Furuncles occur more commonly in males and are generally found in the axillae, anogenital region, and on the back of the neck. The predisposing factors are largely unknown, although they may be precipitated by seborrhoea, malnutrition, diabetes mellitus, and leukaemia. Anaemia, fatigue, and stress have also been implicated.

Symptoms

Furuncles may occur as single or multiple lesions, which are tender and painful, and become pustular with a single head. There is a blood-stained, purulent exudate as the necrotic core is discharged, and scarring may ensue. Fever, pyaemia, and septicaemia may occur in severe cases.

Treatment

Treatment consists of cleansing the affected area with suitable skin disinfecting and cleansing agents (BNF 13.11) and the application of an appropriate anti-infective skin preparation (BNF 13.10). The application of moist heat and magnesium sulphate paste (BNF 13.10.5) may also be beneficial, and patients should be discouraged from squeezing lesions. Penicillinase-resistant penicillins (BNF 5.1.1.2) and surgical drainage may be indicated in severe or recurrent cases. The nares and perianal skin should also be treated in an effort to prevent further infection.

Carbuncles

Definition and aetiology

Carbuncles are formed by the confluence of several furuncles, or by the spread of infection, in the subcutaneous tissues. They tend to occur on the shoulders, hips, thighs, and back of the neck and are most common in middle-aged or elderly men. Predisposing factors may include diabetes mellitus, nephritis, debilitating disease, and prolonged corticosteroid therapy.

Symptoms

Carbuncles are painful and tender with multiple heads. Purulent ulcers are formed (Fig. 5.1) with extensive areas

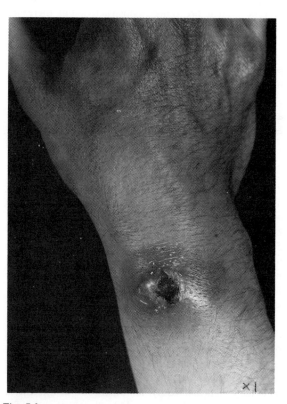

Fig. 5.1
Purulent ulceration caused by a carbuncle.

of necrotic tissue, which separates as a slough. There may be malaise and fever, and in severe cases, septicaemia. Healing is often slow and generally results in scar formation.

Treatment

Treatment comprises the systemic administration of a penicillinase-resistant pencillin (BNF 5.1.1.2).

Gas Gangrene

Definition and aetiology

Gas gangrene (clostridial myonecrosis) is a serious infection of muscle tissue. It is caused by exotoxins produced by various species of *Clostridium* (particularly *C. perfringens*), which are Gram-positive, anaerobic, spore-forming bacilli.

Clostridial species naturally inhabit the soil and gastro-intestinal tract of mammals. They may become pathogenic in the presence of penetrating surgical or traumatic wounds (e.g. after hip or colonic surgery, gunshot wounds, crush injuries, burns, or open fractures). Clostridial growth is facilitated by the hypoxic conditions generated in such wounds by ischaemia, and the presence of necrotic tissue and foreign bodies (e.g. dirt, shrapnel, or pieces of clothing). Very rarely, gas gangrene may occur in an extremity due to secondary spread from an intestinal neoplasm, or as a primary infection in the absence of trauma, usually in the perineum or scrotum.

Symptoms

The incubation period is usually less than four days, but may vary from a few hours to several weeks.

The onset is sudden and characterised by severe pain. The wound becomes oedematous and may ooze a thin serous exudate with a sweet odour. The skin becomes bronze-coloured, and haemorrhagic bullae and necrosis may develop. Subsequently the traumatised area may become extremely tender. In some cases, gas may be present within the tissues as a late symptom. Accompanying constitutional symptoms include fever, sweats, tachycardia, and anxiety. Septicaemia, hypotension, renal failure, and haemolytic anaemia may arise as complications and, if untreated, can be rapidly fatal.

Treatment

Prompt treatment is essential as the mortality may be up to 1 in 3. Complete surgical removal of all affected muscle is necessary and in severe cases involves amputation of a limb. Adjunctive measures include administration of benzylpenicillin (BNF 5.1.1.1) and the use of hyperbaric oxygen. Supportive treatment (e.g. fluid and electrolyte replacement and blood transfusions) may be required in the event of complications.

Gas gangrene may be prevented by antibacterial prophylaxis (BNF 5.1, Table 2) prior to and following surgical operations carrying an associated risk. In the case of traumatic wounds, patients should be evacuated from the accident site and treated as soon as possible. All damaged muscle and skin should be completely excised and wound closure delayed until it is absolutely certain that no infection is present.

Impetigo

Definition and aetiology

Impetigo is a contagious superficial infection (pyoderma) of the epidermis. It is caused most frequently by *Staphylococcus aureus*, less commonly by Group A β-haemolytic streptococci, and in some cases, by the two micro-organisms together.

It may arise as a secondary infection in the presence of eczema, fungal infections, insect bites, pediculosis, or skin trauma. In many cases, however, it occurs in previously healthy skin. Overcrowded and unhygienic conditions may predispose an individual to develop the infection.

Symptoms

Impetigo occurs most often in children. The arms, legs, and face, especially around the nose and mouth, are sites most commonly affected. Vesicles appear initially, rupturing rapidly to release an exudate which dries to form yellow or light brown crusts (Fig. 5.2). Other symptoms include erythema, pruritus, and in some cases, bullae. The lesions spread quickly and, if untreated, the condition may result in further complications (e.g. cellulitis, furunculosis, urticaria, or acute glomerulonephritis). In less severe cases, impetigo may resolve spontaneously in 2 to 3 weeks.

Treatment

Treatment comprises the removal of crusts with soap and water or mild skin disinfecting and cleansing agents (BNF 13.11). Topical administration of an appropriate antibacterial preparation (BNF 13.10.1) may be effective in many cases, although a systemic antimicrobial (BNF 5.1) may be necessary for more severe infections. The nares and perianal skin, which may act as reservoirs of *S. aureus*, should also be treated. Patients should be counselled on personal hygiene to prevent contagion and further attacks.

Legionellosis

Definition and aetiology

Legionellosis is an acute respiratory-tract infection occurring worldwide. It is caused by Gram-negative,

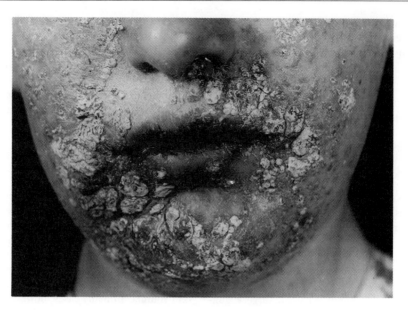

Fig. 5.2
Impetigo. Dried crusts formed in perinasal and peri-oral impetigo.

aerobic, non-sporing bacilli of the genus *Legionella*. Legionnaires' disease, which was first recognised in 1976, is the most serious form of legionellosis. It is caused by *Legionella pneumophila* and often occurs as outbreaks in hospitals (i.e. a nosocomial disease), hotels, or office blocks. Pontiac fever is a much milder form.

The micro-organism has been isolated from water in air-conditioning cooling towers and hot-water systems, and is known to be transmitted by inhalation of water droplets. It is uncertain if infection occurs through the gastro-intestinal tract, and it appears not to be spread from person-to-person. Legionella occur naturally in freshwater ponds, lakes, and in moist soil, particularly when temperatures exceed 25°C, the optimum range for growth being 30°C to 38°C. It is possible that the presence of other micro-organisms in water (e.g. algae, amoebae, and other bacteria) facilitate the growth of legionella.

Individuals most susceptible to developing legionellosis are males between 40 and 70 years of age who smoke or consume excessive quantities of alcohol, those with an underlying disorder (e.g. chronic cardiac, pulmonary, or renal disorders, and diabetes mellitus), or immunosuppressed patients.

Symptoms
About half of those infected develop clinical symptoms. The incubation period is usually 36 hours (range 5 to 66 hours) for Pontiac fever and 5 to 7 days (range 2 to 10 days) for Legionnaires' disease.

Pontiac fever resembles an acute attack of influenza, with common symptoms including fever, headache, myalgia, cough, and nausea and vomiting. Sore throat, diarrhoea, chest pain, and confusion may also occur. It is self-limiting, and patients generally recover within one week. No fatalities have been recorded to date.

Legionnaires' disease is characterised by the development of pneumonia and, in severe cases, the involvement of other organs (e.g. liver, kidney, gastro-intestinal tract, and central nervous system). Initial symptoms include malaise, myalgia, headache, fever, weakness, anorexia, and dry cough. These are followed a few days later by chest pain, dyspnoea, tachypnoea, abdominal pain, and watery diarrhoea. Neurological disturbances which may occur include amnesia, ataxia, slurred speech, and hallucinations. Mild cases may resolve spontaneously after 5 to 7 days, but severe pneumonia or renal failure may be fatal.

Treatment
Pontiac fever is mild and self-limiting and requires no treatment. Erythromycin (BNF 5.1.5) is always indicated in Legionnaires' disease and gives a good prognosis if started early. Premature cessation may precipitate potentially fatal relapses. Supportive treatment may be necessary in severe cases, and includes assisted ventilation and maintenance of adequate fluid and electrolyte levels.

The exact source of the micro-organism in air-conditioning and hot-water systems must be located during outbreaks, and eradication attempted by chlorination or raising the water temperature to at least 55°C. It is uncertain whether chemicals may be an effective means of prevention.

Leprosy

Definition and aetiology

Leprosy (Hansen's disease) is a chronic infectious disease caused by *Mycobacterium leprae*, an acid-fast bacillus. It occurs mainly in tropical climates (e.g. Asia and Africa), but may also occur in some temperate regions (e.g. Japan, Korea, southern Europe, and some southern states of the USA).

The micro-organism is an obligate intracellular parasite, which may be transmitted to new hosts via the nasal secretions from untreated patients. It is also present in the breast milk of infected mothers. The exact mode of entry into the host is, however, unknown.

The prevalence of leprosy is associated with conditions of overcrowding and poor standards of living, and it occurs most commonly between 10 and 30 years of age.

Symptoms

The incubation period is from 3 to 10 years, or even longer in some cases.

Leprosy is characterised by lesions of the skin and peripheral nerves, with the severity of symptoms dependent on the host's resistance.

Indeterminate leprosy occurs most often in children and is marked by 1 to 4 hypopigmented macules with ill-defined margins. There may be reduced sensation and sweating within the macular area. The condition is often self-limiting, although 25% of cases may progress to one of the other forms of determinate leprosy.

Tuberculoid leprosy develops in people with some degree of resistance and is consequently localised in the skin or peripheral nerves. There may be 1 to 3 asymmetric, well-defined, annular lesions showing a hypopigmented flattened centre and an erythematous raised border. There is reduced sensation and sweating, and the nerves supplying the area become thickened. Caseation necrosis may occur within the nerves causing paralysis of extremities. Spontaneous recovery may occur.

Lepromatous leprosy develops in those with low resistance and is a generalised bacteraemic infection. The lesions are small, widespread, ill-defined, symmetric macules or papules; plaques and nodules may also develop. The nasal mucosa thickens, resulting in blockage, production of a discharge, and progressive destruction of nasal cartilage. The skin becomes coarse and thickened, and eyebrows and eyelashes fall out, which combine to cause a change in facial expression. Iritis and keratitis frequently occur and other organs may become involved (e.g. the larynx, pharynx, tongue, and testes). Destruction of dermal nerves leads to loss of sensation of pain, temperature, and touch. As a result, patients are at risk of repeated trauma, secondary infection, and tissue damage.

Borderline leprosy has characteristics of both the tuberculoid and lepromatous forms. The effects of treatment or improvements in the patient's resistance, or both, can cause a regression to the tuberculoid state or, conversely, it may worsen and become lepromatous.

Treatment

Untreated lepromatous leprosy is progressive and, in some cases, fatal, while the other forms often resolve spontaneously.

Treatment of all forms is by the long-term administration of antileprotic drugs (BNF 5.1.10) undertaken in specialist centres. Supportive help includes physiotherapy for patients with paralysed hands or feet, and reconstructive surgery may be beneficial in some cases. Patients should be encouraged to examine anaesthetic limbs regularly for signs of injury or developing infection.

Leprosy may be prevented by identifying and treating infected patients, and isolating lepromatous cases during the active infectious stages.

Leptospirosis

Definition and aetiology

Leptospirosis is an enzootic infection occuring worldwide and caused by *Leptospira interrogans*, an aerobic spirochaete.

The micro-organism is a parasite of many different species, including cattle, dogs, foxes, goats, hedgehogs, and pigs. The main reservoir of infection, however, exists in rodents, particularly rats, who are able to harbour leptospires permanently without any adverse effects. The bacteria are mainly transmitted in the urine of infected animals and humans, although direct contact with infected blood and tissues may also be responsible. Leptospires may survive for weeks in the external environment in moist conditions. They gain entry into a new host via skin abrasions or mucous membranes. Ingestion of contaminated food or penetration of intact macerated skin are also possible mechanisms.

Symptoms

The incubation period is usually from 7 to 14 days, although it may vary from 2 to 20 days. The duration does not affect the severity of the symptoms or the prognosis, which are dependent on inoculum size.

Symptoms vary from a mild self-limiting condition to

severe illness involving the liver and kidneys. The onset is sudden and characterised in the majority of cases by fever, chills, myalgia, and severe headache. In addition, there may be abdominal pain, vomiting, injection of the conjunctiva, pharyngitis, non-productive cough, and haemoptysis. Weil's disease is a severe form of leptospirosis marked by jaundice, hepatomegaly, proteinuria, haematuria, and in some cases, renal failure.

Mild cases resolve within 4 to 9 days and recovery is usually complete. Mortality is generally as a result of hepatic or renal failure and is greatest in the elderly.

Treatment

Appropriate antibacterial treatment must be started within four days of onset of symptoms to be effective and includes the administration of penicillin, chloramphenicol, erythromycin, streptomycin, or tetracycline. The fluid and electrolyte balance should be maintained, and dialysis may be necessary in the event of renal failure.

Leptospirosis may be prevented by controlling the rat population. Penicillin injections should be administered prophylactically to individuals who fall into water containing leptospires.

Listeriosis

Definition and aetiology

Listeriosis is caused by a Gram-positive, facultatively anaerobic, non-sporing bacillus, *Listeria monocytogenes*, and occurs worldwide.

The micro-organism is widely distributed in the environment in water, soil, sewage, and animal fodder (e.g. silage), and colonises many species of mammals, birds, and fish. The exact source of human infection is unclear, but may be from food, which can be contaminated at any stage during agricultural production or during processing. Contamination may also occur via an asymptomatic carrier harbouring micro-organisms in the gastro-intestinal tract. A small inoculum may multiply to form a significant population in food stored in a refrigerator at 4°C to 6°C. Some cases may be sexually transmitted, as *L. monocytogenes* also colonises the genital tract. Transmission from the mother-to-foetus may occur across the placenta, or at birth during passage along an infected birth canal.

Individuals most susceptible to developing listeriosis are neonates, the elderly, those with an underlying disorder (e.g. cirrhosis, diabetes mellitus, and malignant disease), and immunosuppressed patients.

Symptoms

The exact incubation period is unknown, but may vary between 7 and 30 days.

The severity of symptoms ranges from subclinical to mild to fatal. Listeriosis is characterised by formation of micro-abscesses in tissues, which may result in a variety of disorders (e.g. arthritis, cholecystitis, conjunctivitis, endocarditis, lymph node enlargement, peritonitis, osteomyelitis, skin rashes, and chronic urethritis). Meningitis and septicaemia commonly occur in severe cases.

Listeriosis in pregnancy often results in influenza-like symptoms in the mother, with abortion in early infections or prematurity or stillbirth in late infections. Other symptoms experienced by the mother may include diarrhoea, a rash, and convulsions. Surviving neonates may develop septicaemia and pneumonia up to two days after birth. Infection derived from the birth canal usually gives rise to meningitis and, in some cases, hydrocephalus commencing 5 to 7 days after birth.

Treatment

The prognosis of listeriosis depends on the presence of underlying disease or state of immunosuppression. Prompt treatment significantly reduces the mortality, although in neonates this may still be as high as 50% (compared with 90% in untreated cases).

Effective antibacterial drugs are ampicillin or penicillin, combined with an aminoglycoside (e.g. gentamicin or streptomycin) in severe cases.

Listeriosis may be prevented by adopting stringent controls of hygiene in the preparation and storage of food. Prepared food should not be stored for long periods of time prior to consumption.

Lyme Disease

Definition and aetiology

Lyme disease has recently been recognised as a zoonotic infection caused by *Borrelia burgdorferi*, a Gram-negative spirochaete. Cases have been identified in Europe (including the UK and the Republic of Ireland), the USA, and Australia, particularly in forested areas.

The infection is transmitted by ticks, *Ixodes dammini* and *I. pacificus* in the USA, and *I. ricinus* in Europe. Other blood-sucking arthropods (e.g. horseflies and mosquitoes) have also been implicated as vectors. Deer are the most likely reservoir of infection, although smaller mammals (e.g. dogs and raccoons) and passerine birds may also be involved. There is evidence that transmission to the foetus may occur *in utero*.

Symptoms

The exact incubation period is uncertain, but may vary from days to weeks after the initial tick bite. Some patients appear to have no history of a bite.

The majority of patients present with erythema chronicum migrans, which is characterised by a small, erythematous, pruritic, painful, papular or macular lesion at the inoculation site. It has indurated borders and gradually spreads outwards, clearing in the centre. It may be followed by secondary, non-migrating, annular lesions. Accompanying symptoms at this stage may include fever, malaise, headache, fatigue, arthralgia, myalgia, neck stiffness, nausea and vomiting, and lymphadenopathy. Neurological or cardiac complications may arise weeks or months later in some patients and include Bell's palsy, encephalitis, meningitis, an enlarged heart, or atrioventricular block. More than half of all patients develop arthritis, which usually involves the large joints, particularly the knees. It may last for weeks or months and is often recurrent. It may become chronic in some cases and progressively destroy bone and cartilage.

Foetal infection is serious and has resulted in foetal or neonatal death, prematurity, latent development, and blindness.

Treatment

The course of the disease may be halted by prompt treatment with a tetracycline (BNF 5.1.3).

Lymphangitis

Definition and aetiology

Lymphangitis is an inflammation of the lymphatic vessels. It usually arises as a result of infection with *Streptococcus pyogenes* (a Gram-positive aerobe) via an abrasion or wound, often of an extremity.

Symptoms

Lymphangitis is characterised by swelling and tenderness of regional lymph nodes, fever and rigors, headache, and tachycardia. Red streaks along the course of the lymphatic vessels may be visible through the skin. Septicaemia may develop.

Treatment

Treatment consists of the administration of an appropriate antibacterial drug (BNF 5.1).

Mastitis

Definition and aetiology

Mastitis is inflammation of the breast. Acute mastitis usually occurs in lactating females during the first few weeks of nursing a first-born child, and is due to bacterial infection with *Staphylococcus aureus*.

Treatment

Treatment consists of antibacterial drugs (BNF 5.1). Surgical drainage may be necessary if an abscess develops.

Meningococcal Infections

Definition and aetiology

Meningococcal infections are caused by *Neisseria meningitidis*, a Gram-negative, aerobic diplococcus. Epidemics occur every 5 to 10 years in the sub-Saharan belt of Africa, usually during the driest season. Sporadic cases may also occur, and outbreaks are not uncommon in Europe and America, particularly amongst young people living in overcrowded conditions (e.g. hostels and military camps).

The only reservoir of infection is man, and transmission is by inhalation of airborne water droplets from a carrier.

Children under five years of age are most susceptible to developing clinical illness, although during epidemics, older children and adults are also at risk.

Symptoms

Meningococcal infections may result in mild nasopharyngeal symptoms or potentially fatal meningeal infections. The more serious forms may produce meningitis or acute meningococcaemia, although the two forms are not exclusive.

Nasopharyngeal infection may give rise to an asymptomatic carrier state, which may persist for months, or produce clinical symptoms in susceptible individuals following a short incubation period of 1 to 5 days.

Meningitis is produced when the meningococcal micro-organism invades the meninges via the circulation. Initial symptoms include headache, fever, rigors, malaise, vomiting, and neck stiffness. Convulsions may occur in the young, and infants may experience feeding difficulties. A rash may appear after a week, and approximately half of all patients show petechiae in the conjunctiva, skin, or oral mucosa. The condition is fatal in less than 10% of cases, usually the very young. Most patients make a complete recovery, although complications which may occur include arthritis (not usually chronic), permanent deafness, pericarditis, and occasionally pneumonia. Abnormalities may show on the electrocardiogram. Herpes simplex lesions may arise in some cases during the recovery period.

Acute fulminating meningococcaemia without meningitis may be fatal within hours due to peripheral circulatory collapse. The onset is rapid and non-specific, with initial symptoms of fever, malaise, headache, diarrhoea, and vomiting making diagnosis difficult. A rash may appear locally, which rapidly spreads. Occasionally a chronic form persists, characterised by periods of fever, headache, rashes, arthralgia, myalgia, arthritis, and splenomegaly, which may develop into meningitis if untreated.

Treatment

Early administration of an appropriate antibacterial drug (BNF 5.1, Table 1) is essential for meningococcal meningitis as most deaths occur during the initial stages. Rehydration (BNF 9.2), analgesics (BNF 4.7), and anti-epileptics (BNF 4.8) may also be necessary.

Acute meningococcaemia is an emergency. Treatment comprises immediate antimicrobial therapy and supportive measures, preferably in an intensive-care unit. These include maintenance of fluid and electrolyte levels and acid-base balance, and regular monitoring of blood pressure and the electrocardiogram. Corticosteroids (BNF 6.3.4), given early in the course of the disease and in large doses, may be of value to prevent shock.

Patients should be isolated and antibacterial prophylaxis (BNF 5.1, Table 2) administered to close contacts to prevent the spread of infection. Contacts should also be closely monitored during the incubation period for signs of developing disease. A meningococcal polysaccharide vaccine is available against some serotypes of *N. meningitidis*, and mass immunisation may curb an epidemic, although it is not very effective in young children. Living conditions should be improved and overcrowding reduced in institutions to prevent outbreaks.

Ophthalmia Neonatorum

Definition and aetiology

Ophthalmia neonatorum is an acute purulent inflammation of the eyes in the newborn. It arises from maternal infection transmitted to the infant as it passes through the birth canal. The most common infecting micro-organisms are *Chlamydia oculogenitalis* and *Streptococcus pneumoniae*, although gonococci may also be responsible.

Symptoms

Both eyes are usually affected and symptoms may include copious discharge together with local inflammation and swelling. Corneal ulceration may develop in the presence of untreated gonococcal infection.

Treatment

Prevention is of prime importance and any relevant maternal infection should be treated prior to delivery. Maintenance of an aseptic delivery procedure is essential. Nevertheless, if infection is transmitted, prompt administration of an anti-infective preparation (BNF 11.3) is indicated.

Osteomyelitis

Definition and aetiology

Osteomyelitis, which may be acute or chronic, is an infection of bone. It may arise as a result of bone injury or following an acute infection (e.g. otitis media or pneumonia). The most common infecting micro-organism is *Staphylococcus aureus*, but a variety of other micro-organisms may be responsible. Osteomyelitis may be confined to a localised area of bone marrow, although it may spread to affect the whole bone shaft. The tibia or fibula are the most common sites of osteomyelitis. The acute condition affects primarily children between 5 and 14 years of age, with a greater incidence in boys. It may also occur as a sequel to drug abuse.

Symptoms

Acute osteomyelitis is characterised by marked bone pain with tenderness, fever, and restricted mobility of the affected part. Local swelling may develop and adjacent joints can be affected. In some cases, abscess formation may occur and septicaemia may develop. Chronic osteomyelitis arising from the introduction of a prosthetic device may not become symptomatic for many years, although extensive bone destruction may proceed in the intervening period.

Treatment

Treatment comprises the prolonged administration of an appropriate antibacterial drug (BNF 5.1, Table 1). Immobilisation (e.g. splinting) of the affected part may be indicated, and surgical removal of any dead bone or prosthetic device may be necessary in chronic disease.

Pertussis

Definition and aetiology

Pertussis (whooping cough) is an infection of the respiratory tract caused by *Bordetella pertussis*, a Gram-negative, aerobic, non-sporing coccobacillus. It occurs worldwide, particularly in temperate climates during the winter months, and epidemics are common in regions where active immunisation is not practised.

Man is the only known host, and transmission occurs by droplet-spread from an infected patient. Asymptomatic carriers are rare and are not thought to be significant reservoirs of infection.

The infection may occur at any age, but most frequently affects children under 6 years of age. It is particularly serious in infants and the elderly.

Symptoms

An incubation period of 7 to 10 days is followed by the catarrhal stage, which is the most infectious period of pertussis and lasts from 1 to 2 weeks. Non-specific symptoms resembling a viral upper respiratory-tract infection are common, accompanied by a dry cough, which gradually worsens. The paroxysmal stage follows and is marked by the characteristic inspiratory 'whoop' (which may be absent in infants) terminating a succession of short coughs, during the course of which the patient may become cyanosed. A plug of mucus is often expelled and vomiting frequently occurs. The patient is usually exhausted by the end of an attack, although appears well between attacks.

The interval between paroxysms may be as brief as 30 minutes, and they can cause complications (e.g. epistaxis, hernia, rectal prolapse, and conjunctival haemorrhage) due to the effects of increased pressure. Convulsions are common in infants and may arise as a result of cerebral haemorrhage or severe anoxia. Bronchial obstruction by mucus plugs may cause atelectasis, while otitis media and pneumonia may result from secondary infection.

The condition resolves slowly over many weeks or even months, although mild respiratory-tract infections may cause a relapse of the paroxysmal cough until recovery is complete. Complications, particularly in the very young, carry a risk of fatality. One attack often confers life-long immunity.

Treatment
Infants and severe cases should be treated in hospital where effective supportive treatment (e.g. maintenance of adequate fluid and electrolyte levels, and oxygenation) may be carried out. Antibacterial therapy comprises the administration of erythromycin (BNF 5.1.5), which is only effective in shortening the course of the infection if treatment is started during the catarrhal stage. Secondary infections may also require treatment. Antibacterial treatment commenced during the paroxysmal stage will not shorten the course of the infection, but will render the patient non-infectious, and may be administered prophylactically to close contacts.

Pertussis may be prevented by active immunisation of infants (BNF 14.4), which carries a very small risk of causing convulsions and encephalopathy (*see also* Section 17.5). This, however, is much less than the risks of complications associated with pertussis. Infants in whom vaccination may be contra-indicated (i.e. those with brain damage or a familial history of convulsions) may be identified and parents counselled accordingly.

Plague

Definition and aetiology
Plague is a zoonotic infection caused by *Yersinia pestis*, a Gram-negative, aerobic, non-sporing bacillus. The disease is endemic in parts of Asia, Africa, and the Americas (including the USA), and has occurred historically as worldwide pandemics.

The reservoir of infection exists in wild rodents (particularly rats), with their associated fleas acting as the vector; man is an incidental host. Direct transmission may occasionally occur by inhalation of airborne droplets from a patient with pneumonic plague.

Symptoms
The incubation period is 2 to 8 days.

Bubonic plague is the most common form of plague and is characterised by a sudden onset of fever, chills, headache, prostration, and lethargy. Lymph nodes, particularly in the groin and axillae, become swollen, tender, hard, and painful (buboes), and surrounded by oedema. Spread of bacilli to the lungs may cause chest pain, cough, and haemoptysis (secondary pneumonic plague). Infection contracted directly from such patients by droplet-inhalation is termed primary pneumonic plague, which may be fatal within 48 hours of onset. Meningitis is a less common, but serious complication of plague.

Mild cases may resolve spontaneously before bacilli enter the circulation, whereas severe cases may be fatal in 3 to 6 days if untreated.

Treatment
Prompt treatment significantly reduces the mortality of plague. It comprises the administration of streptomycin, tetracycline, sulphonamides, or chloramphenicol (which is particularly useful for meningitis).

Patients with pneumonic plague should be isolated to curb the spread to others, and antibacterial prophylaxis administered to close contacts. Mass immunisation should be undertaken during an epidemic. Plague may be prevented in endemic areas by rat-proofing buildings, using insecticides, and wearing protective clothing to minimise the chance of being bitten.

Prostatitis

Definition and aetiology
Prostatitis is inflammation of the prostate gland. It may be acute or chronic and is usually due to bacterial infection. Common infecting micro-organisms include *Escherichia coli*, and *Klebsiella* and *Proteus* species.

Symptoms
Acute prostatitis is characterised by marked fever, chills, severe perineal pain, and back pain, together with symptoms of urinary-tract infection. Chronic prostatitis is often asymptomatic, although recurrent urinary-tract infection is common and dysuria and urethral discharge may occur.

Treatment
Treatment consists of the administration of an appropriate antibacterial drug (BNF 5.1, Table 1, and 5.1.13) and long-term therapy may be indicated. In severe cases, surgical drainage may be necessary.

Pseudomembranous Colitis

Definition and aetiology
Pseudomembranous colitis is an inflammatory bowel condition caused by *Clostridium difficile*, a Gram-positive, anaerobic, spore-forming bacillus.

Exotoxins produced by the bacilli elicit an inflammatory response in the intestinal walls, which results in the formation of adherent exudative plaques. It is an opportunistic infection and 90% of cases occur in association with the use of antibacterials, particularly ampicillin, cephalosporins, clindamycin, and lincomycin. No age group is exempt, although the condition occurs more commonly in the elderly. It may also infrequently arise secondary to other conditions (e.g. colorectal cancer, colonic obstruction, Hirschprung's disease, ischaemic gastro-intestinal disorders, shigellosis, or uraemia). Cases are usually sporadic, although small outbreaks may occur in institutions or hospitals if the environment becomes contaminated with clostridial spores (which can survive for weeks or months).

Symptoms
Pseudomembranous colitis may present during the course of antibacterial therapy or up to 6 weeks following cessation.

Symptoms, which vary in severity from mild and self-limiting to severe and fulminating, include chills, fever, abdominal pain, leucocytosis, hypoalbuminaemia, and watery or 'porridge-like' diarrhoea. Severe cases may be complicated by fluid and electrolyte imbalance, dehydration, toxic megacolon, and perforation.

Mild cases resolve spontaneously, although symptoms in severe cases may persist for months and prove fatal in some.

Treatment
Withdrawal of the offending antibacterial may allow the condition to resolve. Vancomycin (BNF 5.1.7), metronidazole, or tinidazole (BNF 5.1.11) may be of value in eradication of the bacilli. Fluid and electrolytes (BNF 9.2) may be required in cases of excessive depletion. Colectomy may be necessary in severe cases.

Pseudomembranous colitis may be prevented by avoiding the indiscriminate use in susceptible patients of those antibacterials most often implicated in causing the condition. Patients in institutions should be isolated to prevent spread to others.

Psittacosis

Definition and aetiology
Psittacosis is an infection of the lungs caused by *Chlamydia psittaci*, a weakly Gram-negative, obligate, intracellular parasite. It is mainly a disease of birds (e.g. gulls, pigeons, poultry, and psittacine birds such as parrots), which is transmitted to man by inhalation of dried infected excreta.

Symptoms
The incubation period is 7 to 14 days with a rapid or insidious onset. Common symptoms include high fever, severe headache, chills, anorexia, malaise, nausea and vomiting, myalgia, cough, and haemoptysis. In severe cases, there may be anoxia, dyspnoea, cyanosis, tachycardia, delirium, and stupor.

In untreated psittacosis, the fever may last for 7 days in mild cases and up to 21 days in more severe forms. It slowly abates and is followed by a long convalescence, but relapses may occur even after treatment. Pulmonary complications account for up to 20% of deaths.

Treatment
The prognosis is good with prompt therapy, which reduces the mortality rate to between 1% and 5%.

Treatment is by the administration of tetracyclines (BNF 5.1.3) or erythromycin (BNF 5.1.5), which must be continued for at least 10 days after the fever has subsided to prevent recurrences.

Psittacosis may be prevented by the control and quarantine of imported birds, and the eradication of disease in breeding stock by supplementing food with antibacterials and vitamins. High standards of hygiene should be maintained in areas where birds are kept. Diseased birds should be isolated and adequately treated or destroyed.

Rheumatic Fever

Definition and aetiology
Rheumatic fever is an acute or subacute inflammatory connective tissue disease which follows an upper respiratory-tract infection (usually pharyngitis or tonsillitis). The micro-organism responsible for the initial infection is a Group A β-haemolytic streptococcus (a Gram-positive facultative anaerobe). An abnormal immune reaction may be responsible for initiating the inflammatory response, although the precise mechanism is unknown.

Overcrowded unhygienic living conditions predispose an individual to developing rheumatic fever and there may be a familial tendency. The first attack usually occurs between 5 and 15 years of age, with the possibility of recurrent attacks and chronic complications throughout adult life. Improvements in living conditions and the advent of antibacterials have reduced the UK incidence from 10% of children in the 1920s to current levels of 0.01%.

Symptoms

The onset of rheumatic fever, which may be abrupt or insidious, is usually 1 to 6 weeks after the initial throat infection.

Intermittent fever, arthralgia, and migratory polyarthritis are the earliest symptoms of the acute phase in the majority of patients, affecting the large joints most commonly. The lesions heal in approximately four weeks without any permanent damage.

Carditis, which occurs in up to 40% of patients, may be insidious in onset or even asymptomatic. It is the most serious symptom, as up to 50% may develop rheumatic heart disease in which the valves of the heart become permanently damaged. Endocarditis, myocarditis, and pericarditis may also occur, contributing to the development of heart failure.

Painless subcutaneous nodules may arise over bony surfaces or tendons about three weeks after the onset in a small minority of patients. Their appearance usually accompanies carditis, but they generally disappear within two weeks.

Erythema marginatum often accompanies carditis and subcutaneous nodules. It is an evanescent, non-pruritic, macular or papular rash characterised by spreading erythema with loss of colour from the centre of the lesions.

Sydenham's chorea may develop in a small minority of patients up to 6 months after the onset. In some cases, this may be the only manifestation of rheumatic fever.

Relapses are common following further Group A streptococcal infections, and tend to resemble the symptoms of the first attack. Several streptococcal strains exist as part of the body's normal flora (notably in the mouth), and may be responsible for endocarditis in patients with pre-existing rheumatic heart disease who have recently undergone dental or surgical procedures.

Treatment

An untreated attack of rheumatic fever may last up to three months or in the presence of severe carditis, up to 6 months. Treatment consists of bed rest together with the administration of non-steroidal anti-inflammatory analgesics (BNF 10.1.1) and corticosteroids (BNF 6.3.4) to suppress the inflammatory processes. Heart failure may require further specific therapy, and haloperidol (BNF 4.9.3) may be necessary in severe cases of chorea. Antibacterials (BNF 5.1) may be necessary to eradicate any residual streptococcal infection.

Long-term antibacterial prophylaxis (BNF 5.1, Table 2) is necessary to prevent recurrences of rheumatic fever. Additional chemoprophylaxis is indicated in patients with rheumatic heart disease prior to and following surgery.

Salmonellal Infections

Definition and aetiology

Salmonellal infections are caused by bacteria of the genus *Salmonella*, which are Gram-negative, facultatively anaerobic bacilli. They are responsible for typhoid and the paratyphoid fevers (collectively known as enteric fever), which are systemic infections with widespread tissue involvement, and salmonellosis (food poisoning), an acute gastro-enteritis.

Typhoid Fever

Definition and aetiology

Typhoid fever is caused by *Salmonella typhi*, which is endemic in regions where poor standards of sewage disposal exist. Cases may be sporadic, or epidemics may occur if local water supplies become contaminated. It is uncommon in developed countries, where most infections are imported by returning travellers or immigrants from endemic areas.

S. typhi bacilli are excreted in faeces and, to a lesser extent, urine, and transmitted via contaminated drinking water and food. They are able to withstand freezing and drying, and even remain viable for long periods on soiled clothing or bedding.

The only reservoir of infection is man. Older children and young adults are most frequently affected, although no age is excluded.

Symptoms

The incubation period varies from 5 to 23 days, and is inversely related to the inoculum size (i.e. large dose, short incubation period). The inoculum size does not, however, determine the severity of subsequent symptoms, which is related to the patient's previous general health, nutritional state, and presence of any concurrent disease.

Typhoid fever is marked by phases of approximately one week's duration. The initial phase starts insidiously with a headache, fluctuating fever, and abdominal pain, which coincides with bacterial invasion of the bloodstream. Constipation occurs more frequently than diarrhoea in the early stages, although later the reverse may be true. Accompanying symptoms may include anorexia, non-productive cough, epistaxis, furred tongue, and in many cases, a characteristic, rose-coloured, macular rash on the abdomen. During the second week, the fever becomes persistent, toxaemia may develop, and there may be signs of mental deterioration leading, in severe cases, to delirium and coma. Re-entry of bacilli into the gastro-intestinal tract results in ulceration and necrosis, which may cause greenish diarrhoea (resembling 'pea soup') and melaena. The fever may start to abate after the third week, although intestinal haemorrhage (causing anaemia if severe) or perforation and peritonitis may delay convalescence. Severe cases may be complicated by invasion of other organs, resulting in cholecystitis or pneumonia.

The infection usually resolves after a debilitating course lasting 5 to 6 weeks, or longer if severe. There may be relapses or recrudescences and, in a few cases, complications may be fatal. Convalescent patients remain carriers of the disease for several weeks. Some individuals (who may not have had acute symptoms) exist as chronic carriers. One attack will often confer life-long immunity.

Treatment
Treatment with an appropriate antibacterial drug (BNF 5.1, Table 1) is essential for all patients and carriers. Corticosteroids (BNF 6.3.4) may also be indicated in severe cases of toxaemia. Supportive treatment includes maintenance of adequate fluid and electrolyte levels, and blood transfusions in severe anaemia. Surgery may be necessary to repair perforations.

Typhoid fever may be prevented in endemic areas by improving sanitation, hygiene, and health education. Transmission may be prevented by isolation or barrier nursing of symptomatic patients, and excluding carriers from food handling processes. At least three consecutive stool samples negative for *S. typhi* are required before an individual may be declared free from infection. Travellers may be partially protected by active immunisation (BNF 14.4), but should also boil drinking water and avoid the consumption of raw unpeeled fruit and vegetables.

Paratyphoid Fever

Definition and aetiology
Paratyphoid fever is caused by *Salmonella paratyphi* A, B, or C, and occurs worldwide, especially in developing countries. It is transmitted in a similar way to typhoid fever.

Symptoms
Paratyphoid fever resembles typhoid fever, but with a more abrupt onset, milder symptoms, and a shorter course. Complications, relapses, and fatalities occur less frequently.

Treatment
The treatment is essentially the same as for typhoid fever, although only supportive treatment may be required for mild infections restricted to the gastro-intestinal tract.

Salmonellosis

Definition and aetiology
Salmonellosis is an acute enteritis caused by many species of *Salmonella*, which are enzootic amongst mammals and birds. It is often referred to as food poisoning, but this may also be caused by other bacteria (e.g. *Campylobacter* spp., *Clostridium* spp., *Staphylococcus aureus*, *Vibrio parahaemolyticus*, and *Escherichia coli* (*see* Gastro-enteritis, Section 1.1).

Salmonellae are excreted in faeces. The most important source of human infection is animal-derived products (e.g. meat, particularly poultry, and eggs and milk). Contamination is facilitated by the intensive and crowded farming methods practised in developed countries. Other modes of transmission include direct contact with an infected animal, contamination of food by rodent faeces, or food prepared by an infected person; chronic human carriers are rare. Contaminated food is most likely to cause salmonellosis if it is left for long periods in warm temperatures prior to consumption, allowing multiplication of salmonella.

Achlorhydria, antacid therapy, and gastric surgery render affected individuals particularly susceptible to infection, as salmonella are normally killed by gastric acid. The old, young, and severely debilitated are also at risk.

Symptoms
The number of salmonellae needed to produce clinical symptoms is large. The incubation period reflects the time required for salmonella to multiply further within the gastro-intestinal tract. It is usually 12 to 24 hours, but may vary (i.e. 6 to 48 hours) and is inversely related to the inoculum size. The onset is sudden with symptoms of acute gastro-enteritis, which may be accompanied by headache, chills, muscle cramps, and syncope. In severe cases, mucus and blood may be passed in the stools. Occasionally, septicaemia and symptoms resembling typhoid fever may arise if the bloodstream is invaded.

Salmonellosis is usually self-limiting with a rapid recovery after 2 to 5 days. It may, however, be fatal in severe cases, particularly in infants, the elderly, and dehydrated patients. Convalescent patients excrete salmonellae for a few weeks, but rarely longer than 6 months.

Treatment
Treatment is as for gastro-enteritis. An appropriate antibacterial drug (BNF 5.1, Table 1) may be necessary in severely ill patients, but is not recommended in uncomplicated cases as it prolongs salmonella excretion.

Salmonellosis may be prevented by observing strict hygiene in the processing, preparation, and storage of food. Large frozen joints should be completely thawed before cooking, all food should be thoroughly cooked, and cooked meat should be adequately refrigerated. Milk should be pasteurised, reheating of cooked foods must be thorough and carried out once only, and contact between raw meat and cooked foods should be prevented.

Scarlet Fever

Definition and aetiology
Scarlet fever (scarlatina) follows an attack of pharyngitis caused by erythrogenic toxin-producing strains of Group A β-haemolytic streptococci (which are Gram-positive facultative anaerobes). It is endemic in temperate climates and occurs mainly during the summer and early autumn, although the incidence and mortality has decreased in recent years.

It is transmitted via droplets from an infected person (including carriers) or via contaminated fomites.

Children are most susceptible to developing scarlet fever, the majority of cases occurring in those under five years of age.

Symptoms
The incubation period is usually 2 to 3 days, although it may range from 12 hours to 6 days.

The onset is sudden, and is marked by a sore throat with pain on swallowing, chills, fever, malaise, vomiting, rapid pulse, dry skin, flushed face, and furred tongue with protruding red papillae ('strawberry tongue'). A symmetrical non-pruritic rash appears after 24 to 36 hours, initially on the arms, neck, back, and chest, and later spreads to the remainder of the body. It is characterised by red spots appearing against a background of erythema which blanches on application of pressure. Petechiae may be visible as striations in the skin folds (Pastia's sign), and the face is often flushed with a paler region around the mouth. All symptoms worsen for 2 to 3 days before gradually resolving. During convalescence, desquamation of the skin may occur.

Complications of scarlet fever include bronchitis (which may be fatal) and otitis media in children, arthritis in adults, and adenitis, rhinitis, or nephritis in any age group.

One attack usually confers life-long immunity which is strain-specific, although relapses do occur in approximately 1% of patients.

Treatment
Treatment consists of the administration of pencillins (BNF 5.1.1). Tepid sponging may be of value to reduce fever.

Scarlet fever may be prevented by improvements in living standards and prompt antimicrobial treatment for streptococcal sore throats. Patients should be isolated until at least one negative throat swab has been obtained.

Shigellosis

Definition and aetiology
Shigellosis (bacillary dysentery) is an acute colitis caused by Gram-negative, facultatively anaerobic, non-sporing bacilli of the genus *Shigella. Sh. dysenteriae* is the most virulent species and is responsible for epidemic dysentery in developing countries, where overcrowded conditions exist alongside inadequate sewage disposal. *Sh. flexneri* and *Sh. boydii* infections are of moderate severity, occurring mainly in tropical regions. *Sh. sonnei* causes a mild form of shigellosis, which is endemic in developed countries. Outbreaks occur most frequently in schools and other institutions housing young people.

The only natural reservoirs of infection are man and higher primates. Transmission occurs by the faecal-oral route, usually by ingestion of contaminated food and water. Shigella may survive for several hours on fingers or even days on fomites (e.g. lavatory seats, door handles, and towels) in cold damp conditions. Flies also act as an effective means of transferring bacteria from faeces to food.

Symptoms
The inoculum size required to cause disease is small. The incubation period is short (usually less than three days), although occasionally it may last a week.

The onset of symptoms is generally abrupt, commencing with abdominal pain, headache, tenesmus, vomiting, and watery diarrhoea, which may be almost continuous. In severe cases, there may be passage of pus and blood-stained mucus ('red-currant jelly'), and dehydration may become severe, particularly in infants and the elderly. Other symptoms include anorexia and weight loss. In some, the infection may be very mild or even asymptomatic. After a few days the patient gradually recovers, although shigella continue to be passed in the faeces for several weeks. Serious infections may follow a protracted course which may be fatal in infants, the elderly, and previously debilitated or malnourished individuals.

Complications which may occur with any form of shigellosis include arthritis and haemorrhoids, and in severe cases, peritonitis. Convulsions may occur in children during the early stages.

Treatment
Rehydration is very important and comprises the administration of oral (BNF 9.2.1) or intravenous (BNF 9.2.2) fluids. An appropriate antibacterial drug (BNF 5.1, Table 1) may be necessary in severe cases but is not

recommended in milder self-limiting forms, particularly during epidemics, as antibacterial-resistant strains rapidly emerge. Drugs which reduce intestinal motility should be avoided, as they prolong the course of the infection and excretion of shigella.

Shigellosis may be prevented in endemic areas by improving sanitation and excluding flies from food preparation areas. Spread during an outbreak in institutions may be controlled by isolating infected individuals, thoroughly cleansing the hands after defaecation, regularly disinfecting lavatories, flush handles, door knobs, and taps, and using disposable hand-towels. Infected food handlers should not be allowed to return to work until at least three consecutive stool samples negative for shigella have been passed.

Stye

Definition and aetiology
A stye (hordeolum) is a local pyogenic infection involving the follicle or sebaceous gland of an eyelash, or both. It arises on the outer surface of the eyelid through inflammation of the glands of Zeis or Moll's glands. Its presence on the inner surface caused by inflammation of the Meibomian glands is termed a chalazion. It is most commonly due to staphylococci.

Symptoms
Symptoms of an external stye include painful swelling and inflammation of the edge of the affected eyelid. The swelling 'points' to a head within a few days, and then ruptures (Fig. 5.3) with the discharge of pus and the relief of pain. Recurrence is common.

For symptoms of an internal stye, *see* Chalazion, Section 11.1.

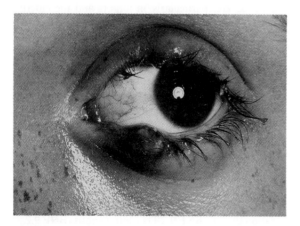

Fig. 5.3
Discharge of pus following rupture of a stye.

Treatment
Treatment consists of the application of hot compresses. An appropriate topical anti-infective preparation (BNF 11.3) may be indicated in recurrent cases, or to prevent the spread of infection.

Sycosis Barbae

Definition and aetiology
Sycosis barbae is an inflammatory infection of the hair follicles in the bearded region caused by *Staphylococcus aureus*. There may be a correlation of incidence with a greasy skin, and recurrence may be caused by emotional disturbances and fatigue.

Symptoms
The condition occurs in males generally between 30 to 40 years of age. It is characterised by red oedematous papules or pustules at the point of emergence of the hair. In chronic forms, larger raised lesions may arise from several confluent infected follicles. Complete follicles may be destroyed resulting in scarring.

Treatment
Treatment is as for folliculitis (*see* Section 13.1), although systemic antibacterial drugs (BNF 5.1) may be necessary in unresponsive cases. The nares, which in some individuals are a possible reservoir of infection, should also be treated.

Tetanus

Definition and aetiology
Tetanus (lockjaw) is caused by a potent exotoxin, tetanospasmin, produced by *Clostridium tetani*, a Gram-positive, anaerobic, spore-forming bacillus. The disease occurs worldwide, although the incidence in developed countries is low due to active immunisation programmes and high standards of hygiene and health-care.

The spores, which are present in soil and in the faeces of many mammmals (including humans), are highly resistant, and remain viable for years under dry conditions and are able to withstand boiling for hours. Spores contaminating a wound germinate if anaerobic conditions prevail (e.g. in deep punctures or in the presence of necrotic tissue or foreign bodies). The infected wound may be minor and ignored by the patient. The toxin produced by vegetative bacilli is carried in the bloodstream and nerve fibres to the central nervous system, where it acts at the presynaptic terminal of inhibitory spinal neurones to prevent the release of inhibitory transmitter. Sensory and autonomic nerves take up some toxin, but the major effect is hyperactivity of motor neurones, which results in muscular rigidity and spasm.

Neonatal tetanus occurs predominantly in under-developed countries, and is caused by infection of the umbilicus due to use of contaminated instruments or dressings. In developed countries, the elderly are most at risk of contracting tetanus, although no age group is exempt. Drug abusers are also susceptible due to contamination of some samples of crude heroin with spores.

Symptoms

The incubation period varies from 1 to 14 days, with an average of 7 days, although some spores may remain dormant for several months.

Tetanus is characterised by muscular rigidity, which may commence with the muscles of the jaw (lockjaw or trismus), and contraction of facial muscles, causing a 'sneering' expression (risus sardonicus). Pain and stiffness in the muscles of the neck and back may cause a 'ram-rod' posture, or backward curvature of the spine (opisthotonos) if there is excessive contraction of the long muscles. The muscles of the abdomen are also rigid. In moderately severe cases, the pharyngeal muscles may be involved and results in dysphagia. Reflex spasms may arise, usually as a result of external stimuli (e.g. movement, injections, sudden noise, or passing a nasogastric tube), which intensify the underlying hypertonia. The spasms become spontaneous in severe tetanus, and increase in intensity and frequency. Complications arising as a result include spinal fractures due to extreme opisthotonos, and respiratory failure due to respiratory-muscle spasm. Other respiratory complications include atelectasis and broncho-pneumonia. The autonomic nervous system is also frequently involved in severe cases, causing a fluctuating blood pressure, high fever, peripheral vasoconstriction, increased cardiac output, arrhythmias and, if persistent, cardiac arrest.

Most deaths are due to cardiac or pulmonary complications and occur during the first 8 days. Surviving patients usually show a gradual but complete recovery in 4 to 6 weeks.

Treatment

The prognosis is poor in severe tetanus, with 50% mortality rising to 90% in neonatal tetanus. Less than 10% of milder cases are fatal.

Treatment comprises the administration of a benzylpenicillin (BNF 5.1.1.1) to eliminate bacteria, passive immunisation with tetanus immunoglobulin of human origin (HTIG) (BNF 14.5) to neutralise toxin circulating in the bloodstream, and a skeletal muscle relaxant (BNF 10.2.2). Thorough cleansing and debridement of the wound after administration of the antitoxin may also be of value in eradicating a known focus of infection.

Intensive supportive measures are necessary in moderate and severe cases until the disease has run its course, as toxin cannot be removed from the CNS. These include endotracheal intubation, tracheostomy, and enteral (BNF 9.4.2) and intravenous (BNF 9.3) nutrition. Respiratory complications may require assisted ventilation in conjunction with peripheral neuromuscular blockade. A beta-adrenoceptor blocking drug with alpha-blocking activity (BNF 2.4) or an opioid analgesic (e.g. morphine, BNF 4.7.2) may be indicated for cardiovascular complications. It may also be necessary to monitor the fluid and electrolyte balance.

The most effective means of preventing tetanus is by active immunisation with tetanus vaccine (BNF 14.4) in infancy, followed by regular booster doses throughout adult life (see also Section 17.5). Any wound contaminated with soil or faeces should be treated promptly and HTIG administered if the patient's immunity is in doubt. A course of tetanus vaccine should also be administered to all patients with tetanus as an attack does not confer immunity. Neonatal tetanus may be prevented by immunisation of pregnant women and use of sterile equipment and dressings at delivery.

Toxic Shock Syndrome

Definition and aetiology

Toxic shock syndrome (TSS) is due to the effects of a toxin produced, in the majority of cases, by *Staphylococcus aureus*. It is rarely the result of bacteraemia.

It occurs most frequently in association with the use of highly-absorbent tampons by menstruating women. The synthetic material contained in these tampons is broken down by specific enzymes produced by host and bacterial cells, which may be found in the vagina under normal circumstances. The end-product of degradation is glucose, providing an ideal source of nutrient for toxin-producing strains of *S. aureus*, which may be present in up to 17% of women. Less than 10% of cases have been reported as occurring in men, children, and non-menstruating women. In these cases, the primary focus of infection may be an abscess or empyema, or colonisation of surgical sutures or contraceptive diaphragms and sponges.

Symptoms

TSS has an abrupt onset and is characterised by high fever, myalgia, nausea and vomiting, and watery diarrhoea. Other symptoms may include conjunctivitis, headache, lethargy, sore throat, and intermittent confusion. A rash resembling sunburn appears, which desquamates, particularly on the palms of the hands and soles of the feet, after 3 to 7 days. The condition may rapidly progress to hypotension and shock, which may be fatal if untreated. Complications involving any organ may occur due to the effects of shock (e.g. acute renal failure and adult respiratory distress syndrome). Recurrences are common for up to 6 months in 10% of patients continuing to use tampons.

Treatment
The treatment is supportive, as described under shock. Antibacterial drugs (BNF 5.1) will not modify the course of the syndrome, but may be of value in removing the primary focus of infection and preventing recurrences.

TSS may be prevented in menstruating women by avoiding the continual use of tampons, particularly those with high absorbency.

Trachoma

Definition and aetiology
Trachoma is a chronic inflammatory disease of the conjunctiva and cornea due to infection with *Chlamydia trachomatis*, a weakly Gram-negative, obligate, intracellular parasite. It is endemic in many under-developed parts of the world (e.g. in rural areas of Africa, Asia, the Middle East, and South and Central America), and is the most common worldwide cause of blindness.

The infection is transmitted by contact with infected conjunctival secretions via fingers, fomites, and flies. It may also be transmitted sexually, the main reservoir of infection being the cervix in the female genital tract. The sexually-transmitted form is a common cause of trachoma in urban areas of developed countries. Neonatal trachoma arises as a result of passage through an infected birth canal.

Symptoms
The exact incubation period is unknown, but may be between 1 and 3 weeks. Neonatal trachoma usually arises between 5 and 14 days after birth, whereas sexually-transmitted infections may present with symptoms in less than two weeks.

Trachoma is usually bilateral and is characterised by local inflammation, lachrymation, pain, discharge, erythematous and swollen eyelids, ptosis, and photophobia. As the disease progresses, follicles develop in the conjunctiva and papillary hyperplasia occurs. Eventually, vascularisation of the cornea (i.e. pannus formation) occurs and ulceration and scarring may result. The degree of visual impairment may vary, but in severe cases, blindness may follow. Re-infection is common, as is secondary bacterial infection.

The symptoms of neonatal trachoma are similar, although the cornea may be unaffected. Adult sexually-transmitted trachoma is often unilateral.

Treatment
Treatment includes the topical (BNF 11.3.1) or systemic (BNF 5.1.3) administration of a tetracycline, or both. A systemic sulphonamide (BNF 5.1.8) may also be effective. Erythromycin (BNF 5.1.5) should be used in children. Surgery may be necessary in severe cases.

Trachoma may be prevented in endemic areas by mass therapy using topical anti-infective preparations (BNF 11.3.1), and improvements in living standards and encouragement of scrupulous hygiene. Topical erythromycin administered prophylactically may be of value in preventing neonatal trachoma.

Tuberculosis

Definition and aetiology
Tuberculosis is a chronic infectious disease usually caused by *Mycobacterium tuberculosis*, an acid-fast bacillus. Other species (e.g. *M. bovis*) may also be responsible. It is prevalent in developing countries, particularly where conditions of poor housing, overcrowding, poverty, poor nutrition, and inadequate medical care prevail.

The micro-organism is an obligate parasite, which is transmitted from person-to-person by inhalation of airborne droplets. Ingestion of unpasteurised milk from infected cows is a mode of transmission which is of historic interest only in developed countries, but accidental skin inoculation in laboratory personnel is a possibility. Disease develops in only 5% to 15% of infected people and is dependent on various factors (e.g. inoculum size, virulence of infecting strain, the host's age, inherent resistance, and state of health and nutrition). It most commonly affects the respiratory tract (pulmonary tuberculosis) and may be primary or post-primary. It is characterised by inflammatory infiltrations, tubercle formation, caseation, fibrosis, and calcification. In up to one-third of patients, the micro-organism may spread in the blood circulation and lymphatics to other organs (e.g. lymph nodes, heart, gastro-intestinal or genito-urinary tracts, meninges, bones, joints, and skin), and several organs may be affected simultaneously (miliary tuberculosis).

Primary Pulmonary Tuberculosis

Definition and aetiology
Primary pulmonary tuberculosis occurs in previously uninfected subjects and is most common in children. It is usually caused by droplet inhalation and it results in pulmonary inflammation and exudate production. Although necrosis and cavitation of the lungs do not frequently occur, calcification is common.

Symptoms

It is usually a mild disease and is often asymptomatic. Nevertheless, common symptoms include cough (usually non-productive), fever, malaise, wheezing, anorexia with weight loss, and occasionally erythema nodosum. In severe cases, respiratory distress may occur. The primary disease usually resolves spontaneously within a few weeks, although it may occasionally become progressive and affect other organs.

Treatment

See Post-primary Pulmonary Tuberculosis below.

Post-primary Pulmonary Tuberculosis

Definition and aetiology

Post-primary pulmonary tuberculosis occurs as a result of reactivation of latent primary infection and is more common in the elderly. Other contributory factors include diabetes mellitus, administration of drugs affecting the immune response, and poor nutrition. It results in pulmonary caseation, with extensive necrosis and cavitation followed by fibrosis. It may be acute or chronic and may become progressive.

Symptoms

Post-primary disease has an insidious, often asymptomatic, onset. Early symptoms, however, include anorexia with weight loss, fever, and malaise. Other common symptoms are cough with the production of purulent sputum, chest pain, haemoptysis, night sweats, anxiety, depressive disorders, resistant pneumonia, and chronic ill-health.

Treatment

The treatment of both primary and post-primary tuberculosis consists of the long-term administration of anti-tuberculous drugs (BNF 5.1.9). Bronchoscopy may occasionally be required to clear diseased airways, and surgical drainage, excision of lesions, or reconstruction may be necessary in rare cases.

The spread of tuberculosis may be prevented by the identification, using the Mantoux test (BNF 14.4), and treatment of all infected individuals. Close contacts of patients should receive antibacterial prophylaxis (BNF 5.1, Table 2), and all tuberculin-negative children should be actively immunised with the Bacillus Calmette-Guérin vaccine (BNF 14.4). Host resistance in endemic areas may be increased by improvements in living conditions, nutrition, and medical care.

Typhus Fevers

Definition and aetiology

Typhus fevers are caused by species of *Rickettsia*, which are Gram-negative, pleomorphic, obligate intracellular parasites. These fevers are now uncommon in developed countries, although they have been associated historically with periods of famine, mass poverty, or war.

R. prowazekii is responsible for classical epidemic typhus, which is transmitted to man in the faeces of the human body louse (*Pediculus humanus corporis*). The micro-organism gains entry via skin abrasions (including the louse-bite site), or the respiratory tract if dried faeces are inhaled. The louse acquires the infection during a blood meal on a patient with typhus. Brill-Zinsser disease is a milder form of epidemic typhus occurring as a recrudescence of the primary infection due to the persistence of bacteria within the tissues. The milder form may occur many years after the primary infection.

Murine (endemic) typhus and scrub typhus are zoonotic infections involving rodents (e.g. rats) as the reservoir of infection, and fleas or mites respectively as vectors, with man an incidental host.

Symptoms

The incubation period of epidemic typhus fever is between 5 and 14 days.

The onset is sudden and is characterised by sustained fever, rigors, severe and persistent headache, facial flushing, myalgia (particularly in the back and legs), prostration, and a dulled mental state. A macular rash may become petechial in severe cases. Later symptoms include deafness, incontinence, restlessness, delirium, profound prostration, and stupor.

Mortality is greatest in untreated patients over 40 years of age. Death is usually due to peripheral vascular collapse, renal failure, or pulmonary complications. Surviving patients start to recover after approximately two weeks of fever.

The symptoms of murine typhus are similar but milder, and the course is shorter and mortality rate lower. Lymph nodes become enlarged and other constitutional symptoms similar to those of epidemic typhus fever develop.

Treatment

Treatment is effective and can dramatically reduce the mortality rate.

Tetracyclines (BNF 5.1.3) are appropriate antibacterial drugs used in the treatment of rickettsial diseases. Chloramphenicol and corticosteroids may be used in severely ill patients.

Patients should be deloused and all clothes and bedding decontaminated to curb further spread. Wider measures to prevent typhus fevers include the control of rat and flea populations, and wearing clothes treated with insect repellents in endemic areas. A vaccine (BNF 14.4) is available for travellers likely to be at risk of contracting epidemic (not scrub) typhus (e.g. those coming into close contact with the indigenous population).

5.3   VIRAL INFECTIONS

(Background information on viruses can be found in Section 14.3.)

Acquired Immunodeficiency Syndrome

Definition and aetiology
Acquired immunodeficiency syndrome (AIDS) arises as an end-stage manifestation of infection by human immunodeficiency virus type 1 (HIV-1), and is prevalent worldwide. Human immunodeficiency virus type 2 (HIV-2) will also cause AIDS, and is thought to be spreading from West Africa. HIV-infection results in the reduction of the number of T-cells, particularly helper T-cells (*see* Section 15.6), although other leucocytes are also susceptible (e.g. B-cells, monocytes, and macrophages).

Primary manifestations of HIV-infection are progressive immunodeficiency (particularly affecting cell-mediated immunity), diminished immunosurveillance, and the direct effects of HIV on tissues (e.g. the central nervous system and gastro-intestinal tract). Secondary manifestations of HIV-infection occur as a result of impaired immunity and include malignant disease and infections.

In the absence of other causes of immunodeficiency, diagnosis of HIV-infection is based upon the presence of circulating HIV-antibodies. HIV-infection can be transmitted if the virus gains entry into the blood circulation. This can occur through sexual intercourse (heterosexual and homosexual), transplantation of infected organs and tissues, transfusion of infected blood or blood products, contaminated equipment (e.g. during parenteral drug abuse), and from an infected mother to child *in utero*, during childbirth, or possibly during breast-feeding.

Symptoms
Symptoms of HIV-infection depend upon the clinical stage of the infection. Progression from infection by HIV to development of AIDS may take months or years. It is unpredictable and patients may remain asymptomatic for many years. Following infection there is a latent period of between 4 to 12 weeks which, on rare occasions, can be longer. During this time, there is no immune response, and the infection cannot, therefore, be detected. This period is followed by acute HIV-infection, with the formation of HIV-antibodies (seroconversion). Most patients are asymptomatic, but non-specific symptoms can occur and are generally self-limiting. These include arthropathy, diarrhoea, fever, headache, malaise, myalgia, nausea and vomiting, and photophobia. Transient lymphadenopathy, rashes, convulsions, and coma may also occur.

Progression to chronic HIV-infection may be asymptomatic, or may result in persistent generalised lymphadenopathy. During the later stages the patient may develop the AIDS-related complex (ARC), which is characterised by fever, lethargy, malaise, night sweats, persistent diarrhoea, and weight loss. Minor opportunistic infections may also occur, including folliculitis, herpesvirus infections, oral candidiasis, oral hairy leucoplakia, tinea infections, and warts.

Further progression to AIDS (end-stage disease or full-blown AIDS) occurs when immunity is severely impaired. Patients usually develop life-threatening opportunistic infections or malignant disease. These most commonly include *Pneumocystis carinii* pneumonia or Kaposi's sarcoma, which may occur together. Other opportunistic infections may also occur, including cerebral toxoplasmosis, cytomegalovirus infection, meningitis, and pulmonary tuberculosis. Other malignant disease may be present (e.g. non-Hodgkin's lymphoma and cerebral lymphoma).

Neurological disease associated with HIV-infection may occur with varying severity and at any stage. It includes dementia, encephalopathy, and neuropathy, and is thought to be caused by the direct effect of the virus.

Treatment
There is no effective treatment or prophylaxis of HIV-infection. Patients usually require counselling and regular monitoring of health. Antiviral drugs (BNF 5.3) may be indicated together with appropriate treatment for secondary manifestations.

Prevention of further transmission comprises the primary basis of management of HIV-infection. This includes screening donor blood, organs, and tissues; heat-treatment of blood products; adoption of safer sexual activities; and avoidance of contaminated equipment. In addition, women within high-risk groups (e.g. drug abusers) who are pregnant or who may be planning a pregnancy should be screened and counselled.

Self-help organisations
Haemophilia Society
Terrence Higgins Trust

Common Cold

Definition and aetiology

The common cold (acute coryza or infective rhinitis) is caused by infection of the nose, nasopharynx, and upper respiratory tract, mainly by rhinoviruses. However, a wide variety of other viruses including coronaviruses, adenoviruses, and myxoviruses are also responsible. The infection occurs worldwide, particularly during the autumn and winter months in temperate climates.

Infection spreads rapidly (especially in crowded conditions) via nasopharyngeal droplets, which may be inhaled directly or passed indirectly on fingers. The latter mode of transmission may be more significant than formerly thought; saliva does not appear to be an important means of viral transmission. The major portals of entry are the nasal mucosa and conjunctiva.

Children are particularly susceptible and may have several colds each year, although physical resistance in any age group may be lowered by physical or emotional disturbances, or ill-health. Exposure to low temperatures does not cause the common cold and appears to have little effect on lowering host resistance.

Symptoms

The incubation period is 1 to 4 days, with the period of greatest infectivity starting about 24 hours before, and lasting for up to five days after, the onset of symptoms.

The onset is abrupt and is characterised by discomfort in the eyes, nose, and throat, with nasal congestion and discharge. There may also be sore throat and cough. Mild fever occasionally occurs in children, but is uncommon in adults, and this is an important means of differentiating a common cold from influenza. There is usually complete recovery within 4 to 10 days of onset, although complications (e.g. laryngitis, sinusitis, and otitis media) may develop, and secondary bacterial infection may follow.

Treatment

Treatment is symptomatic and may include the administration of non-opioid analgesics (BNF 4.7.1), systemic (BNF 3.10) or topical (BNF 12.2.2) nasal decongestants, and antitussives (BNF 3.9). Aromatic inhalations (BNF 3.8) may be useful.

Production of an effective vaccine is unlikely, as many strains of different viruses are responsible. Spread of the common cold within households may be prevented by regular handwashing, avoiding hand-to-face contact, and taking measures to curtail droplet spread.

Definition and aetiology

Encephalitis is inflammation of the brain, usually arising from a viral infection. A wide variety of viruses may be responsible, but paramyxoviruses (e.g. measles and mumps viruses) are commonly implicated, together with arboviruses and herpesviruses. The infecting virus may vary according to geographical location.

Symptoms

The onset may be sudden or insidious and is characterised by an alteration in consciousness, which may vary from lethargy to coma and headache. Other symptoms include convulsions, fever, neck stiffness, raised intracranial pressure, and motor and sensory disturbances. Confusion and behavioural disturbances may occur. Encephalitis may be fatal, and surviving patients may suffer permanent disability (e.g. epilepsy or intellectual impairment).

Treatment

Treatment is supportive with the administration of analgesics (BNF 4.7) for headache, tepid sponging for fever, and the maintenance of an adequate fluid intake. Corticosteroids (BNF 6.3.4) and antiviral drugs (BNF 5.3) have been used. Antiepileptics (BNF 4.8) may be necessary. Neurosurgical decompression may be indicated.

Subacute Sclerosing Panencephalitis

Definition and aetiology

Subacute sclerosing panencephalitis is a rare form of encephalitis found in children and young adults, and is due to a persistent measles virus infection, first contracted at an early age.

Symptoms

The onset of symptoms is insidious, usually occurs around 6 years after primary infection with the measles virus, and is initially characterised by general lethargy. Weeks or months later, clumsiness and involuntary movements develop. Visual disturbances are common and, as the disease progresses, intellectual impairment, spasticity, and rigidity occur. Death usually follows within two years.

Treatment

No effective treatment exists.

Herpesvirus Infections

Definition and aetiology

Herpesviruses are widely distributed throughout the animal kingdom, although some (e.g. cytomegalovirus) are highly specific for a particular host. It is common for the virus to become latent after the primary infection, with reactivation of disease occurring in response to a variety of stimuli despite the presence of circulating antibodies. Most infections are mild and non-life-threatening, although serious and fatal disease may occur in infants or immunocompromised hosts and by viruses not normally specific for humans.

Herpes Simplex Virus Infections

Definition and aetiology

Herpes simplex virus (HSV) infections are transmitted directly from person-to-person via oral secretions (usually HSV type 1) or genital secretions (usually HSV type 2). Transmission does not always take place in the presence of active lesions, and asymptomatic carriers may represent an important reservoir of infection. In some cases, auto-infection may occur.

Herpes labialis (cold sore or fever blister) occurs as a recurrence of an HSV 1 infection. The latent virus, present in ganglia of the trigeminal nerve, may be reactivated by emotional disturbances, fever, menstruation, sunlight, or local trauma.

Symptoms

The incubation period is from 2 to 12 days for HSV 1 infections and 2 to 7 days for HSV 2 infections.

Primary infection with HSV 1 may be asymptomatic or can present with prodromal symptoms that include fever, malaise, gingivitis, pharyngitis, and generalised adenopathy (especially in the cervical region). Vesicles appear within the mouth and on the lips, rupturing to form painful ulcers. Accompanying symptoms in some are excessive salivation and halitosis. The condition is self-limiting and untreated ulcers heal without scarring within 14 days.

Herpes labialis is characterised by the appearance of vesicular eruptions on the edges of the lips, preceded by a prodromal phase during which the patient experiences localised burning and itching sensations. Eruptions develop singly or in crops and persist for up to 10 days, during which time they rupture and become encrusted. Local inflammation often occurs and secondary bacterial infection may develop. Recurrence may occur, usually at the same site, over a period of many years.

HSV 2 infections are characterised by painful vesicular lesions appearing in the anogenital region. Accompanying constitutional symptoms include anorexia, fever, malaise, and lymphadenopathy. Dysuria or urinary retention may occur in females and the infection may be transferred to neonates during delivery. Lesions may take several weeks to heal. Recurrent infections are generally less severe and extensive, and the lesions may be preceded by burning or itching sensations.

Other sites may be involved in primary infections with both types of virus. Herpetic whitlows occur on fingers and are often seen in medical and dental personnel. Infections of the eye result in keratoconjunctivitis, which may be recurrent. Encephalitis is an uncommon, but potentially fatal, complication, particularly in neonates.

Treatment

Herpes simplex virus infections respond well to systemic antiviral drugs (BNF 5.3). Additional local measures include ophthalmic anti-infective preparations (BNF 11.3.1), antiviral skin preparations (BNF 13.10.3), or an oropharyngeal anti-infective mouth-bath (BNF 12.3.2).

Spread of infection may be prevented by avoiding contact with active lesions. Caesarean delivery may be necessary for babies born to infected mothers, and chemoprophylaxis with antiviral drugs (BNF 5.3) may be administered to immunocompromised hosts.

Varicella-zoster Virus Infections

Definition and aetiology

The primary infection in non-immune individuals caused by the varicella-zoster virus is chickenpox (varicella), an acute highly contagious disease. Following recovery, the virus remains latent within sensory root ganglia and may be reactivated by stimuli (e.g. malignancy, irradiation with X-rays or ultraviolet light, immunosuppressant therapy, or trauma), resulting in herpes zoster (shingles). In many cases, there appears to be no obvious stimulus.

Chickenpox is transmitted between individuals via airborne droplets or by contact with active lesions. Contrary to popular belief, it is unlikely that herpes zoster arises as a result of contact with a chickenpox sufferer (i.e. it is not a reinfection). However, a non-immune subject may develop chickenpox following contact with a herpes zoster patient.

Chickenpox is primarily a disease of the young and is prevalent in children between 2 and 8 years of age. Herpes zoster may occur at any age, although the greatest incidence is in the elderly. Second attacks of either disease are uncommon.

Symptoms

The incubation period of chickenpox is usually between 14 to 16 days, although the range may extend from 10 to 23 days. The infection is most contagious during the period immediately before the rash starts, and infectivity lasts until the vesicles have formed crusts.

Prodromal symptoms, which may be absent or only mild in the very young, include fever, malaise, and anorexia. These symptoms are more severe in adults, who may also suffer with headache, back pain, myalgia, chills, and vomiting. The lesions, which commonly appear on the trunk and scalp, are macular, develop rapidly into vesicles, and finally become pustular and encrusted. Successive crops appear over several days, but rarely spread to the limbs. Accompanying pruritus may allow development of secondary infections, particularly with staphylococci, through scratching.

Mucous membranes (e.g. conjunctiva, the buccal mucosa, pharynx, and vagina) may also be involved. Pneumonitis is a potentially fatal complication, which occurs in up to one-third of adult patients. Encephalitis may occur in any age group, but is uncommon.

Herpes zoster is characterised by a unilateral rash, which generally follows the course of sensory nerves (Fig. 5.4) innervating those areas where the chickenpox rash is most commonly seen (i.e. the trunk and along the trigeminal nerve). The lesions are similar in nature to those seen in chickenpox, although they are usually accompanied by paraesthesia, neuralgia, and in some cases lymphadenopathy. Paralysis of motor nerves may occasionally occur, although this is not permanent in the majority of cases.

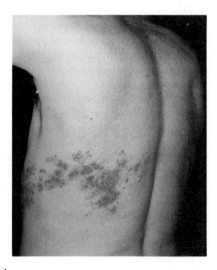

Fig. 5.4
A unilateral rash occurring along the course of sensory nerves, and characteristic of herpes zoster infection.

Ophthalmic zoster (involving the eye) is a serious complication, which may cause blindness if untreated. Some patients, particularly the elderly, suffer persistent pain (post-herpetic neuralgia) for many months or years after the lesions disappear.

Treatment
Treatment of chickenpox is usually symptomatic, comprising the administration of antipruritic preparations (BNF 13.3) and non-opioid analgesics other than aspirin (BNF 4.7.1). Specific antiviral therapy (BNF 5.3) is usually reserved for those at risk of developing serious disease (e.g. immunocompromised patients).

Herpes zoster may be treated with a combination of systemic antivirals (BNF 5.3), antiviral skin preparations (BNF 13.10.3), and analgesics (BNF 4.7). Institution of early therapy is essential and may help to reduce the incidence of post-herpetic neuralgia. Antiviral ophthalmic ointments (BNF 11.3.1) are indicated for eye infections, for which patients are referred to a specialist.

All patients should be discouraged from scratching lesions, to reduce the chance of secondary bacterial infection and scarring on healing.

Spread of infection may be prevented by avoiding contact with active lesions. Anti-varicella-zoster immunoglobulin injection (BNF 14.5) is also available as prophylaxis for highly susceptible groups.

Cytomegalovirus Infection

Definition and aetiology
Cytomegaloviruses are widely distributed throughout the animal kingdom, although individual members of this group are host-specific. Human cytomegalovirus, which is found worldwide, is transmitted by close contact with body tissues and fluids. As with other herpesviruses, latent infections may be reactivated after the primary infection.

In adults, the infection is common and, in most cases, trivial. Neonates with congenital infections and immunocompromised patients (e.g. those with AIDS) are most susceptible to developing serious disease.

Symptoms
Acquired infections in otherwise healthy individuals are often asymptomatic or present with mild, non-specific, self-limiting symptoms. More serious symptoms may include hepatosplenomegaly, lymphadenopathy, pneumonia, ulcerative colitis, and encephalitis. Some patients may present with a syndrome resembling infectious mononucleosis (*see below*).

Congenital infections may cause cerebral palsy, hepatosplenomegaly, jaundice, microcephaly, and purpura and, to a lesser extent, chorioretinitis, sensorineural deafness, and epilepsy. In some cases, there may be no detectable symptoms at birth, although available data indicates that such infants may later have learning and developmental difficulties.

Treatment
The prognosis for immunocompromised hosts varies considerably from complete recovery to death.

There is as yet no effective antiviral agent available to treat cytomegalovirus infections, although ganciclovir (BNF 5.3) may be used in immunocompromised patients.

Reduction in the level of immunosuppressants may be of value in reducing the severity of infection in graft patients.

Infectious Mononucleosis

Definition and aetiology
Infectious mononucleosis (glandular fever) is caused by the Epstein-Barr virus, which is distributed worldwide. Infection with the virus is associated with conditions of overcrowding and poor hygiene, and is almost universal amongst children in underdeveloped countries. It is less prevalent in developed countries, although more likely to cause clinical illness, especially amongst young people living together in groups (e.g. military recruits and college students).

The exact mode of transmission is unknown, but is likely to be via oropharyngeal secretions. Infected individuals may excrete the virus for up to a year.

Symptoms
Many cases are asymptomatic, but in those that do develop symptoms the incubation period is from 5 to 7 weeks.

There may be a prodromal period of 4 to 5 days with symptoms of headache, fatigue, and malaise followed by fever, sore throat, and cervical adenopathy. Additional symptoms may include oedema of the oronasopharyngeal region, resulting in dysphagia, periorbital oedema, and petechiae and vesicles on the palate. There may be a non-pruritic maculopapular rash in a few cases. Splenomegaly frequently occurs and in rare cases may lead to rupture. Other complications include jaundice, myocarditis, pneumonitis, meningo-encephalitis, Bell's palsy, Guillain-Barré syndrome, and aplastic or haemolytic anaemia.

The acute phase generally lasts for 4 to 6 weeks, although fatigue and lethargy often persist during convalescence and may continue for many months afterwards.

One attack usually confers lifelong immunity, although immunosuppression at a later date may initiate reactivation.

Treatment
There is no specific treatment for infectious mononucleosis. Patients should be advised to rest and be reassured that the illness is self-limiting. Antipyretics (BNF 4.7.1) may be of value in alleviating fever. Corticosteroids (BNF 6.3.4) have been used in cases where complications become life-threatening.

Influenza

Definition and aetiology
Influenza is an acute infection of the respiratory tract caused by influenza viruses A, B, and C, which occur worldwide and are responsible for causing epidemics and pandemics. The highest incidence in the UK is between December and May, with a peak during February and March.

Influenza virus A is the least stable antigenically and is usually responsible for epidemics and pandemics. Type B also causes epidemics, but they are less frequent and more localised as the virus is more stable. Type C is the most stable and least pathogenic serotype, and generally produces mild or subclinical infections.

Influenza is highly contagious and transmitted by droplet inhalation. Elderly and debilitated individuals are particularly susceptible and infection may be life-threatening in such patients.

Symptoms
The incubation period is 1 to 3 days. The patient is most infectious from the day preceding symptoms until 3 to 7 days after onset.

Influenza may be differentiated from the common cold by fever and a sudden onset of symptoms, which may include rigors, headache, myalgia, vertigo, and back pain. Dry cough, nasal congestion, and sore throat are common respiratory symptoms, and anorexia, depression, and nausea and vomiting may also occur. In mild cases, symptoms may last for only 24 hours. However, the more usual course for uncomplicated influenza is a gradual improvement after 4 to 5 days, with full recovery 7 to 10 days from onset. In some, cough and malaise may persist for longer. Secondary bacterial invasion may cause more serious respiratory-tract infections (e.g. pneumonia), and is a common cause of death, particularly in elderly patients. There may also be cardiac complications (e.g. myocarditis) and a worsening of other chronic conditions (e.g. diabetes mellitus). Convulsions and croup may occur in young children, and Reye's syndrome is a rare but serious complication.

Treatment
Treatment consists of bed rest and the administration of adequate fluids and antipyretic non-opioid analgesics (BNF 4.7.1). Oxygen therapy (BNF 3.6) and assisted ventilation may be required in severe cases of pneumonia.

An influenza vaccine (BNF 14.4) is available for prophylaxis in susceptible individuals, and amantadine (BNF 5.3) has also been used.

Lassa Fever

Definition and aetiology
Lassa fever, caused by the Lassa virus, was first identified in 1969 in Nigeria, and subsequent outbreaks have occurred in Liberia and Sierra Leone.

Mastomys natalensis, a rat commonly found in regions south of the Sahara, acts as the reservoir of infection. The rodent is unaffected by the infection, but passes the virus in urine and other body fluids throughout life. Man primarily becomes infected as a result of contact with infected rat urine, although the exact portal of entry is unknown. Lassa fever is highly contagious. Viral transmission usually occurs via the patient's body fluids, and contacts (including attendant medical staff) may become secondarily infected. Many of the outbreaks have been nosocomial, and fatal infections in laboratory personnel have also occurred.

Symptoms

The incubation period is between 3 and 16 days. Subclinical infections may occur or symptoms can vary in severity from mild to fulminating and fatal.

The onset is usually insidious, with non-specific symptoms of malaise, myalgia, and chills followed by fever, headache, and sore throat. Symptoms gradually worsen as fever and prostration increase. Exudative pharyngitis is characteristic and other symptoms may include diarrhoea, dysphagia, nausea and vomiting, injection of the conjunctiva, chest pain, and cough. Capillaries become damaged, resulting in increased permeability, which causes haemorrhage, hypotension, and hypovolaemic shock. Severe cases show a sudden worsening of symptoms during the second week, and death due to cardiac arrest, respiratory insufficiency, or shock may follow. Vertigo and deafness can occur, and the latter may be permanent.

Excretion of the virus may continue for up to 5 or 6 weeks after recovery.

Treatment

Patients must be barrier-nursed in isolation, taking stringent precautions against contagion. Supportive therapy, including maintenance of fluid and electrolyte levels and other measures to control shock, is necessary. Lassa-immune plasma taken from convalescent patients and administered to others early in the course of infection has been of value. It may, however, exacerbate some cases, as it is believed symptoms may be caused in part by antigen-antibody complexes. Ribavarin has been successful in some cases as an antiviral agent.

There is as yet no vaccine available, and the only means of control are rapid identification and isolation of patients and control of the rat population in endemic areas.

Marburg Disease and Ebola Fever

Definition and aetiology

Marburg Disease (green monkey or vervet monkey disease) and Ebola fever are haemorrhagic fevers caused by Marburg and Ebola viruses respectively. These viruses are morphologically identical, but differ antigenically. The first cases of Marburg disease were reported in 1967 amongst laboratory personnel in Europe, who contracted the infection from imported vervet monkeys. Subsequent outbreaks have originated in the equatorial belt of Africa, although it is unclear exactly where the reservoir of primary infection lies. Person-to-person transmission occurs mainly by contact with infected blood, although sexual transmission has also been documented. The first cases of Ebola fever were reported in the Sudan and Zaire in 1976.

Both viruses cause pathological changes in the liver, lymph nodes, and spleen, while the Ebola virus has a predilection for the gastro-intestinal tract, lungs, and genitalia.

All ages are susceptible to contracting the infection, although there appears to be a greater likelihood in adults.

Symptoms

The incubation period for the Marburg virus is 3 to 9 days, and 4 to 16 days for the Ebola virus.

Both viruses produce a similar clinical illness in man and monkeys. The onset may be abrupt or insidious, usually commencing with a severe headache and fever. Myalgia and especially back pain, prostration, watery diarrhoea, and nausea and vomiting are also common. A non-pruritic maculopapular rash (which is less obvious on black skins) may develop, followed by desquamation after 3 to 4 days. In addition, chest pain, cough, sore throat, and scrotal and labial inflammation are common in Ebola fever. Severe internal bleeding usually starts within 5 to 7 days, characterised by haematemesis, melaena, epistaxis, subconjunctival haemorrhage, and petechiae. There may also be bleeding from the gums, vagina, and needle-puncture sites. In some cases, disseminated intravascular coagulation and renal failure may develop.

Severe blood loss results in death due to shock within 16 days, particularly in primary infections. Patients with secondary infections are more likely to survive, although recovery is slow.

Treatment

The mortality may be as high as 90% in rural areas of underdeveloped countries where modern methods of intensive supportive care are not available.

There is no specific antiviral therapy, but administration of plasma obtained from convalescent patients has been of value in some cases. Disseminated intravascular coagulation may be prevented by the early administration of heparin (BNF 2.8.1) under strict supervision.

Spread of the infection may be prevented by barrier-nursing patients in isolation and decontamination of all excreta and fomites.

Measles

Definition and aetiology
Measles (morbilli or rubeola) is an acute infection caused by the measles virus. It occurs worldwide, although the morbidity and mortality are greater in developing countries where overcrowded and poor socio-economic conditions prevail (e.g. west Africa).

The disease is epidemic every 3 to 5 years in remote rural villages of Third World countries, but has become endemic in urban areas. In the northern hemisphere, it has traditionally occurred as a biennial epidemic lasting 3 to 4 months during the winter and spring, although immunisation programmes have modified this picture in some countries.

The measles virus is transmitted from person-to-person in airborne droplets (e.g. by coughing or sneezing), and gains entry via the respiratory tract or the conjunctiva. It is highly contagious, infecting up to 90% of close contacts.

Those most susceptible in developed countries are children starting school. Maternal antibodies protect infants under 6 months of age and the majority of adults have acquired immunity through active immunisation or previous infection. In developing countries, younger children are most at risk.

Symptoms
The incubation period is usually about 10 days, although it may range from 8 to 14 days or even be up to three weeks in adults.

The onset is often abrupt, with prodromal symptoms of fever, sneezes, cough, nasal discharge, conjunctivitis, photophobia, and myalgia. This catarrhal stage is the most infectious. Characteristic white spots surrounded by a red ring (Koplik's spots) appear on the buccal mucosa in the region of the lower molars. After about four days, the fever abates and the Koplik's spots disappear as a maculopapular rash erupts. The rash starts on the neck and face and spreads to the rest of the body. Initially, the lesions are reddish-brown and blanch on pressure, but finally become coalescent and non-blanching. The disappearance of the rash after about five days is marked by desquamation. Further symptoms include bronchitis, laryngitis, and occasionally diarrhoea.

Convalescence is rapid in uncomplicated measles. In severe cases, secondary infections may give rise to otitis media, enteritis, ulcerative herpes simplex lesions, and bronchopneumonia (the most common cause of death).

Corneal ulceration in vitamin A-deficient children may result in impaired vision. Encephalitis is a rare but serious complication.

Subacute sclerosing panencephalitis is a rare but fatal disorder caused by persistence of the measles virus in the brain.

Treatment
There is no specific antiviral therapy for measles. Appropriate antibacterial drugs should be administered for secondary infections, while symptomatic treatment may include administration of non-opioid analgesics and antipyretics (BNF 4.7.1). Patients should be confined to bed, preferably in a darkened room if suffering with photophobia.

A measles vaccine (BNF 14.4) is available for active immunisation and is thought to confer life-long immunity with a single dose (see also Section 17.5). Passive immunisation using normal immunoglobulin (BNF 14.5) may be offered to contacts most at risk (e.g. pregnant women, immunocompromised individuals, and tuberculosis patients).

Mumps

Definition and aetiology
Mumps (epidemic parotitis) is an acute infection caused by the mumps virus, and occurs worldwide with a peak incidence in winter and spring. The infection is endemic in urban areas and also gives rise to epidemics.

Mumps virus is transmitted in airborne droplets and enters a new host via the respiratory tract. The infection occurs most commonly in children between 5 and 15 years of age, only rarely affecting infants.

Symptoms
The incubation period is 14 to 18 days, and the patient becomes infectious about four days before symptoms develop. Many infected individuals are asymptomatic, although still infectious.

The onset of mumps is marked in most cases by pain and swelling of the salivary glands (most commonly the parotid), which occur unilaterally or bilaterally. The patient may have a dry mouth as a result of blockage of saliva flow, and other symptoms include malaise, fever, and chills.

Mumps virus frequently penetrates the central nervous system and can cause mild meningitis, which does not usually leave any permanent sequelae. Encephalitis is less common, but more serious, and may cause convulsions. Orchitis may develop in males infected after puberty and is characterised by headache, fever, chills, lower abdominal pain, and a swollen and tender scrotum. One or both testes may be affected, causing varied degrees of testicular atrophy on recovery which, contrary to popular belief, only rarely leads to infertility. Other complications can include pancreatitis, oophoritis, vertigo, and deafness, which may be permanent.

Mumps is rarely fatal. In most cases, there is complete recovery and life-long immunity.

Treatment
There is no specific antiviral therapy, but symptomatic treatment may include administration of analgesics (BNF 4.7). The patient should be confined to bed and may appreciate a diet of soft or semi-solid foods. Inflamed testes should be well-supported, but not encased in tight bandages.

A mumps vaccine (BNF 14.4) (*see also* Section 17.5) is available for active immunisation as part of the Mumps, Measles, and Rubella vaccine.

Poliomyelitis

Definition and aetiology
Strains of poliovirus are responsible for causing poliomyelitis (infantile paralysis or polioencephalitis), occurring worldwide with a peak incidence during the summer and autumn. In areas where conditions of overcrowding and poor sanitation prevail, individuals become infected in early childhood and generally suffer only mild illness. A large proportion of the adult population is thus immune to further infection, although the immunity is strain-specific. As living conditions are improved, the age of first exposure rises and this usually results in more serious infections and epidemics. This situation has been brought under control in developed countries by the introduction of routine active immunisation programmes, but epidemics still occur in developing countries. Poliovirus type 1 is often responsible for endemic and epidemic cases, while type 3 is usually the cause of the sporadic cases in a vaccinated population. Type 2 is the least virulent strain.

The virus is transmitted from person-to-person via nasopharyngeal secretions and the faecal-oral route.

Symptoms
The incubation period varies from 4 to 12 days, and may even be as long as 35 days. The most infectious stage commences about five days before the onset of symptoms and lasts about 10 days. Many infected individuals remain asymptomatic, although still capable of transmitting the virus.

Initial symptoms are non-specific and include fever, sore throat, diarrhoea, anorexia, and nausea and vomiting. Some patients may recover after a few days, while others may progress (in some cases, following a period of

remission) to show signs of neurological involvement. These include headache, anxiety, irritability, neck and back stiffness, and drowsiness. About two-thirds of these patients do not recover at this stage and progress to develop flaccid paralysis. There may be varying degrees of improvement over weeks or months in some patients, while in others the paralysis is permanent. Complete recovery from this stage is unusual.

Paralysis of muscles involved in respiration is life-threatening, and bronchopneumonia is a common cause of death. Paralysed muscles in growing children may result in shortened limbs and other deformities.

Treatment
There is no specific antiviral therapy, but antipyretics and non-opioid analgesics except aspirin in children (BNF 4.7.1) may be administered symptomatically. Paralysed muscles should be kept warm and prevented from being stretched. Strenuous exercise, injection of vaccines, and tonsillectomy (or other surgery) during the course of the disease should be avoided as they have been linked to exacerbations of the extent of paralysis.

A vaccine (BNF 14.4) is available for active immunisation (*see also* Section 17.5), and should be included in the vaccination programme for all children. Travellers to endemic areas should also be immunised. Patients in vaccinated communities should be isolated during the infectious period, and all body discharges handled with care to prevent the spread of infection. Isolation is not an effective means of control in endemic areas.

Self-help organisations
Disabled Living Foundation
Equipment for the Disabled

Postviral Fatigue Syndrome

Definition and aetiology
Postviral fatigue syndrome (myalgic encephalomyelitis) is an ill-defined condition which occurs predominantly following a viral infection. It affects mainly adults, with a greater proportion of women reporting symptoms. Although a wide range of causes and aetiological factors have been postulated, the chronic presence of enteroviruses in muscle and gut is the most likely cause, but has not been conclusively demonstrated.

Symptoms
Symptoms often appear after an upper respiratory-tract infection and may last for months or years. The dominant features of the syndrome are muscular fatigue and emotional disturbances. Fatigue is aggravated by exercise, even to the extent that it may last for weeks following a single session of activity. Emotional disturbances may be apparent in the presence of disturbed

sleep patterns, inability to concentrate, anxiety, and depressive disorders. A wide range of other symptoms have also been associated with the syndrome (e.g. headache, neck pain, paraesthesia, cold extremities, muscle weakness, and blurred vision).

Treatment

There is no proven treatment for the condition other than complete rest. Symptomatic treatment may be beneficial and includes non-opioid analgesics (BNF 4.7.1). In cases of underlying emotional disturbances and with appropriate professional support, anxiolytics (BNF 4.1.2) and antidepressant drugs (BNF 4.3) may be useful.

Self-help organisation

Myalgic Encephalomyelitis Association

Rabies

Definition and aetiology

Rabies (hydrophobia) is a zoonotic infection of warm-blooded animals caused by the rabies virus. The disease occurs worldwide, except in Australia and Antarctica, but has been successfully eliminated from some geographically isolated countries as a result of eradication programmes (e.g. Japan and the UK).

The virus is present in saliva and other body fluids and transmitted to man in most cases via bites. In developed countries, rabies control measures have confined the reservoir of infection to wild animals, the species involved varying between regions (e.g. skunks, raccoons, and foxes in the USA, vampire bats in Latin America, and foxes in Europe). In these areas, man contracts the infection in 90% of cases from domestic animals who have had contact with wild animals. Rabies has also been transmitted by inhalation of infected secretions in bat caves. Man-to-man transmission rarely occurs, although rabies has been reported in patients receiving infected corneal transplants. In underdeveloped countries, rabies is endemic in urban areas and thus poses a greater threat to humans.

Symptoms

The incubation period is usually between 1 and 2 months, although longer periods have been reported. Only about 1 in 6 humans bitten by rabid animals develop the disease. The risks are greater the closer the location of the bite to the head, which also tends to shorten the incubation period.

The onset is marked by a prodrome of non-specific symptoms, which include anorexia, malaise, fatigue, fever, myalgia, and headache. The bitten area, which may already have healed, becomes painful and irritable. As the virus enters the nervous system, there may be behavioural changes (e.g. a wish to be alone) and feelings of apprehension, anxiety, depression, or agitation. Further symptoms include hallucinations, convulsions, paralysis, and short periods of aggressive behaviour (e.g. thrashing or biting), which may arise as a reaction to various stimuli (e.g. noise, water, or air draughts). Between attacks, the patient is lucid. Hydrophobia is a characteristic symptom of rabies, marked by laryngeal spasm in response to sight, sound, or feel of water. The patient may die of cardiac arrest or respiratory failure during a spasm, or progress to paralysis, coma, and death. This sequence of events is termed furious rabies and is the most common form in man.

Paralytic (dumb) rabies occurs in less than 20% of cases, and is particularly associated with infection contracted from vampire bats or in patients who have received post-exposure rabies vaccine. Hydrophobia does not usually occur following the prodromal period, but flaccid paralysis dominates the course, and is terminated by coma and death.

Treatment

Rabies is invariably fatal once the virus enters the nervous system. There is no specific antiviral therapy and only a very small number of patients have survived as a result of intensive supportive care.

Rabies may be prevented from developing by thorough cleansing and careful management of the wound, commenced as soon as possible after the bite. Rabies vaccine (BNF 14.4) may be administered during the incubation period as post-exposure treatment, together with antirabies immunoglobulin (BNF 14.5).

Rabies vaccine may be offered as pre-exposure prophylaxis to individuals at risk (e.g. veterinary surgeons, employees in quarantine stations, wild animal collectors, and dog catchers). In endemic areas, spread of rabies may be prevented by vaccination of domestic animals and destruction of strays. Control of wild animal reservoirs is more difficult. In rabies-free areas, strict regulations governing import and quarantine of animals is required.

Rubella

Definition and aetiology

Rubella (German measles) is caused by the rubella virus, and occurs worldwide with a peak incidence in spring and early summer in temperate climates.

The virus resides in the upper respiratory tract and is transmitted from person-to-person by droplets.

Rubella occurs most commonly in children, particularly those under 9 years of age, although non-immune young adults living together in groups (e.g. college students and military recruits) are also susceptible.

Symptoms

The incubation period is usually 17 days, although it can range from 14 to 21 days. The most infectious period commences about one week before the rash appears and lasts about 11 days.

Rubella is a mild self-limiting infection characterised by a rose-coloured, evanescent, papular rash spreading from the face to the trunk and finally the limbs. It may be accompanied by mild constitutional symptoms of malaise, slight fever, headache, conjunctivitis, and lymphadenopathy. Arthritis occurs frequently in adults (particularly women), but is rarely permanent.

The rash usually lasts for a maximum of three days. It is followed by a rapid and complete recovery, with life-long immunity against subsequent attacks. In some cases, rubella may occur without the rash, making accurate diagnosis difficult.

Rubella occurring during pregnancy (particularly the first trimester) poses a threat to the foetus, and may result in abortion, stillbirth, or congenital malformations, some of which may not present until later in life. Cataracts, heart defects, and deafness are common disorders. Hepatitis and hepatosplenomegaly, visual defects, meningo-encephalitis, microcephaly, and osteopathy may also occur.

Treatment

There is no specific antiviral therapy and symptomatic treatment is rarely required. Women contracting rubella early in pregnancy may wish to consider therapeutic abortion. Alternatively, passive immunisation with normal immunoglobulin (BNF 14.5) may afford some protection to the foetus.

Rubella vaccine (BNF 14.4) is available for active immunisation of non-immune females to prevent congenital rubella infections in subsequent pregnancies (*see also* Section 17.5). It is a component of MMR vaccine.

Self-help organisation
National Rubella Council

Smallpox

Definition and aetiology

The world was officially declared free from smallpox in 1980, more than two years after the last reported endemic case in Somalia in 1977.

Smallpox was caused by the variola virus and, before eradication, was endemic in parts of Africa, south-east Asia, and Brazil, although no country was free from the risk of imported cases.

Transmission of infection occurred from person-to-person via the respiratory tract. There was no known animal reservoir, the infection did not become latent in surviving patients, and there were no chronic carriers. Spread of infection was slow and resulted in highly localised incidence. The combination of these factors made eradication possible.

Symptoms

The incubation period was about 12 days, during which time the patient was not infectious.

The onset was abrupt with symptoms of fever, prostration, headache, aching, and nausea and vomiting. A characteristic maculopapular rash appeared after 3 to 5 days as the fever abated. The lesions became vesicular and then pustular, forming scales, and finally separating after about three weeks, leaving hypopigmented areas. Smallpox lesions were all at the same stage of development, unlike those of chickenpox, which appear in crops. The patient was infectious until the rash subsided. The severity of symptoms depended to a great extent on the host's resistance, and varied from subclinical non-infectious cases to haemorrhagic smallpox, which was invariably fatal.

Death generally occurred during the second week of the rash. Surviving patients were usually marked by dermal pits and scars and many suffered loss of vision.

Treatment

There was no specific treatment for smallpox. Early administration of smallpox vaccine (BNF 14.4) or immunoglobulins or methisazone to contacts prevented development of the disease or converted it to a milder form.

Routine active immunisation against smallpox is no longer practised in any country. The vaccine is held in selected centres and only deemed necessary for laboratory personnel working with orthopoxviruses.

Eradication of the disease was effected by a worldwide campaign begun in 1967. Mass immunisation in endemic areas was undertaken, and the chain of transmission broken by seeking and isolating infected patients and vaccinating contacts. The search continued for two years after the last reported case in each area to ensure complete eradication.

Warts

Definition and aetiology

Warts (verrucae) are circumscribed, benign, contagious, epithelial growths induced by human papillomavirus. Viral entry is effected through damaged or moist skin.

Symptoms

Warts occur most frequently in older children and are generally uncommon in infants and the elderly. The lesions are firm and may be single or multiple, flesh-coloured, brown, grey, yellow, or black. They often regress spontaneously within 6 to 24 months.

Common warts (verruca vulgaris) occur most frequently. They are usually located on the hands and fingers, less commonly on the elbows and knees. They may be irregularly shaped or round with a rough surface. Peri-ungual warts occur around the nails, are usually associated with nail biting, and are often painful. Verruca plana are warts occurring on the face. Plantar warts (verruca plantaris) are commonly referred to as verrucae, and occur on the soles of the feet, usually in the weight-bearing regions (Fig. 5.5). They are flattened by pressure and are often tender and painful. Small black pinpoints representing thrombosed blood vessels may be seen on paring away the surface. Mosaic warts are groups of plantar warts occurring close together or becoming confluent. Condylomata acuminata (anogenital warts) are sexually-transmitted warts and are usually moist and soft.

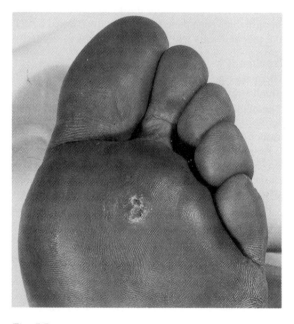

Fig. 5.5
Confluent plantar warts.

Treatment
In most cases, warts will disappear spontaneously. Where indicated, treatment may involve the use of a keratolytic preparation for warts and calluses (BNF 13.7). For common and plantar warts, this may be followed by careful removal of dead tissue. Soaking the affected foot in a solution of formaldehyde may be of value in treating mosaic warts. Physical means of removal (e.g. cauteris-

ation, curettage, electrodesiccation, liquid nitrogen, and solid CO_2), may be be necessary in resistant cases.

Prevention of transmission of warts can be encouraged by avoiding barefooted communal activities (e.g. swimming in public baths) and ensuring personal use of towels and bath mats. An occlusive dressing may also minimise the risks of transmission.

Yellow Fever

Definition and aetiology
Yellow fever is a haemorrhagic fever, endemic in tropical areas of Africa and South and Central America, and caused by the yellow fever virus.

The vector of the infection is a mosquito (*Aedes* spp.), which maintains a cycle with man in urban areas. In forested regions, yellow fever is a zoonotic infection involving monkeys, mosquitoes, and man.

Symptoms
The incubation period is 3 to 6 days. The severity of symptoms varies from mild to fulminating and fatal, often being more severe in travellers than the indigenous population. Yellow fever has an abrupt onset with fever, headache, rigors, myalgia, back pain, and nausea and vomiting. The face is often flushed and oedematous, with swollen lips and gums and injection of the conjunctiva. Bleeding from the nose and gums may also occur. A period of remission usually occurs after 1 to 3 days, during which time the fever and other symptoms subside. Mild cases may start to recover at this stage, but in severe cases the symptoms reappear in a more exaggerated form. Jaundice may become obvious, and more serious bleeding results in melaena, haematemesis ('coffee grounds' or black vomit), petechiae, and ecchymoses. Renal damage may occur, causing albuminuria and a reduction in urine output.

The overall mortality rate of yellow fever is 5%, although 50% of severe cases may be fatal with death almost always occurring before the tenth day. Relapses in surviving patients are uncommon.

Treatment
There is no specific treatment for yellow fever.

Supportive treatment includes maintenance of fluid and electrolyte levels, blood transfusion, dialysis, and intensive monitoring of all vital functions.

An effective and safe vaccine (BNF 14.4), which confers long-lasting immunity, is available and mandatory for travellers to many countries. Spread of yellow fever in endemic areas may be controlled by the use of nets and screens to prevent mosquitoes from gaining access to patients. Mass immunisation and control of the mosquito population using insecticides should be undertaken during epidemics.

5.4 FUNGAL INFECTIONS

(Background information on fungi can be found in Section 14.4.)

Aspergillosis

Definition and aetiology

Aspergillosis is an opportunistic fungal infection caused by *Aspergillus* species, which may be found worldwide in a variety of habitats including soil, vegetation, grain, and materials used for construction. The most common species to cause disease is *A. fumigatus*, although *A. flavus* is often a cause of infections of the upper respiratory tract and *A. niger* a cause of infections involving the external ear.

Inhaled airborne spores colonise lung tissue which has been damaged by other chronic respiratory disease (e.g. bronchitis or tuberculosis). Antimicrobial therapy predisposes susceptible hosts to developing the disease, and immunocompromised patients are also at risk. Transmission of infection from animals or man-to-man is unlikely.

An allergic reaction to spores or fungi in the respiratory tract (allergic bronchopulmonary aspergillosis) may also occur, particularly in asthma patients.

Symptoms

An aspergilloma (fungal ball) consisting of tangled hyphae and other debris may develop in lung cavities previously created by an unrelated disorder (e.g. tuberculosis or bronchiectasis). They rarely invade and may spontaneously resolve or be expectorated. The only symptoms may be cough and occasionally haemoptysis.

Invasion of tissues may occur in transplant patients and other immunocompromised individuals, and can be fatal. In most instances, it remains confined to the lungs, although spread to other sites via the circulation (e.g. to the brain, liver, skin, or gastro-intestinal tract) is a possibility. The infected tissue becomes necrotic and suppurative. Symptoms of invasive chronic pulmonary aspergillosis include fever and productive cough.

Patients with allergic reactions may have symptoms of wheezing, dyspnoea, and productive cough, and may develop permanent pulmonary fibrosis and bronchiectasis. The condition can be recurrent.

Treatment

Surgery may be necessary for serious life-threatening aspergillomas. Invasive aspergillosis requires prompt treatment, usually by the parenteral administration of amphotericin B (BNF 5.2). Treatment of allergic bronchopulmonary aspergillosis consists of corticosteroids (BNF 6.3.4), which may be required indefinitely for re-current cases. Bronchodilators (BNF 3.1) may also be of value.

Candidiasis

Definition and aetiology

Candidiasis (moniliasis or thrush) is an acute or chronic fungal infection caused by species of *Candida*, particularly *C. albicans*. It occurs worldwide and is the most common opportunistic mycosis.

The micro-organism is a yeast-like fungus, which exists as part of the normal human flora of the mouth, gastro-intestinal tract, and vagina. Species other than *C. albicans* may also colonise the skin. Certain factors (e.g. antimicrobial therapy, pregnancy, and diabetes mellitus) increase the number of micro-organisms present, predisposing the host to the condition. Debilitated and immunocompromised individuals are also susceptible. Trauma and maceration allow development of infections of the nails (*see* Paronychia) and skin. The latter commonly occur in moist areas, especially folds and other apposed surfaces (e.g. axillae, groin, under the breasts, and napkin area). Trauma due to ill-fitting dentures may result in oral candidiasis. Most infections arise endogenously, but transmission can occur to man from animals or from person-to-person. Oral candidiasis is common in neonates and arises as a result of passage along an infected birth canal. Inhaled corticosteroids may cause infection of the mouth, pharynx, or oesophagus.

Systemic candidiasis occurs in seriously ill hospitalised patients receiving antimicrobial therapy. It may occur in the presence of indwelling catheters or intravascular lines, or following gastro-intestinal surgery.

Chronic mucocutaneous candidiasis is an uncommon condition characterised by persistent infection at several sites. Susceptibility can be inherited, or cases can be associated with an underlying endocrine disorder (e.g. hypothyroidism or diabetes mellitus). There appears to be an immunological abnormality.

Symptoms

Oral candidiasis is characterised by the appearance of creamy white raised patches on the oral mucosa. These patches may be painful and often bleed if removed. It is most common in young children and often recurs. The infection can be an early symptom of AIDS.

Vaginitis is characterised by a thick creamy white discharge, pruritus, and an inflamed mucosa with white plaques. The irritation may be exacerbated by sexual intercourse, urination, or hot baths. Male genital infection may be asymptomatic or result in balanitis, but it does not occur as frequently as vaginitis in women.

Initial symptoms of skin candidiasis are erythema and pruritus, which may become intense. Wet pustular or dry scaly lesions with well-defined edges and satellite vesicles may develop.

Infections involving the gastro-intestinal tract are often asymptomatic, but represent an important source for systemic invasion in immunosuppressed patients.

Systemic candidiasis is rare, but serious and often fatal. Organs which may become involved include the kidneys, brain, liver, bone and joints, spleen, thyroid, lungs, and heart. Blindness may develop as a result of systemic spread to the eye.

Treatment
Any underlying condition should be corrected, in addition to the administration of appropriate antifungal drugs (BNF 5.2).

Oral candidiasis may be treated with oropharyngeal antifungal preparations (BNF 12.3.2), and good oral hygiene should be encouraged to prevent further attacks.

Vaginal candidiasis is usually treated with an antifungal pessary or cream (BNF 7.2.2). Washing the affected area with warm water may provide relief during an attack of vaginitis, although overwashing and the use of irritant toiletries (e.g. soap, talc, or deodorants) should be avoided. It may be necessary to treat sexual partners concurrently to prevent reinfection. Vaginitis may be prevented by good personal hygiene to avoid contamination of the genital area with faecal matter. Tight-fitting garments made from synthetic fabrics should be avoided.

Chronic mucocutaneous candidiasis can rarely be cured, but may respond to antifungal therapy. However, relapses are common if therapy is stopped.

Cryptococcosis

Definition and aetiology
Cryptococcosis is caused by the yeast *Cryptococcus neoformans*. It occurs worldwide, but particularly in the USA and Australia.

The most common source of the micro-organism is pigeon excreta, although the birds themselves do not suffer from the infection. Man becomes infected by inhalation of micro-organisms, but is not infectious to others. Immunosuppressed patients or those with pre-existing pulmonary disease are particularly at risk of developing infection.

Symptoms
The initial site of infection is the lung, and common symptoms include fever, malaise, cough, haemoptysis, and chest pain. Cavitation may occur and the condition frequently becomes chronic. Some cases, however, resolve spontaneously.

The infection may spread from the lungs, most commonly to the meninges, although other sites (e.g. kidney, liver, bone, skin, and spleen) may be involved. Cryptococcal meningitis is characterised by headache. Accompanying symptoms may include lethargy, confusion, agitation, behavioural changes, blurred vision, photophobia, and nausea and vomiting. The course may be chronic and progressive. Most cases prove fatal within two years if untreated.

Treatment
Treatment, consisting of systemic antifungal drugs (BNF 5.2), is only required for progressive cases of pulmonary cryptococcosis or in the presence of underlying disorders or immunosuppression. Meningitis and any other signs of extrapulmonary infection always require therapy.

Pityriasis Versicolor

Definition and aetiology
Pityriasis versicolor (tinea versicolor) is a chronic skin infection caused by *Malassezia furfur* (*Pityrosporum orbiculare*), which is a commensal yeast found on skin. The condition occurs more commonly in tropical regions. In temperate zones, cases occur most frequently during the warmer months.

The infection may affect any age group, although it is most commonly seen in young adults.

Symptoms
Pityriasis versicolor is characterised by oval, slightly wrinkled, well-defined macules, which may coalesce (Fig. 5.6). They may be pink, white, or brown and do not tan on exposure to ultraviolet radiation. They occur most frequently on the upper part of the trunk, although spread may occur to the neck, upper arms, and abdomen. There may be mild irritation, and fine scales are shed on scratching. Spontaneous resolution occasionally occurs in cooler climates, but the infection is more likely to persist for years if untreated. In some cases, non-scaly depigmented areas may remain for some months after treatment. Relapse is not uncommon, particularly in tropical climates.

Treatment
Topical application of suspensions containing selenium sulphide (BNF 13.9) or pyrithione zinc may be effective. In resistant or recurrent cases, an appropriate systemic antifungal drug (BNF 5.2) may be indicated.

Sporotrichosis

Definition and aetiology
Sporotrichosis is a fungal infection of the skin and lymphatics caused by *Sporothrix schenkii*. It frequently occurs in central America and Brazil, but is no longer common in Europe.

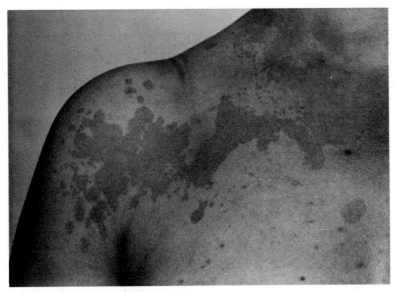

Fig. 5.6
Pigmented areas of coalesced macules in pityriasis versicolor.

The micro-organism is present in soil, plants, and bark and represents a source of infection for those whose occupation brings them into close contact with timber and vegetation (e.g. wood cutters, farmers, or horticulturists). The portal of entry is likely to be an abrasion, scratch, or insect bite. Inhalation of spores may cause pulmonary infection, although this is uncommon.

Symptoms
Sporotrichosis occurs most commonly as a subcutaneous infection. Ulceration of the primary nodule at the inoculation site is followed days or weeks later by secondary nodules, which appear along the course of the lymph channels draining the region. These may also ulcerate through the skin. 'Fixed' infections are confined to the inoculation site only, and are characterised by a single lesion, which may ulcerate. Sporotrichosis may be progressive or resolves spontaneously. Remissions and relapses over a period of years is, however, the common course.

Pulmonary sporotrichosis is usually chronic and symptoms may resemble pulmonary tuberculosis. It is often fatal if untreated. Dissemination to other sites is rare, but usually involves bone and joints.

Treatment
Cutaneous and pulmonary sporotrichosis may be treated by the oral administration of a saturated solution of potassium iodide. Amphotericin B may be of value for pulmonary and disseminated infections, but surgery may be necessary for cases of pulmonary cavitation.

Tinea Infections

Definition and aetiology
Tinea infections (dermatophyte infections or ringworm) are common fungal infections of the skin, hair, and nails caused by species belonging to the genera *Trichophyton, Epidermophyton,* and *Microsporum.* The infections occur worldwide, although the species responsible may vary from region to region.

The micro-organisms have a variety of habitats. Geophilic infections are transmitted to man from soil, zoophilic from animals (e.g. dogs, cats, or cattle), and anthropophilic from other humans. Human infections derived from animals are generally more inflammatory than those from other humans.

The micro-organisms colonise keratin and invasion is facilitated by heat, moisture, and occlusion.

Tinea Capitis

Definition and aetiology
Tinea capitis is an infection of the scalp, which is rare in adults but occurs most frequently in children. The most common causative micro-organism in the UK is *Microsporum canis,* derived from dogs and cats. *M. audouinii* is spread from child-to-child, giving rise to epidemics in schools, mainly in tropical regions. *Trichophyton* species (e.g. *T. tonsurans* and *T. violaceum*) are also responsible for scalp infections. Transmission of micro-organisms may occur by direct contact, or indirectly by means of shared towels, combs, brushes, and hats.

Symptoms

Symptoms of tinea capitis may include patchy alopecia, pruritus, and scaling, which can progress to involve the whole scalp. The hair breaks off above the scalp to leave stumps, rather than total loss of the hair follicle. Some species of fungi cause the hair to break at scalp level (black dot ringworm). *M. canis* may produce inflammation and kerions. The infection may resolve spontaneously at puberty.

Treatment

Treatment of tinea capitis consists of the administration of systemic antifungal drugs (BNF 5.2). Infected patients should not share towels or hairdressing implements with others, and in severe cases it may be necessary to cover the head.

Tinea Corporis

Definition and aetiology

Tinea corporis is ringworm of the body caused most frequently by *Trichophyton rubrum*. It is transmitted from man or animals directly by contact with infected lesions or indirectly by skin or scalp scales.

Symptoms

The characteristic ring-shaped lesion (Fig. 5.7) is initially flat, round, and red, clearing from the centre as it

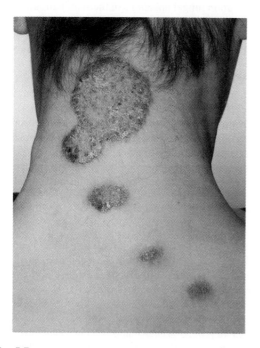

Fig. 5.7
The characteristic annular lesion of tinea corporis, with raised and reddened borders.

expands. The borders are often raised and may be scaly or blistered. There is seldom more than one lesion, which may occur at any non-hairy site on the trunk, limbs, or face. There may be pruritus, especially in animal-derived infections, and this can be further complicated by kerions.

Treatment

Tinea corporis may be treated with topical antifungal preparations (BNF 13.10.2), although refractory cases may require systemic antifungal drugs (BNF 5.2). Patients should be particularly careful about personal hygiene to prevent passing the infection to others.

Tinea Cruris

Definition and aetiology

Tinea cruris (dhobie itch) is ringworm of the groin, frequently caused by *Trichophyton rubrum* or *Epidermophyton floccosum*. It is common in all climates, although in Europe it affects men more often than women.

Symptoms

Tinea cruris is characterised by ring-like erythematous lesions with raised edges. Pruritus is often a problem and there may be inflammation, maceration, or scaling. Both groins are typically affected and the infection may spread to the upper thighs and buttocks. In tropical regions, it may be more extensive and involve the waist. Secondary bacterial infections or candidiasis may develop. Recurrences commonly occur, particularly during the summer.

Treatment

Treatment consists of the application of topical antifungal preparations (BNF 13.10.2), although in refractory cases systemic antifungal drugs (BNF 5.2) may be required. The affected area should be kept as dry as possible, and this may be facilitated by applying a non-perfumed talc. Tight clothing should be avoided.

Tinea Pedis

Definition and aetiology

Tinea pedis (athlete's foot) is a common infection of the feet, most often caused by *Trichophyton rubrum* and *T. interdigitale*, and to a lesser extent by *Epidermophyton floccosum*. It occurs worldwide, with a greater frequency and severity during the warmer months of the year. A similar infection affects the hands (tinea manuum) and often develops in the presence of existing foot infection. It occurs more commonly in adult men, especially in the presence of excessive perspiration and occlusive footwear.

Transmission may be direct from person-to-person or indirect via infected skin scales on towels, shoes, socks, or floors, particularly in communal washing areas.

Symptoms

Tinea pedis usually starts in the fourth toe cleft, and the skin initially appears cracked and scaly. It may become white and macerated, with developing blisters. Pruritus is often a problem and the skin may become inflamed. Blisters may ooze, forming crusts, and there may be secondary bacterial infection. Spread of infection may involve the rest of the foot, and in severe cases, the nail becomes distorted and thickened (tinea unguium) (Fig. 5.8). Recurrences are common.

Treatment

Treatment comprises the application of topical antifungal preparations (BNF 13.10.2) and attention to foot care. Patients should wash feet daily, drying thoroughly. Socks (preferably cotton) should be changed daily and occlusive footwear avoided. Dusting footwear with an antifungal powder may be beneficial. Systemic antifungal drugs (BNF 5.2) may be necessary in severe or chronic cases, and are always indicated if the nails are infected.

Spread of infection may be prevented by regular and thorough cleansing of floors in communal changing rooms. Patients should take care not to contaminate areas used by other people.

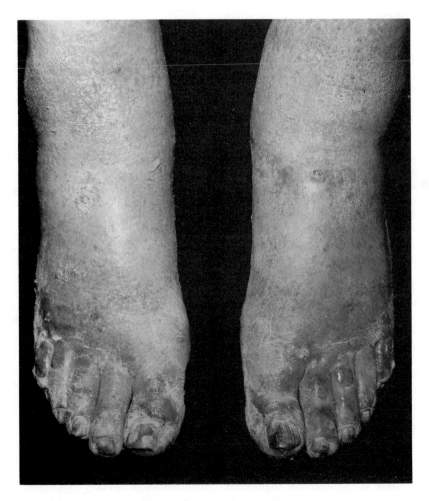

Fig. 5.8
A severe form of tinea pedis. The skin is highly macerated and blistered, and the nails are thickened and distorted.

5.5 PROTOZOAL INFECTIONS

(Background information on protozoa can be found in Section 14.5.)

Amoebiasis

Definition and aetiology

Amoebiasis (amoebic dysentery) is a protozoal intestinal infection caused by *Entamoeba histolytica*. It occurs worldwide, although most commonly in warm humid climates.

The source of the infection is faecal matter containing the encysted form of the parasite, and transmission occurs by ingestion of contaminated food or water. Direct transmission during sexual activity may also occur. The ingested cysts release trophozoites, which feed on bacteria in the colon. As they pass along the colon, they develop into cysts, which are excreted in the faeces to continue the cycle. Under certain conditions (e.g. a change in the resistance of the host, malnutrition, or immunodeficiency), the commensal relationship between parasite and host is disturbed and tissue invasion occurs, resulting in amoebic colitis.

Symptoms

Symptoms of amoebiasis may arise at any time from a few days to several years after infection, although they occur most commonly during the first four months.

Onset may be sudden or insidious and symptoms vary in severity from mild diarrhoea to dysentery. Spread to other organs may occur via the circulation, particularly to the liver causing amoebic liver abscesses. Complications of chronic infection include anaemia, emaciation, peritonitis, fibrous strictures (leading to obstruction), and irritable bowel syndrome. The infection resolves spontaneously in some individuals, while others experience relapses over several years. Many infected individuals are asymptomatic, although they excrete cysts which are the infective form of the parasite. Patients with diarrhoea are non-infectious, since they excrete only trophozoites which do not survive in the external environment.

Treatment

The prognosis is good if the infection is uncomplicated and is treated early in its course. Treatment of amoebiasis comprises the administration of amoebicides (BNF 5.4.2). Asymptomatic cyst carriers should also be treated to control spread of the infection. Supportive treatment may be necessary in patients with complications (e.g. fluid and electrolyte replacement, or blood transfusion) and aspiration of large liver abscesses may be indicated.

Amoebiasis may be prevented by improving sanitation and observing strict standards of hygiene in food handling. In endemic areas, drinking water should be boiled, and only peeled fruit and vegetables or cooked food consumed.

Giardiasis

Definition and aetiology

Giardiasis is a protozoal intestinal infection caused by *Giardia lamblia*. It occurs worldwide, most commonly in the tropics and subtropics, although endemic giardiasis is also found in some industrialised areas (e.g. Leningrad and south and eastern Europe).

The source of the infection is human faeces containing the encysted form (the infective form) of the parasite. Ingested cysts release trophozoites which colonise the small intestine. They encyst on passing into the colon and are excreted in the faeces to continue the cycle. It is possible that humans may also be susceptible to *Giardia* species harboured by other mammals. Transmission usually occurs by ingestion of food or water contaminated with faecal matter, although direct transmission from person-to-person may also occur. Those particularly susceptible to infection include children (especially if malnourished), immunodeficient individuals, and travellers to endemic areas.

Symptoms

The incubation period varies from a few days to several weeks. Giardiasis may be acute or chronic and symptoms vary in severity from asymptomatic to marked diarrhoea accompanied by malabsorption and weight loss. There may be abdominal pain and distension, flatulence, anorexia, steatorrhoea, nausea, and lethargy. Stools are usually yellow, frothy, and malodorous. Children often fail to thrive. Acute giardiasis may resolve spontaneously after 2 to 3 weeks (some individuals, however, continue to excrete cysts) or it may become chronic. Many infected individuals are asymptomatic and pass cysts from the onset of infection.

Treatment

Treatment comprises the administration of antigiardial drugs (BNF 5.4.4). It is essential that asymptomatic cyst carriers (pregnant women excluded) are also treated to curb spread of the infection.

Giardiasis may be prevented by improving standards of sanitation and hygiene, particularly with respect to food preparation. In endemic areas, drinking water should be boiled and only cooked food consumed where possible. Raw vegetables and fruit should always be peeled.

Leishmaniasis

Definition and aetiology

Leishmaniasis is a zoonotic infection caused by protozoa of the genus *Leishmania*. It occurs in the semi-arid and desert regions of Africa, central Asia, China, India, the Mediterranean basin, and the Middle East (Old World leishmaniasis), and the tropical forests of central and South America (New World leishmaniasis).

Vertebrate reservoirs of infection include wild and domestic canines, hyraxes, rodents, and sloths; man is generally an incidental host. Transmission is effected by sandflies (*Phlebotomus* spp. in the Old World, and *Lutzomyia* and *Psychodopygus* spp. in the New World) during a blood meal. There are 12 species known to infect man, the target cells being those within the reticulo-endothelial system. Infection may occasionally be acquired as a result of sexual or congenital transmission, or blood transfusion.

Cutaneous Leishmaniasis

Definition and aetiology

Cutaneous leishmaniasis (oriental sore or tropical sore) is due to infection with *L. major* (rural), *L. tropica* (urban), and *L. aethiopica* (highland regions of Ethiopia and Kenya) in the Old World, and *L. mexicana* and *L. brasiliensis* in the New World.

Symptoms

The incubation period varies from days to many months. Papular lesions, which may be single or multiple, appear at the inoculation site, usually on exposed parts of the body. They slowly develop into encrusted nodules and finally into ulcers, which may be wet or dry. The lesions heal spontaneously within 18 months, leaving a depressed depigmented scar. New World leishmaniasis tends to be more ulcerative and destructive than the Old World variety. Infections caused by *L. brasiliensis* may, after some years, involve the oronasopharynx, resulting in gross deformity (mucocutaneous leishmaniasis). Infection with *L. tropica major* results in immunity, and deliberate infection of the leg with local live strains of *L. tropica major* has been practised as a means of preventing unsightly lesions on the face.

Treatment

Treatment is essential in areas where *L. brasiliensis* occurs, to avoid mucocutaneous complications which may result in death due to aspiration pneumonia or obstruction. Old World cutaneous leishmaniasis is self-limiting and usually requires no treatment unless the ulcers are potentially disfiguring or disabling (e.g. a large ulcer sited over a joint or invasion of cartilage occurs). Treatment consists of the systemic administration of leishmaniacides (BNF 5.4.5). Ulcers may also be treated locally by cryotherapy, curettage, or surgery.

Prevention may be effected by using insecticides to control the sandfly population and wearing protective clothing.

Visceral Leishmaniasis

Definition and aetiology

Visceral leishmaniasis (kala-azar) is caused by *L. donovani* and affects mainly the bone marrow, liver, and spleen. Children and young adults are particularly susceptible.

Symptoms

The incubation period varies from 10 days to more than a year. The onset is usually insidious in endemic areas and characterised by intermittent fever, weakness, sweats, diarrhoea, weight loss, non-productive cough, and discomfort due to an enlarging spleen. Occasionally, there may be spontaneous recovery early in the disease. The usual course, however, is a chronic progression over several years marked by anaemia and leucopenia, hepatosplenomegaly, bleeding from mucous membranes, and emaciation leading to a final cachectic state. Intercurrent infections (e.g. dysentery, pneumonia, and septicaemia) are common and a frequent cause of death. Visitors to endemic areas often experience an abrupt onset of symptoms which may include high fever, weakness, dyspnoea, acute anaemia, and septiciaemia, with rapid progression of the disease.

Some patients in certain geographical locations (e.g. India) develop subcutaneous nodules containing large numbers of parasites following recovery from visceral disease (post kala-azar dermal leishmaniasis). It may lead to a relapse of the visceral infection. These patients possibly act as the main reservoir of infection in local areas.

Treatment

Visceral leishmaniasis is invariably fatal if untreated. Treatment comprises bed rest and the administration of leishmaniacides (BNF 5.4.5). Intercurrent infections should also be treated with an appropriate antibacterial drug (BNF 5.1). Patients benefit from a protein-rich diet and correction of other nutritional deficiencies. Further supportive treatment (e.g. correction of fluid and electrolyte balance and blood transfusion) may be indicated.

There is no effective chemoprophylaxis and the only means of prevention is eradication of reservoir hosts, and vectors where possible. This may be achieved by detection and treatment of human hosts, destruction of infected dogs, and use of insecticides. Individuals in endemic areas should wear protective clothing and sleep under nets.

Malaria

Definition and aetiology

Malaria (ague or jungle fever) is a protozoal infection caused by four species of *Plasmodium* pathogenic to man, *P. falciparum*, *P. malariae*, *P. ovale*, and *P. vivax*. It is widespead in the tropical areas of Africa, India, South America and south-east Asia.

Natural transmission in man occurs by inoculation with sporozoites from the salivary glands of female anopheline mosquitoes during a blood meal. The sporozoites migrate almost immediately to the liver where they undergo asexual division to form merozoites. These leave the liver and infect erythrocytes, and undergo further asexual division. When lysis of erythrocytes occurs, merozoites are released and infect new host cells. Some merozoites develop into gametocytes, which can be ingested by mosquitoes. Sexual reproduction takes place within the vector, producing sporozoites which continue the cycle. Infection may also be acquired as a result of congenital transmission, transfusion of blood from an infected donor, or sharing syringes and needles.

Symptoms

The incubation period varies from 10 days to many months and is determined by species of parasite and chemoprophylaxis, which may mask the initial phase.

The clinical symptoms are entirely due to the asexual blood forms, with the synchronous lysis of erythrocytes causing characteristic periodic paroxysms. There is a prodromal phase marked by influenza-type symptoms which include anorexia, headache, malaise, myalgia, and mild fever. The first paroxysm follows and is characterised by violent shivering and feelings of intense cold, which may be accompanied by nausea and vomiting and diarrhoea. After 1 to 2 hours, the patient suffers a throbbing headache, hot flushes, palpitations, tachypnoea, postural syncope, vomiting, and prostration. A high fever culminates in a drenching sweat, after which the exhausted patient sleeps. Following an initial phase of irregular fever, regular paroxysms occur every 48 hours with *P. ovale* and *P. vivax* infections and every 72 hours with *P. malariae*. The patient generally feels well between attacks. Periodic paroxysms are unusual with *P. falciparum*. *P. ovale* and *P. vivax* cause relapses over 2 to 8 years due to dormant sporozoites in the liver. *P. falciparum* and *P. malariae* cause recrudescent infections, which may persist for years, or in the case of *P. malariae* for decades. Possible complications, particularly with falciparum malaria, include cerebral malaria, anaemia, jaundice, hypoglycaemia, hepatosplenomegaly, acute renal failure, and blackwater fever (haemolytic anaemia and haemoglobinuria).

Immunity, which is species specific, may develop in endemic areas following prolonged or repeated infections. It usually renders an infected host asymptomatic rather than preventing the disease, and such individuals continue to act as reservoirs of the infection.

Treatment

Falciparum malaria is the most serious form and should be treated as an emergency; cerebral complications account for most fatalities. Treatment of all forms of malaria comprises administration of antimalarials (BNF 5.4.1), bed rest, temperature control, and appropriate treatment of complications.

Malaria may be prevented by chemoprophylaxis (BNF 5.4.1), and must be continued for an adequate interval after departing from the endemic area. The changing patterns of drug resistance demand that all advice is completely up-to-date. The spread of the disease may be controlled by destroying mosquito breeding sites, using residual insecticides in buildings, wearing protective clothing, sleeping under nets, and detecting and treating hosts.

Pneumocystis carinii Pneumonia

Definition and aetiology

Pneumocystis carinii pneumonia is an uncommon infection caused by *Pneumocystis carinii*, a micro-organism of uncertain classification but thought to be a protozoan.

Pneumocystis spp. are harboured by many mammals (e.g. dogs, goats, horses, rodents, rabbits, sheep, and humans). However, there does not appear to be any evidence that animals act as reservoirs for human infections. Transmission between humans is possibly by an airborne route or may occur from mother-to-foetus. The lungs represent the major target organ, although the micro-organisms have been found in rare cases in lymph nodes, bone marrow, and the spleen. Those most susceptible to developing disease are malnourished or premature infants and immunocompromised hosts, especially those suffering with AIDS.

Symptoms

A large proportion of healthy individuals are infected with *P. carinii* without showing any clinical signs. *P. carinii* pneumonia is characterised by dyspnoea, tachypnoea, and a non-productive cough, often accompanied by fever and cyanosis, and culminating in respiratory insufficiency and death. The course is variable, arising insidiously over weeks or months (characteristic of AIDS patients and children suffering with congenital immunodeficient disorders) or progressing rapidly.

Treatment

The disease is always fatal if untreated. Treatment is usually successful, especially if started early, although some recurrences do occur, particularly with AIDS patients. It consists of the administration of co-trimoxazole (BNF 5.1.8), which may also be used as chemoprophylaxis in patients with a high risk of developing active disease.

Primary Amoebic Meningo-encephalitis

Definition and aetiology
Primary amoebic meningo-encephalitis is a rare protozoal infection of the brain and meninges caused by some species of free-living amoebae.

Naegleria fowleri infection appears to be contracted during swimming in contaminated freshwater lakes or pools. The micro-organism enters via the nose and crosses the cribriform plate of the ethmoid bone to invade the central nervous system. *Acanthamoeba* and *Hartmannella* spp. are associated with subacute infections in immunocompromised individuals. The pathogenesis is unknown, although it is possible that *Acanthamoeba* spp. gain entry via abrasions on the skin or cornea. They may also be inhaled or swallowed, as they exist as windborne cysts.

Symptoms
Both forms of the infection give rise to fever, meningitis, and haemorrhagic encephalitis. *N. fowleri* infections are more fulminant and result in death in a few days.

Treatment
Early treatment is essential, especially for *N. fowleri* infections, and consists of the intravenous and intrathecal administration of amphotericin B.

Toxoplasmosis

Definition and aetiology
Toxoplasmosis is a common protozoal infection caused by *Toxoplasma gondii*. It is a worldwide zoonosis involving birds and mammals (including man), with the domestic cat as the definitive host.

Sexual reproduction takes place in the intestinal epithelial cells of the cat forming oocysts, which are excreted and may remain viable for many months in warm moist soil (Fig. 5.9). The infection is acquired by ingestion of oocysts, present in cat faeces only, or tissue cysts in undercooked meat. Trophozoites are released, invade the intestinal mucosa, and spread to other organs via the circulation. They reproduce asexually until the host develops immunity and cysts are formed within the tissues, particularly in cardiac and skeletal muscle, lymph nodes, the retina, and brain. Insects may play a role in transferring oocysts to food. Transmission may also occur from mother-to-foetus and in organ transplants from infected donors. Children are particularly at risk of becoming infected when playing in soil or sand contaminated with cat faeces.

Symptoms
The majority of patients infected with *T. gondii* are asymptomatic, although cysts may lie dormant in living tissues for years and only cause active disease if the host's immunity is compromised (e.g. those taking immunosuppressant drugs or suffering from AIDS or Hodgkin's disease). Commonly occurring symptoms in mild infections include fever, malaise, and lymphadenopathy, and may be accompanied by fatigue, myalgia, and a maculopapular rash. There is usually complete recovery after several weeks or months. Fulminating disseminated toxoplasmosis, which may be fatal, occurs in immunodeficient hosts. Symptoms include hepatitis, hepatosplenomegaly, meningo-encephalitis, myocarditis, and pneumonitis.

Congenital transmission only occurs if the mother (who may remain asymptomatic) acquires the infection immediately prior to or after conception. The consequences for the foetus are most severe if the disease is contracted during the first trimester, and may result in abortion or stillbirth. Symptoms of varying severity which arise at birth or later include hepatosplenomegaly, hydrocephalus, microcephaly, convulsions, mental retardation, spasticity, and deafness. Chorioretinitis develops in adulthood and, if recurrent, may lead to loss of vision.

Treatment
Treatment (BNF 5.4.7) is only necessary in the presence of complications and for immunodeficient patients. Treatment of pregnant women is complicated by the risk of teratogenesis. There is no drug available to eradicate tissue cysts.

Toxoplasmosis may be prevented by avoiding the consumption of rare meat, especially pork and lamb. Children should be discouraged from sucking their fingers, particularly when playing outside, and instructed to always wash their hands before eating. Cat-litter trays should be cleansed daily and sterilised with boiling water.

Trichomoniasis

Definition and aetiology
Trichomoniasis is a common protozoal infection of the genital tract caused by *Trichomonas vaginalis*. It is sexually transmitted in the majority of cases and occurs most commonly in females during the reproductive years. Males are often asymptomatic carriers of the micro-organism.

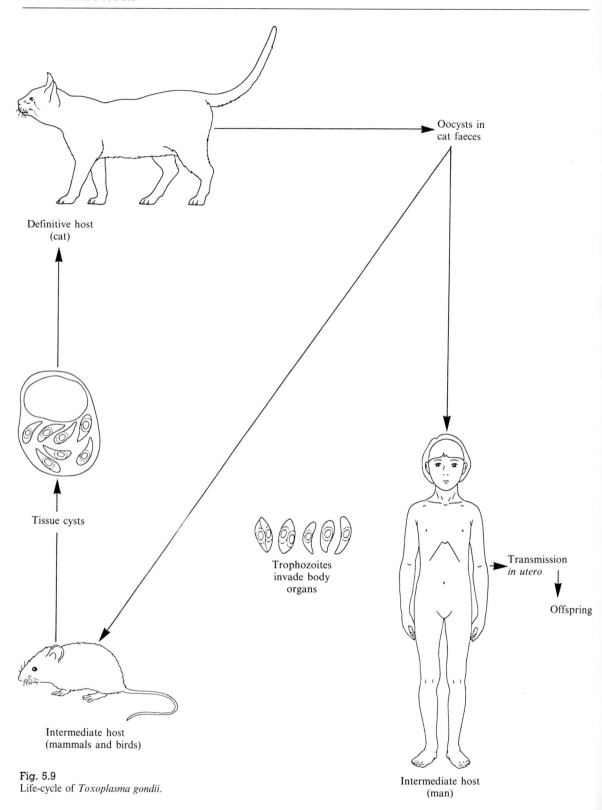

Fig. 5.9
Life-cycle of *Toxoplasma gondii*.

Definitive host
(cat)

Oocysts in
cat faeces

Tissue cysts

Trophozoites
invade body
organs

Transmission
in utero

Offspring

Intermediate host
(mammals and birds)

Intermediate host
(man)

Symptoms

Symptoms in females vary from mild to severe vaginitis, with a scanty or profuse, frothy, yellow discharge with an offensive odour. Accompanying symptoms include pruritus vulvae, vulval swelling, cystitis, and dyspareunia. Males may develop urethritis, cystitis and prostatitis. Trichomoniasis is often associated with other sexually-transmitted diseases (e.g. gonorrhoea) because *T. vaginalis* may carry pathogenic bacteria on its surface.

Treatment

Trichomoniasis should be treated promptly and investigations undertaken to detect any other sexually-transmitted disease. Treatment consists of the administration of trichomonacides (BNF 5.4.3).

It may be prevented from further spread by concurrent treatment of sexual partners and refraining from sexual intercourse until cured.

Trypanosomiasis

Definition and aetiology

Trypanosomiasis is an infection caused by protozoa of the genus *Trypanosoma*. There are two different forms of the disease, African trypanosomiasis (sleeping sickness) and American trypanosomiasis (Chagas' disease).

African Trypanosomiasis

Definition and aetiology

African trypanosomiasis occurs in the tropical regions of Africa and is caused by two subspecies of *T. brucei* pathogenic to man, *T. b. gambiense* (Gambian sleeping sickness, occurring in west and central Africa) and *T. b. rhodesiense* (Rhodesian or east African sleeping sickness).

The infection is transmitted as a zoonosis between various mammalian hosts by flies of the genus *Glossina* (tsetse flies). Trypanosomes ingested by a fly during a blood meal from an infected host develop within the vector for 2 to 5 weeks, and are then passed on to a new host in the fly's saliva. The natural host for Gambian sleeping sickness is man, although animals (e.g. pigs and sheep) may also enter the cycle. Wild game (e.g. antelopes) are the main reservoirs of *T. b. rhodesiense* infection, which is transmitted to humans entering endemic areas. Infection may also arise as a result of laboratory accidents with infected specimens, blood transfusion, and occasionally by congenital transmission.

Symptoms

Gambian sleeping sickness is a chronic disease and develops slowly over 2 to 3 years. There is an initial nodular lesion (chancre) at the inoculation site which may remain unnoticed. Spread to lymph nodes and the bloodstream occurs some weeks or months later and may give rise to intermittent fever, malaise, headache, lymphadenopathy, urticaria, and anaemia. An asymptomatic period lasting months or years may follow before invasion of the central nervous system occurs. There is a progressive neurological degeneration, characterised by personality changes, delusions, hallucinations, mania, drowsiness, and convulsions. Severe pruritus, headache, and back pain may also occur. A deterioration in the level of consciousness leads to coma. Death is often brought about by a secondary infection (e.g. pneumonia).

The symptoms of Rhodesian sleeping sickness are similar to Gambian, but proceed with a more rapid and severe course and less clearly defined stages. Death often occurs within a year due to heart failure, before invasion of the CNS has occurred. Patients do not develop immunity to African trypanosomiasis.

Treatment

Once invasion of the CNS has occurred, death is inevitable unless the disease is treated. Most cases respond well to treatment, especially in the early stages. Treatment (BNF 5.4.6) should be undertaken by specialists. Any underlying nutritional deficiencies should be corrected and complications (e.g. anaemia and intercurrent infection) treated. Preventive measures include reducing the human reservoir of infection by detecting and treating infected individuals early.

American Trypanosomiasis

Definition and aetiology

American trypanosomiasis is a protozoal infection caused by *Trypanosoma cruzi* and is endemic in remote rural areas of Central and South America.

Reservoirs of infection include the cat, dog, armadillo, opossum, rodents, and man. The vectors are bugs of the family *Reduviidae*, several species of which have adapted to cohabit with man, living in cracks in the walls of poorly constructed houses. The bug ingests trypanosomes during a blood meal from an infected host. The trypanosomes multiply within the vector and are passed on to a new host during defaecation after feeding. The parasite gains entry into the new host through skin abrasions, mucous membranes, or the conjunctiva and multiplies in myocardial cells and smooth muscle cells of the gastro-intestinal tract.

Symptoms

The incubation period is 4 to 12 days, although many patients show no detectable signs of disease. The majority of those presenting with an acute phase illness are children, approximately half of whom develop a visible lesion at the inoculation site. Subsequent symptoms, which persist for 2 to 4 months, include fever, weakness, facial oedema, lymphadenopathy, and hepato-splenomegaly. The ensuing intermediate phase may last for decades in some individuals before signs of chronic disease become apparent. The usual manifestations of chronic disease are cardiomyopathy or dilatation of the oesophagus or colon (mega syndromes). The course of the disease and prognosis are variable. A small propor-tion of patients die of myocarditis or acute meningo-encephalitis in the acute phase, although some in-dividuals never develop chronic complications. If chronic organ damage does occur, it is irreversible.

Treatment
All acute cases should be treated, as this stage deter-mines the subsequent course of the disease. Treatment (BNF 5.4.6) should be undertaken by specialists and comprises the administration of nifurtimox and benznidazole, which are of value in the acute phase only. Chronic cardiomyopathy requires symptomatic treat-ment and surgery may be necesary for the mega syndromes. Infected adults showing no abnormalities on the electrocardiogram should be reassured that they may not necessarily develop chronic complications.

American trypanosomiasis may be prevented by improving housing conditions, health education, using insecticides in homes, and detecting and treating infected individuals early in an effort to eliminate the reservoir of infection.

5.6   HELMINTHIC INFECTIONS

(Background information on helminths can be found in Section 14.6.)

Cestode Infections

Definition and aetiology
Dwarf tapeworm infection is caused by *Hymenolepis nana* and occurs in warm dry climates (e.g. Africa, the Middle East, South America, and south and east Europe). It occurs most commonly in children, as host resistance improves with age and the adult tapeworm survives for only a few months. No intermediate host is required and the infection may be passed from person-to-person by faecal contamination of food and water. Auto-infection may also occur, internally or by hand-to-mouth transmission.

Fish tapeworm infection is caused by *Diphyllobothrium*

latum, which is the largest tapeworm infecting man (up to 10 m long). It is prevalent in areas where raw or under-cooked freshwater fish are consumed (e.g. Alaska, Fin-land, Japan, Siberia, and Sweden). The first intermediate host is a copepod (a minute aquatic arthropod), which is ingested by freshwater fish (e.g. perch, pike, turbot, and salmon). The adult tapeworm may survive for up to 20 years.

Hydatid disease is an infection with larval forms of *Echinococcus granulosus*, which occurs worldwide, parti-cularly in sheep-rearing areas. The definitive host is the domestic or wild dog, with sheep acting as the main inter-mediate host. Man is an incidental host and contracts the infection by ingesting eggs present in contaminated food and water or by close contact with infected dogs.

Taeniasis is caused by *Taenia saginata* (beef tapeworm) or *T. solium* (pork tapeworm) and occurs worldwide in areas where poor standards of sewage disposal exist. Man is the only definitive host, contracting the infection by ingesting raw or undercooked beef or pork containing cysticerci (Fig. 5.10). The adult tapeworm can survive for years in the small intestine, reaching a length of 2 to 4 m (*T. solium*) or 4 to 10 m (*T. saginata*). **Cysticercosis** occurs if humans ingest eggs and thus become infected with larval forms of *T. solium*, which may migrate to any body tissue but particularly muscle, subcutaneous tissue, and the central nervous system. The infection is contracted by consumption of contaminated food or water. It may also be due to auto-infection with eggs in an individual already harbouring an adult tapeworm, either by the hand-to-mouth route or by the passage of eggs to the stomach by reverse peristalsis (e.g. vomiting).

Symptoms
Infections with adult tapeworms are often asymptomatic unless the worm load is heavy, when mucosal irritation may lead to gastro-intestinal disturbances (e.g. abdomi-nal discomfort, diarrhoea, and nausea and vomiting). Other symptoms include weight loss, nervousness, diz-ziness, fatigue, urticaria, allergic reactions, and pruritus ani. Patients suffering with taeniasis are often aware of a 'crawling' sensation as gravid proglottides are shed from the anus. The fish tapeworm may cause pernicious anaemia.

Infections with larval forms (i.e. hydatid disease and cysticercosis) are generally more serious, and symptoms, which may not appear for several years, are due to the effects of enlarging cysts on surrounding tissue (e.g. atro-phy, compression, or obstruction). Hydatid cysts occur most commonly in the liver and lungs. Symptoms of cysticercosis usually occur when the cysts die and calcify, and are most severe if the brain is involved re-sulting in some cases in epilepsy and psychotic changes.

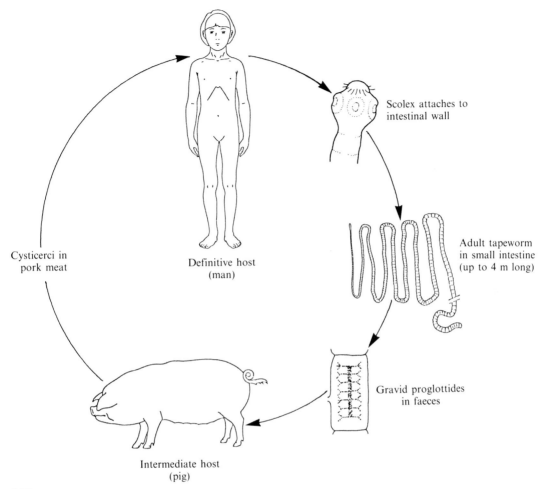

Fig. 5.10
Life-cycle of *Taenia solium*.

Scolex attaches to intestinal wall

Adult tapeworm in small intestine (up to 4 m long)

Gravid proglottides in faeces

Intermediate host (pig)

Cysticerci in pork meat

Definitive host (man)

Treatment
Treatment of most cestode infections comprises the administration of taenicides (BNF 5.5.3), while surgical aspiration or excision may be necessary for hydatid cysts. Symptomatic treatment may be required for allergic reactions or epilepsy.

Prevention and control may be effected by ensuring high standards of sewage disposal and general hygiene, and deep freezing or thoroughly cooking fish and meat. Dogs should be prevented from gaining access to uncooked sheep meat in areas endemic for hydatid disease.

Nematode Infections

Ascariasis

Definition and aetiology
Ascariasis (roundworm infection) is caused by the com-
mon roundworm *Ascaris lumbricoides* and occurs world-wide, particularly in warm climates.

Eggs ingested in faecal-contaminated food and water hatch in the intestine. The larvae pass into the lymphatics and the bloodstream, and migrate to the small intestine via the liver, lungs, trachea, and oesophagus. Mature female worms, which may be up to 30 cm long, produce eggs which are passed in the faeces and may remain viable in the soil for several years.

Symptoms
Ascariasis occurs more frequently in children than adults. Symptoms caused by migration of larval forms may include fever, cough, dyspnoea, eosinophilia, and urticaria, particularly if they die *en route*, and set up foreign-tissue reactions. Light intestinal infections with adult worms are usually asymptomatic, but large worm loads may lead to colic, diarrhoea, melaena, and intes-

tinal obstruction. Worms may occasionally be vomited. Development in children may be retarded. The disease may be fatal if ectopic migration of worms occurs to the appendix, common bile duct, and pancreatic duct.

Treatment

Treatment of ascariasis is essential to prevent the possible occurrence of ectopic migration, and consists of the administration of ascaricides (BNF 5.5.2). Surgery may be necessary to relieve intestinal obstruction.

Transmission of the infection may be prevented by improving sanitation, avoiding the use of human faeces as fertiliser, boiling drinking water, and consuming only cooked food in endemic areas. Regular mass chemotherapy may help to break the cycle.

Dracontiasis

Definition and aetiology

Dracontiasis occurs in rural areas of India and west Africa and is caused by *Dracunculus medinensis* (guinea worm).

A minute aquatic crustacean (*Cyclops* spp.) acts as an intermediate host. Infected cyclops, present in drinking water, release larval forms in the intestinal tract of the definitive host, which migrate to subcutaneous tissues (usually of the leg or scrotum) where they mature into adult worms. The adult female, which may be up to 1 m in length, protrudes a little way through the skin and discharges embryos when the skin is cooled. Those emerging in freshwater enter cyclops and develop into infective larvae.

Symptoms

Generalised symptoms include diarrhoea, eosinophilia, urticaria, and vomiting. A painful ulcer often develops at the site of protrusion and can be complicated by secondary infection (e.g. tetanus). Dead worms may calcify under the skin if not removed.

Treatment

The worm must be extracted by surgery or by slowly and carefully winding it out, which is facilitated by first killing it (BNF 5.5.7). Antibacterial drugs (BNF 5.1) may be required to treat secondary infection. (For treatment of ulcers, *see* Chapter 13.)

Transmission of infection may be prevented by filtering or boiling drinking water in endemic areas, and preventing contamination of water supplies by people with guinea-worm ulcers.

Enterobiasis

Definition and aetiology

Enterobiasis (threadworm infection) is a common infection caused by *Enterobius vermicularis* (pinworm or threadworm), occurring worldwide in urban and rural areas.

No intermediate host is required and person-to-person transmission or auto-infection occurs. Eggs, which are ingested in contaminated food or from fingers, hatch and mature in the small intestine. After copulation, the female worms migrate to the caecum and colon and travel to the anus at night to lay eggs in the perianal region. Their presence results in intense irritation causing the patient to scratch and pick up eggs on the fingers. Some eggs hatch *in situ* and the larvae return to the rectum to mature.

Symptoms

Children are affected more frequently than adults. The principal symptom is pruritus ani, and intense scratching may lead to secondary infection. Other symptoms include anorexia, emotional disturbances, insomnia, and weight loss. Occasionally, ectopic migration may cause appendicitis and in females, salpingitis. Female worms (8 to 13 mm in length) may be observed moving in faeces.

Treatment

Treatment of enterobiasis consists of the administration of drugs for threadworms (BNF 5.5.1), combined with measures to break the cycle of auto-infection. These include wearing close-fitting undergarments in bed to reduce the number of eggs shed onto bedding, a bath on rising to wash away eggs deposited during the night, daily changing of bedding and night clothes until the infection is cleared, keeping nails trimmed and well-scrubbed, and always washing hands after using the toilet and before eating or handling food. All the members of a household should be treated at the same time.

Filariasis

Definition and aetiology

Filariasis is a disease caused by filarial worms, 8 species being responsible for infection in man. They all rely on arthropods as intermediate hosts and vectors. Larvae are transferred to man during a blood meal and mature into adult forms which inhabit the lymphatic system, subcutaneous tissues, or connective tissues, depending on the species. After fertilisation, the female continuously produces microfilariae (motile prelarval forms), which circulate in the bloodstream or skin. When ingested by a suitable arthropod, they undergo further development to the infective larval stage. Adult worms of some species may survive for as long as 15 years.

Wuchereria bancrofti and *Brugia malayi* are lymphatic dwelling filariids. The infection is transmitted by mosquitoes in tropical and subtropical regions.

Onchocerca volvulus relies on the female black-fly (*Simulium* spp.) as an intermediate host (Fig. 5.11) and causes onchocerciasis (river blindness), a subcutaneous infection occurring in tropical regions of Africa, Mexico, and parts of South America.

Loa loa (eye worm) causes loiasis, which is transmitted by deerflies or red-flies (*Chrysops* spp.) in the rain-forest regions of Africa. The adult worms move freely in the subcutaneous tissues and the conjunctiva.

Symptoms

Initial symptoms of lymphatic filariasis, which may not appear until up to two years after infection, include fever, malaise, chyluria, lymphangitis, and back pain. Lympha-tic blockage causing distension of distal lymph vessels and subsequent inflammation (elephantiasis) may also occur, with the legs and male genital tract most frequently affected. Light infections may be asymptomatic.

In onchocerciasis, the adult worms inhabit subcutaneous fibrous nodules or occasionally deeper nodules in the muscles or joint capsules. Their presence rarely causes symptoms, unlike the skin-inhabiting microfilariae. The incubation period may be as long as 18 months before the initial symptoms of pruritus and maculopapular rash appear. Heavy infection leads to depigmentation, scarring, and loss of elastic tissue. Ocular involvement causes keratitis, which leads to loss of vision if untreated.

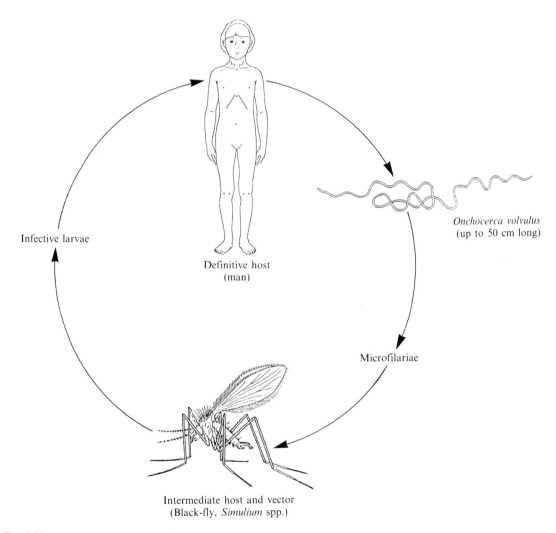

Infective larvae

Onchocerca volvulus
(up to 50 cm long)

Definitive host
(man)

Microfilariae

Intermediate host and vector
(Black-fly, *Simulium* spp.)

Fig. 5.11
Life-cycle of *Onchocerca volvulus*.

The characteristic symptom of loiasis is the Calabar swelling, which develops at least three months after infection. The swelling often develops on the face, particularly close to the eye, and over medium-sized joints. It lasts about 2 to 3 days and may be associated with fever, malaise, and eosinophilia. The adult worms may be seen migrating through the skin or across the conjunctiva, felt as a prickling sensation under the skin, or as deeper aches with paraesthesia.

Treatment

Treatment of all types of filariasis comprises the administration of filaricides (BNF 5.5.6). Antihistamines (BNF 3.4.1) and, in severe cases, corticosteroids (BNF 6.3.4) may be necessary to control the allergic reaction and the initial exacerbation of symptoms caused by destruction of microfilariae.

Prevention of infection may be effected by wearing protective clothing and by sleeping under nets in endemic areas.

Hookworm Infection

Definition and aetiology

Hookworm infection is an intestinal infection caused by *Ancylostoma duodenale* (Old World hookworm), occurring in warm, humid, temperate, and tropical climates, and *Necator americanus* (New World hookworm), occurring in the tropics.

No intermediate host is required. Larvae present in soil penetrate the host's skin (usually the feet), enter the circulation, and migrate to the intestines via the heart, lungs, trachea, and oesophagus. Infection may also be contracted by ingestion of larvae in contaminated drinking water. Mature female worms produce eggs for many years, which are passed in the faeces and hatch in warm moist soil.

Symptoms

There may be an initial reaction at the site of entry (ground itch). The adult worm feeds upon blood and interstitial fluid in the intestinal wall. Heavy infections produce serious symptoms which include anaemia, abdominal pain, gastro-intestinal disturbances, hypoalbuminaemia, oedema, palpitations, and retarded growth in children; light infections are usually asymptomatic. Larvae migrating through the lungs in sufficient numbers may result in symptoms of bronchitis.

Treatment

Treatment comprises the administration of drugs for hookworms (BNF 5.5.4). It may also be necessary to treat severe anaemia.

The cycle of transmission may be broken by improving standards of sanitation, boiling drinking water, and always wearing shoes outdoors in endemic areas.

Strongyloidiasis

Definition and aetiology

Strongyloidiasis is an intestinal infection caused by *Strongyloides stercoralis*, which occurs in humid tropical climates.

Infective larval forms present in faecal-contaminated soil penetrate man's skin (usually the feet) and migrate to the small intestine via the lungs, trachea, and oesophagus. They mature into adult worms, which inhabit the mucosa and submucosa. Eggs produced by the female worms hatch within the host, the non-infective larvae passing in the faeces to the external environment where they develop into infective forms. Occasionally, their development may take place in the bowel, thus allowing auto-infection and a build-up of large numbers of worms. The infection may persist for more than 30 years.

Symptoms

Strongyloidiasis is usually asymptomatic if worm loads are light, although there may be an initial reaction (ground itch) at the site of entry. Heavy infection may result in abdominal pain, diarrhoea and, in severe cases, malabsorption. Larvae migrating through the lungs may cause cough, pneumonitis, and sometimes death due to alveolar haemorrhage. Occasionally, larvae may migrate through the skin (cutaneous larva migrans) and cause pruritus and urticaria.

Treatment

Treatment is by the administration of drugs for strongyloidiasis (BNF 5.5.8). Vitamin supplements (BNF 9.6) and iron with folic acid (BNF 9.1.1) may be indicated in patients with chronic disease.

The infection may be prevented by avoiding skin contact with soil in endemic areas and improving standards of sewage disposal.

Toxocariasis

Definition and aetiology

Toxocara canis and less commonly *T. cati* are roundworms of dogs (mainly puppies) and cats respectively. They cause toxocariasis in man, who is not a definitive host.

The infection is contracted mainly by children ingesting eggs in faecal-contaminated soil. It is also possible to pick up eggs from the coat of an infected dog or from food to which eggs have been transferred by flies. The eggs hatch in the intestine, releasing larvae which may pass to any body tissue via blood and lymph (visceral larva migrans).

Symptoms

Toxocariasis is often asymptomatic unless the larvae penetrate vital organs, in which case even light infections are potentially serious. General symptoms may include cough, eosinophilia, fever, and malaise, while specific symptoms caused by burrowing larvae and granulomatous reactions to dead larvae depend on the site involved. These may include asthma, bronchitis, epilepsy, hepatomegaly, and loss of vision. The larvae survive for one year only and the infection resolves spontaneously in the absence of reinfection. Irreparable damage may, however, occur within that time.

Treatment
Diethylcarbamazine is used in the treatment of toxocariasis, but treatment must be started early to prevent permanent damage. Relapses may occur.

The disease may be controlled by prohibiting dog-owners from allowing their pets to foul public parks and children's playgrounds. All dogs (and especially puppies) should be routinely wormed and puppy faeces incinerated. Disinfectants are of little value in destroying the eggs. Children should be encouraged to wash their hands before eating, and discouraged from sucking their fingers or ingesting soil when playing outside.

Trichiniasis

Definition and aetiology
Trichiniasis (trichinosis) is an intestinal infection caused by a small roundworm, *Trichinella spiralis*, occurring worldwide, particularly in temperate zones.

There are many definitive hosts, including man, and the infection is contracted by ingestion of undercooked infected meat (e.g. pork); no intermediate host is required. Larvae within cysts are released in the small intestine and mature into adult worms. These in turn produce larvae, which are carried in blood and lymph to striated muscle (particularly abdominal muscles, the diaphragm, tongue, larynx, and larger voluntary muscles) where they encyst and remain viable for years.

Symptoms
Light infections are often asymptomatic, but heavy infections produce symptoms which depend on the parasite's stage of development and the site involved.

Young adult worms burrowing into the intestinal wall may cause abdominal pain, diarrhoea, fever, and nausea and vomiting during the first week. Later symptoms are due to larvae migrating to the muscles and include eosinophilia, fever, facial oedema, and myositis. Invasion of the diaphragm may cause dyspnoea, while involvement of the tongue or larynx may lead to aphonia. Larvae may invade myocardial muscle and cause arrhythmias. After about three weeks, the patient usually starts to recover as cyst formation commences, although fatal complications may arise due to involvement of myocardial tissue, the lungs, and the central nervous system.

Treatment
Treatment comprises the administration of thiabendazole (BNF 5.5.8) and symptomatic relief for complications.

The spread of infection may be prevented by thoroughly cooking pork, freezing raw meat at $-18°C$, and improving the standards of pig-rearing (e.g. by carefully controlling their diet).

Trichuriasis

Definition and aetiology
Trichuriasis is an infection of the large intestine caused by the whipworm, *Trichuris trichiura*, and occurs in warm humid regions (e.g. south-east Asia).

No intermediate host is necessary. Infection is contracted by ingestion of contaminated food and water containing eggs, which hatch in the small intestine. Mature worms inhabit the caecum or colon and pass eggs in the host's faeces. The eggs become infective after three weeks in appropriate soil conditions.

Symptoms
Light infections are usually asymptomatic, but heavy infections may cause abdominal pain, anaemia (due to intestinal bleeding), colitis, diarrhoea, melaena, and weight loss. Occasionally, worms in the appendix may cause appendicitis, and rectal prolapse is a common complication in children.

Treatment
The infection is difficult to eradicate. Drugs in use include mebendazole (BNF 5.5.1) and thiabendazole (BNF 5.5.8).

Prevention may be effected by improving sanitation, avoiding the use of human faeces as fertiliser, and consuming only boiled water and cooked foods in endemic areas.

Trematode Infections

Definition and aetiology
Schistosomiasis (bilharziasis) is a chronic blood fluke infection caused by *Schistosoma haematobium*, *S. japonicum*, and *S. mansoni*, and occurs in Africa, Asia, and South America. The primary definitive host is man, who contracts the infection by contact with contaminated fresh water and passes eggs in urine and faeces.

Intestinal fluke disease occurs in south-east Asia and the Far East. The largest intestinal fluke is *Fasciolopsis buski*, whose main definitive host is the pig. Man may contract the infection in endemic areas by consumption of raw contaminated aquatic vegetation (e.g. water chestnuts). Eggs are passed in the faeces.

Liver fluke disease is caused by several species, the most important being *Clonorchis sinensis* (Chinese liver fluke), prevalent in China and south-east Asia. The infection is contracted by the consumption of raw or undercooked freshwater fish (e.g. carp or salmon). *Fasciola hepatica* is a common parasite of sheep in areas of wet pasture, but man may also contract the infection by ingestion of contaminated aquatic plants (e.g. watercress). The eggs of both species of helminth are passed in faeces.

Lung fluke disease is most commonly due to *Paragonimus westermani* (Oriental lung fluke) and is widespread in Asia. The infection is contracted by the ingestion of raw freshwater crustaceans. The eggs are passed by coughing up and spitting out sputum or in the faeces if the sputum is swallowed.

Symptoms

The onset of schistosomiasis is usually insidious, although some individuals may present with early symptoms of 'swimmer's itch', a papular pruritic rash caused by cercariae burrowing into the skin. There may be acute symptoms several weeks after infection (Katayama fever), which include anorexia, diarrhoea, hepatosplenomegaly, fever, cough, and urticaria. Chronic manifestations may not appear until several years later and are related to the site of the veins infected, which is species specific. Usually those of the intestines or urinary bladder are involved. Symptoms are caused by formation of granulomas around eggs trapped in tissues, and include portal hypertension, cirrhosis of the liver, splenomegaly, melaena, and obstruction of urine outflow. Some patients with light infections may be asymptomatic.

Most hermaphroditic fluke infections are asymptomatic or present with mild symptoms only and are rarely life threatening; spontaneous recovery may even occur. Heavy worm loads produce symptoms related to the site of infection. Heavy intestinal infections may be marked by diarrhoea, nausea and vomiting, abdominal pain, haemorrhage and, in severe cases, ascites and obstruction. Symptoms of liver fluke disease may include abdominal discomfort, diarrhoea, nausea and vomiting, hepatomegaly, jaundice and, in severe cases, cholangitis. Lung fluke infection may result in a productive cough, haemoptysis, dyspnoea, and chest discomfort.

Treatment

Treatment of trematode infections is by the administration of praziquantel (BNF 5.5.5).

Infections may be prevented by ensuring high standards of sanitation, changing particular eating habits, and treatment of all infected individuals in endemic areas. Skin contact with fresh water should be avoided as far as possible, and drinking water should be boiled in areas where schistosomiasis is prevalent.

5.7 ECTOPARASITIC INFESTATIONS

Myiasis

Definition and aetiology

Myiasis is an infestation of living tissue of vertebrates by larvae (maggots) of several species of fly (e.g. greenbottle, bluebottle, or house flies). It occurs most commonly in warm climates and eastern Europe.

The condition is uncommon in humans and is usually the result of accidental inoculation of sleeping, debilitated, or bedridden individuals. Poor living conditions and low standards of hygiene predispose to infestation. People working closely with animals (e.g. cattle or sheep) may also be at risk.

Symptoms

Symptoms vary according to the species of fly and site of body involved. The most common lesions are nonspecific and may be asymptomatic if larvae are confined to superficial wounds. Dermal invasion may result in furuncular lesions, which are swollen and painful as a result of the larvae moving under the skin and feeding on tissue fluid.

Larvae may invade orifices and produce a variety of symptoms. Pain and discharge are symptoms of involvement of the ear, with two-thirds of such patients developing otitis media. Infestation of the eye (e.g. by sheep bot fly) may cause conjunctivitis, photophobia, and swollen lids. Other sites of infestation include mouth, nose, and anogenital orifices. Accidental ingestion of larvae in food may give rise to intestinal myiasis, although in some cases, the discomfort may only last until the larvae are passed in stools.

Creeping eruptions are caused by larvae migrating under the skin, usually in the search for an exit site to continue the next phase of the life-cycle. Warble fly larvae migrate through the body dorsally and may cause serious damage or even death.

Many flies carry pathogenic micro-organisms, and secondary infections may complicate myiasis.

Treatment

The larvae may be removed by gentle compression and extraction with forceps, preferably using a local anaesthetic. Surgery or irrigation may be necessary to remove larvae from orifices. Application of an anti-infective skin preparation (BNF 13.10) may be necessary to treat secondary infections.

Myiasis may be prevented by improving living conditions and standards of hygiene, including frequent dressing changes. People at risk should protect themselves against contact with flies (e.g. by using eye shields or sleeping nets).

Pediculosis

Definition and aetiology
Pediculosis is an infestation with lice, which are blood-sucking arthropods. Three different species affect different sites of the body.

Pediculosis Capitis

Definition and aetiology
Pediculosis capitis is infestation of the scalp by *Pediculus humanus capitis*, which is transmitted by close personal contact or fomites (e.g. hats, pillows, combs, or brushes). Contrary to popular belief, lice do not jump from one person to another.

The adult louse is between 2.5 and 3.5 mm in length, greyish in colour, and inhabits the scalp attached to the base of a hair. The average number per head is 10. Eggs (nits), which are yellowish-white in colour and approximately 0.8 mm long, are laid close to the hair base. They hatch in 3 to 14 days, the length of time increasing as environmental temperature decreases. The eggs cannot be dislodged, and remain on the hairs as empty opalescent shells after hatching. With hair growth of about 1 cm per month, the distance of the nit from the scalp thus indicates the time of initial infestation. Lice survive for approximately three days away from the body and die quickly if damaged (e.g. by combing).

The condition is common in schoolchildren and is not particularly associated with social class, standards of cleanliness, or length of hair.

Symptoms
Pediculosis capitis mainly affects the scalp, although other areas of facial hair (e.g. eyebrows, eyelashes, or beard) may also be involved. The eggs are easier to see than the adult lice, and are found most frequently above the ears and close to the nape of the neck.

Symptoms of infestation include pruritus and cervical adenopathy. Severe excoriation may produce secondary bacterial infection (e.g. furunculosis or impetigo), although the lice themselves do not carry pathogenic micro-organisms.

Treatment
Pediculosis capitis is treated by the topical administration of lotions of malathion or carbaryl (BNF 13.10.4).

It is recommended that local policies should be adopted whereby only one of these insecticides is used for a given period, alternating with the other to prevent the emergence of resistant strains. Patients should be advised to follow instructions carefully to avoid the use of sublethal doses which encourage resistant strains; similarly, lotions or shampoos should not be used prophylactically.

Lice and eggs may be removed after treatment using a special nit comb with close-set teeth. All family and social contacts should be inspected and treated if infested. Fomites should also be disinfected. Vacuuming carpets may help to remove shed hairs with attached eggs.

The condition may be prevented by avoiding close head contact or sharing hats, towels, or hairdressing implements with others. Thorough combing of hair every night may damage any lice present and prevent egg laying.

Pediculosis Corporis

Definition and aetiology
Pediculosis corporis is infestation of the body by *Pediculus humanus corporis* (Fig. 5.12a), which is associated with overcrowding and poor standards of hygiene.

The eggs and adults are similar in appearance to the head louse, although the adult body louse is slightly larger (3 to 4.5 mm long). The eggs hatch within 6 to 15 days. They inhabit clothing fibres more frequently than body hairs, particularly clothes which are in close contact with skin.

The body louse also acts as a vector for some micro-organisms that cause disease (e.g. epidemic typhus fever).

Symptoms
Symptoms include pruritus and urticaria, particularly on the shoulders, abdomen, and buttocks. Small red punctate marks may be seen at the bite site.

Treatment
The treatment of pediculosis corporis is as for pediculosis capitis (*see above*). Resistant strains of the body louse are less common, and benzyl benzoate or lindane may also be effective.

Contacts should similarly be inspected and treated if necessary, and all bedding and clothing laundered in hot water and ironed.

Pediculosis Pubis

Definition and aetiology
Pediculosis pubis (crabs) is infestation of the hairs in the pubic and anogenital region by *Phthirus pubis* (Fig. 5.12b). The eyelashes may also be affected.

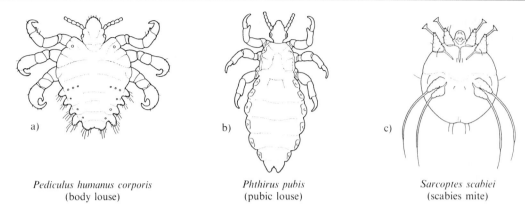

Pediculus humanus corporis
(body louse)

Phthirus pubis
(pubic louse)

Sarcoptes scabiei
(scabies mite)

Fig. 5.12
Examples of ectoparasites: a) *Pediculus humanus corporis*; b) *Phthirus pubis*; and c) *Sarcoptes scabiei*.

It is generally transmitted by sexual contact, and only rarely by fomites, as the adult louse does not leave the body unless damaged.

The adult is approximately 1 to 2 mm in length and breadth and grey-white or yellow-brown in colour.

Symptoms
Pediculosis pubis is characterised by small, non-pruritic, greyish-blue macules, irregular in outline. However, the condition itself may be irritating and excoriation may give rise to erythematous pustules.

Treatment
Treating and preventing further infestation is as for the other forms of pediculosis.

Scabies

Definition and aetiology
Scabies is a contagious skin infestation caused by a mite, *Sarcoptes scabiei* (Fig. 5.12c). It is transmitted mainly by close personal contact as the mite does not survive for more than 2 to 3 days away from the host. The incidence of scabies is not significantly linked to poor living conditions.

The female mite, which is approximately 300 μm in breadth and 400 μm in length, burrows in the stratum corneum at a rate of 2 mm a day, and lays eggs. The larvae hatch in 3 to 4 days and mature about 10 days later.

Symptoms
Scabies is characterised by severe pruritus, particularly at night. Pruritus does not commence until at least two weeks after initial infestation, and is probably an allergic reaction to the presence of the mite. A variety of lesions may arise as a result of scratching including urti-carial papules, macules, vesicles, pustules, or haemo-rrhagic crusts. Eczema may develop and be particularly severe in infants; secondary infection may also complicate scabies.

The actual burrow can easily be overlooked in the presence of other lesions. It is grey in colour, slightly raised, often curved, and between 3 to 15 mm long. Common sites include finger webs, hands, wrists, elbows, ankles, and feet. The nipples in women and male penis may be similarly affected. Palms and soles are less frequently affected in adults and the face and scalp only in infants.

Treatment
Treatment consists of the application of an appropriate parasiticidal preparation (BNF 13.10.4). Pruritus may persist for several weeks after eradication of the mite, but the patient should be advised not to reapply the parasiticide. Administration of oral antihistamines (BNF 3.4.1), the application of a topical antipruritic preparation (BNF 13.3), or both may be of value. Secondary infections may need treatment with appropriate antibacterial drugs (BNF 5.1).

All family and social contacts should be inspected and treated if necessary. Clothing and bedding should be laundered in the usual manner.

5.8 SEXUALLY-TRANSMITTED DISEASES

Chancroid

Definition and aetiology
Chancroid is a bacterial infection caused by *Haemophilus ducreyi*, a Gram-negative bacillus. It is endemic in parts

of Africa and Asia and occurs sporadically throughout the rest of the world. Its incidence appears to be associated with poor living conditions and low standards of hygiene.

The infection is transmitted sexually, invading the host through small abrasions. The incidence is greatest in men, although the exact number of cases in women is difficult to assess as lesions are less obvious.

Symptoms
The incubation period is usually less than a week, but may be as long as 2 to 3 weeks.

A small painful papule develops at the inoculation site (usually in the perianal or genital area), and rapidly develops into a pustular vesicle which ulcerates. The ulcer is shallow, painful, and tender with ragged margins and an erythematous border; there is a purulent necrotic base. Lesions may be multiple, arising as a result of auto-infection. In over 50% of cases, there may also be unilateral enlargement of the inguinal lymph nodes, which may fuse to form painful buboes. Large buboes may spontaneously suppurate through a sinus.

The lesions may persist for several months, causing tissue destruction which may be exacerbated by secondary infection. The condition is, however, often self-limiting and the ulcers heal with scar formation.

Treatment
Treatment consists of the administration of co-trimoxazole (BNF 5.1.8), erythromycin (BNF 5.1.5), or a tetracycline (BNF 5.1.3). Buboes may require aspiration.

All sexual contacts should be screened and treated if necessary. Use of condoms during sexual intercourse, or thorough cleansing of genitalia subsequently may help to prevent chancroid developing.

Condylomata Acuminata

Definition and aetiology
Condylomata acuminata (anogenital warts) are caused by the human papillomavirus, which is usually transmitted sexually. There may be an association between some subtypes of this virus and cervical cancer.

Symptoms
The average incubation period is 2 to 3 months, with a range of 3 weeks to 9 months.

Condylomata acuminata may occur anywhere in the genital or perianal area of males and females. They are small, soft, pointed, pink, fissured lesions of varying shape. They grow rapidly, become pedunculated and, because several usually occur at the same site, can resemble a cauliflower; single lesions are infrequent. They may become more widespread during pregnancy, which

favours even more rapid growth. Spontaneous resolution may occur.

Treatment
Treatment consists of the topical application of preparations containing podophyllin for warts and calluses (BNF 13.7), cryosurgery, or surgical removal.

All sexual contacts should be treated, although up to one-third of patients may relapse, but not necessarily as a result of reinfection.

Gonorrhoea

Definition and aetiology
Gonorrhoea is a bacterial infection caused by *Neisseria gonorrhoeae*, a Gram-negative aerobic diplococcus. Man is the natural host and the disease occurs worldwide.

In addition to sexual transmission, gonorrhoea may be acquired by an infant from an infected mother during birth. It is rarely transmitted via fomites, as the micro-organism does not survive for long outside the body.

Symptoms
The incubation period is shorter in men (range 2 to 14 days) than women (range 7 to 21 days).

Gonorrhoea is frequently asymptomatic, particularly in women who may remain carriers for weeks. Almost all infected males present with symptoms, the most common complaint being urethritis, characterised by dysuria, frequency, and urgency. A yellowish, purulent, urethral discharge may also occur. Complications are rare if treatment is prompt, but may include epididymitis, prostatitis, and urethral stricture. Post-gonococcal urethritis may develop after successful treatment.

The most common site of infection in females is the endocervix, and symptoms include vaginal discharge and occasionally abnormal menstrual bleeding. Symptoms of gonorrhoea in women may be masked by those of trichomoniasis, with which it is often associated. The most serious complication is salpingitis, which may lead to pelvic inflammatory disease and infertility. Other sites which may become infected in both sexes include the rectum and pharynx, and in females, the urethra.

Disseminated gonococcal infection is a serious complication affecting women more than men. Symptoms vary in severity from mild fever and arthralgia to destructive arthritis and prostration. Bacteraemia may lead to further complications (e.g. hepatitis, meningitis, endocarditis, myocarditis, and pericarditis).

The eyes are most frequently affected in neonates (*see* Ophthalmia Neonatorum), although other sites may include the pharynx, larynx, and rectum.

Treatment

The prognosis of gonorrhoea in the absence of serious complications is good. The infection may resolve spontaneously without treatment, although lasting immunity does not develop.

Treatment comprises the administration of appropriate antibacterial drugs (BNF 5.1, Table 1 and BNF 5.1.1.1) or, if the micro-organism has developed a resistance to penicillin, by administration of spectinomycin (BNF 5.1.7).

Complete control of gonorrhoea is difficult due to the large numbers of asymptomatic carriers. Diagnosis and treatment should be undertaken at specialist centres and sexual contacts traced and treated. Further spread may be prevented by abstaining from sexual intercourse until treatment is complete. Use of condoms during sexual intercourse may afford some protection against infection; counselling may also be of value.

Syphilis

Definition and aetiology

Syphilis is a chronic, contagious, bacterial infection caused by *Treponema pallidum*, a microaerophilic spirochaete. The disease occurs worldwide, although in western countries the number of cases in the late stages is declining. The number of patients presenting with early syphilis is, however, increasing.

The micro-organism gains entry into a new host via mucous membranes and skin, and rapidly disseminates throughout the body. Transmission in blood transfusions is a possibility, although other mechanisms (e.g. fomites) are rare as the micro-organism cannot survive for long outside the body. Congenital transmission across the placenta does occur, although the incidence is waning as a result of antenatal screening and treatment.

Symptoms

The incubation period is usually about three weeks, although it may be as long as three months depending on inoculum size.

The first stage of syphilis (primary syphilis) is characterised by a lesion (the chancre) appearing at the inoculation site, which is usually the genitalia although other sites (e.g. mouth, finger, or anus) may be involved. Initially, it is a painless papule which becomes ulcerated with hardened edges, and heals spontaneously within 2 to 6 weeks. The chancre may be accompanied by enlarged lymph nodes.

The secondary stage follows several weeks later, or in some cases, after several months. Conversely, some individuals may show an overlap between these first two stages. There is a macular or papular, non-pruritic, symmetrical rash characteristically covering the palms and soles; it is also evident on the trunk and limbs. Accompanying symptoms include enlarged lymph nodes, malaise, nausea, fatigue, mild fever, headache, anorexia, arthralgia, and myalgia. Condylomata lata are highly infectious, papular, pinkish-grey, discoid lesions arising in areas where two skin surfaces are in contact (e.g. axillae, perineum, and under the breasts). Greyish-white infectious mucous patches, surrounded by a red margin, develop in the oropharynx and on the genitalia. Other organs which may also be affected during secondary syphilis are the eyes, liver, spleen, kidneys, and meninges. The secondary stage resolves after a few months, although recurrences may occur in 20% of patients. Most patients enter a latent period after one year and are generally not infectious, although women who become pregnant may transmit the infection to the foetus.

After several years, some patients progress to a late non-infectious tertiary stage, whose manifestations are currently changing and becoming atypical. The classical benign lesion, which is now less commonly seen, is the gumma. This is a granulomatous lesion appearing on the face, legs, buttocks, and upper trunk as single or multiple punched-out ulcers. Mucosal gummas in the oropharynx may destroy the hard palate and nasal septum. Periostitis may affect bones and cause pain, particularly at night.

Cardiovascular syphilis may arise 20 to 30 years after infection. The most common manifestations are aortic aneurysm and insufficiency of the aortic valve, resulting in congestive heart failure and death.

The earliest manifestation of neurosyphilis, appearing five years after infection, is meningovascular syphilis. Characteristic symptoms include headache, dizziness, neck stiffness, blurred vision, papilloedema, insomnia, poor concentration, and confusion. Thrombosis and infarction may occur.

General paresis, occurring after 10 to 20 years, is now very rare. It is the result of meningo-encephalitis and has an insidious onset. It starts with fatigue, headache, irritability, personality changes, confusion, delusions, and convulsions. Patients gradually deteriorate physically and mentally until they are completely unable to look after themselves.

Tabes dorsalis is a degenerative condition commencing 20 to 30 years after infection. It is gradually progressive with an insidious onset. The first symptom is often severe repetitive lightning pains in the legs and feet, which cease as abruptly as they start. There may also be severe abdominal pain, loss of sensation in the feet, ataxia, optic atrophy, destruction of the large joints, faecal or urinary incontinence, and impotence.

The symptoms of congenital syphilis increase in severity the more recent the mother's infection. Symptoms appearing within 2 to 10 weeks of birth represent early congenital syphilis; after two years of age, the condition is referred to as late congenital syphilis. Symptoms at birth are rare, but if present, offer a poor prognosis. Early symptoms resemble the secondary stage of acquired syphilis in adults, although the lesions (which are infectious) are often bullous. In addition, there may be lymphadenopathy, hepatosplenomegaly, rhinitis, failure to thrive, and osteochondritis causing immobility in the limbs.

Many children do not develop late symptoms but remain in the latent period for the rest of their lives. In late congenital syphilis, cardiovascular symptoms do not occur, but neurological symptoms are more common than in adults. These may include interstitial keratitis, deafness, and optic atrophy. General paresis can occur between 8 and 15 years of age, although tabes dorsalis rarely occurs. Periostitis may cause misshaping of bone, resulting in bowed tibia, bossed frontal and parietal skull bones, and a saddle nose. The maxillae remain underdeveloped, and mucocutaneous gummas may cause destruction of the palate and nasal septum.

Permanent teeth show a characteristic central notch and are widely spaced (Hutchinson's teeth).

Treatment
All stages of syphilis and congenital syphilis may be treated by the administration of penicillin (BNF 5.1, Table 1). In late cases, treatment may prevent further damage but cannot reverse that already done. Follow-up examinations are required for up to a year in primary and secondary stages of syphilis, into adult life for congenital cases, and possibly for life in late cases.

Diagnosis and treatment should be undertaken at specialist centres and sexual contacts traced and treated. Further spread may be prevented by abstaining from sexual intercourse until treatment is complete. Use of condoms during sexual intercourse may afford some protection against infection; counselling may also be of value. Individuals at greatest risk (e.g. prostitutes and homosexuals) should be encouraged to attend for regular check-ups.

All pregnant women should be routinely screened and treated if necessary to minimise the effects on the foetus. Treatment before 16 weeks of pregnancy may totally prevent any damage.

Chapter 6

ENDOCRINE DISORDERS

6.1 PITUITARY AND HYPOTHALAMIC DISORDERS

Acromegaly

Definition and aetiology

Acromegaly is a rare disorder in which there is hyper-secretion of growth hormone, usually caused by a pituitary adenoma.

Symptoms

It is characterised by enlargement of the hands and feet, and coarsening of the facial features (e.g. large nose, full lips, large tongue, prominent brow, and protrusion of the jaw). The onset is usually insidious and the presenting symptoms may be arthralgia, sweating, paraesthesia, or pain and stiffness in the hands and feet. Headache and visual disturbances may be caused by the pituitary tumour. Other symptoms may include deepening of the voice, diabetes insipidus, hirsutism, hypertension, impaired glucose tolerance or occasionally diabetes mellitus, kyphosis, muscle weakness, progressive heart failure, skin thickening and seborrhoea, and thyroid disorders.

Treatment
Treatment consists of surgery (hypophysectomy), external irradiation, implantation of radioactive materials, or the administration of bromocriptine (BNF 6.7.1).

Diabetes Insipidus

Definition and aetiology
Diabetes insipidus results from impaired water reabsorption by the kidney which is caused by a deficiency of vasopressin (cranial diabetes insipidus) or, occasionally, to insensitivity of the renal tubules to vasopressin (nephrogenic diabetes insipidus).

Cranial diabetes insipidus may be idiopathic or caused by trauma, pituitary surgery, or cranial tumours or metastases. Rarely it may be caused by granulomas, infections (e.g. meningitis and encephalitis), or vascular lesions. Nephrogenic diabetes insipidus may be caused by hypercalcaemia, hypokalaemia, hydronephrosis, pyelonephritis, or may be drug-induced (e.g. by lithium or demeclocycline). Diabetes insipidus may be chronic or temporary.

Symptoms
It is characterised by polyuria with the loss of fluid ranging from 3 to 20 litres daily. This results in excessive thirst, and nocturia is also common. Dehydration occurs if patients are deprived of water.

Treatment
Treatment is directed towards removing the underlying cause. Cranial diabetes insipidus may be treated by replacement therapy with vasopressin and its analogues (BNF 6.5.2). Thiazide and related diuretics may be used in the treatment of cranial and nephrogenic diabetes insipidus (BNF 6.5.2). Chlorpropamide and carbamazepine have also been used for partial cranial diabetes insipidus (BNF 6.5.2).

Growth Hormone Deficiency

Definition and aetiology
A lack of growth hormone secreted by the anterior pituitary in childhood results in dwarfism. It is commonly caused by pituitary tumours, but is not often recognised until the child starts school and comparisons with other children are made.

Symptoms
Size at birth is usually normal, but growth rate is slower during childhood. Hypoglycaemic episodes may accom-

pany the short stature, and other outward signs include plump and immature features, and small hands, feet, and genitalia. Normal muscular development is often retarded, with 'baby fat' being more persistent.

If the condition remains untreated, puberty may be delayed, but unlike other causes of dwarfism intelligence is not impaired.

Treatment
Treatment comprises the administration of somatrem or human growth hormone (BNF 6.5.1). Therapy must continue until an acceptable adult height is reached.

Self-help organisation
Association for Research into Restricted Growth

Hyperprolactinaemia

Definition and aetiology
Hyperprolactinaemia is excessive secretion of prolactin and increased plasma-prolactin concentrations.

Hyperprolactinaemia may be of non-pathological origin (e.g. pregnancy, breast feeding, sleep, or emotional disturbances) or may be due to hypothalamic or pituitary tumours (e.g. prolactinomas), or granulomatous disease (e.g. sarcoidosis). It may also be iatrogenic (e.g. caused by phenothiazines, haloperidol, methyldopa, cimetidine, metoclopramide, or oestrogens) or idiopathic (functional hyperprolactinaemia). Other causes include hyperthyroidism and chronic renal failure.

Symptoms
It is more common in women, and is characterised by amenorrhoea or oligomenorrhoea, galactorrhoea, infertility, and hirsutism. In men, symptoms include impotence, galactorrhoea, oligospermia, infertility, and feminine-type distribution of body fat.

Treatment
Treatment consists of surgery (hypophysectomy) to remove any underlying prolactinoma, and radiotherapy or medical treatment with bromocriptine (BNF 6.7.1), or both.

Hypopituitarism

Definition and aetiology
Hypopituitarism is reduced or absent function of the pituitary gland. There may be a deficiency of only one or of all pituitary hormones (panhypopituitarism).

Hypopituitarism in the adult usually occurs as a result of destruction of the pituitary gland by a pituitary or local tumour, or metastases. Associated pressure on the optic chiasma may result in visual impairment. Pituitary damage may also be caused by infections (e.g. tuberculosis and syphilis), granulomatous disease (e.g. sarcoidosis), or trauma. It may also follow pituitary surgery, radiotherapy, or prolonged treatment with target-organ hormones (e.g. steroids and thyroxine), or occur secondary to hypothalamic disease. In women, pituitary infarction and necrosis may occur in association with postpartum haemorrhage, and results in lack of prolactin. When hypopituitarism occurs before puberty, it is usually partial rather than complete, and is dominated by growth hormone deficiency, which causes short stature. Additionally the onset of puberty is delayed or may not occur: the cause may be congenital.

Symptoms
Deficiency of a single pituitary hormone will result in deficient function of the target organ of that hormone. Panhypopituitarism results in a syndrome characterised by the total lack of pituitary hormones and of the hormones from the target glands. Lack of thyrotrophin results in fatigue and cold intolerance (*see* Hypothyroidism). Lack of adrenocorticotrophin (ACTH) results in secondary adrenocortical insufficiency, hypotension, fluid retention, pallor, and a tendency to develop coma through hypoglycaemia. Lack of gonadotrophins (i.e. follicle-stimulating hormone and luteinising hormone) results in loss of libido, impotence, infertility, atrophy of the genitalia, and loss of body hair (*see* Hypogonadism). Lack of vasopressin results in the passage of large volumes of dilute urine (*see* Diabetes Insipidus). Lack of prolactin results in failure of lactation. Patients become weak and easily fatigued, and personality changes may occur.

Treatment
Hypopituitarism is treated by replacement therapy (BNF 6.3.1, 6.4.2, and 6.5.1) and surgical removal of any underlying tumour or treatment of causal infection.

6.2 THYROID AND PARATHYROID DISORDERS

Hyperparathyroidism

Definition and aetiology
Hyperparathyroidism is the excessive secretion of parathyroid hormone by one or more parathyroid glands. Primary hyperparathryoidism is usually caused by an adenoma of a parathyroid gland, but may also be due to hyperplasia and rarely carcinoma of the glands. It usually occurs in patients over 50 years of age and is more common in women. Secondary hyperparathyroidism arises as a result of an abnormal physiological state (e.g. deficiency of vitamin D, vitamin D-resistant osteomalacia or rickets, malabsorption of calcium, chronic renal disease, or renal tubular acidosis) which leads to hypocalcaemia. The hypocalcaemia results in hyperplasia of the parathyroid glands. Occasionally (e.g. in renal transplant patients, or patients with chronic malabsorption or chronic renal failure), long-standing hypocalcaemia may give rise to autonomous parathyroid secretion and hypercalcaemia (tertiary hyperparathyroidism).

Symptoms
Primary hyperparathyroidism is characterised by hypercalcaemia and hypophosphataemia, although some patients may be normocalcaemic. A large proportion of patients are asymptomatic. General symptoms include depressive disorders, malaise, and hypertension. Reabsorption of calcium from bones is increased and results in skeletal rarefaction, the formation of cysts, and weakness of the bones; bone pain and tenderness may occur but are more common in secondary hyperparathyroidism. Kidney involvement may be marked by renal calculi and polyuria.

Treatment
Hyperparathyroidism is treated by surgical removal of parathyroid tissue (parathyroidectomy) or treatment of any underlying condition.

Hyperthyroidism

Definition and aetiology
Hyperthyroidism (thyrotoxicosis) results from an excess of circulating thyroxine or liothyronine, or both. It is usually due to diffuse hyperplasia and hypertrophy of the thyroid gland (Graves' disease), which is associated with circulating thyroid-stimulating immunoglobulins. Less commonly, it is caused by a single toxic adenoma or by multiple toxic nodular goitres (Plummer's disease). Rarely, hyperthyroidism may be caused by a well-differentiated thyroid cancer, Hashimoto's thyroiditis, or subacute thyroiditis.

Symptoms
Hyperthyroidism is characterised by an increased metabolic rate, which causes weight loss, increased appetite, fatigue, emotional disturbances, heat intolerance and sweating, diarrhoea or increased frequency of defaecation, muscle weakness, and tachycardia or atrial fibrillation. Ocular symptoms (e.g. retraction of the upper eyelid, exophthalmos, and eyelid lag) are common especially in Graves' disease. Hyperthyroidism is

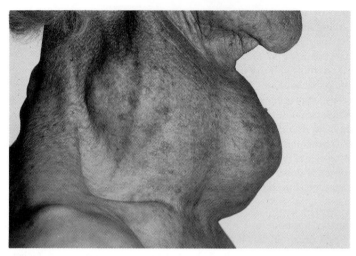

Fig. 6.1
A nodular goitre present in hyperthyroidism.

associated with a goitre (Fig. 6.1) in most patients. Other symptoms include alopecia, angina pectoris, heart failure, nausea and vomiting, and tremor. Menstrual disorders (e.g. oligomenorrhoea) or gynaecomastia may also occur.

Treatment
Hyperthyroidism is treated by the administration of anti-thyroid drugs (BNF 6.2.2), radioactive sodium iodide, or by surgery (thryoidectomy). Certain beta-adrenoceptor blocking drugs (BNF 2.4) are used pre-operatively and in the treatment of 'thyroid storm'.

Hypoparathyroidism

Definition and aetiology
Hypoparathyroidism is a reduced secretion of para-thyroid hormone and is characterised by hypocalcaemia and hyperphosphataemia. It is usually the result of removal of parathyroid tissue during thyroidectomy, parathyroidectomy, or laryngeal surgery, but may also be idiopathic (e.g. due to auto-immune disease of the parathyroid glands, congenital absence of parathyroid tissue, or may be familial). It may also be a consequence of severe and prolonged magnesium depletion. Neo-natal hypoparathyroidism occurs as a result of maternal hypercalcaemia. Idiopathic hypoparathyroidism may also be associated with Addison's disease, candidiasis, malabsorption syndromes, osteomalacia, and mega-loblastic anaemia.

Symptoms
Hypoparathyroidism results in a decreased reabsorption of skeletal calcium and a reduced absorption of calcium from the intestine. The immediate effect of hypopara-thyroidism is hypocalcaemia. Longer term consequences include mental disorders, epilepsy, cataracts, alopecia, brittle deformed nails, and dry skin. Papilloedema and other signs of raised intracranial pressure indicate calcification of the basal ganglia. Mental retardation and dental abnormalities may occur in children.

Treatment
Severe hypocalcaemia due to hypoparathyroidism is treated initially by intravenous injection of calcium gluconate (BNF 9.5.1.1). Plasma calcium is maintained in the long term by the administration of vitamin D pre-parations (BNF 9.6.4).

Hypothyroidism

Definition and aetiology
Hypothyroidism is a deficiency of circulating thyroid hormones. It may occur congenitally (cretinism) or may arise later in life. Adult hypothyroidism is often termed myxoedema. Cretinism may be caused by iodine defi-ciency, absence of the thyroid gland, a defect in hormone synthesis, or maternal ingestion of antithyroid drugs. Hypothyroidism in later life may be primary, due to disease of the thyroid gland (e.g. Hashimoto's thyroiditis or idiopathic atrophy), or to prolonged treatment with antithyroid drugs, sodium aminosalicylate, or lithium salts. It may also arise secondary to pituitary and hypothalamic disorders. Hypothyroidism may also be caused by excessive thyroidectomy or irradiation of the thyroid. Myxoedemic coma may be precipitated by exposure to cold, infections, and drugs (e.g. phenoth-iazines, opioid analgesics, or anaesthetics).

Symptoms
Early symptoms of hypothyroidism in neonates are non-specific and vague, but include constipation, lethargy, feeding difficulties, jaundice, and respiratory distress. Later symptoms include a bloated face, large tongue, umbilical hernia, and dry skin and hair. If untreated, cretinism leads to physical and mental retardation.

Onset of hypothyroidism in later life is insidious and is characterised by a gradual increase in fatigue and cold intolerance, weight gain, and constipation. There may also be swelling of the skin with mucinous infiltration (myxoedema), characterised by coarsening of the features and puffy eyes. Other symptoms may include alopecia, angina pectoris, anaemia, arthralgia, bradycardia, depressive disorders, coarsening of the voice, dry skin and hair, goitre, heart failure, menorrhagia, and myalgia.

Treatment
Hypothyroidism is treated by replacement therapy with thyroid hormones (BNF 6.2.1). Myxoedemic coma is treated by intravenous injection of liothyronine (BNF 6.2.1), and appropriate adjunctive therapy.

Cretinism is prevented by routine screening of neonates for thyroid function.

Thyroiditis

Definition
Thyroiditis is inflammation of the thyroid gland which may be acute (rare), subacute, or chronic (e.g. Hashimoto's thyroiditis).

Subacute Thyroiditis

Definition and aetiology
Subacute thyroiditis (de Quervain's thyroiditis) is a disease of unknown aetiology, although a viral origin has been proposed.

Symptoms
It is characterised by an acutely tender goitre, fever, and sweating. It most commonly affects young women and may start insidiously with features of an upper respiratory-tract infection, occasionally with dysphagia. Hyperthyroidism may develop, and very rarely the disease may progress to permanent hypothyroidism as a result of destruction of the gland.

Treatment
Subacute thyroiditis is usually self-limiting and may be treated symptomatically with non-opioid analgesics (BNF 4.7.1). More severe disease may require treatment with corticosteroids (BNF 6.3.4).

Hashimoto's Thyroiditis

Definition and aetiology
Hashimoto's thyroiditis (lymphocytic thyroiditis) is a very common chronic auto-immune disease. It is often familial and women are affected more frequently than men.

Symptoms
It is characterised by a firm, well-defined goitre or hypothyroidism, or both. Very rarely, Hashimoto's thyroiditis may be associated with clinical hyper-thyroidism. Other auto-immune diseases may occur concurrently.

Treatment
Treatment consists of replacement therapy with thyroid hormones (BNF 6.2.1).

6.3 ADRENAL DISORDERS

Addison's Disease

Definition and aetiology
Addison's disease (primary adrenocortical insufficiency) is chronic insufficiency of the adrenal cortex, resulting in the reduced secretion of glucocorticoids, mineralocorticoids, and sex hormones. The adrenocortical insufficiency is usually caused by idiopathic atrophy often attributable to auto-immune processes, or to destruction of adrenal glands (e.g. by tuberculosis or metastases). Total adrenalectomy for the treatment of Cushing's syndrome may also result in Addison's disease. Secondary adrenocortical insufficiency is usually caused by corticosteroid therapy or hypopituitarism. It results in a deficiency of glucocorticoids and androgenic secretions, but not of aldosterone.

Symptoms
Addison's disease is characterised by progressive fatigue and weakness, weight loss, hypotension, and gastro-intestinal disturbances (e.g. abdominal pain, anorexia, nausea and vomiting, and diarrhoea). Skin pigmentation or vitiligo are classical symptoms, but are not always present. The symptoms of secondary adrenocortical insufficiency are similar to, though milder than, those of Addison's disease, and pigmentation of the skin does not occur.

Treatment
Addison's disease is treated by replacement therapy with hydrocortisone (BNF 6.3.4) and a mineralocorticoid (e.g. fludrocortisone, BNF 6.3.1). Mineralocorticoids are not required in secondary adrenocortical insufficiency.

Adrenal Virilisation

Definition and aetiology
Adrenal virilisation is virilisation produced by an excess of adrenal androgens. It may be caused by adrenal hyperplasia (either congenital or acquired, as in Cushing's syndrome) or by virilising adrenal adenomas or adenocarcinomas. Mild hirsutism and virilisation may also be produced by the polycystic ovary syndrome.

Symptoms
Symptoms depend on the sex and age of the patient at the onset of the disease. Virilisation is not usually noticeable in male adults. In adult females, symptoms include hirsutism, alopecia, acne, amenorrhoea, deepening of the voice, atrophy of the uterus, clitoral hypertrophy, decreased breast size, and increased muscularity. In mild cases, hirsutism may be the only feature. Congenital adrenal hyperplasia may cause masculinisation of the female external genitalia or enlargement of the penis in boys. Affected children grow at an accelerated rate, and show advanced skeletal maturation and precocious puberty in boys. Females undergo slow and progressive virilisation.

Treatment
Treatment depends on the underlying cause. Surgery may be required for adrenal adenomas. Dexamethasone and betamethasone (BNF 6.3.4) are used in the treatment of congenital adrenal hyperplasia.

Adrenocortical Insufficiency, Acute

Definition and aetiology
Acute adrenocortical insufficiency is an acute deficiency of corticosteroid hormones caused by an exacerbation of Addison's disease by stress or infections, abrupt withdrawal of maintenance corticosteroid therapy, or attributed to adrenal haemorrhagic necrosis caused by an overwhelming infection (e.g. meningococcal septicaemia). It may also occur as a complication of anticoagulant therapy, or be precipitated by abrupt or too fast withdrawal of corticosteroids used in the treatment of other conditions.

Symptoms
The condition is rapid in onset and is characterised by extreme weakness, apathy, abdominal pain, hypotension, myalgia, nausea and vomiting, diarrhoea, and shock followed by oliguria. In the absence of treatment, death will follow.

Treatment
Immediate intravenous administration of corticosteroids (BNF 6.3.4) and intravenous fluid replacement (BNF 9.2.2) are required. Replacement therapy with corticosteroids (BNF 6.3.1) may subsequently be required. During surgery or infection and in times of stress, the physiological requirements for corticosteroids are increased, and maintenance dosage should therefore be raised accordingly.

Cushing's Syndrome

Definition and aetiology
Cushing's syndrome is a chronic overproduction of hydrocortisone by the adrenal gland which occurs most commonly in women. Most cases are caused by bilateral adrenal hyperplasia, which arises through excessive secretion of adrenocorticotrophin by a pituitary tumour (Cushing's disease). Cushing's syndrome may also be caused by benign or malignant adrenocortical tumours or the production of adrenocorticotrophin by carcinomas, but it most commonly arises through the administration of high doses of corticosteroids.

Symptoms
Cushing's syndrome is characterised by obesity of the trunk and neck, facial rounding (mooning) and reddening, muscle weakness and atrophy, skin atrophy, livid striae, spontaneous bruising, and osteoporosis. Growth arrest and obesity are characteristic in children. Other common symptoms include acne, hypertension, impaired glucose tolerance or diabetes mellitus, hirsutism, oedema, oligomenorrhoea, and psychiatric disturbances.

Treatment
Adrenal hyperplasia may be treated by irradiation of the pituitary by X-rays or heavy particles, by implantation of radioactive materials, by pituitary surgery, or by total adrenalectomy. Tumours of the adrenals may be removed, and iatrogenic Cushing's syndrome may be treated by reducing the dose of corticosteroid. Cushing's syndrome may also be treated with metyrapone (BNF 6.3.1), aminoglutethimide (BNF 8.3.4), or trilostane (BNF 6.7.4).

Primary Aldosteronism

Definition and aetiology
Primary aldosteronism (Conn's syndrome) is characterised by excessive production of the adrenocortical hormone aldosterone. The condition may be classified as aldosterone-producing adenoma, idiopathic hyperaldosteronism (commonly due to adrenal hyperplasia), and glucocorticoid-remediable hyperaldosteronism. All three classifications produce a similar spectrum of symptoms, although their treatment is varied.

Symptoms

Primary aldosteronism may initially present with hypertension which may be severe and associated with renal damage, retinal damage, and hypokalaemia. Normally, aldosterone causes the retention of sodium and the loss of potassium in the distal kidney tubules. Excess retention of sodium causes an expansion of the plasma volume which results in hypertension. Depletion of body potassium levels produces muscular weakness, which may manifest as tetany, cramp, paraesthesia, and paralysis. An inability to concentrate urine results in polyuria and polydipsia. Personality disturbances, hyperglycaemia, and glycosuria may also occur.

Treatment

Removal of the adenoma by surgery will reverse hypertension and hypokalaemia in 50% to 60% of cases. In idiopathic hyperaldosteronism, potassium-sparing diuretics (BNF 2.2.3) will correct electrolyte abnormalities and improve hypertension. Glucocorticoid-remediable hyperaldosteronism may be treated with dexamethasone (BNF 6.3.4), possibly in conjunction with potassium-sparing diuretics (BNF 2.2.3). Trilostane (BNF 6.7.4) may be of value.

6.4   PANCREATIC DISORDERS

Diabetes Mellitus

Definition and aetiology

Diabetes mellitus is characterised by persistent hyperglycaemia, usually with glycosuria, caused by a deficiency, or diminished effectiveness, of insulin. The condition may be of multifactorial origin in which hereditary factors, age, sex, pregnancy, obesity, autoimmune factors, infections, and emotional disturbances may be important. It may be precipitated by pancreatic disorders, hormonal disorders (e.g. acromegaly and Cushing's syndrome), or by administration of drugs (e.g. corticosteroids or diuretics, especially thiazides). Diabetes mellitus is classified as Type I and Type II, although the clinical distinction may be blurred.

Type I Diabetes

Definition

Type I diabetes (insulin-dependent diabetes or juvenile-onset diabetes) usually develops during the first 30 years of life, but can occur at any age.

Symptoms

The onset of symptoms is frequently abrupt, but may be insidious. Classical symptoms include polydipsia, polyuria and nocturia, dehydration, fatigue, and weight loss. Blurred vision, paraesthesia in the hands and feet, nocturnal leg cramps, and constipation may occur. Some patients develop a craving for sweet foods. Pruritus vulvae is common. The presence of ketonuria is an early indication of progression towards diabetic ketoacidosis and hyperglycaemic coma. Ketones, which arise as a result of abnormal breakdown of fats by the liver, accumulate in the blood. They are excreted in the urine and on the breath which develops a sweet, sickly smell. Ketonuria may be associated with a dry furred tongue, cracked lips, rapid pulse, and hypotension. Mental confusion and apathy may also be present.

Treatment

Type I diabetes is treated by long-term replacement therapy with insulin (BNF 6.1.1) and a controlled diet. Diabetic ketoacidosis and hyperglycaemic coma are treated by intravenous or intramuscular administration of insulin (BNF 6.1.3) and intravenous fluid replacement (BNF 9.2.2). Hypoglycaemia is treated by administration of glucose or glucagon (BNF 6.1.4). Diabetics should be counselled about diet control, insulin administration, urine testing, and the symptoms of hypoglycaemia.

Type II Diabetes

Definition and aetiology

Type II diabetes (non-insulin-dependent diabetes or maturity-onset diabetes) develops most commonly in middle-aged or elderly patients, who are often obese. There is a marked familial tendency.

Symptoms

The onset is insidious and the disease is usually mild. Ketoacidosis and other classical symptoms are often absent, but there may be pruritus vulvae. The presence of chronic recurrent infections, neuropathy, and retinopathy may be indicative of long-standing diabetes.

Treatment

Type II diabetes may be controlled by diet alone, but if this is unsuccessful it may be possible to obtain control by diet together with the administration of oral antidiabetic drugs (BNF 6.1.2).

Self-help organisations

British Diabetic Association
Diabetes Foundation

Hypoglycaemia

Definition and aetiology

Hypoglycaemia is an abnormally low plasma-glucose concentration. It occurs commonly in diabetes mellitus as a complication of insulin therapy and occasionally of therapy with oral antidiabetic drugs, but is otherwise uncommon in adults. Spontaneous hypoglycaemia may be precipitated by fasting for several hours, following which symptoms commonly occur during the night or on waking. It may also occur in severe hepatic disease or as a consequence of insulinoma. Alcohol can induce hypoglycaemia in fasting alcoholics. Rarely, spontaneous hypoglycaemia can arise in patients with Addison's disease or hypopituitarism, or as a result of large extrapancreatic sarcomas.

Reactive (postprandial) hypoglycaemia occurs 2 to 5 hours after eating. It may be idiopathic or occurs as an early symptom in patients with mild Type II diabetes.

Symptoms
Hypoglycaemia produces adrenergic symptoms (e.g. pallor, sweating, tachycardia, tremor, weakness, hunger, and nervousness) and neurological symptoms (e.g. confusion, lack of co-ordination, mental and visual disturbances, and transient stroke). The neurological symptoms may progress to loss of consciousness, convulsions, coma, and if untreated, death.

Treatment
Treatment of acute hypoglycaemia consists of oral or intravenous admininistration of glucose or glucagon injected by any route (BNF 6.1.4). Any underlying cause should also be treated. Diazoxide (BNF 6.1.4) may be useful in the management of chronic intractable hypoglycaemia (e.g. due to a non-operable insulinoma). All Type I diabetics should carry a readily absorbed form of glucose.

6.5 GONADAL DISORDERS

Hypogonadism

Definition and aetiology
Hypogonadism is the deficiency or absence of testicular function in men, or of ovarian function in women. It may be hereditary (e.g. caused by Turner's or Klinefelter's syndromes), caused by the destruction of the gonads by irradiation, caused by infections (e.g. tuberculosis, syphilis, or mumps), or by surgical removal of the gonads. It may also be secondary to a hypothalamic disease or hypopituitarism, in which lack of gonadotrophins results in gonadal atrophy. A reversible state of hypogonadism also occurs in patients with anorexia nervosa.

Symptoms
If hypogonadism occurs before puberty, the expected pubertal changes do not take place during adolescence.

If it occurs in the adult, there is regression of some of the secondary sexual characteristics.

In the prepubertal female, hypogonadism results in primary amenorrhoea, the absence of mammary development or growth of body hair, and failure of the bony epiphyses to close resulting in excessive growth of the long bones. In the adult female, there is atrophy of the breasts and external genitalia, loss of libido, amenorrhoea, and infertility.

In the prepubertal male, hypogonadism results in non-development of the genitalia or muscles, the absence of erection or ejaculation, failure of the voice to break, absence of facial and body hair, and failure of the bony epiphyses to close. In the adult male, there is regression of muscle development, smoothing of the skin, loss of beard and body hair, atrophy of the external genitalia, loss of libido, infertility, and the development of obesity and mental lethargy.

Treatment
Hypogonadism is treated by replacement therapy with androgens (BNF 6.4.2) or oestrogens (BNF 6.4.1.1) as appropriate. This will promote pubertal changes or the return of secondary sexual characteristics, but will not confer fertility. If hypogonadism is due to hypothalamic or pituitary disorders, fertility may be restored by treatment with gonadotrophins (BNF 6.5.1).

Precocious Puberty

Definition and aetiology
Precocious puberty is the premature occurrence of puberty. It may be complete (true precocious puberty) or incomplete (e.g. pseudoprecocious puberty, in which testicular enlargement or ovulation does not occur). The onset of menstruation (menarche) in girls, or the development of secondary sexual characteristics in boys, before 9 years of age is abnormal. Precocious puberty is commonly idiopathic (especially in girls), but may also be caused by lesions affecting the hypothalamus, intracranial tumours, hypothyroidism, adrenal virilisation, ovarian tumours or testicular cancer, or ingestion of oestrogens, androgens, or anabolic steroids. Iatrogenic precocious puberty may also be precipitated in boys treated with large doses of chorionic gonadotrophin for cryptorchidism.

Symptoms
In boys, precocious puberty is characterised by the development of facial, axillary, pubic, and body hair, penile growth, and deepening of the voice. In girls, it is characterised by growth of pubic and axillary hair, development of the breasts and external genitalia, and menarche. Initially, rapid linear growth may occur in

both sexes, but premature closure of the bony epiphyses results in short adult stature.

Treatment
Treatment is dependent on the underlying cause. Idiopathic precocious puberty may be treated with danazol (BNF 6.7.3) or cyproterone acetate (BNF.6.4.2). Danazol may also be useful for precocious puberty in which the underlying cause cannot be treated.

6.6 ANATOMY AND PHYSIOLOGY OF THE ENDOCRINE SYSTEM

The endocrine system consists of a group of diverse tissues located throughout the body that exert their effects on metabolism through the secretion of hormones. The hormones interact with specific target structures, triggering reactions within that structure.

The integration of the activity of the endocrine glands is carried out by the hypothalamus, which forms part of the floor of the third ventricle. The hypothalamus secretes 'releasing factors', which are secreted into the hypophyseal portal veins and carried to the anterior pituitary (adenohypophysis). The output of the anterior pituitary gland is regulated by the action of hypothalamic releasing factors. The secretion of releasing factors from the hypothalamus is modulated by a negative feedback mechanism. When the levels of circulating hormone released from the target gland reach a certain concentration in the plasma, the hypothalamus responds by decreasing its output of the corresponding releasing factor (*see* Fig. 16.12).

The Pituitary Gland

The pituitary gland (hypophysis) is located on the underside of the brain immediately above the sphenoidal sinus (*see* Fig. 12.3), and in close anatomical relationship with the hypothalamus. The posterior portion of the gland (neurohypophysis) secretes hormones produced by the hypothalamus (vasopressin and oxytocin). However, the posterior pituitary is normally considered part of the nervous system rather than of the endocrine system.

The anterior pituitary consists of three types of cells. The chromophobes are resting cells. The trophic hormones, which act on the target endocrine glands, are secreted by the basophils, while the acidophils produce prolactin and growth hormone. The trophic hormones released by the anterior pituitary are:

- thyrotrophin (thyroid-stimulating hormone)
  Acts on the thyroid gland to increase the rate of secretion of thyroid hormones.
- adrenocorticotrophin (ACTH)
  Stimulates the release of cortisol from the adrenal cortex.
- the gonadotrophins, luteinising hormone (LH) and follicle-stimulating hormone (FSH)
  Act on the ovaries and testes to stimulate the release of oestrogens, progesterone, and testosterone. FSH also assists in the development of the ova and initiates spermatogenesis. In the female, LH induces the release of an ovum from the ovary and prepares the uterine structure to receive the fertilised ovum.

Two other hormones are secreted by the anterior pituitary, but are not classed as trophic hormones as they exert their effects directly on the target sites and not through intermediate glands. Prolactin acts on the mammary glands to produce enlargement and induce milk production during pregnancy and lactation. Growth hormone stimulates the growth activity of cells, particularly skeletal and soft tissues. This is achieved through influencing the rate of protein synthesis, the breakdown of fat, and the conversion of glycogen into glucose.

The Thyroid Gland

The two lobes of the thyroid gland are situated on both sides of the upper trachea (Fig. 6.2). The lobes are joined by a central isthmus, which lies in front of the trachea, and they receive an abundant blood supply from the superior and inferior thyroid arteries. The gland is made up of follicles whose interior is lined by a unicellular wall which extracts iodine from the blood. The central cavity of each follicle is filled with thyroglobulin, which stores the thyroid hormones. The combination of iodine and the amino acid tyrosine within thyroglobulin produces liothyronine (tri-iodothyronine or T_3) and thyroxine (T_4). The complex of thyroglobulin and thyroid hormones are stored as the thyroid colloid. The release of liothyronine and thyroxine into the bloodstream is under the control of thyrotrophin secreted from the anterior pituitary. Excessive concentrations of circulating thyroid hormones decrease the amount of thyrotrophin produced by the pituitary.

Thyroxine is widely distributed within the body and acts to increase the rate of metabolism of all tissues. In the young, its presence is essential for the development and maturation of the nervous system and for normal growth. In adults, it is required for continued normal mental and physical activity.

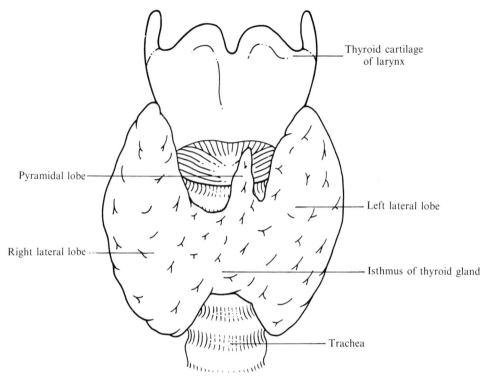

Fig. 6.2
Anterior view of thyroid gland.

The cells which fill the spaces between the follicles have been shown to release the hormone calcitonin, which acts to increase the uptake of calcium into bone, and consequently decrease plasma-calcium concentrations.

The Parathyroid Glands

The four approximately spherical parathyroid glands are symmetrically located on the posterior surface of the thyroid gland (Fig. 6.3). The glands secrete parathyroid hormone which has the overall effect of increasing the plasma-calcium concentration. This is achieved by increasing the reabsorption of calcium from bone, decreasing the amount of calcium excreted by the kidneys, and stimulating an increased absorption of calcium from the gastro-intestinal tract. The release of parathyroid hormone is regulated by the parathyroid glands themselves which monitor the concentrations of circulating calcium (there is no direct pituitary involvement in the maintenance of hormone secretion). Normal physiological plasma-calcium concentrations are maintained by the balance between the secretion of parathyroid hormone and calcitonin.

The Adrenal Glands

The two adrenal (suprarenal) glands, which lie adjacent to the upper surface of the kidneys (Fig. 6.4), are anatomically and functionally divided into two regions.

The outermost tissue, the adrenal cortex, is composed of three unequal layers. The external layer, the zona glomerulosa, consists of aggregates of small cells which secrete mineralocorticoids. The centrally sited zona fasciculata, which covers the largest area, is composed of columns of cells which produce glucocorticoids and small quantities of sex hormones. The internal layer, the zona reticularis, contains 'reserve' cells whose secretory activity may be called upon when the capacity of the other cells is overstretched.

The hormones secreted by the adrenal cortex are all derived from cholesterol. The mineralocorticoids, of which aldosterone is the most important, regulate the permeability of cell membranes to the passage of electrolytes, especially sodium and potassium ions. In the kidney, aldosterone increases the reabsorption of sodium ions and decreases the reabsorption of potassium ions into the bloodstream, and thereby regulates ionic and water homoeostasis. This regulation is achieved by

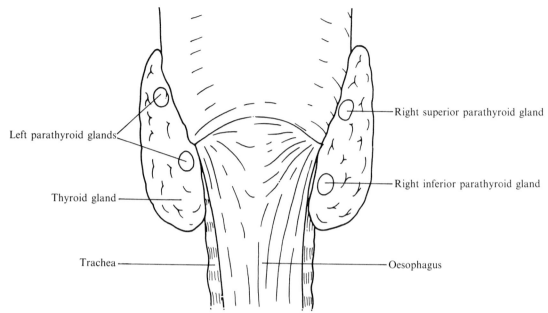

Fig. 6.3
Posterior view of thyroid and parathyroid glands.

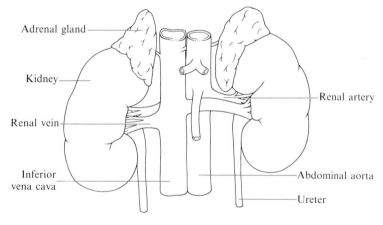

Fig. 6.4
Position of adrenal glands.

several mechanisms. Ionic exchange of plasma hydrogen ions for sodium ions maintains the electrostatic equilibrium, but decreases blood acidity. The movement of sodium ions generates a positively-charged environment in the blood vessels in the kidney tubules. As a result, anions (e.g. chloride and bicarbonate ions) are drawn from the urine into the blood. The increase in plasma-sodium concentration leads to the flow of water from urine into the blood by osmosis.

The control of the release of aldosterone is a complex process, involving the adrenal glands and the kidneys. When the blood pressure falls (e.g. as a result of haemorrhage, dehydration, or hyponatraemia), the kidney secretes an enzyme, renin, into the bloodstream. Renin converts angiotensinogen, a plasma protein, into angiotensin I, which is further modified to angiotensin II by a pulmonary plasma enzyme. Circulating angiotensin II stimulates the release of aldosterone from the adrenal cortex, producing retention of sodium and water to restore blood volume. The complex control system is described as the renin-angiotensin system.

The glucocorticoids are a triad of hormones, hydrocortisone (cortisol), corticosterone, and cortisone, of which hydrocortisone is the dominant member. The hormones increase the rate of catabolism of protein, converting the resultant amino acids to energy if the stores of fat and glycogen are low (gluconeogenesis). Other fat stores are also mobilised to provide energy (e.g. fatty acids). The provision of an adequate energy source is critical for normal body metabolism, and may also assist the body to respond to stress (e.g. surgery, severe infection, extreme cold, and fright). The vasoconstrictor effects of the glucocorticoids may be of benefit if the induced stress is as a result of haemorrhage.

The glucocorticoids suppress inflammatory and allergic responses through a range of mechanisms (e.g. stabilisation of lysosomal membranes and reduction in the secretion of histamine). However, excessive secretion of these hormones may retard wound healing and suppress immune responses.

The adrenal medulla is both an endocrine gland and an important part of the sympathetic nervous system. It secretes the catecholamines adrenaline and noradrenaline into the bloodstream from chromaffin cells. Adrenaline stimulates the breakdown of muscular and hepatic glycogen, providing an important source of energy in an emergency. Noradrenaline and adrenaline increase the metabolic rate of certain organs of the body, and supplements the activity of the sympathetic nervous system.

The Pancreas

The pancreas is both an endocrine and exocrine organ. It is divided into a head, tail, and body, the head portion lying closest to the junction with the duodenum (see Fig. 1.4). Exocrine secretions from the pancreas are transported to the duodenum through the pancreatic duct. The bulk (99%) of the pancreas is composed of exocrine cells, the acini, which secrete pancreatic juice (see Section 1.10). The endocrine secretions of the pancreas are produced by the islets of Langerhans which are subdivided as alpha, beta, and delta cells according to their secretions.

The largest cells, the alpha cells, secrete glucagon, a polypeptide whose principal action is to increase the level of circulating glucose. This is achieved by stimulating the hepatic formation of glucose from glycogen (glycogenolysis), and amino acids, lactic acid, and glycerol (gluconeogenesis). The release of glucagon is controlled by a negative feedback mechanism which monitors plasma-glucose concentrations.

The beta cells secrete insulin. Insulin is a hypoglycaemic agent by virtue of its effects on the transport and utilisation of glucose. It increases the rate of uptake of glucose from the blood into tissues, and the conversion of glucose into glycogen. Insulin also prevents glycogenolysis and gluconeogenesis (see above). Fatty acid formation (lipogenesis) and protein synthesis are promoted in the presence of insulin. The secretion of insulin is regulated directly by plasma-glucose concentrations, but indirect control may also be exerted by the action of other hormones. Growth hormone secretion and the release of glucocorticoids caused by the secretion of ACTH induce hyperglycaemia, which in turn increases the secretion of insulin.

The delta cells of the pancreas secrete growth hormone inhibiting factor (somatostatin), but are not normally considered an integral part of the endocrine system.

The Gonads

The gonadal endocrine glands in the female are the ovaries (see Fig. 7.2 and Section 7.6), and in the male, the testes. The ovaries are the primary reproductive organs of the female, responsible for the secretion of oestrogens and progesterone and the production of ova. The oestrogens, of which oestradiol is the most important, are responsible for the development and maintenance of the female secondary sexual characteristics (e.g. the shape of the pelvis, the pitch of the voice, and the distribution of body fat). They exert control over the menstrual cycle (e.g. by stimulating the production of luteinising hormone from the anterior pituitary) and increase the likelihood of successful fertilisation (e.g. by decreasing the viscosity of cervical mucus at the time of ovulation). If conception is successful, the oestrogens assist in the maintenance of pregnancy and the preparation of the mammary glands for lactation.

The release of progesterone is responsible for the preparation of the endometrium on the assumption that fertilisation will occur. Its release and steady accumulation from day 14 of the menstrual cycle increases the vascularity and thickness of the lining of the uterus to receive the fertilised ovum. If fertilisation and implantation of the ovum does not occur, the continued secretion of progesterone inhibits the release of luteinising hormone. Consequently, the concentrations of oestrogens and progesterone decline through the destruction of their source and lead to shedding of the proliferative endometrium (menstruation).

The release of progesterone assumes greater importance in the event of fertilisation and implantation. It reduces the risk of premature labour by preventing uterine contractions, and, in combination with oestrogen, inhibits further ovulation during the pregnancy. Progesterone is also secreted from the developing placenta.

The male gonadal glands, the testes, are suspended in two scrotal sacs outside the abdominal wall. The sperm are produced within the tightly-coiled seminiferous tubules. Interstitial Leydig cells are located within the spaces between the seminiferous tubules, and are responsible for the secretion of testosterone, the male sex hormone. Like oestrogen in the female, testosterone is necessary for the development of male secondary sexual characteristics (e.g. deepening of the voice, muscular and skeletal development, and the production and distribution of facial, body, and pubic hair). The production of testosterone is controlled by the secretion of luteinising hormone from the anterior pituitary.

Chapter 7

OBSTETRIC, GYNAECOLOGICAL, RENAL, AND UROGENITAL DISORDERS

7.1 OBSTETRIC DISORDERS

Abortion

Abortion is the termination of pregnancy before the foetus is considered viable legally (i.e. before the 28th week of pregnancy).

Spontaneous abortion occurs without external stimuli. During the first trimester of pregnancy, spontaneous abortion is usually due to foetal abnormalities, but in later weeks it is commonly due to maternal factors (e.g. abnormalities of the genital tract).

Habitual abortion is repeated spontaneous abortion. The usual criterion is the occurrence of three consecutive, unexplained abortions, usually in a subject who has never had a successful pregnancy. Causes of habitual abortion include endocrine and metabolic disease (e.g. hypothyroidism or hyperthyroidism, diabetes mellitus, or chronic renal failure), anatomical uterine abnormalities, and incompetence of the cervix. Defective function of the corpus luteum is a common cause. Progestogens (BNF 6.4.1.2) have been used to maintain the endometrium, but their efficacy is doubtful. Suturing of the cervix may prevent abortion in cases of cervical incompetence.

Threatened abortion is uterine bleeding in the presence of an apparently intact pregnancy. The usual treatment is bed rest for several days or until the bleeding stops, and avoidance of coitus.

Inevitable abortion occurs when, in addition to vaginal bleeding in early pregnancy, there are uterine contractions accompanied by pain and passage of foetal or placental tissue. Abortion occurs soon after the onset of symptoms. If abortion is incomplete (i.e. products of conception remain in the uterus), it may be completed by curettage.

Missed abortion is the retention of the products of conception within the uterus for a prolonged period after the death of the foetus. There is cessation of growth or diminution in the size of the uterus. The pregnancy test becomes negative, but there is no expulsion of uterine contents. Complete abortion is achieved by stimulation of the uterus with prostaglandins and oxytocics (BNF 7.1.1), or by curettage.

Septic abortion occurs when the contents of the uterus become infected by bacteria before, during, or usually after, an abortion. Chills, fever, septicaemia, and peritonitis may occur and septic shock may develop. It is treated with antibacterial drugs (BNF 5.1).

Therapeutic abortion is the elective termination of pregnancy. Very early abortion can be carried out using a fine cannula passed into the uterine cavity, and sucking out the contents. After 14 weeks gestation, instillation of prostaglandins (BNF 7.1.1) via the cervix or injection into the amniotic cavity results in evacuation, usually within 8 to 18 hours. Oxytocin infusion (BNF 7.1.1) may also be required, and retained uterine contents must sometimes be removed under anaesthetic. Rarely pregnancy may be terminated by hysterotomy.

Self-help organisations
Birth Control Trust
British Pregnancy Advisory Service
Marie Stopes House
Pregnancy Advisory Service

Ectopic Pregnancy

Definition and aetiology
An ectopic pregnancy is a pregnancy in which a fertilised ovum implants and begins to develop outside the endometrium. The majority occur within the Fallopian tubes, although other possible sites include the ovaries, cervix, and peritoneal cavity. Tubal ectopic pregnancies occur more commonly in patients with partial tubal obstruction, usually as a consequence of salpingitis. The incidence of ectopic pregnancy is also increased in women who become pregnant in the presence of an intra-uterine device and in those who have had a previous ectopic pregnancy.

Symptoms
Symptoms may include slight vaginal bleeding ('spotting') and colicky lower abdominal pain. This is usually followed by abrupt severe lower abdominal pain, marked vaginal bleeding, and syncope caused by rupture of the Fallopian tube and intra-abdominal haemorrhage; hypotension and shock may develop.

Treatment

Treatment consists of surgical removal of the foetus, placenta, and part or all of the affected tube. Transfusion may be required.

Hydatidiform Mole

Definition and aetiology

Hydatidiform mole is a benign tumour of the trophoblastic tissue. It occurs in abnormal pregnancies when a degenerating ovum fails to abort spontaneously. The trophoblastic tissue continues to proliferate, resulting in a fleshy tumour in which the villi are grossly distended with fluid (hydropic). Hydatidiform mole occurs most commonly in females over 40 years of age.

Symptoms

It is characterised by abnormally rapid uterine enlargement, severe nausea and vomiting, and vaginal bleeding, eventually followed by spontaneous abortion. Patients with hydatidiform mole may later develop choriocarcinoma. In other patients, the mole may be locally invasive and there may be distant spread. Metastases formed as a result may regress after removal of the mole. Other complications include intra-uterine infections, haemorrhage, septicaemia, and pre-eclampsia.

Treatment

Abortion may be induced with prostaglandins (BNF 7.1.1) or by suction curettage. Patients require careful follow-up to detect choriocarcinoma. Antimetabolites (BNF 8.1.3) or cytotoxic antibiotics (BNF 8.1.2), or both, may be required in the treatment of invasive moles.

Postpartum Haemorrhage

Definition and aetiology

Primary postpartum haemorrhage is characterised by significant blood loss (at least 500 mL) occurring after birth and within 24 hours. It may be caused by an atonic uterus, retained products of conception, lacerations, or hypofibrinogenaemia. It usually occurs soon after parturition and before complete delivery of the placenta, but may occur as long as one month after delivery.

Secondary postpartum haemorrhage occurs after 24 hours and usually within several weeks. Its aetiology may be the same as the primary form, or it can be caused by uterine infection.

Treatment

Postpartum haemorrhage may be prevented or controlled by the routine administration of ergometrine and oxytocin (BNF 7.1.1). The placenta should be examined for completeness and any retained products of conception removed from the uterus. If haemorrhage does occur, the risk of serious blood loss may be reduced by intravenous injection of ergometrine, by intravenous oxytocin infusion when the patient does not respond to ergometrine, and repair of lacerations. Hypotension should be treated promptly to prevent pituitary necrosis. Antibacterial drugs (BNF 5.1) may be required for infection.

Pre-eclampsia and Eclampsia

Definition and aetiology

Pre-eclampsia (toxaemia of pregnancy) is characterised by hypertension, proteinuria, and oedema. Its presence results in increased foetal and, to a lesser extent, maternal morbidity and mortality. Pre-eclampsia usually occurs in the latter half of the pregnancy and resolves soon after delivery. It occurs more frequently in first pregnancies, older women, and in multiple pregnancies, although its aetiology is uncertain. Eclampsia refers to convulsions in late pregnancy, labour, or the puerperium and can lead to coma. It is often preceded by pre-eclampsia. Foetal morbidity and mortality is very high.

Symptoms

The only symptoms of pre-eclampsia are oedema and weight gain. In impending eclampsia, headache, visual disturbances, and vomiting can occur. There may also be epigastric pain and reduced urinary volume.

Treatment

Pre-eclampsia responds to rest and careful observation. Hospitalisation is necessary for all cases considered more than mild, in an attempt to prevent eclampsia. Should it develop, early delivery may be required. Antihypertensive therapy (BNF 2.5), antiepileptics (BNF 4.8), and hypnotics and anxiolytics (BNF 4.1) may be necessary.

7.2 GYNAECOLOGICAL DISORDERS

7.2.1 GENERAL DISORDERS

Endometriosis

Definition and aetiology

Endometriosis is a condition in which functioning endometrial tissue is found in an abnormal location. It occurs most commonly between 30 and 40 years of age. Common sites for the ectopic endometrium include the ovary, Fallopian tubes, vagina, myometrium, uterine ligaments, uterorectal pouch, rectum, and sigmoid colon

(Figs. 7.1 and 7.2). The endometrial tissue may form a small nodule often with surrounding fibrosis. In the ovaries, lesions are commonly cystic and respond to the cyclic changes in oestrogen and progesterone by repeated swelling (causing pain) and bleeding (causing fibrosis) at the time of menstruation. In ovarian cysts some of the fluid may be of a chocolate and tarry consistency, and the cyst may grow as large as an orange. Its rupture may result in multiple adhesions.

Symptoms

The symptoms of endometriosis are varied, depending upon location, but usually include dysmenorrhoea, dyspareunia, menorrhagia, intermenstrual pelvic pain, and back pain. Infertility occurs in about 30% to 40% of patients. If the rectum or sigmoid colon is involved, there may be cyclic rectal pains, pain on defaecation, and occasionally mild diarrhoea and tenesmus. Dysuria may occur if the bladder is involved.

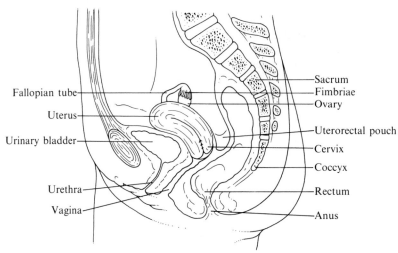

Fig. 7.1
Female pelvic organs (sagittal section).

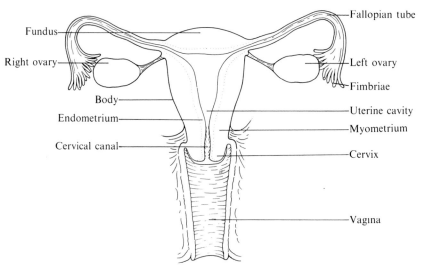

Fig. 7.2
Female reproductive system.

Treatment

Treatment depends on the severity of symptoms and the age and parity of the patient. Endometriosis is suppressed by pregnancy and the menopause. Progestogens (BNF 6.4.1.2) may be given continuously for several months; alternatively cyclical or continuous treatment with combined oral contraceptives (BNF 7.3.1) or danazol (BNF 6.7.3) may be useful. Fertility may be enhanced on the withdrawal of such treatment. Surgery (usually hysterectomy) may be required in more severe cases.

Hirsutism

Definition and aetiology

Hirsutism is excessive facial and body hair growth, especially in women. It may be idiopathic or caused by increased testosterone production, usually as a result of polycystic ovary syndrome. Rarer causes include adrenal or ovarian tumours, Cushing's disease, acromegaly, and juvenile hypothyroidism. Hirsutism may also be induced by drugs (e.g. anabolic steroids, androgens, corticosteroids, phenytoin, diazoxide, and minoxidil).

Treatment

Treatment is dependent on the underlying cause. Idiopathic hirsutism may be treated by local removal of unwanted hair. Severe cases may be treated with cyproterone acetate (BNF 6.4.2) or combined oral contraceptives (BNF 7.3.1).

Infertility

Definition and aetiology

Infertility is the reduced or absent ability to conceive children, which affects 10% to 15% of couples and may be caused by abnormalities in either partner. It may also be psychogenic. Failure to conceive after 12 months is considered abnormal as 90% of fertile couples achieve conception within that time.

In males, infertility may occur as a result of impaired spermatogenesis caused by endocrine disturbances (e.g. hyperprolactinaemia, hypogonadism, hypopituitarism, prolonged fever, testicular infection or injury, cryptorchidism, or varicocoele). Spermatogenesis may also be affected by drug administration (e.g. testosterone) or environmental toxins (e.g. heavy metals). Infertility may also arise from obstruction of the seminal ducts due to congenital abnormalities, infection, stricture, or surgery. In addition, sperm may not be deposited in the vagina as a result of certain disorders (e.g. impotence or premature ejaculation).

In females, infertility may arise through abnormal ovarian function as a result of endocrine disorders and polycystic ovary syndrome. Fallopian tube defects may be present as a consequence of congenital abnormalities

or infection (e.g. salpingitis). Congenital uterine defects may also exist or conditions in the cervix may not be ideal for the transmission of sperm.

Treatment

Treatment is aimed at the underlying cause. Corrective surgery may be necessary in the case of anatomical abnormalities, and *in-vitro* fertilisation may be considered in selected cases.

Self-help organisations

British Pregnancy Advisory Service
Family Planning Association
Infertility Advisory Centre
Marie Stopes House
National Association for the Childless

Menopause

Definition and aetiology

The menopause (climacteric) is the cessation of menstruation. It usually occurs between 45 and 55 years of age, during which time the ovaries progressively secrete less oestrogen and progesterone. This results in increased plasma-gonadotrophin concentrations and menstrual irregularities, culminating in the cessation of menstruation.

Symptoms

Clinical features of the menopause are primarily due to oestrogen deficiency. They include vasomotor symptoms (e.g. hot flushes, sweating, and headache), insomnia, irritability, loss of libido, anxiety, and depressive disorders. Long-term effects of endocrine changes, which may appear in post-menopausal women combined with the effects of ageing, include osteoporosis and atrophy of the breasts, endometrium, myometrium, vagina, and vulva. Atrophy of pelvic muscles and ligaments may lead to uterine prolapse. The incidence of ischaemic heart disease is increased post-menopausally.

Treatment

Symptomatic treatment with clonidine (BNF 4.7.4.2) for hot flushes, and anxiolytics (BNF 4.1.2) and antidepressant drugs (BNF 4.3) may be necessary. Symptoms may also be treated by hormone replacement therapy, with oestrogens given cyclically with a progestogen (BNF 6.4.1.1 and 6.4.1.2) or combined preparations (BNF 6.4.1.3). Hormone implants may also be used. The majority of women, however, may be successfully treated by counselling and reassurance alone.

Polycystic Ovary Syndrome

Definition and aetiology

The polycystic ovary syndrome (Stein-Leventhal syndrome) is characterised by the presence of multiple bilateral ovarian cysts and stromal hyperplasia. It may be associated with the conditions of hypersecretion of androgens (e.g. congenital adrenal hyperplasia and Cushing's syndrome).

Symptoms
It usually occurs in young women and is characterised by menstrual irregularities (e.g. secondary amenorrhoea or oligomenorrhoea) and impaired fertility. Hirsutism and obesity commonly occur and occasionally other signs of virilisation may be present.

Treatment
Infertility arising from the polycystic ovary syndrome may be treated by administration of clomiphene or chorionic gonadotrophin (BNF 6.5.1), or both.

Turner's Syndrome

Definition and aetiology
Turner's syndrome is a form of defective gonadal development in females associated with the complete or partial absence of the second X-chromosome.

Symptoms
It is characterised by primary amenorrhoea, short stature, and numerous skeletal abnormalities (e.g. webbing of the neck, shield-like chest, metacarpal abnormalities, and cubitus valgus). Other signs include poorly developed secondary sexual characteristics, hypertension, lymphoedema, a low posterior hairline, and multiple naevi. Cardiovascular and renal abnormalities are common. Turner's syndrome is associated with an increased incidence of Hashimoto's thyroiditis, diabetes mellitus, and infertility.

Treatment
Treatment consists of replacement therapy, initially with ethinyloestradiol (BNF 6.4.1.1) for several months and subsequently with a combined oral contraceptive (BNF 7.3.1); infertility is irremediable. Antihypertensive therapy (BNF 2.5) may be required.

Vaginitis

Definition and aetiology
Vaginitis is inflammation of the vagina which may be infectious or atrophic.

Infective Vaginitis

Definition and aetiology
Infective vaginitis may be caused by a variety of microorganisms (e.g. *Chlamydia trachomatis*, *Candida albicans*, *Trichomonas vaginalis*, and *Neisseria gonorrhoeae*) or may be non-specific. Vaginal candidiasis may be pre-

cipitated by diabetes mellitus, pregnancy, or the administration of antibacterials, corticosteroids, and possibly combined oral contraceptives. Non-specific vaginitis is thought to be due to infection with *Gardnerella vaginalis*, although other causes include foreign bodies (e.g. retained tampons) and local irritants (e.g. douches, deodorants, or spermicides).

Symptoms
In vaginal candidiasis the discharge is usually thick, white, and caseous and is accompanied by vulvitis and marked pruritus. In vaginal trichomoniasis the discharge is usually offensive, yellowish, and may be frothy and profuse with soreness and pruritus. In non-specific vaginitis the discharge is usually greyish, frothy, and malodorous (fishy smell).

Treatment
Treatment is dependent on the underlying cause. Vaginal candidiasis is treated with anti-infective drugs (BNF 7.2.2). Vaginal trichomoniasis and *Gardnerella* infections are treated systemically with metronidazole or tinidazole (BNF 5.1.11), or nimorazole (BNF 5.4.3).

Atrophic Vaginitis

Definition and aetiology
Atrophic (senile) vaginitis occurs in post-menopausal women and is associated with oestrogen deficiency; the discharge is usually thin and watery. Abnormal vaginal discharge may also be caused by malignancy, foreign bodies, cervical erosions or strictures, radiotherapy, or sexually-transmitted diseases.

Symptoms
Atrophic vaginitis may be asymptomatic in many. Some patients do, however, experience pruritus and discharge, and soreness may cause pain during sexual intercourse.

Treatment
Atrophic vaginitis may be treated with topical oestrogens (BNF 7.2.1) or, in severe unresponsive cases, by systemic hormone replacement therapy with oestrogens and progestogens (BNF 6.4.1).

Vulvitis

Definition and aetiology
Vulvitis is inflammation of the vulva. It may accompany atrophic or infective vaginitis or may be due to local allergic reactions, poor hygiene, bacterial, fungal, parasitic, or viral infections, or malignant or sexually-transmitted diseases.

Symptoms
It is characterised by local erythema and oedema, burning pain, and pruritus vulvae. Ulceration may be present and atrophy (kraurosis vulvae) may occur in post-menopausal women.

Treatment
Treatment is dependent on the underlying cause. Topical corticosteroids (BNF 13.4) may be required for local allergic reactions; local anaesthetic and antipruritic preparations (BNF 13.3) may provide symptomatic relief; topical hormones (BNF 7.2.1) may be indicated for kraurosis vulvae; anti-infective drugs (BNF 7.2.2) may be required for vulval infections.

7.2.2 BREAST DISORDERS

Benign Mammary Dysplasias

Definition and aetiology
Benign mammary dysplasias (cystic mastopathy or chronic cystic mastitis) are a group of benign breast changes which frequently occur in pre-menopausal women and are the commonest cause of breast lumps.

Symptoms
The changes occur mainly in the lobular and terminal ducts and include formation of cysts, epitheliosis (hyperplasia of the ductular epithelium), adenosis, and fibrosis. Any one of these changes may predominate and they may occur in any combination. Cysts are usually multiple and bilateral, although solitary cysts may occur.

Treatment
Treatment is not usually required, although aspiration and biopsy may be necessary to differentiate the condition from breast cancer.

7.2.3 MENSTRUAL DISORDERS

(The menstrual cycle in the absence of fertilisation is illustrated in Fig. 7.3.)

Amenorrhoea

Definition and aetiology
Amenorrhoea is the absence of menstruation. In primary amenorrhoea the menarche fails to occur by 16 years of age. Secondary amenorrhoea is the absence of menstruation for 6 months or longer in a female who has

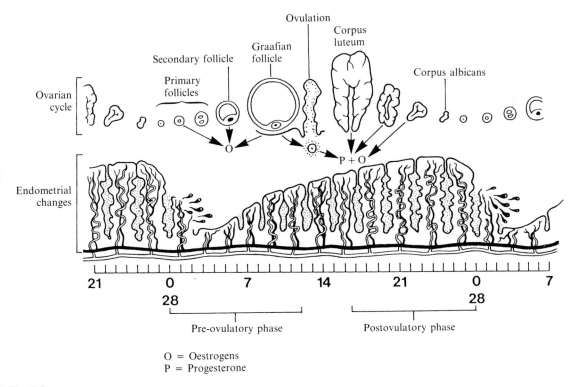

O = Oestrogens
P = Progesterone

Fig. 7.3
Menstrual cycle (in the absence of fertilisation).

previously been menstruating. It may be physiological (e.g. due to pregnancy, lactation, or the menopause) or pathological. Amenorrhoea is usually a symptom of an underlying disorder and can be caused by disturbances of the hormonal regulation of the menstrual cycle. It is commonly associated with endocrine disease. Primary causes include pituitary or hypothalamic disorders (e.g. hyperprolactinaemia and hypopituitarism). Secondary causes include other endocrine pathology, ranging from thyroid disorders (e.g. hyperthyroidism) and adrenal disorders (e.g. adrenal virilisation) to gonadal disorders (e.g. hypogonadism). Amenorrhoea may also be associated with anorexia nervosa and obesity. Emotional disturbances, excessive exercise, and severe systemic illness (e.g. malignant disease) may also cause amenorrhoea. Amenorrhoea may also be drug-induced (e.g. due to antipsychotic drugs or corticosteroids) or may follow discontinuation of oral contraception. Rarely, primary amenorrhoea may be due to structural uterine or vaginal abnormalities.

Treatment
Treatment is dependent on the underlying cause. Oestrogens (BNF 6.4.1.1) may be used to induce artificial menstruation in primary amenorrhoea. They are usually given cyclically with a progestogen (BNF 6.4.1.4), or a combined oral contraceptive (BNF 7.3.1) may be used. Clomiphene or cyclofenil (BNF 6.5.1) may be used to induce ovulation in patients with idiopathic secondary amenorrhoea or amenorrhoea caused by the polycystic ovary syndrome.

Dysmenorrhoea

Definition
Dysmenorrhoea is painful menstruation which may be primary or secondary.

Primary Dysmenorrhoea

Definition and aetiology
Primary (spasmodic) dysmenorrhoea is caused by uncoordinated uterine contractions which occur as the endometrium is shed and expelled. There is increasing evidence of a role for prostaglandins in its aetiology.

Symptoms
It is common in young nulliparous women, and is characterised by colicky lower abdominal, back, and leg pain which usually starts on the first day of menstruation and lasts for up to 48 hours. Occasionally, the pain may precede menstruation. Dysmenorrhoea may be associated with abdominal distension, nausea and vomiting,

diarrhoea, headache, premenstrual syndrome, and urinary frequency.

Treatment
It may be treated with anti-inflammatory non-opioid analgesics (BNF 4.7.1), myometrial relaxants (BNF 7.1.2), or in severe cases with progestogens (BNF 6.4.1.2) or combined oestrogen/progestogen preparations (BNF 6.4.1.3 and 7.3.1). Application of local heat, adequate rest, and regular exercise may also be beneficial.

Secondary Dysmenorrhoea

Definition and aetiology
Secondary (congestive) dysmenorrhoea is pain secondary to various disorders (e.g. endometriosis, fibroids, salpingitis, or chronic pelvic inflammatory disease).

Symptoms
The pain usually occurs as a dull ache in the lower abdomen and back, commencing several days before menstruation and often relieved within 24 hours of its onset, although it may persist throughout menstruation. Abdominal distension and the premenstrual syndrome may also occur.

Treatment
Treatment should be directed at the underlying cause. Measures indicated in primary dysmenorrhoea may also be useful.

Premenstrual Syndrome

Definition and aetiology
Premenstrual syndrome usually starts 7 to 10 days before menstruation and commonly disappears a few hours after the onset of menstruation.

Symptoms
It is characterised by emotional lability, irritablity, nervousness, depressive disorders, weight gain, abdominal distension, and breast tenderness. Headache, fatigue, and oedema may also occur.

Treatment
A wide variety of treatment measures have been tried. Many women benefit from explanation and reassurance. A wide variety of drugs have been used, with varying degrees of success. These include pyridoxine (BNF 9.6.2), diuretics (BNF 2.2), progestogens (BNF 6.4.1.2), and combined oral contraceptives (BNF 7.3.1). Bromocriptine may relieve breast tenderness, and antidepressant drugs have been used for emotional instability.

7.3   MALE GENITAL DISORDERS

Benign Prostatic Hypertrophy

Definition and aetiology
Benign prostatic hypertrophy is a non-malignant condition in which the prostate gland becomes large and nodular. It is common in men over 50 years of age and results in varying degrees of urethral obstruction. Its cause is unknown, but it is thought to be associated with the endocrine disturbances of ageing.

Symptoms
The symptoms are associated with obstruction of the urethra. Difficulty in urination is common in conjunction with a decrease in the volume and force of the urine flow, terminal dribbling, and incomplete bladder emptying. Urinary frequency and nocturia usually follow. Urinary retention may become total and severe pain develops as a result of pressure build-up. Urinary-tract infection is a common complication. If urinary retention is prolonged, renal failure may develop.

Treatment
Catheterisation may be performed in order to drain the bladder. Surgical resection (prostatectomy) may be necessary either via the urethra (transurethral resection) or by an abdominal incision.

Cryptorchidism

Definition and aetiology
Cryptorchidism is a developmental defect in which one or both testes fail to descend into the scrotum, but remain in the abdominal cavity or inguinal canal (normal descent commonly occurs before birth or during the first two years of life). The cause is not known, but endocrine or anatomical abnormalities may be responsible. Infertility caused by impaired spermatogenesis is likely to develop, particularly if the defect persists after five years of age. There is also a greater likelihood of malignant disease in undescended testes.

Treatment
Chorionic gonadotrophin and gonadorelin (BNF 6.5.1) have been used in the treatment of cryptorchidism. The standard treatment is surgical relocation and fixation in the scrotum (orchidopexy). If the defect persists after puberty, orchidectomy may be carried out because of the risk of malignancy.

Klinefelter's Syndrome

Definition and aetiology
Klinefelter's syndrome is a familial condition in males associated with the presence of one or more extra X-chromosomes in at least one cell line.

Symptoms
It is characterised by infertility due to azoospermia or oligospermia, small firm testes, and variable degrees of masculinisation; hypogonadism and gynaecomastia may occur. Patients are often tall with long limbs, and mental retardation is common; skeletal abnormalities may occur. There is an increased incidence of breast cancer compared to other males, and an increased frequency of impaired glucose tolerance and diabetes mellitus.

Treatment
Hypogonadism may be treated by replacement therapy with androgens (BNF 6.4.2), but infertility is irremediable.

Torsion of the Testis

Definition and aetiology
Torsion of the testis occurs when a testis twists on the spermatic cord within the membranous covering (tunica vaginalis) of the testis. This may occur spontaneously and at any age, although it is more common during puberty. It may follow vigorous physical activity, particularly if there is a pre-existing anatomical defect. Torsion results in venous obstruction which may lead to local oedema, haemorrhage, arterial obstruction, and infarction.

Symptoms
Symptoms include extreme pain and tenderness in the testis, and the patient may be unable to walk. The scrotum and testis become inflamed and swollen. Fever, nausea and vomiting, and very occasionally dysuria and frequency, may develop.

Treatment
Surgical investigation of any suspected torsion must be urgently carried out. Delay reduces the chances of the testis remaining viable. In severe cases, orchidectomy may be indicated.

Varicocoele

Definition and aetiology
Varicocoele is a varicose condition of the veins within the scrotum. It is usually left-sided.

Symptoms

It is characterised by scrotal swelling (often described as a 'bag of worms') which disappears on lying down. The swelling is often accompanied by a constant, dragging, dull pain and blue discoloration may be visible through the scrotal skin. Varicocoele is a common cause of infertility.

Treatment

A scrotal support (or similar garment) may be all that is required. Surgery, by ligation of the spermatic vein, may be necessary if infertility develops or the symptoms are unacceptable.

7.4   RENAL DISORDERS

Glomerulonephritis

Definition

Glomerulonephritis (Bright's disease) is characterised by inflammation of renal glomeruli which may be acute or chronic. (The structure of a healthy nephron is illustrated in Fig. 7.4.)

Acute Glomerulonephritis

Definition and aetiology

Acute (postinfectious) glomerulonephritis is usually preceded by a Group A β-haemolytic streptococcal infection, often of the pharynx or skin. It is associated with the laying down of antigen-antibody complexes in the glomeruli.

Symptoms

It is most common in children and young adults. The onset is usually sudden in children, occurring 2 to 3 weeks after the infective episode, but slower in adults. Symptoms include fever, headache, malaise, nausea and vomiting, and oedema with hypertension and dyspnoea. Proteinuria and haematuria are almost always present, and abdominal and back pain may occur. The probability

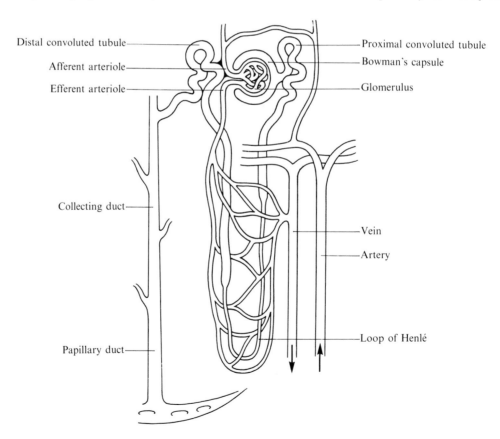

Distal convoluted tubule

Afferent arteriole

Efferent arteriole

Proximal convoluted tubule

Bowman's capsule

Glomerulus

Collecting duct

Vein

Artery

Loop of Henlé

Papillary duct

Fig. 7.4
Nephron.

of recovery is favourable, especially in children, although progressive renal impairment may develop in some and culminate in renal failure.

Treatment
Treatment consists of bed rest and, in the presence of residual streptococcal infection, the administration of an appropriate antibacterial drug (BNF 5.1). Diuretics (BNF 2.2) and antihypertensive therapy (BNF 2.5) may be necessary. An adequate fluid intake should be maintained and dietary protein and sodium restricted.

Chronic Glomerulonephritis

Definition and aetiology
Chronic glomerulonephritis is a syndrome which may follow any one of a number of inflammatory glomerular disorders. A history of acute glomerulonephritis is, however, uncommon.

Symptoms
The onset is insidious and usually occurs in adults. Persistent proteinuria and haematuria are usually present and common symptoms, associated with renal impairment, include dyspnoea, fatigue, nausea and vomiting, and pruritus. Oedema may occur and hypertension is common. Death may occur as a result of renal failure.

Treatment
Treatment is generally ineffective. Antihypertensive therapy (BNF 2.5) may be useful and dialysis may be necessary in severe renal failure. Dietary sodium and protein should be restricted, while maintaining an adequate fluid intake.

Self-help organisation
British Kidney Patients Association

Interstitial Nephritis

Definition and aetiology
Interstitial nephritis is characterised by inflammation of the renal interstitial tissue, including the tubules. It may be acute or, more commonly, chronic. It has a wide variety of causes including toxicity due to drugs (e.g. analgesics and antibacterials or heavy metals (e.g. lead), metabolic disorders (e.g. hypokalaemia and gout), immunological disorders (e.g. systemic lupus erythematosus), urinary-tract infection, obstruction, and vascular abnormalities (e.g. renal artery obstruction). It may also be idiopathic.

Symptoms
The acute form of the disease, which is most often due to drug toxicity, may present with oliguria, fever, and occasionally arthralgia. Renal failure may develop. In chronic interstitial nephritis, there are few symptoms before the onset of renal failure and uraemia. Subsequent symptoms include anaemia, anorexia, fatigue, nausea and vomiting, and weight loss. Hypertension may occur in severe cases. Renal failure is a common complication which may prove fatal.

Treatment
Treatment in acute disease comprises the administration of corticosteroids (BNF 6.3.4). In the chronic form, treatment is aimed at the underlying cause. Antibacterial drugs (BNF 5.1) may be used in the presence of infection, and surgery may be indicated in the presence of urinary-tract obstruction. In both forms of the disease, dialysis or transplantation may be necessary if chronic renal failure develops.

Nephrotic Syndrome

Definition and aetiology
The nephrotic syndrome is characterised by increased glomerular permeability to protein, resulting in more than 3 to 5 g in the urine each day. The most common cause is glomerulonephritis, but occasionally diabetes mellitus, malignant disease, or systemic lupus erythematosus may be responsible. It may also arise as an adverse effect of drug administration (e.g. penicillamine and sodium aurothiomalate).

Symptoms
The onset is usually insidious and symptoms include persistent severe proteinuria and hypoproteinaemia, leading to salt and water retention, and marked generalised oedema. An increased susceptibility to infection is common, and other complications include hypertension and renal failure.

Treatment
Treatment consists of bed rest and a high-protein low-sodium diet. Specific treatment depends on the underlying disorder. Diuretics (BNF 2.2) may be administered and corticosteroids (BNF 6.3.4) may be helpful. Cyclophosphamide has also been used. Antibacterial drugs (BNF 5.1) and antihypertensive therapy (BNF 2.5) may be necessary.

Oedema

Definition and aetiology
Oedema is the presence of abnormally large amounts of fluid in the intercellular tissue spaces of the body. It is usually detected by the accumulation of fluid in the subcutaneous tissues and is accompanied by retention of sodium and chloride ions. It may be localised, caused by venous (*see* Embolism) or lymphatic obstruction, or to

increased vascular permeability. It may also be generalised, caused by systemic heart disease, hepatic disease, or renal disease.

Symptoms
It is commonly characterised by an increase in weight, facial puffiness, and swelling of other parts of the body (e.g. ankles, hands, and wrists, Fig. 7.5). Effusions into body cavities may occur (e.g. ascites).

Treatment
Treatment is directed at the underlying disease, and the administration of diuretics (BNF 2.2) may be indicated.

Polycystic Kidney Disease

Definition and aetiology
Polycystic kidney disease is an autosomally dominant inherited disease in which normal kidney tissue is replaced by cysts. Its cause is unknown.

Symptoms
The onset of the disease usually occurs between 30 and 40 years of age, and common symptoms include abdominal and back pain, haematuria, hypertension, and urinary-tract infections. Polycystic kidney disease is a common cause of chronic renal failure. Hepatic cysts may accompany the renal cysts.

Treatment
No specific treatment exists, although drug treatment is indicated in the presence of hypertension and urinary-tract infection. Patients with chronic disease may eventually require dialysis or transplantation.

Renal Calculi and Colic

Definition and aetiology
Renal calculi (kidney or urinary stones) are abnormal hard concretions, composed mainly of mineral salts. The calculi are formed in the kidney and may be found in any part of the urinary tract (i.e. kidney, ureter, bladder, and urethra). Calcium calculi are most common and may be associated with dehydration, hypercalcaemia, or hypercalciuria. A low urinary pH or gout may result in the formation of uric acid calculi, and calculi of mixed composition (e.g. calcium phosphate and magnesium ammonium phosphate) may arise due to high urinary pH or after urinary-tract infection.

Symptoms
The presence of large calculi retained in the kidney may be asymptomatic. Most very small calculi are spontaneously voided in the urine. Calculi in the kidney may

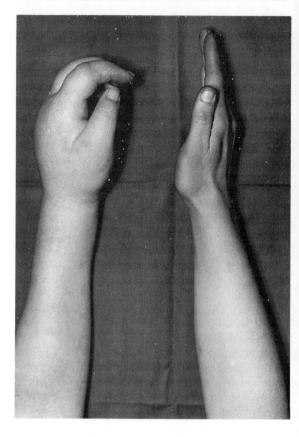

Fig. 7.5
Oedema of hand and wrist, preventing full extension of the fingers.

however cause loin pain, and a ureteric calculus may produce severe colicky pain (ureteric or renal colic) radiating from loin to groin. Bladder calculi may produce strangury, and urine flow may be interrupted by urethral calculi. Other symptoms include dysuria and frequency, haematuria and proteinuria, and recurrent urinary-tract infections. The pain of renal colic is very severe and often accompanied by retching and vomiting.

Treatment
Calculi associated with urinary-tract obstruction and infection should be surgically removed (lithotomy). Extraction via the urethra may be possible, and ultrasonic destruction (lithotripsy) may be used. In other cases, treatment is conservative. Any identifiable cause should be treated and patients should be maintained on a high fluid intake. Drugs which alter urinary pH (BNF 7.4.3) may be of value. An opioid analgesic (BNF 4.7.2) may be required for renal colic and an injectable non-steroidal anti-inflammatory drug has been shown to be of benefit.

Renal Failure

Definition

Renal failure is the failure of the kidney to excrete metabolic waste products or to maintain plasma electrolytes at normal concentrations in the presence of normal dietary intake. It may be acute or chronic. In either case it is characterised by the development of uraemia. Drugs which are excreted by the kidney (e.g. many antimicrobials) will remain in the body for longer than is normal, and when used in renal failure their dosage will require adjustment (BNF – Prescribing in Renal Impairment).

Uraemia

Definition

Uraemia is a clinical state associated with advanced renal impairment and retention of nitrogenous waste products in the blood.

Symptoms

Initially it is characterised by fatigue, insomnia, lethargy, and general malaise. This is followed by gastro-intestinal symptoms (e.g. anorexia, diarrhoea, gastro-intestinal bleeding, hiccup, and nausea and vomiting). If water intake is reduced, dehydration may occur because urine of a fixed osmolality is produced. Conversely, water retention may arise if fluid intake is increased. Hypertension together with sodium and water retention are common, and may lead to heart failure and resultant peripheral and pulmonary oedema. There may be pericarditis, and anaemia is a common sign. Neurological symptoms include confusion with loss of concentration, muscle twitching, and peripheral neuropathy. Convulsions and coma may develop. Infection, particularly of the urinary tract, is a common complication and may lead to septicaemia. Metabolic acidosis can occur and hyperphosphataemia may lead to hypocalcaemia. Hyperkalaemia may develop and result in sudden death.

Treatment

Haemodialysis or peritoneal dialysis will remove nitrogenous waste products from the blood and delay the onset of uraemia.

Acute Renal Failure

Definition and aetiology

Acute renal failure is an acute severe deterioration in renal function resulting in acute uraemia. Acute failure may be caused by hypovolaemic shock, acute tubular necrosis, interstitial nephritis, acute glomerulonephritis, renal vascular abnormalities, or urinary-tract obstruction. It may also arise as a result of drug administration (e.g. analgesics and antibacterials), septicaemia, or heavy metal poisoning (e.g. lead). Other causes include burns, crushing injuries, malignant hypertension, or heart failure. It may also occur after surgery.

Symptoms

The onset of acute renal failure is sudden. The only initial symptoms may be oliguria, back pain, and tenderness, but this is followed by anuria and uraemic symptoms.

Treatment

Acute renal failure is a medical emergency. The underlying cause should be treated if possible. Hyperkalaemia must be treated immediately and a calcium salt (BNF 9.5.1.1) or glucose (BNF 9.2.2), or both, with or without insulin, may be given intravenously. In addition, an ion-exchange resin (BNF 9.2.1.1) may be used. A loop diuretic (BNF 2.2.2) may be administered, although fluid replacement may be necessary if the patient becomes dehydrated. Metabolic acidosis should be treated with an infusion of sodium bicarbonate with isotonic sodium chloride (BNF 9.2.2). Antiepileptics (BNF 4.8) and antihypertensive therapy (BNF 2.5) may be necessary. The patient should be maintained on a low-protein diet (BNF Appendix 3) with fluid and electrolyte intake regulated. Dialysis may be indicated.

Chronic Renal Failure

Definition and aetiology

Chronic renal failure is a chronic reduction in renal function which is characterised by the progressive development of uraemia. It commonly arises as a result of glomerulonephritis, interstitial nephritis, or pyelonephritis. Other causes include urinary-tract obstruction, hereditary abnormalities (e.g. polycystic kidney disease), or systemic disorders (e.g. diabetes mellitus, gout, or systemic lupus erythematosus). It may also be due to nephrotoxic drugs (e.g. analgesics and antibacterials) or heavy metals (e.g. lead).

Symptoms

Initially, compensation for the loss of renal function may occur and the only symptoms of failure may be an impaired power of urine concentration and clearance, resulting in polyuria, nocturia, and thirst. Pruritus and increased skin pigmentation may occur. Only when excretion fails to keep pace with production does uraemia develop.

Treatment

Treatment is as for acute renal failure (*see above*). Phosphate-binding agents (BNF 9.5.2.2) may be required to treat hyperphosphataemia, and a vitamin D analogue (BNF 9.6.4) to prevent renal osteodystrophy. Long-term dialysis or renal transplantation may prevent the fatal outcome of chronic renal failure.

Self-help organisation
British Kidney Patients Association

Renal Osteodystrophy

Definition and aetiology
Renal osteodystrophy (renal rickets) is a collective term for a group of skeletal disorders which occur as a result of chronic renal failure. These disorders include osteitis fibrosa, osteomalacia, and osteoporosis. They may occur singly or in combination, and are due to the development of hyperphosphataemia and hypocalcaemia together with hyperparathyroidism, and disturbed vitamin-D metabolism. All of these can occur as a result of chronic renal failure. Renal osteodystrophy may be exacerbated by corticosteroid administration, and by aluminium retention resulting from dialysis.

Symptoms
Symptoms include bone pain and tenderness, fractures, joint disease, skeletal deformity, and soft-tissue calcification. Growth retardation (renal dwarfism) may occur in children.

Treatment
Treatment consists of the administration of a phosphate-binding agent (BNF 9.5.2.2) and a vitamin D preparation (BNF 9.6.4). Calcium (BNF 9.5.1.1) and vitamin supplements without vitamin A (BNF 9.6) may be required. A reduction in dialysis fluid aluminium concentration may be helpful. If drug treatment is ineffective, parathyroidectomy may be considered.

7.5   URINARY-TRACT DISORDERS

Urinary Incontinence

Definition and aetiology
Urinary incontinence is characterised by constant or frequent involuntary urination.

Urge incontinence is involuntary urination which occurs as soon as the desire to urinate becomes apparent. It may be a consequence of dementia, stroke, urinary-tract infection, or caused by an instability of bladder smooth muscle (unstable detrusor muscle).

Stress incontinence occurs more commonly in women and is characterised by the leakage of urine as a result of stress (e.g. coughing, laughing, or lifting). It is usually due to weakness of the pelvic floor muscles and may occur as a result of childbirth, the menopause, pregnancy, or uterine prolapse. It may occur in men subsequent to prostatectomy.

Urinary incontinence may also occur as a result of drug administration (e.g. diuretics and hypnotics), neurological disorders (e.g. multiple sclerosis), or spinal cord injury (e.g. neurogenic bladder).

Treatment
Treatment comprises bladder training, the use of incontinence aids, and physiotherapy to strengthen the pelvic floor muscles. Catheterisation may be indicated in severe cases. Anticholinergic drugs or certain tricyclic antidepressants (BNF 7.4.2) may be helpful in urge incontinence, and surgery may be required in severe cases of stress incontinence.

Nocturnal Enuresis

Definition and aetiology
Nocturnal enuresis is persistent involuntary urination during sleep. It occurs normally in young children, but is abnormal if it continues after the age at which control is usually achieved. It is most common in boys and a family history often exists. It is often associated with deep sleep and may be due to some underlying physical cause (e.g. phimosis, spina bifida, or urethral stricture). Urinary-tract infection (e.g. cystitis and urethritis) may be responsible and it may be psychogenic.

Treatment
Appropriate antibacterial therapy (BNF 5.1) is indicated in the presence of urinary-tract infection. Enuretic alarms may be used, psychotherapy is beneficial in some patients, and surgical correction is required in others. In refractory cases, drug treatment comprises the administration of certain anticholinergic, sympathomimetic, or tricyclic antidepressant drugs (BNF 7.4.2). Bladder training, however, may be all that is required.

Self-help organisations
Disabled Living Foundation
Equipment for the Disabled

7.6   ANATOMY AND PHYSIOLOGY OF THE GENITAL, RENAL, AND URINARY-TRACT SYSTEMS

The Male and Female Genital Systems

The female reproductive organs   The female reproductive system (*see* Fig. 7.2) consists of the ovaries, the

Fallopian tubes (oviducts), the uterus (womb), the vagina, and the external organs. The breasts are also considered to be part of the system.

The two ovaries, located one on each side of the uterus in the pelvic cavity, are the primary organs of the female system and are responsible for the maturation of the ova and the secretion of the reproductive hormones, the oestrogens and progesterone. Approximately 18 000 primary oocytes (the precursor cells from which the ova develop) are formed by the third month of foetal development and stored within the ovaries. The ovaries are suspended by ligaments immediately outside the open ends of the Fallopian tubes. The two Fallopian tubes provide the channels along which the ovum is transported from the ovary to the uterus. The movement of the ovum is assisted by peristaltic contractions of the muscular layer and surface cilia of the Fallopian tubes.

The uterus is the central feature of the female reproductive system. It is the site of origin of the elements in menstrual flow, the site of implantation and nurture of a fertilised ovum, and the tissue which expels the developed foetus from the mother's body. It is anatomically divided into the innermost fundus, the central tube-shaped body, and the outermost narrow neck of the uterus (the cervix). The outer surface of the uterine wall forms part of the peritoneum. The uterovesical and uterorectal pouches denote the front and rear projections of the peritoneum over the bladder and rectum respectively (see Fig. 7.1). The muscular central portion of the uterus wall is the myometrium. The inner surface of the uterus (the endometrium) is highly vascularised and undergoes cyclical changes to its structure and thickness (see below).

The uterine orifice at the cervix is held tightly closed except during childbirth, although the opening is sufficient to allow the passage of sperm. The channel from the cervix to the exterior is formed of a muscular passageway (the vagina) which can dilate to accommodate the penis during sexual intercourse and to allow the passage of the foetus at birth.

The outermost organ of the female reproductive system is the vulva which comprises the clitoris, the labia majora and minora, and the prepuce.

The menstrual and ovarian cycles   The ovum is produced within the ovary from the primary oocyte by meiosis (oogenesis). At puberty and cyclically until the menopause, an ovum develops each month during the first two weeks of the menstrual cycle (see Fig. 7.3). The ovum is formed within a fluid-filled Graafian follicle and at ovulation it is released from the follicle into the pelvic cavity. The ovum is guided into the funnel-shaped infundibulum of the Fallopian tube by finger-like ciliary projections (the fimbriae). The remnants of the Graafian follicle in the ovary multiply rapidly and form the yellow, highly vascularised corpus luteum. The corpus luteum secretes oestrogens and progesterone, which act on the endometrium to increase its blood supply and thickness in preparation for the receipt of a fertilised ovum. If the ovum is not fertilised, the corpus luteum degenerates. The resultant decline in progesterone and oestrogen levels leads to menstruation through the breakdown and shedding of the endometrium (see also Section 6.6).

The mammary glands   The development of the mammary glands at puberty is stimulated by increased secretion of oestrogens and the presence of progesterone. Each gland (Fig. 7.6) consists of 15 to 20 lobes separated by adipose tissue, the quantity of which determines the size of the breast. The lobes are subdivided into lobules consisting of connective tissue in which clusters of milk-secreting cells (the alveoli) are embedded. Milk is transported from the alveoli through the mammary ducts to storage compartments, the ampullae, and is then released to the nipple through lactiferous ducts.

The male reproductive organs   In the male, the organs analogous to the female ovaries are the testes. They are formed on the foetal posterior abdominal wall and descend before birth into a sac (the scrotum) located outside the body cavity (Fig. 7.7). The position of the testes in an environment maintained 3 or 4°C below body temperature is important for the production and survival of sperm.

The testes are internally divided into 200 to 300 lobules, which each contain 1 to 3 highly convoluted seminiferous tubules of up to 60 cm length. The spaces between the tubules are occupied by the interstitial cells of Leydig which secrete testosterone. The process of sperm production (spermatogenesis) starts at puberty and continues throughout life. It begins in the basement membrane of the seminiferous tubules with the formation of the spermatogonia, which become primary spermatocytes on detachment from the membrane. Meiotic division results in the formation of spermatids which develop into spermatozoa. The spermatozoa are transported from the seminiferous tubule to the epididymis where they undergo final maturation. Approximately 300 million spermatozoa reach full maturity each day.

The epididymis, which lies on the rear surface of the testis (Fig. 7.8), consists of a tightly coiled tube which may extend to up to 6 metres in length. Spermatozoa may reside within the tube for up to four weeks but if they are not ejected within this period they are reabsorbed.

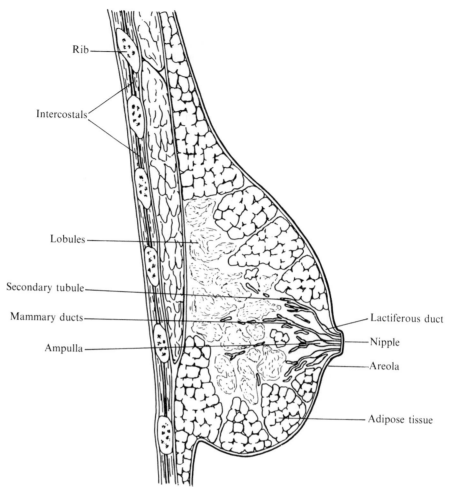

Fig. 7.6
Breast (sagittal section).

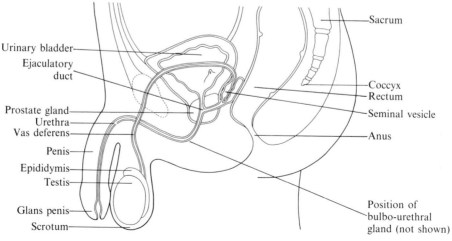

Fig. 7.7
Male pelvic organs.

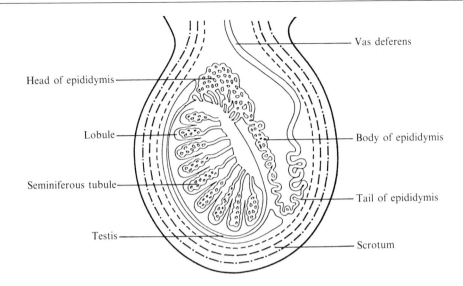

Fig. 7.8
Cross-section of a testis.

Sperm are transported from the epididymis along the vas deferens (ductus deferens) into the ejaculatory duct located at the back of the bladder. The vas deferens is supported and protected by the spermatic cord (comprising arteries, veins, nerves, lymphatic vessels, and muscle). From the ejaculatory duct, sperm enter the urethra which passes through the prostate gland and into the penis.

The sperm are maintained within a fluid which is secreted by the prostate gland, the seminal vesicles, and the bulbo-urethral (Cowper's) glands. The prostate gland encircles the neck of the bladder and its alkaline secretions, which impart a milky appearance to seminal fluid, are added to the spermatozoa through numerous ducts into the prostatic portion of the urethra.

The seminal vesicles are a pair of sac-like structures lying on each side of the lower surface of the bladder. Their secretions, which include fructose in an alkaline medium, are added to the sperm in the vas deferens immediately before they enter the ejaculatory duct.

The bulbo-urethral glands are located underneath the prostate gland and secrete an alkaline fluid into the urethra.

The Renal and Urinary-tract Systems

The kidneys are located within the rear of the abdominal cavity on either side of the vertebral column and are partially protected by the lowest pairs of ribs (Fig. 7.9). They lie outside the peritoneal cavity (i.e. retroperitoneally) and are surrounded by a protective mass of fat, the adipose capsule.

Internally, the kidney consists of the renal parenchyma which is divided into an outer cortex and an inner medulla. The medulla contains from 5 to 14 pyramidal structures. The base of each pyramid forms the boundary between the cortex and medulla and the apex points towards the renal pelvis. The pyramids appear striated due to the presence of linear blood vessels and tubules. The renal pelvis is the collecting chamber for urine which subsequently drains into the ureters, bladder, and urethra.

Each kidney contains approximately one million nephrons which are the basic functional units. The head of the nephron is formed of a cup-shaped tubule (the Bowman's capsule) which embraces a capillary network (the glomerulus). Nephrons may be classed as cortical if the glomerulus lies in the outer cortex, or as juxtamedullary if the glomerulus lies within the cortex but close to the cortico-medulla border.

Beyond the Bowman's capsule the nephron consists sequentially of the proximal convoluted tubule, the loop of Henlé, the distal convoluted tubule, and the collecting duct (see Fig. 7.4).

The kidney receives approximately 25% of the blood output of the heart and is abundantly supplied with blood vessels. Blood enters the kidneys via the renal artery which subdivides into individual afferent arterioles for the glomerulus of each nephron. The network of capillaries which comprise the glomerulus rejoin to form the efferent arteriole (not an efferent venule). Capillaries branch off from the efferent arteriole to produce a meshwork of blood vessels around the

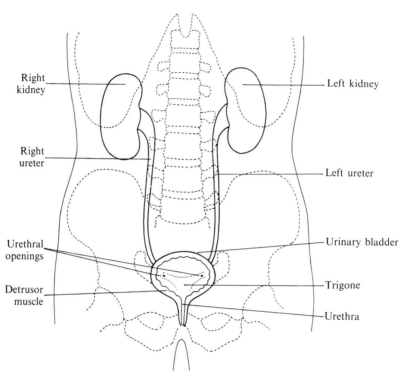

Fig. 7.9
Position of kidneys and bladder.

convoluted tubules and loop of Henlé. These peritubular capillaries eventually reunite to pass blood to the renal vein which leaves the kidney near the renal pelvis.

The kidney carries out its roles of controlling blood volume and solute concentration, regulation of blood pH, and removal of toxic waste materials by the processes of glomerular filtration, tubular reabsorption, and tubular secretion. Approximately 10% of the 1300 mL of blood which enters the glomerulus each minute is forced through the glomerular-Bowman's capsule interface. The pressure for filtration derives primarily from the hydrostatic pressure within the blood vessel but is opposed by osmotic pressure generated by the presence of plasma protein and the pressure of fluid already within the kidney tubule. Under normal circumstances, the filtrate consists of all blood components with the exception of blood cells and the larger proportion of plasma protein. In a healthy adult, the glomerular filtration rate is approximately 125 mL per minute, but of this only 1% is excreted as urine.

As the fluid passes along the nephron, essential materials are conserved through their transfer into the peritubular capillaries by the processes of diffusion, active reabsorption, and electrostatic attraction. Under normal circumstances, all the glucose, amino acids, and potassium ions present in the filtrate are actively reabsorbed in the proximal convoluted tubule.

Sodium ions are actively transported by the 'sodium pump' from the nephron, mainly in the proximal convoluted tubule and the loop of Henlé but also in the distal convoluted tubule. The passage of sodium ions into the blood creates a temporary electropositive environment which is balanced by the reabsorption of chloride ions from the nephron.

The return of sodium ions into the plasma leads to the reabsorption of an iso-osmotic equivalent of water, and accounts for the reabsorption of approximately 80% of all water retained. The remainder is reabsorbed in the distal and collecting tubules under the influence of vasopressin, and it is this component which significantly affects the blood volume.

The homoeostatic regulation of blood pH is achieved by the secretion of potassium and hydrogen ions in the distal convoluted tubule. Hydrogen ions, commonly in combination with ammonia produced by the deamination of amino acids, are secreted in exchange for the reabsorption of sodium ions, causing the pH of blood to rise. (Urea, another deamination waste product, is also excreted by the nephron.)

Hydrogen ions are also removed from the blood through the formation of carbonic acid. Carbon dioxide from the plasma diffuses into the cells lining the distal and collecting duct tubules. In these cells, it combines with water to form carbonic acid which can then dissociate to produce hydrogen ions and bicarbonate ions. If the pH of the blood is low (i.e. there is a high hydrogen-ion concentration), a diffusion concentration gradient is established between the capillaries and the tubule, and hydrogen ions enter the urine. The electrostatic balance in the tubule cells is maintained by the reabsorption of a cation, usually sodium, from the urine. Sodium ions then combine with bicarbonate ions in the tubule cell and the product is absorbed into the blood. As a result, the pH of the blood is raised and the presence of sodium bicarbonate acts as a buffer to prevent a further fall in blood pH.

The end-product of the processes of filtration, reabsorption, and secretion which occur in the kidney is urine. The volume of urine excreted each day varies from 1 to 2 litres and is influenced by many factors (e.g. blood pressure, temperature, and fluid intake). Urine passes from the collecting ducts of each nephron into the renal pelvis. From the pelvis, a funnel-like neck narrows to form the ureter, a long muscular tube, which leads to the urinary bladder.

Urine flows down the ureter partially by gravity, but its passage is considerably assisted by peristaltic contractions of the muscular wall of the ureter. The waves of contraction cause the urine to enter the bladder in spurts occurring every 10 to 60 seconds.

The bladder is a muscular reservoir which in the male lies directly in front of the rectum, and in the female is situated in front of the vagina and below the uterus. The ureters have to pass beneath the bladder to reach the openings, which arise on its floor in a triangular non-elastic muscular region, the trigone. This anatomical arrangement means that, despite the absence of reflux valves, the backflow of urine towards the kidneys is prevented by the pressure of the expanding bladder on the underlying ureters. The ureteral openings are situated at the two rear apices of the trigone, and the urethral orifice lies at the front apex.

As the bladder fills with urine, the muscular layer within its wall, the detrusor muscle, relaxes. When the volume within the bladder exceeds approximately 200 to 400 mL, stretch receptors in the detrusor muscle are stimulated leading to the desire to void urine (micturition). The bladder initiates emptying by contraction of the detrusor muscles and relaxation of the internal bladder sphincter. Urine is voided by the conscious relaxation of the external sphincter which lies in the urogenital diaphragm (pelvic floor) and is composed of skeletal muscle.

The urethra is the vessel which carries urine from the base of the bladder to the outside. In males, it is approximately 20 cm in length, but is much shorter in females (approximately 4 cm).

Chapter 8

MALIGNANT DISEASE

8.1 MALIGNANT NEOPLASMS OF THE GASTRO-INTESTINAL TRACT

(For a detailed explanation of the morphological characteristics of malignant tissue, *see* Section 15.7.)

Cancer of the Gall Bladder and Bile Ducts

Definition and aetiology
Cancer of the gall bladder is uncommon, but occurs more frequently in the elderly, particularly women. There may be an association with obesity and the presence of gallstones.

Bile-duct cancers are most commonly adenocarcinomas, slow-growing, and arise predominantly in the middle-aged and the elderly. An increased incidence may be associated with chronic ulcerative colitis.

Symptoms
In gall-bladder cancer, periodic pain and dyspepsia may be present for several years prior to diagnosis. Later symptoms, which indicate an advanced stage of the disease, may include weight loss, severe pain particularly located in the right upper abdominal quadrant, and jaundice. A firm tender mass may also be felt at the site of the pain. Confirmation of diagnosis may be achieved with ultrasound or computerised tomography (CT).

Cancer of the bile ducts may produce symptoms of progressive obstruction. Jaundice, pruritus, and weight loss may occur, together with dark urine and pale stools. Vomiting, and diarrhoea or constipation may also develop.

Treatment
The prognosis is poor in cancer of the gall bladder, but can be variable in cancer of the bile ducts. Surgical removal of the gall bladder and liver resection may be attempted in cancer of the gall bladder, often with very limited success. It is not usually possible to excise the slower growing bile-duct tumour, although drainage of bile can be facilitated by the insertion of prostheses.

Cancer of the Liver

Definition and aetiology
Cancer of the liver is a disease with a grim outlook, which commonly occurs secondary to cancer in another organ and only infrequently as a primary malignancy (hepatocellular carcinoma).

Metastatic Carcinoma of the Liver

Definition and aetiology
The passage of blood through the liver may act as a source of metastases, particularly from the gastro-intestinal tract and respiratory system. The breast may also be a primary source of the cancer. Initial diagnosis of the primary cancer, particularly in the elderly, may be shown through the presence of liver metastases.

Symptoms
Non-specific symptoms include weight loss, anorexia, and fever. The degree of hepatomegaly may correspond to the stage of advancement of the disease. Splenomegaly and ascites may also occur and, in later stages, jaundice may develop. Liver-function tests may initially remain normal, although alkaline phosphatase levels may rise steadily as the disease progresses.

Treatment
Treatment is often ineffective.

Hepatocellular Carcinoma

Definition and aetiology
Hepatocellular carcinoma is a primary malignant disease, and is less common than metastatic carcinoma of the liver. The condition is comparatively rare in the western world, but has a higher incidence in Africa and southeast Asia. It is most commonly associated with pre-existing cirrhosis, although hepatitis B virus infections have also been implicated.

Symptoms
The onset may be insidious, and presenting symptoms include right upper abdominal pain, fever, and weight loss. Abdominal swelling may be caused by hepatomegaly, in the presence or absence of ascites. The tumour may rupture, causing intraperitoneal bleeding.

Treatment
The mean survival time is limited to several months. Improvement in survival time may only be achieved by transplantation or complete resection, although surgical resection is frequently hampered by the presence of cirrhosis. Chemotherapy may be beneficial, with a positive response sometimes obtained following intravenous administration of doxorubicin (BNF 8.1.2).

Cancer of the Stomach

Definition and aetiology
Stomach cancer is commonly an adenocarcinoma. It has a varied geographical distribution, and has been tentatively linked to genetic factors because of a higher incidence in people of blood group A. Environmental and

dietary factors are more important, and proposed factors include ingestion of pickled foods and alcohol, and inhalation of smoke and dust particles. Interest has been expressed in the levels of nitrates in water or food, as they are converted to potentially carcinogenic nitrosamines by bacteria in the intestine.

Stomach cancer is predominantly a condition of ageing, with the highest incidence in those of 60 to 70 years of age. It is the third most common fatal cancer in the UK. Its incidence appears to be declining, although the reason for this is unknown.

Symptoms

Early disease may be asymptomatic, and many patients do not present until the condition is advanced. Dyspepsia, epigastric pain, and a feeling of fullness after eating may be early signs which are difficult to distinguish from peptic ulceration. Later signs may include anorexia, nausea and vomiting, and weight loss, resulting in weakness. Anaemia may also occur as a result of occult blood loss. Metastases may cause abdominal swelling due to ascites, or jaundice due to liver involvement. Metastases may also arise in bone, brain, and lungs.

Treatment

Early surgical removal of the tumour (partial gastrectomy) provides the best prognosis, giving a 5-year survival rate of 90%. However, few tumours are diagnosed sufficiently early. The survival rate in advanced disease is considerably reduced. Total parenteral nutrition (BNF 9.3) may be required. Chemotherapy has been used with limited success.

Carcinoid Syndrome

Definition and aetiology

The carcinoid syndrome (argentaffinoma syndrome) comprises a varied and complex group of symptoms occurring in patients with malignant carcinoid tumours (argentaffinoma). The primary tumour may originate in the argentaffin cells of the gastro-intestinal tract (most commonly in the terminal ileum, appendix, and rectum), lung tissue, ovaries, and testes. Most patients with carcinoid tumours do not, however, get the syndrome. Whereas symptoms of the syndrome may be produced by primary lung and gonadal tumours, they do not develop from primary gastro-intestinal tumours unless hepatic metastases have arisen. This is because the biologically-active agents (e.g. serotonin and prostaglandins) released from these tumours are metabolised in the hepatic-portal system before they can reach the general circulation.

Symptoms

The syndrome is characterised classically by flushing. This may be accompanied by a sensation of intense heat, hypotension, and tachycardia. The flush, which ranges from redness to cyanosis, typically affects the head and neck, but in severe cases may spread to the trunk and limbs. The duration of the flush ranges from minutes to almost continuous. Flushing may be precipitated by alcohol, caffeine, food, emotional disturbances, and other forms of stress. Other symptoms include bronchospasm, diarrhoea (which is often severe and may be associated with abdominal pain), nausea and vomiting, weight loss, and wheezing. Complications include obstruction of the small intestine, pellagra, and pulmonary and tricuspid stenosis, causing dyspnoea and oedema as a result of right ventricular failure.

Treatment

Treatment is directed towards alleviating the symptoms. Surgical removal of the primary tumour is indicated only if it is situated in the lungs, ovaries, or testes. Surgery to remove liver metastases or selective embolisation via the hepatic artery may help relieve symptoms. Flushing may be controlled by avoidance of precipitating factors, and by the administration of alpha-adrenoceptor blocking drugs (BNF 2.5.4), or phenothiazines (BNF 4.2.1). Antihistamines (BNF 3.4.1) and H_2-receptor blocking drugs (BNF 1.3) may also be used. The use of corticosteroids (BNF 6.3.4) is reserved for severe and protracted attacks. Diarrhoea may be treated with antidiarrhoeal drugs which reduce motility (BNF 1.4.2); cholestyramine (BNF 1.5) may reduce bile acid-induced diarrhoea in patients with a resected ileum. Specific serotonin antagonists such as cyproheptadine (BNF 3.4.1) or methysergide (BNF 4.7.4.2) may be effective in controlling intractable diarrhoea and flushing, but methysergide should be used with caution in view of the risk of retroperitoneal fibrosis. Nicotinamide (BNF 9.6.2) is used for the prevention and treatment of pellagra.

Colorectal Cancer

Definition and aetiology

Cancers in the large intestine may be classified as adenomas found as polyps, which are frequently precancerous, and adenocarcinomas found in colorectal cancer.

A significant proportion of cancers of the large intestine occur in the rectum and sigmoid colon. Colonic cancer is more common in women, whereas rectal cancer is twice as common in men. Most cancers are adenocarcinomas, slow-growing, and form discrete anatomical entities that can be easily removed. Metastases may develop in the liver and bladder.

The incidence has been related to the intake of fat, meat, processed foods, and alcohol, with diets high in fibre producing a low incidence. Ulcerative colitis may also be a predisposing factor. With the exception of those cases associated with genetic factors (e.g. familial adenomatous polyposis, *see* Polyps), most cases of colorectal cancer arise in the middle-aged and the elderly.

Symptoms
Symptoms in the early stages may include occult blood in the stools, fatigue, and weakness. Patients may also report a change in bowel habits. Late symptoms may occur (e.g. pain and weight loss) and a detectable mass may be caused by the tumour or blockage of faeces.

Treatment
Surgery is the primary form of treatment. Colorectal carcinomas may be surgically excised and the large intestine resected. If the anal sphincter is involved, the formation of a colostomy is required. Radiotherapy may be beneficial, particularly for patients who are experiencing significant pain. Some patients may respond to chemotherapy with fluorouracil (BNF 8.1.3).

Oesophageal Cancer

Definition and aetiology
Malignant tumours in the oesophagus arise predominantly in the middle and lower portions. They are commonly squamous cell carcinomas, although a small proportion may be adenocarcinomas. Oesophageal tumours have been associated with heavy alcohol and tobacco consumption. Poisoning with corrosive agents may also increase the likelihood of cancer due to oesophageal damage. Achalasia has also been linked with oesophageal cancer.

Symptoms
The commonest symptom is dysphagia, initially only present on ingestion of solids, but subsequently also associated with fluid intake. The presence of persistent chest pain warns of infiltration, with metastases commonly arising in the liver, gastric glands, lungs, and aorta. Weight loss and anorexia may develop, possibly associated with difficulty in swallowing. In advanced stages of the disease, anaemia may also occur.

Treatment
Symptomatic relief may be obtained by oesophageal dilatation. Surgery may be useful, particularly in adenocarcinoma, but is often associated with a high incidence of mortality. Chemotherapy is of little value, but

radiotherapy and laser photocoagulation may provide temporary relief. The prognosis is poor following diagnosis, with an expected 5-year survival rate of less than 5%.

Pancreatic (Exocrine) Cancer

Definition and aetiology
Pancreatic (exocrine) cancer is an invariably fatal disease and is usually an adenocarcinoma. Most malignancies arise in the head of the gland although, because early diagnosis is difficult, dissemination to many sites may occur prior to initial identification. Metastases to the lung and liver are common.

Pancreatic cancer occurs most commonly in patients of 50 years of age and over and is more common in smokers than non-smokers. A high incidence has also been correlated with a high dietary fat content, alcohol intake, and with diabetes mellitus.

Symptoms
The predominant symptom is usually pain, commonly arising in the upper abdomen. The pain may be aggravated by food and relieved by changes in posture. Obstructive jaundice may develop due to blockage of the bile duct or gall bladder. Other non-specific symptoms may include a progressive loss of weight, anorexia, and lassitude. If the tumour is initially localised to the body or tail of the gland, gastric and oesophageal varices may occur in association with splenomegaly and gastrointestinal haemorrhage.

Treatment
Most measures which may be taken after diagnosis are palliative only. Surgery (e.g. total pancreatectomy) may be carried out but must be followed by pancreatin supplements (BNF 1.9.4) and insulin therapy (BNF 6.1.1). Chemotherapy has not proved effective, although in combination with radiotherapy a slight improvement in life expectancy has been shown. However, most patients do not survive beyond 9 months.

8.2 MALIGNANT NEOPLASMS OF THE RESPIRATORY SYSTEM

Cancer of the Pleura and Peritoneum

Definition and aetiology
Cancer of the pleura and peritoneum may arise as a primary malignancy or as a metastasis. Primary cancer, which usually takes the form of a mesothelioma, commonly arises through exposure to asbestos. Unlike lung

cancer, it is not related to smoking. The mesothelioma usually arises in the pleura, but it may also originate in the peritoneum.

Metastatic pleural cancer can occur as a consequence of cancer of the lung, breast, and ovaries, and may develop unilaterally or bilaterally.

Symptoms

Symptoms of primary malignancy may be ill-defined and include dyspnoea, dull chest pain, and weakness. Cough, pyrexia, and weight loss are less common symptoms. Radiography may reveal massive pleural effusions.

Treatment

Surgery is not feasible, whereas radiotherapy and chemotherapy may be beneficial in a minority of early cases. The accumulation of pleural fluid may be retarded by intrapleural injection of tetracycline, bleomycin, or thiotepa. These irritant substances produce adhesion between the inner surfaces of the pleural membranes and are injected following drainage of the pleural fluid. The prognosis is grim, with an average survival of 8 to 10 months.

Lung Cancer

Definition and aetiology

Lung cancer (bronchial carcinoma) may arise primarily in the bronchi, or as a secondary growth from other parts of the body (e.g. pancreas, breast, colon, and bone). It occurs most frequently between 50 and 70 years of age and is the most common cause of death from cancer in males in the UK. The incidence is increasing in women.

Well-documented statistical studies have linked the development of lung cancer to various factors, the most common being smoking (cigarette, cigar, and pipe). The incidence may be related to the amount smoked each day, the depth of inhalation, number of puffs, and the type of tobacco smoked. All tobacco smoking can cause lung cancer, but the incidence is greatest in cigarette smoking. There is also a correlation between the degree of risk and how young the individual is when smoking is started. Individuals subjected to continual smoke-filled atmospheres also have a higher risk of developing lung cancer through 'passive' smoking.

Other causes of lung cancer include ionising radiations, asbestos, and possibly air pollution. Occupations associated with a high risk of lung cancer include workers exposed to tar in steel and aluminium industries, and environments where a high level of polycyclic hydrocarbons may be introduced into the atmosphere.

The classification of lung cancers has been devised by the World Health Organization (WHO). Epidermoid (squamous) cell cancers give rise to bulky tumours and are commonly attributable to smoking. They occur predominantly in the larger bronchi and are spread through the lymphatic system. Small (oat) cell cancers are undifferentiated cells which may arise anywhere within the proximal large bronchi. The cells are rapid-growing, are commonly induced by ionising radiations, and are highly invasive. Adenocarcinomas, which appear in the periphery of the lung and are spread through the bloodstream, are less directly the consequence of smoking. The remainder of the cell types which appear in lung cancer are grouped under the classification of large cell carcinomas. They are commonly caused by smoking and, like adenocarcinomas, are spread through the bloodstream.

Symptoms

The symptoms of lung cancer are varied and depend on the type of cancer cell; the direct spread of the tumour to adjacent tissues and indirect metastasis via the blood and lymphatic system; and the secretion of hormones and other agents from the tumour which may give rise to metabolic, endocrine, and neurological symptoms.

Cough is commonly the primary symptom. A smoker may cough as a result of chronic bronchitis, and a change in the nature and severity of the cough may be an important indication of the development of cancer. Excess sputum in the bronchial tree (produced as a direct consequence of the tumour, from infection due to blockage, or the presence of the tumour itself) may cause the entrapment of air in the alveoli, leading to wheezing and atelectasis. Haemoptysis, commonly seen as streaking in the sputum, may occur in up to 50% of patients. Less clearly defined symptoms, but whose presence may indicate a deterioration in general health, include chest pain or ache, dyspnoea, weight loss, lack of energy, and a loss of interest.

Complications may develop from the pressure of the growth on adjacent structures or from the presence of metastases. The superior vena cava may become compressed, resulting in distension of the veins of the neck, thorax, and upper arms. Associated symptoms may include oedema of the face and neck, headache, and pleural effusions. Speech impairment may be a consequence of compression of the laryngeal nerve, and dysphagia can occur as a result of oesophageal constriction. Metastases are common in the skeleton (e.g. the humerus, ribs, and vertebrae), liver, and brain.

Endocrine complications occur due to the production of polypeptides which mimic the action of endogenous hormones (e.g. vasopressin, adrenocorticotrophin, parathormone, and gonadotrophin).

Treatment

With the exception of the majority of small cell lung cancers, surgery is the most effective means of treatment. Surgical excision (thoracotomy) of a well-formed mass may give a better prognosis, although surgery may be contra-indicated in patients with cardiac or respiratory impairment, and in those with distant metastases.

Radiotherapy is used primarily for the relief of symptoms, although it has been employed as an adjunct before and after surgery. It is effective in reducing the pain of bone and brain metastases.

Chemotherapy is used predominantly for the treatment of small cell lung cancers. Drugs are most effective when used in combinations of up to four agents (BNF 8.1) comprising members from each of the classes of cytotoxic drugs. Survival times for patients with localised small cell cancer may be up to 18 months and for patients with extensive disease up to 12 months.

Other drugs may be required to treat the complications of lung cancer. Antibacterial drugs (BNF 5.1) may be used for respiratory infections and dexamethasone for the control of cerebral oedema from brain metastases.

8.3 MALIGNANT NEOPLASMS OF THE CENTRAL NERVOUS SYSTEM

Intracranial Tumours

Definition and aetiology

Intracranial tumours constitute a wide variety of cell types which produce a broad spectrum of disease. The classification of malignant and benign is less important in the brain than in other tissues of the body, as the ability of the brain to accommodate any growth is extremely limited.

Tumours may arise from the meninges, the skull, or any component of the central nervous tissue. Primary tumours predominate, although approximately 25% of all intracranial tumours may arise as metastases from the lungs, kidneys, breast, thyroid, and melanomas. Central nervous tissue is the second most common site for primary tumours in childhood. No causative agents have been discovered, but certain primary tumours (e.g. meningioma and optic glioma) have been associated with von Recklinghausen's neurofibromatosis.

The commonest intracranial tumours develop from neural tubes and are classed as **gliomas**. These are further subdivided as astrocytomas, oligodendrogliomas, and medulloblastomas. Astrocytomas may be benign or malignant and occur at any age. They may be well circumscribed and slow-growing, producing few early clinical symptoms, or rapidly proliferating and invasive and causing significant cerebral oedema. Oligodendrogliomas are extremely slow-growing and only appear in adulthood. Medulloblastomas usually develop in the roof of the fourth ventricle, are extremely malignant, and appear in childhood. Unlike the majority of other intracranial tumours, they form metastases in bone and bone marrow.

The second largest group of tumours is classed as **meningiomas**. They occur predominantly in adults of 40 to 60 years of age, are commonly benign, and usually develop from arachnoid cells to appear on the dorsal surface of the brain and the base of the skull. If there is a rich vascular supply to the tumour, it may be described as angioblastic, and on enlargement may cause erosion of the skull.

Schwannomas (neurilemmomas or neurinomas) are derived from Schwann cells (which supply the myelin sheath) and are benign. The presence of a Schwannoma on the acoustic nerve may affect hearing as a result of pressure on the nerve.

Pituitary tumours may develop from the remnants of the pituitary stalk (craniopharyngiomas) and cause compression of the optic nerve and chiasma, hypopituitarism, and hydrocephalus. Pituitary adenomas are more common and usually benign. They may be secreting, producing a range of pituitary hormones (e.g. adrenocorticotrophin, growth hormone, and prolactin), or non-secreting, causing compression of normal pituitary tissue and resulting in hypopituitarism.

Haemangioblastomas are benign tumours of uncertain origin, but are normally classed as vascular tumours. They are commonly found in the cerebellum of adolescents and young adults, and usually arise singly and are cystic.

Other less common forms of intracranial tumours include colloid cysts and choroid plexus papillomas.

Symptoms

The symptoms of an intracranial tumour vary according to its size, location, morphological characteristics, and rate of growth. Symptoms may be attributed to raised intracranial pressure, epilepsy, and localised neurological changes.

Intracranial pressure produces headache, vomiting, drowsiness, and visual disturbances. Headache commonly occurs early in the morning or may wake the patient from sleep. It may be aggravated by factors which further increase intracranial pressure (e.g. coughing). In the presence of a tumour in the fourth ventricle, vomiting may occur on its own or as a precursor to headache. Drowsiness, increased lethargy, and tiredness indicate depression of the central nervous system and are signs of severe worsening of the patient's condition. Deterioration in vision, commonly due to enlargement of the blind spot as a result of papilloedema, also requires urgent investigation.

The development of epilepsy or changes in the nature of epileptic attacks, particularly when accompanied by changes in behaviour, are positive warnings of intracranial tumours. Seizures may be generalised or focal, and the type of seizure may provide an indication of the site of the lesion.

Localised neurological changes may be subtle and identified only by those who have irregular contact with the patient. The most common changes include reduced memory, increased irritability, reduction in co-ordination, dizziness, fatigue, and lethargy. Personality changes may be apparent and, in the later stages of the condition, stupor, confusion, and dementia may develop.

Other symptoms may reflect the changes in pituitary function (e.g. acromegaly, amenorrhoea, and hyper-prolactinaemia) and hypothalamic function (e.g. diabetes insipidus and disturbed temperature regulation).

Treatment
Suspected intracranial tumours may be investigated by computerised tomography (CT) scanning, radioisotopic brain scanning, and nuclear magnetic resonance (NMR) scanning. Treatment may involve relieving severe symptoms or specific measures to remove as great a proportion of the tumour tissue while preserving brain function intact.

Non-specific emergency measures may include the use of intravenous antiepileptics (BNF 4.8) and the administration of dexamethasone (BNF 6.3.4) to counteract cerebral oedema. Headache may be treated with non-opioid (BNF 4.7.1), or non-depressant opioid (BNF 4.7.2), analgesics.

Surgery may be used to completely remove the tumour or to relieve intracranial pressure. Complete excision may be impracticable due to the diffuse boundary between tumour and healthy tissue, and the need to limit the damage to surrounding structures. Hydrocephalus produced as a result of raised pressure within the cerebral ventricles may be relieved by insertion of a ventriculo-atrial or ventriculo-peritoneal shunt.

External irradiation may be carried out over a period for the treatment of malignant primary and secondary tumours, although meningiomas are insensitive to radiotherapy. Improved results may be obtained with less malignant growths and in patients who have previously had intracranial pressure reduced surgically.

Chemotherapy is ineffective for the treatment of primary intracranial tumours, but may be used in secondary deposits.

Spinal Cord Tumours

Definition and aetiology
Tumours within the spinal cord may be classified as extramedullary, occurring outside the spinal cord but within the surrounding membranes, or intramedullary. All tumours of the spinal cord are rarer than intracranial tumours and tend to develop in middle life. The majority are extramedullary, malignant, and spread rapidly. Primary tumours include neurofibromas (which develop from the Schwann cells of the spinal roots), meningiomas, and astrocytomas. Metastatic tumours are also common and may develop from almost any site (e.g. breast, lung, or from lymphomas).

Symptoms
Most symptoms of spinal cord tumours arise as a result of compression of the spinal cord and spinal nerve roots. Initial symptoms, which include pain and paraesthesia, may develop insidiously and commonly occur in areas below the site of the lesion. Pain may be localised, mild or severe, and located to one or both sides of the spine. Sensory loss, muscle weakness, and muscle wasting along the distribution of the affected nerves may ensue. Progressive growth of the tumour may lead to spasticity, and loss of control of bladder and bowel function. Intramedullary tumours may produce symptoms which mimic syringomyelia. Some secondary tumours can produce paraplegia within hours or days.

Treatment
Surgical excision may be possible for extramedullary primary tumours, although only partial excision may be practicable to retain function. Radiotherapy may be necessary postoperatively. Intramedullary and non-operable extramedullary tumours may benefit from radiotherapy in isolation or following surgical decompression. Dexamethasone (BNF 6.3.4) may be used to reduce spinal cord oedema.

8.4 ENDOCRINE MALIGNANT NEOPLASMS

Pancreatic Endocrine Tumours

Definition
Pancreatic endocrine tumours must be differentiated from pancreatic cancer, which involves the exocrine

functions of the pancreas. Endocrine tumours may secrete a particular hormone in isolation (*see below*) or in combination (multiple endocrine adenomatosis), giving rise to varied clinical syndromes. The tumours commonly occur in association with other forms of neoplasm (e.g. pituitary adenomas).

Insulinoma

Definition and aetiology

Insulinomas are rare adenomas of the beta-cells of the pancreas and are responsible for the continued secretion of insulin even in the presence of fasting. The tumour is usually small and slow-growing and may develop in any part of the pancreas. The condition can develop at any age but there is a peak incidence between 40 and 60 years of age. Only approximately 10% of cases are malignant.

Symptoms

Symptoms are related to the development of hypoglycaemia and may be especially prominent several hours after a meal or on exercise. Central nervous system symptoms include headache, drowsiness on waking, confusion, and lightheadedness. Palpitations, sweating, and hunger may also develop. In severe forms, unconsciousness, convulsions, and coma may develop. Some patients may become obese as frequent meals prevent symptoms, although most patients do not experience a change in weight.

Malignant insulinomas may produce metastases (e.g. in the liver) and uncontrollable hypoglycaemia may be fatal.

Treatment

Surgical excision is the treatment of choice. Deep-set adenomas may require distal subtotal pancreatectomy. If symptoms persist, total pancreatectomy may be necessary. Diazoxide (BNF 6.1.4) is used to treat hypoglycaemia. Streptozocin, fluorouracil, or doxorubicin, alone or in combination, may be used for treatment of metastases.

Glucagonoma

Definition and aetiology

Glucagonoma is a rare alpha-cell tumour of the pancreas, which occurs in adulthood with a mean onset at 50 years of age. The majority of tumours occur in women and are malignant.

Symptoms

Patients commonly present with insulin-dependent diabetes mellitus and a distinctive rash. A chronic necrolytic migratory rash may occur on the extremities and the perineum, and is accompanied by bullae which break down, heal, and subsequently recur at a different position. The lesions are reddish-brown and exfoliating. Other symptoms include a vermilion tongue, cheilitis, weight loss, diarrhoea, and crumbling nails.

Treatment

Reversal of the rash and diabetic symptoms may be obtained by surgical excision of the tumour. If metastases have been produced or the tumour is not resectable, streptozocin may be useful. The rash may also respond to administration of oral corticosteroids (BNF 6.3.4) and oral tetracycline (BNF 5.1.3).

Zollinger-Ellison Syndrome

Definition and aetiology

The Zollinger-Ellison syndrome is a condition in which there is an increased plasma-gastrin concentration and hypersecretion of gastric acid. Peptic ulceration or diarrhoea, or both, may also occur. The increased plasma gastrin is usually due to a gastrin-secreting tumour of the pancreas (gastrinoma) which may be malignant.

Symptoms

The syndrome is characterised by diarrhoea, and abdominal pain due to peptic ulceration; steatorrhoea may sometimes occur. Multiple ulcers are frequently present, but occasionally diarrhoea may occur in the absence of ulceration. Haemorrhage or perforation occurring soon after gastric surgery is characteristic of the syndrome.

Treatment

Treatment involves administration of H_2-receptor antagonists (BNF 1.3), together with an antimuscarinic (BNF 1.2) if necessary. Resection of the tumour and selective vagotomy may be carried out, and total gastrectomy may be required if medical treatment is ineffective.

Phaeochromocytoma

Definition and aetiology

A phaeochromocytoma is a catecholamine-producing tumour arising from chromaffin tissue usually in the adrenal medulla but sometimes in other sites; the tumours are usually benign. Phaeochromocytomas are often familial and may be associated with other disorders (e.g. von Recklinghausen's neurofibromatosis).

Symptoms

Phaeochromocytoma is characterised by hypertension, which may be paroxysmal or sustained, with exacerbations occurring during paroxysmal attacks. In a minority of patients, hypotension may develop, often following a paroxysmal hypertensive attack. Severe headache, tachycardia, pain in the chest and abdomen, sweating, apprehension, nausea and vomiting, orthostatic hypotension, weight loss, hyperglycaemia, and glycosuria may occur. Paroxysmal attacks may occur several times a day or sometimes less frequently. They usually last between 15 and 60 minutes and are followed by exhaustion, weakness, and aching muscles. Pallor commonly occurs but may be followed by cyanosis. Paroxysmal attacks may be precipitated by changes in posture, emotional stress, exercise, straining during defaecation, abdominal pressure, and administration of anaesthetics.

Treatment
Phaeochromocytoma is treated by the surgical removal of the tumour. Alpha-adrenoceptor blocking drugs (BNF 2.5.4) are used in conjunction with beta-adrenoceptor blocking drugs (BNF 2.4) for short-term management of paroxysmal attacks. Metirosine (BNF 2.5.7) may be used alone or in combination with an alpha-adrenoceptor blocking drug in pre-operative treatment and in patients with inoperable tumours.

Thyroid Cancer

Definition and aetiology
Thyroid cancer is a comparatively rare form of cancer of uncertain aetiology. Its incidence has been related to the former practice of irradiation of the head, neck, and upper thorax for the treatment of minor illnesses of childhood (e.g. thymic enlargement, tonsillitis, and acne), although the time lag between irradiation and the development of thyroid cancer may be up to 30 years.

The majority of primary thyroid malignancies are papillary carcinomas. These are slow-growing, and may infiltrate the local lymph nodes, neck muscles, lungs, bone, and the trachea. Follicular carcinomas occur later in life, predominantly in women, and have a greater malignant potential than papillary carcinomas. They may spread to the lungs and bone through the blood. Other rarer forms of thyroid cancer are medullary and anaplastic carcinomas.

Symptoms
The presence of thyroid cancer may be asymptomatic apart from the presence of a palpable mass in the neck region. The distinction between a thyroid nodule and the presence of thyroid cancer may be difficult.

Treatment
Small discrete papillary carcinomas may be surgically excised, although the amount of tissue removed from larger tumours may be determined by the degree of spread of the carcinoma. Unilateral lobectomy is preferred but greater tissue involvement may require total or subtotal thyroidectomy. Follicular carcinoma invariably requires total thyroidectomy.

Thyroxine (BNF 6.2.1) may be administered to suppress regrowth and to reduce the secretion of thyroid-stimulating hormone. Radioactive iodine (^{131}I) may be used to ablate remaining thyroid tissue, in which case subsequent thyroxine administration is essential. The prognosis for papillary and follicular carcinomas is good, although the outlook for rarer forms is less good.

8.5 MALIGNANT NEOPLASMS OF THE GYNAECOLOGICAL AND GENITO-URINARY SYSTEMS

8.5.1 GYNAECOLOGICAL MALIGNANT NEOPLASMS

Breast Cancer

Definition and aetiology
Breast cancer is the most common fatal cancer in women, accounting in the developed world for approximately 20% of all female deaths from cancer. It is rare in women under 30 years of age, but its incidence increases with age particularly after the menopause. Breast cancer is commonly an adenocarcinoma.

The incidence of breast cancer has been linked to hormonal and genetic factors. The combination of an early menarche and late menopause, and the greater the age at the time of the first pregnancy, have been associated with increased rates. Breast feeding does not protect against the development of breast cancer, although the age at which lactation is initiated may be important. The risk is approximately trebled if there is a family history of breast cancer, suggesting an aetiological role for genetic factors.

Breast cancer may also occur rarely in men (e.g. in Klinefelter's syndrome and other male genital disorders).

Clinically, breast cancer may be classified as Stage I (early stages of the disease with negligible lymph node involvement) through to Stage IV (the presence of tumours of greater than 5 cm diameter and metastases). Tumours may also be categorised as oestrogen-receptor protein positive or negative, depending on their ability to bind radiolabelled oestradiol, and this may be important for drug therapy (*see below*).

Metastases are common (e.g. in the liver, pleura, and bone) and may arise by direct invasion of localised tissue or via the lymphatics and bloodstream.

Symptoms
The detection of a slow-growing, single, painless lump in the breast, especially in women in high-risk groups, is often presumed to indicate breast cancer until proved otherwise. There may be vague discomfort, but more serious signs include a retracted nipple, bleeding from the nipple, distorted breast contour, oedema of the skin of the breast, skin dimpling and ulceration above the site of the lesion, and enlargement of localised lymph nodes. The breast mass may become attached to the surrounding chest wall. Diagnosis may be aided by mammography.

Treatment
Radical mastectomy (in which pectoral muscles are removed as well as mammary tissue and axillary lymph nodes) is now less widely used. It has been superseded by the cosmetically more acceptable modified radical mastectomy in which the pectoral muscles are retained, although 10-year survival rates for both procedures are less than 50%.

Conservative surgery (partial mastectomy) may be possible for primary Stage I and II tumours, followed by radiotherapy. This gives excellent cosmetic results, and is replacing both forms of radical mastectomy. Radiotherapy may also be used following surgery if metastases of the lymphatic system are found.

Chemotherapy is reserved for advanced and recurrent cases. A wide range of cytotoxic drugs (BNF 8.1) may be employed singly, or in combination with corticosteroids (BNF 8.2.2) or hormonal agents.

Hormonal therapy may be used to relieve the symptoms and retard the development of the disease. It may be combined with radiotherapy in recurrent cases following surgery, or in advanced disease. Oestrogens (BNF 8.3.1) may be used in postmenopausal women and are particularly effective in those who are oestrogen-receptor protein positive. Progestogens (BNF 8.3.2) may be reserved for refractory cases. The most successful form of hormonal treatment in pre- and postmenopausal women is the use of tamoxifen (BNF 8.3.4), although the majority of successful cases are oestrogen-receptor protein positive.

Cervical Cancer

Definition and aetiology
Cervical cancer is the second most common cancer of the female reproductive tract and the incidence appears to be increasing, particularly in young women. There is a higher incidence in women from a poor social back-ground and a number of other risk factors have been identified. There may be a higher risk in women who have had a large number of sexual partners, and the disease has been tentatively linked to the presence of sexually-transmitted disease, commonly a human papillomavirus or herpes simplex virus type 2. There may be an association between the development of the disease and the use of oral contraceptives and with heavy smoking.

Cervical carcinoma is commonly a squamous cell carcinoma, with a minority appearing as adenocarcinomas. Early pathological changes may be detected by the proliferation of cells in the lower third of the cervical epithelium (minimal cervical dysplasia) and these may be detected by cervical smear testing. Many of these abnormalities may spontaneously regress, but some may progress to carcinoma *in situ*. The further spread of these cells may occur to adjacent organs.

A positive diagnosis is staged as a means of indicating the spread of the cancer.

Stage	Spread of cancer
0	Pre-invasive
I	Confined to the cervix
II	Spread beyond cervix, but not onto pelvic wall
III	Spread onto pelvic wall
IV	Widespread dissemination

Symptoms
Early disease may be asymptomatic, and the disease is usually well advanced before symptoms arise. These may include malodorous vaginal discharge, bleeding that can often occur after intercourse, abdominal pain, dyspareunia, and low back pain. Following widespread dissemination, urinary and rectal symptoms may develop.

Treatment
The treatment depends on the stage of the disease and the age of the patient. Early stages may be managed by cryotherapy, laser treatment, and diathermy. Hysterectomy at this stage may be reserved for women who have completed a family, or those who are likely to be unreliable in attending follow-up examinations. Radiotherapy, surgery, or both, may be used for more extensive forms, particularly when there is lymph node involvement, although proctitis and cystitis are major complications. Chemotherapy is of limited value, and drug administration may be reserved for the treatment of pain.

Prophylaxis by cervical screening (Pap test) of all sexually active women has reduced the development of the disease by increased early detection. Screening is carried out every 3 years although high-risk groups may need more frequent checks.

Choriocarcinoma

Definition and aetiology
Choriocarcinoma is a rare malignant tumour of the trophoblastic (placental) tissue which characteristically secretes chorionic gonadotrophin. The term choriocarcinoma is also applied to certain types of testicular teratomas and ovarian cancers that secrete chorionic gonadotrophin. Most cases occur in females as a result of malignant degeneration of a hydatidiform mole, but the tumour may also develop after spontaneous abortion or after a period of months or years as a sequel to normal pregnancy.

Symptoms
Choriocarcinoma may present with abnormal uterine bleeding, rapid uterine enlargement, or symptoms of disseminated disease. The tumour produces metastases at an early stage via the circulation to the lungs, liver, brain, or vaginal wall. Pulmonary embolism or pulmonary hypertension may occur. In males, choriocarcinoma may present with testicular pain, accidental discovery of a hard testicular mass, or signs of disseminated disease.

Treatment
Choriocarcinoma is treated with the administration of antimetabolites (BNF 8.1.3). Surgery, radiotherapy, and chemotherapy may be indicated for testicular or ovarian tumours.

Endometrial Cancer

Definition and aetiology
Endometrial cancer is the third most common malignancy affecting women (after breast and colorectal cancers). It is commonly an adenocarcinoma and is more prevalent in developed societies. Unlike cervical cancer, women who have not had children are at greatest risk, but it is unrelated to the number of sexual partners. There is a peak incidence postmenopausally between 50 and 60 years of age. A higher incidence has been linked to an early menarche and late menopause (as in breast cancer).

The condition has been linked to the secretion of oestrogen predominantly in the absence of progestogen secretion. Hypersecretion of oestrogen may occur in oestrogen-secreting tumours and polycystic ovary syndrome. Predisposition to endometrial cancer may occur in other conditions in which oestrogen secretion can be unopposed (e.g. diabetes mellitus, hypertension, and obesity).

Symptoms
The presence of unexpected uterine bleeding between menstrual periods (in premenopausal women) and in others postmenopausally is a potent indicator of endometrial abnormalities. Bleeding may be preceded by a watery discharge. Diagnosis may be confirmed by fractional curettage.

Treatment
Surgery may be possible in many cases and involves hysterectomy and removal of the Fallopian tubes and ovaries. Progestogens (BNF 8.3.2) may be used indefinitely for advanced disease or relapses and may prove effective in retarding the development of metastases. Combined cytotoxic (BNF 8.1) and progestogen therapy may also be beneficial in the treatment of metastases. The 5-year survival rate is approximately 60%, although age and staging of the disease may significantly affect the prognosis.

Ovarian Tumours

Definition and aetiology
Cancer of the ovaries comprises a range of histological entities, the most common of which are adenocarcinomas. Approximately 75% are benign, although the proportion which are malignant increases with age. The incidence of the cancer increases with high standards of living and with an early menarche linked to a late menopause. A decreased incidence has been associated with increased parity and oral contraceptive use.

There may be a familial history of the cancer in up to 40% of patients, and its development with breast cancer has also been noted.

Symptoms
The tumour may be asymptomatic until it has spread to other structures within the pelvis. The presence of a palpable mass may indicate the presence of a tumour, but cysts must also be considered. Early signs may be non-specific and include vague abdominal discomfort and gastro-intestinal disturbances. Ascites, anaemia, and pelvic pain may be associated with late stages of the disease. Rarely, tumours may secrete one or more hormones. The secretion of oestrogens may lead to precocious puberty in girls and endometrial proliferation in postmenopausal women. Other hormones secreted may include serotonin, thyroxine, and chorionic gonadotrophin.

Treatment
Treatment depends upon the stage of the disease. Localised tumours may be surgically excised conservatively, preserving reproductive function. In advanced disease, hysterectomy, and salpingo-oophorectomy with omentectomy, may be necessary. Three or more cytotoxic drugs may be used in combination, and the addition of a progestogen (BNF 8.3.2) may improve the outcome. The 5-year survival rate may range from 15% to 45%.

8.5.2   GENITO-URINARY SYSTEM MALIGNANT NEOPLASMS

Bladder Cancer

Definition and aetiology
Bladder cancer is usually a transitional cell carcinoma, which may be localised or highly invasive. Squamous cell carcinoma, which has a poor prognosis, occurs less frequently and may be associated with parasitic infection.

Aetiological factors which have been identified include smoking, occupational exposure to aromatic amines used in the dyeing, cable, and rubber industries, and administration of cyclophosphamide. Parasitic infection (e.g. with *Schistosoma haematobium*) may produce cancer as a result of chronic irritation.

Symptoms
Haematuria without pain is the initial presenting symptom, and is accompanied by dysuria, urinary frequency, and pyuria. Pain in the lower abdomen may develop in the later stages of the disease.

Treatment
Superficial lesions of the bladder wall may be surgically excised by endoscopic resection, although the procedure may need repeating. Partial or total cystectomy may be necessary for tumours which have infiltrated the bladder wall. Urostomy formation is required in total cystectomy. Local cystodiathermy is also widely used.

Radiotherapy may be beneficial postoperatively and can be curative on its own. Chemotherapy is of limited use, although direct instillation of alkylating drugs (BNF 8.1.1) and cytotoxic antibiotics (BNF 8.1.2) into the bladder has been attempted.

Prostatic Cancer

Definition and aetiology
Cancer of the prostate gland is invariably an adenocarcinoma and most cases occur in men over 50 years of age. Metastases may frequently be present on diagnosis, commonly occurring in the lymph nodes, bone, lung, and liver.

The identification of androgen receptors in approximately 75% of patients may be a useful marker to predict the effectiveness of hormonal therapy.

The incidence is increasing due to the larger numbers of elderly people. No definite causative factors have been identified but an increased incidence has been associated with sexually-transmitted diseases, sedentary occupations, and sexual activity. A hormonal link has been suggested on the basis that castrated males do not develop the disease.

Symptoms
Early stages of the disease may be asymptomatic. Later symptoms may only develop once the disease is well advanced and include urinary outflow obstruction and, less commonly, haematuria and pyuria. In some patients, the presenting symptom may be bone pain caused by metastases. Rectal examination may identify the presence of a firm nodule.

Treatment
Localised disease may be managed symptomatically, especially as the mean age of presentation is 70 years and other pathology is invariably present. In more diffuse disease, and in the absence of lymph node involvement, treatment by prostatectomy or radiotherapy may be attempted. However, elderly patients may suffer more from the complications of treatment (e.g. urinary incontinence and diarrhoea) than from the tumour itself.

A significant proportion of patients have metastases at presentation and they may benefit from hormonal therapy and orchidectomy. Oestrogens (BNF 8.3.1) suppress plasma levels of testosterone. Medical orchidectomy may also be carried out by the administration of gonadorelin analogues (BNF 8.3.4).

Renal Cancer

Definition
Renal cancer is very common, comprising 1% to 2% of adult cancers. The classification is based upon the cell types. Renal tubule epithelium cells may give rise to renal cell carcinomas (hypernephromas). A tumour arising from the embryonic renal tissue is described as a Wilms' tumour (nephroblastoma). Urothelial tumours arise from transitional cells, and rarely from squamous cells.

Renal Cell Carcinomas

Definition and aetiology
Renal cell carcinoma occurs predominantly in adults, with a higher incidence in males. Its occurrence has been tentatively linked to smoking. The tumour may occur singly or as multiples in one or both kidneys. It is encapsulated, but metastases may occur via the bloodstream to the lungs, liver, and bone and by direct invasion into adjacent tissues.

Symptoms
Initial non-specific symptoms may include weakness, anorexia, and weight loss. The classical symptoms are pain, haematuria, and the presence of a palpable mass. Pain may be experienced as a dull ache in the loin. Other symptoms may be due to substances released by the tumour or by invasion of other structures. Fever may be

produced by the secretion of pyrogens, while the secretion of renin can lead to hypertension. Endocrine effects may occur (e.g. hypercalcaemia caused by the secretion of parathormone, and polycythaemia due to the secretion of an erythropoietin-like substance). Varicocoele may develop as a result of dissemination of the tumour into the renal vein and the resultant occlusion of the testicular vein.

Treatment
Nephrectomy may be carried out if only one kidney is affected. If both are involved, partial nephrectomy may be attempted. The use of radiotherapy, chemotherapy, and immunotherapy has not proved beneficial. The 5-year survival rate may be as high as 60% in localised disease.

Wilms' Tumour

Definition and aetiology
Wilms' tumour is a solid tumour of childhood, with the majority identified before three years of age. The tumour consists of connective tissue, epithelial cells, and muscle cells and is rapid-growing, often reaching enormous proportions. Tumours usually arise unilaterally, but may also occur bilaterally. Metastases (e.g. to the lungs, liver, and bone) may be formed at an early stage via the bloodstream, and by direct local invasion.

Symptoms
A palpable mass may be found in the abdomen and is associated with abdominal pain, nausea and vomiting, anorexia, fever, haematuria, and weight loss.

Treatment
The tumour, which is commonly encapsulated, may be surgically removed or nephrectomy carried out. Radiotherapy may be used pre-operatively to promote shrinkage of the tumour or postoperatively to treat any leakage of cells. Vinca alkaloids (BNF 8.1.4) and cytotoxic antibiotics (BNF 8.1.2) may be administered following nephrectomy. 5-year survival rates are approximately 65%.

Urothelial Tumours

Definition and aetiology
Urothelial tumours may occur not only in the renal pelvis, but also in the epithelium of the ureter, urethra, and urinary bladder (*see also* Bladder Cancer). Those of the renal pelvis and ureter are usually only of low-grade malignancy and they may be papillary or solid. They have been linked to occupational exposure (e.g. to aromatic amines used as dyes), the ingestion of phenacetin, to schistosomiasis, and to chronic inflammation (e.g. caused by indwelling catheters).

Symptoms
The most prominent symptom is haematuria. Obstruc-

tion to the outflow of urine may produce renal colic, but the tumour only rarely becomes large enough to be palpable. If the tumour develops in the ureter, the presence of only a small mass may cause urinary obstruction.

Treatment
Complete removal of the kidney and ureter may be necessary, although local dissection of the tumour may be effective in some cases. Radiotherapy may be used postoperatively. Tumours may give a 5-year survival rate of 50% overall, ranging from 90% for localised tumours to virtually zero for those which have spread to tissues around the ureter.

Testicular Cancer

Definition and aetiology
Although testicular cancer is rare, it is the most common cancer in young men, and consists of two cell types. Teratomas, which are of uncertain origin, have a peak incidence at approximately 20 years of age. Seminomas, which arise from the germinal cells, occur most commonly at approximately 30 years of age. Tumours may rarely occur in older men and are usually lymphomas.

The disease has been associated with a high standard of living, and predisposing factors include undescended testes and testicular feminisation syndrome.

Symptoms
The presence of an enlarging firm mass in the scrotum may cause discomfort. If bleeding into the tumour develops, the mass may be tender with extreme local pain. Metastases to the lymph nodes, lungs, and liver may occur.

Treatment
Identification of the cell type provides the basis for treatment. Seminomas may respond to radiotherapy and have a 5-year survival rate of at least 80%. Teratomas and other cell types may require lymph node dissection and combination chemotherapy with cytotoxic drugs (BNF 8.1), and have a poorer prognosis than seminomas.

8.6 HAEMATOLOGICAL MALIGNANT NEOPLASMS

Leukaemias

Definition and aetiology
Leukaemias are characterised by the uncontrolled proliferation of blood-forming elements arising from pro-

genitor bone-marrow cells. The normal bone marrow is replaced and the production of normal cellular components is reduced, leading to anaemia, thrombocytopenia, and neutropenia.

Leukaemias are classified as acute or chronic, depending on the maturity of the cell populations. In acute forms, immature leucocytes proliferate and fail to reach maturity. In chronic forms, mature leucocytes are not removed from the circulation but accumulate. Leukaemia is also classified by the identity and origins of the dominant cell as lymphoid (lymphocytic, lymphatic, or lymphogenous) or non-lymphoid (myeloid, granulocytic, myelocytic, or myelogenous). Care must be taken in the use of classifications as there is little consistency in nomenclature (*see* Table 8.1).

The aetiology of the leukaemias is unknown in the majority of cases, although a higher incidence has been linked to a number of factors. Exposure to environmental or occupational radiation may predispose to leukaemia. Occupational contact with benzene, administration of some cytotoxic drugs (e.g. alkylating drugs), and exposure to viruses may also contribute to the development of leukaemia. Genetic defects (e.g. Down's syndrome) may produce a higher incidence.

The acute forms are considered jointly, but the more clinically variable chronic forms are discussed separately.

Acute Leukaemias

Definition and aetiology
Acute leukaemias may be classified as acute lymphatic leukaemia (ALL) (acute lymphoblastic leukaemia) and acute non-lymphoid leukaemia, which includes acute myeloid leukaemia (AML). ALL occurs predominantly in boys between 5 and 14 years of age, and it is the most common form of cancer in childhood. A smaller peak of incidence, which is equivalent in males and females, occurs between 55 and 75 years of age.

AML occurs at all ages, but is the more common form of acute leukaemia in adults.

Symptoms
Non-specific early symptoms may include the progressive development of pallor, weakness, and lethargy. The predominant features relate to the replacement of normal bone marrow with malignant cells.

Infection, haemorrhage, and anaemia are common. Infection may arise in any tissue but occurs most commonly in the lungs, mucous membranes, and skin. Skin lesions may be extremely slow to heal and, if infected, may be characterised by the absence of pus. Septicaemia may suddenly develop and prove rapidly fatal. The presence of herpes and candidal infections may complicate the development of fulminant oral aphthae. Haemorrhagic lesions are common. Petechiae, bruising, and purpura may develop spontaneously and persistent epistaxis can occur.

Bone pain may be a prominent feature, caused by the presence of a tumour mass or infarction in the bone marrow. Later symptoms may be due to infiltration of the central nervous system and include irritability, headache, and vomiting.

Treatment
Prior to treatment, laboratory assessment of blood is essential to differentiate between ALL and AML. The aim of treatment is to remove the leukaemic cells from the blood and bone marrow and to allow its repopulation by normal cells. Chemotherapy is the mainstay of

TABLE 8.1
Classification of leukaemias

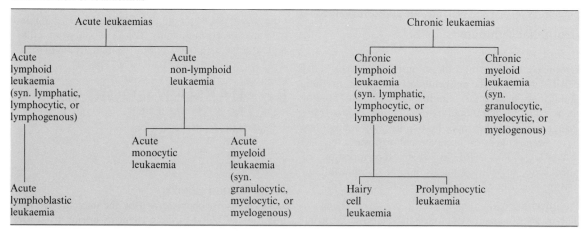

treatment, and is sometimes used in conjunction with radiotherapy, but all schedules are complex and undergoing continual revision. The results from bone-marrow transplantation have been encouraging.

In ALL, combined corticosteroids (BNF 8.2.2) and the vinca alkaloids (BNF 8.1.4) have proven successful in inducing remission. The addition of colaspase may increase the period of remission. Once an improved blood profile has been achieved, methotrexate (BNF 8.1.3), and possibly radiotherapy, may be used in the prophylaxis of CNS complications. Varying periods of maintenance therapy using antimetabolites (BNF 8.1.3) may be administered to minimise the occurrence of relapses. Relapses may occur in the bone marrow, CNS, and testes, of which the most serious is the bone marrow. The 5-year survival rate is 50%, although the prognosis is worse in boys because of the risk of testicular relapses, and is dependent on the leucocyte cell-count on diagnosis.

The initial treatment of AML is similar to that of ALL described above even though the course of the condition is different. The range of drugs which are effective in AML is narrower than in ALL. Those that are effective invariably cause myelosuppression and, as a result, the patient is initially at increased risk of succumbing to infection and may clinically worsen before improvements are noted. Maintenance therapy may include the alternation of a wide range of drugs which have been shown to be effective in AML, although CNS prophylaxis is usually omitted.

Chronic Lymphoid Leukaemia

Definition and aetiology
The presence of small immature lymphocytes in the bone marrow and blood is indicative of chronic lymphoid leukaemia (CLL)(chronic lymphatic leukaemia). Its incidence increases with age and it affects 2 to 3 times as many men as women.

Other closely related, but much rarer, forms of leukaemia are hairy cell leukaemia and prolymphocytic leukaemia.

Symptoms
Approximately 25% of cases may be asymptomatic. In patients with symptoms, there may be an insidious development. Non-specific symptoms can include anaemia, weight loss, anorexia, fever, dyspnoea on exertion, and a sense of abdominal fullness. Lymphadenopathy and splenomegaly may be present. Macules and plaques can develop during the course, and these may ulcerate. Later symptoms include petechiae, bruising, and bleeding.

Complications can arise from the increased susceptibility to infection. Herpes zoster infection and recurrent chest infections are a major cause of morbidity and mortality. Haemolytic anaemia may occur as a result of an auto-immune reaction.

Treatment
Patients diagnosed with CLL who are asymptomatic do not require treatment. Treatment may be indicated in the presence of bone-marrow failure, lymphadenopathy, systemic symptoms, or the appearance of complicating symptoms.

Radiotherapy may be used for treatment and the relief of symptoms (e.g. lymphadenopathy and splenomegaly). Alkylating drugs (BNF 8.1.1) may be administered, although they must be used with caution in the presence of thrombocytopenia and anaemia. Advanced stages of CLL and certain complications may be treated by the administration of corticosteroids (BNF 8.2.2).

Chronic Myeloid Leukaemia

Definition and aetiology
Chronic myeloid leukaemia (chronic myelocytic leukaemia, chronic granulocytic leukaemia, or chronic myelogenous leukaemia) is a rare form of leukaemia which predominantly affects those over 40 years of age. It may be associated with exposure to ionising radiations or to chemicals (e.g. benzene). The condition has been linked to a chromosomal abnormality (the Philadelphia chromosome).

Symptoms
The progression of chronic myeloid leukaemia may be considered to consist of two stages. The chronic phase is of widely variable duration and the symptoms may be controlled by treatment. The accelerated phase represents a considerable worsening of the condition which may be associated with dissemination of the tumour to other sites (e.g. skin and bone), although the transition in symptoms between the two phases may be ill-defined.

The condition may be characterised by the insidious onset of non-specific symptoms. These may include anaemia, a sense of abdominal fullness, anorexia, weight loss, and night sweats. Abdominal pain may occur due to infarction of the spleen, and splenomegaly may be severe and accompanied by hepatomegaly. Later symptoms may include the development of large haematomas.

Treatment
The condition cannot be cured and treatment is intended to arrest its development. This may be possible during the chronic phase with the administration of busulphan (BNF 8.1.1) or hydroxyurea (BNF 8.1.5). Radiotherapy of the spleen may be used as an adjunct to chemotherapy, but resistance to irradition may develop. Bone-marrow

transplantation may be attempted in the chronic phase in patients under 50 years of age. There is no effective treatment of the accelerated phase of the condition.

Lymphomas

Definition
Lymphomas are neoplasms of the lymphoid tissue which are progressive, destructive, and invasive, and which cause swelling of the lymph nodes and spleen. They are differentiated from infections which may also cause swelling of lymphoid tissue. Lymphomas give rise to approximately 5% of all cancers.

Hodgkin's Disease

Definition and aetiology
Hodgkin's disease rarely occurs before 10 years of age and has peak incidences in early adulthood and in middle to old age. Its aetiology is uncertain, although certain infections have been implicated. The disease may be caused by chromosomal abnormalities, but no specific characteristics have been universally noted.

The disease is clinically staged through localised involvement (Stage I) to widely-disseminated disease (Stage IV), and subclassified according to the presence of systemic symptoms.

Symptoms
Early disease may be characterised by enlarged lymph nodes (e.g. in the neck and axillae) which are usually painless. As the disease spreads through the reticuloendothelial system, systemic symptoms may appear. Severe pruritus may be an early symptom that may lead to extensive excoriation. More widespread disease may be indicated by night sweats, fever, and weight loss, which may be caused by involvement of internal lymph nodes (e.g. in the retroperitoneum), bone marrow, or liver. Bone pain may be a consequence of bone infiltration.

The presence of an enlarged lymphoid mass may cause obstruction of other tissues and organs. Oedema of the face and neck may result from superior vena cava obstruction, and bile-duct obstruction may cause jaundice. Advanced disease may be characterised by hepatomegaly.

The progressive deterioration in cell-mediated immunity may predispose patients with advanced disease to opportunistic infectious diseases (e.g. herpes zoster and *Pneumocystis carinii* pneumonia).

Treatment
Radiotherapy may be used to treat patients with localised disease. Adjacent uninvolved lymph nodes may also be irradiated. Chemotherapy is used in other cases of localised disease and in all disseminated states. Combination therapy with cytotoxic drugs (BNF 8.1) is used, with 28- or 42-day cycles of treatment repeated up to 6 times to ensure remission. Chemotherapy may also be used in the event of relapse following initial radiotherapy or chemotherapy.

Complications of successful chemotherapy and radiotherapy may occur with the development of secondary malignancies (e.g. acute non-lymphoid leukaemia). The 5-year survival rate for Hodgkin's disease without treatment was approximately 10%. With the introduction of chemotherapy, this has increased to approximately 75%, and most patients do not suffer relapses.

Non-Hodgkin's Lymphoma

Definition and aetiology
Non-Hodgkin's lymphoma comprises a diverse range of lymphomas. The incidence is greater than Hodgkin's lymphoma and it is predominantly a disease of the elderly. It is of unknown aetiology although viral associations have been suggested. The conditions are staged similarly to Hodgkin's lymphoma (i.e. Stage I through Stage IV) and the classification of the disease ranges from low-grade with reasonable prognosis to high-grade with potentially poor prognosis.

Symptoms
Lymphadenopathy characterised by the presence of large rubbery nodes may be the only presenting symptom (Fig. 8.1). The distribution of nodal involvement may be similar to that in Hodgkin's disease, although popliteal nodes and pharyngeal lymphoid tissue may also be affected. Extranodal tissue is also commonly involved (e.g. the skin, bone marrow, and gastrointestinal tract) and may produce varied symptoms (e.g. malabsorption syndrome). Anaemia, neutropenia, and thrombocytopenia may occur, and night sweats, weight loss, and fever may indicate disseminated disease.

Central nervous system disease may develop due to spinal cord compression, especially in high-grade lymphomas. Depressed immunoglobulin production may predispose to infection.

Treatment
Most patients will have high-grade disease at presentation and, despite appropriate treatment, the prognosis is poor. Treatment is directed towards relief of symptoms and prolongation of life. Localised low-grade disease may be treated by radiotherapy, although relapse to other sites is common. Disseminated low-grade disease may be treated with a single agent or combination therapy with cytotoxic drugs (BNF 8.1). Advanced disease may respond to treatment with interferons (BNF

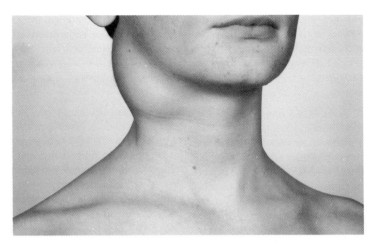

Fig. 8.1
Enlarged lymph nodes in non-Hodgkin's lymphoma.

8.2.4), although high-dose multiple drug regimens may also be used.

The prognosis of non-Hodgkin's lymphoma is poorer than Hodgkin's lymphoma. The prognosis for high-grade lymphomas has improved with the introduction of aggressive chemotherapy, and cure may be possible.

Myeloma

Definition and aetiology
Myeloma is a paraproteinaemia in which the plasma concentration of a single immunoglobulin is increased due to the monoclonal proliferation of B-cells. It is characterised by the presence of plasma-cell tumours in the bone marrow. It affects predominantly those of 40 or more years of age, with an average age at diagnosis of 62. The disease has a slow course.

Symptoms
Patients may be asymptomatic apart from a general malaise. The most common early symptom is bone pain, which may affect predominantly the back and the ribs and may be aggravated by movement. Diffuse osteoporosis or erosion of the skeleton may be caused by the tumour or a tumour secretion (osteoclast-activating factor), and may lead to vertebral collapse or pathological fracture. Hypercalcaemia may be associated with bone erosion, leading to depression, vomiting, and anorexia. Gradual renal impairment may be due to the deposition of immune complexes within the renal tubules. Spontaneous bleeding may be caused by impairment of renal and platelet function. Hyperviscosity of the circulation due to the excess presence of immuno-globulins may cause neurological disturbances (e.g. vis-ual disturbances, headache, and peripheral neuropathy). The patient may be predisposed to the development of infections caused by depressed immunoglobulin function.

Treatment
Treatment is symptomatic. Localised myeloma may be treated by radiotherapy, but most cases are disseminated and require chemotherapy. Alkylating drugs (BNF 8.1.1) are given singly, although the addition of cortico-steroids (BNF 8.2.2) may improve the response. Bone-marrow transplantation may be successful in a minority of cases. Interferons (BNF 8.2.4) may achieve limited remission when used as a first-line treatment.

General measures include the use of radiotherapy in the relief of bone pain, and the patient should be encouraged to remain ambulant. Improvement in renal function may be noted if the fluid intake is greatly increased, particularly in the presence of hypercalcaemia. Opportunistic infections should be immediately treated with antibacterial drugs (BNF 5.1).

8.7 MALIGNANT NEOPLASMS OF THE SKIN

Basal Cell Carcinoma

Definition and aetiology
A basal cell carcinoma (rodent ulcer) is the commonest malignant disease of the skin, arising from the basal layer of the epidermis. It rarely forms metastases but is capable of invading and destroying local tissues. It may

occur in areas damaged by ionising radiation or ultra-violet light, or in scar tissue (e.g. from burns and vaccinations). It is more common in males and usually occurs after middle-age, although it is also common in young immunocompromised patients.

Symptoms
Basal cell carcinomas occur more frequently in fair-skinned people, the commonest sites being the face, head, and neck. The appearance may take several forms, but they are most commonly seen in early stages as small, firm, pearly, raised nodules (Fig. 8.2) that are covered by a thin epidermis. The thin epidermis may rupture, resulting in ulceration, and later stages are characterised by a pearly border with superficial telangiectasia surrounding the ulcer. Death may result in rare cases due to an untreated basal cell carcinoma destroying underlying structures (e.g. cartilage or bone).

Treatment
Treatment comprises removal by chemosurgery, cryosurgery, radiotherapy, or surgery. It is essential that the excision is complete to prevent recurrence.

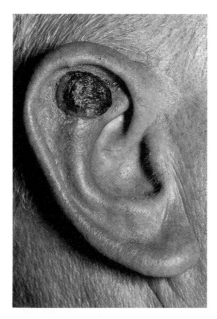

Fig. 8.2
A basal cell carcinoma. The raised nodule has a central area of necrosis which may ulcerate.

Kaposi's Sarcoma

Definition and aetiology
Kaposi's sarcoma is a form of vascular tumour which arises in the dermis and may spread to the epidermis. It may present as an indolent form, but an aggressive form has become more widespread due to its association with acquired immune deficiency syndrome (AIDS). In this form, it becomes widely disseminated to the gastrointestinal tract, lymph nodes, and brain.

Symptoms
The indolent form may be characterised by the formation of a nodule, often appearing on the leg or foot, or by the presence of a brown, plaque-like lesion which may penetrate soft tissue and enter bone. Kaposi's sarcoma in AIDS may produce red or pink plaques or papules, initially occurring on the upper torso but rapidly spreading to other parts. Mucous membranes may also be involved.

Treatment
Radiotherapy may be used to treat indolent forms of the disease, depending on the depth of the lesions. Chemotherapy using vinblastine (BNF 8.1.4) or combinations of up to six cytotoxic drugs (BNF 8.1) may be used in aggressive forms of the disease. The tumour may respond to treatment with interferons (BNF 8.2.4).

Melanoma

Definition and aetiology
Melanoma (malignant melanoma) is a malignant disease of the skin arising from melanocytes in the epidermis. Approximately 50% of all melanomas arise from an existing lentigo, mole, or naevus, while the rest occur in previously unblemished skin. Ultraviolet light (e.g. through chronic sun exposure) appears to be the most likely significant causative agent. Melanomas are more common in females and prognosis is related to the stage of the disease, thickness of the tumour, and its site.

Symptoms
Melanomas occur in various forms and all have the ability to invade and form metastases. The only common symptom is mild pruritus and a tingling sensation. They may be classified according to their appearance and behaviour.

Nodular melanoma, which usually occurs in middle-age, may be dark brown, greyish-black, or virtually colourless. The initial nodule is raised and rapidly invades the dermis with little lateral growth. The lesion is usually asymptomatic until ulceration occurs.

Superficial spreading melanoma (Fig. 8.3) develops most frequently on female legs and on the male torso, occurring commonly at middle-age. The lesion is slightly raised with a well-defined but irregular margin, brown or black with red, white, or blue spots, and spreads horizontally. Peripheral inflammation may also be present. Vertical dermal invasion may eventually occur and result in bleeding and crusting.

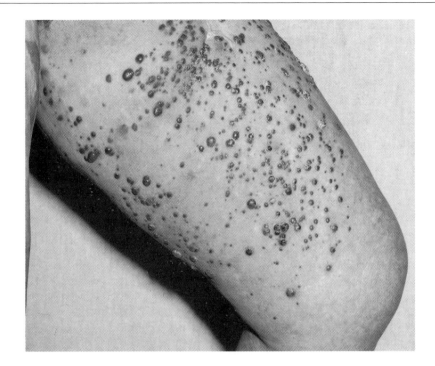

Fig. 8.3
Superficial spreading melanoma.

Lentigo maligna melanoma arises from flat uniformly brown lesions (lentigo maligna) and occurs on the face in elderly patients. As malignancy develops, the margins become irregular and the colour changes to brownish-black and blue. Dermal invasion may occur after years of lateral growth and results in a raised nodule.

Treatment
Successful treatment relies upon early diagnosis and consists of wide surgical excision with, in some cases, skin grafts. Lymphadenectomy may be necessary when deep invasion and metastasis has occurred. Chemotherapy with cytotoxic drugs (BNF 8.1) may also be of value.

8.8 MISCELLANEOUS NEOPLASMS

Cancer of the Bone

Definition and aetiology
Cancer of the bone may arise as a primary tumour or as a metastasis. Primary bone tumours are rare and occur predominantly in children and young adults, whereas metastatic bone tumours are more common in adults. Immunodeficiency may be a causative factor and the degree of immunocompromise may have a bearing on the course of the disease.

The most common forms of primary malignant bone tumour are osteosarcoma (osteogenic sarcoma), Ewing's sarcoma (Ewing's tumour), and chondrosarcoma. Osteosarcomas may occur at any age but have the greatest incidence at 10 to 20 years of age. Metastases to the lung are common. Ewing's sarcoma has a similar age profile and has a higher incidence in males. Chondrosarcoma is a cartilaginous sarcoma and occurs in an older age group, with peak incidence occurring in patients of 40 to 60 years of age.

Symptoms
Osteosarcoma occurs predominantly around the knee and is characterised by the presence of pain and swelling. The mass may be firm and tender and its presence may restrict joint movement. Similar symptoms may be present in Ewing's sarcoma, which occurs commonly in the femur and the pelvis. Accompanying symptoms may include fever and weight loss. Chondrosarcomas are slow-growing and commonly arise in the pelvis and less frequently in the femur, humerus, ribs, and scapula.

Early disease may be asymptomatic, although pain and swelling may arise as the disease progresses.

Treatment

In osteosarcoma, amputation of the limb may be required although more conservative measures may be attempted initially. These include removal of the tumour and insertion of prostheses. Cytotoxic antibiotics (BNF 8.1.2) and cisplatin (BNF 8.1.5) may be used pre- and postoperatively and may be effective at preventing metastases. Ewing's sarcoma may be treated by a combination of surgery, radiotherapy, and intensive chemotherapy and may give 5-year survival rates of 30% to 60%. Chondrosarcomas appear to be resistant to radiotherapy and chemotherapy and therefore must be treated by surgical removal or amputation.

Cancer of the Head and Neck

Definition and aetiology

Cancer of the head and neck constitutes a diverse group of cancers of the upper respiratory and gastro-intestinal tracts. Many individual conditions are uncommon but as a group they form approximately 4% of all cancers. The most common aetiological factor is tobacco and alcohol consumption. Poor dental and oral hygiene may also be contributory factors. The majority are squamous cell carcinomas.

Cancer of the Larynx

Definition and aetiology

Cancer of the larynx forms the largest single group of head and neck cancers. A strong causative link with smoking and alcohol intake has been established. It is commonly caused by a squamous cell carcinoma and the site of origin is predominantly the glottis.

Symptoms

A common early symptom is hoarseness. Other and subsequent symptoms are linked to the presence of the tumour above or below the glottis. If the tumour arises above the glottis, dysphagia may occur. Subglottal carcinoma may be accompanied by dyspnoea and stridor.

Treatment

Treatment of localised glottal cancer consists of a combination of radiotherapy, and where necessary, surgery. For advanced disease, laryngectomy may be required, although voice preservation or substitution is often attempted. Speech therapy is also necessary for many patients.

Cancer of the Mouth

Definition and aetiology

Cancer of the mouth encompasses all tumours which arise on the lip, tongue, gingiva, floor and inner lining of the mouth, and hard and soft palate. The incidence of disease increases with age and is twice as common in males. The incidence has been linked to smoking (with pipes and cigars more strongly implicated than cigarettes), poor oral hygiene, and regular alcohol consumption. Infective agents may also be important in the development of the disease, and leucoplakia may be a predisposing factor. Local infiltration of lymph nodes may occur to produce metastases.

Symptoms

An early warning of cancerous changes in the mouth may be the development of a dry mouth, although some patients, especially those with large tumours, may salivate excessively. Cancer of the lip, gingiva, and tongue may be characterised by an ulcerated lesion with an indurated base, which can be extremely reluctant to heal. Cancer of the tongue may cause pain and earache. Alternatively, an oral tumour may present as a single or multiple firm mass which gradually increases in size and interferes with eating and speech.

Treatment

Good results may be obtained by surgical removal of the lesion and surrounding tissues. Radiotherapy may be used as a primary treatment for cancer of the lip or as an adjunct to surgery or in refractory cases. Chemotherapy may also be successful in management of the condition. The patient should be advised to stop smoking, and improved oral hygiene should be recommended. The prognosis is variable depending on the site. The 5-year survival rate for cancer of the lip is 80%, while the prognosis of other forms may range from 20% to 50%.

Cancer of the Pharynx

Definition and aetiology

Cancer of the nasopharynx is largely localised to Chinese populations, including those who have settled in the west. The unusual distribution may be attributed to dietary factors or localised infective agents. It occurs equally in children and adults but has a higher incidence in males.

Oropharyngeal cancer occurs predominantly in patients over 50 years of age and has a significant male preponderance. Smoking or chewing tobacco have been identified as causative factors. Hypopharyngeal carcinomas have a similar aetiology.

Many pharyngeal neoplasms are non-Hodgkin's lymphomas, and these may spread to other tissues (e.g. paranasal sinuses and the stomach).

Symptoms

Cervical lymph node involvement is often the presenting symptom in cancer of the nasopharynx. Unilateral nasal obstruction may also occur, and sero-mucinous otitis media may lead to deafness as a result of Eustachian tube obstruction. Pain may be produced by involvement of the cranial nerves which pass through the sinuses.

Oropharyngeal cancer may produce tonsillar enlargement which causes dysphagia, and occasionally dysarthria may arise if the posterior tongue is affected. Pain may be referred to the ear, and ulceration may produce blood-stained saliva.

Cancer of the hypopharynx may cause dysphagia and referred earache. Spread of the tumour may lead to hoarseness, dyspnoea, stridor, or anorexia.

Treatment

The mainstay of treatment and the relief of symptoms is intensive radiotherapy. Surgery is reserved for advanced stages of disease and in patients who are refractory to radiotherapy. The overall prognosis is poor, with 5-year survival rates of approximately 30%.

Cancer of the Salivary Glands

Definition and aetiology

Cancer of the salivary glands is of unknown aetiology and occurs largely in the parotid glands, although the minor salivary glands (e.g. in the cheeks, lips, and palate) may also be affected. They may be benign (mainly pleomorphic adenomas) or malignant (e.g. muco-epidermoid carcinomas). The disease occurs primarily in patients over 50 years of age.

Symptoms

The gradual development of a painless encapsulated mass may lead to facial distortion. The presence of facial palsy may indicate infiltration of the facial nerve by a malignant growth, and acute swelling of the parotid gland may cause discomfort.

Treatment

The tumour is removed by surgery. For malignant tumours, surgery may be followed by radiotherapy if complete excision is not possible or a recurrent tumour is undergoing removal. Radiotherapy may also be used as a primary therapy for malignant tumours if surgery is contra-indicated (e.g. in the elderly).

Chapter 9

BLOOD, NUTRITIONAL, AND METABOLIC DISORDERS

9.1 BLOOD AND LYMPH DISORDERS

9.1.1 GENERAL DISORDERS

Agranulocytosis

Definition and aetiology
Agranulocytosis is characterised by a marked decrease in the number of granulocytes, which results in an increased susceptibility to infection. It may be acute or chronic, and is due to decreased production of granulocytes in the bone marrow, or to increased destruction or utilisation. Impaired production invariably results from the toxic effects of certain drugs (e.g. phenylbutazone, antithyroid drugs, cytotoxic drugs, phenothiazines, or sulphonamides) on the bone marrow. In addition, production may be impaired by irradiation or malignant bone-marrow disease. Agranulocytosis may also be inherited.

Symptoms
Symptoms are a direct consequence of an increased susceptibility to bacterial and fungal infection. The mouth and throat appear to be particularly at risk and ulceration and dysphagia are common. Initial symptoms may include fever, rigors, and prostration. Localised infections of the gastro-intestinal and respiratory systems and the skin may also occur and, if untreated, may progress to septic shock and death.

Treatment
The offending agent should be withdrawn immediately

and any serious infection treated by the administration of an appropriate antimicrobial drug (BNF 5.1 and 5.2). Antimicrobials may also be given as prophylaxis. Corticosteroids (BNF 6.3.4) may be given to treat shock, and lithium carbonate has been used in attempts to stimulate granulocyte production. Mouth ulcers may require local treatment (BNF 12.3).

Amyloidosis

Definition and aetiology
Amyloidosis is an uncommon disorder characterised by the deposition of a glycoprotein, amyloid, in a wide variety of body tissues. Amyloid is synthesised by reticuloendothelial cells and is not normally found in the body in significant amounts. In amyloidosis, amyloid invades and displaces parenchymal cells and thus impairs the function of the affected organ. Amyloidosis may be idiopathic, but is often associated with chronic infections and inflammatory or malignant diseases (e.g. Hodgkin's disease, myeloma, rheumatoid arthritis, ankylosing spondylitis, and tuberculosis). It may be inherited.

Symptoms
Symptoms are related to the site of amyloid deposition, and include arrhythmias, heart failure, nephrotic syndrome, renal failure, macroglossia, hepatomegaly, splenomegaly, diarrhoea, and haemorrhage in the gastro-intestinal tract. Amyloid may also accumulate in skin.

Treatment
The underlying disease should be treated. There is no specific treatment for amyloidosis, although colchicine,

corticosteroids, cytotoxic drugs, and dimethyl sulphoxide have been used.

Embolism and Venous Thrombosis

Embolism

Definition and aetiology
An embolism is an obstruction of a blood vessel by a mass of undissolved material or gas (an embolus) which has been transported from another part of the circulation.

An embolus may consist of a thrombus (thromboembolus) or may be composed of gas, fat, or tumour cells. Thromboemboli usually arise in the leg veins (*see* Deep Vein Thrombosis below) or in the heart. Air emboli may be introduced into the circulation during surgical procedures. Gas embolism may also be caused by bubbles of nitrogen appearing in the circulation of subjects who undergo rapid decompression (e.g. divers). Fat embolism may occur as a result of bone marrow entering the circulation following the fracture of a long bone. Malignant cells from a tumour may enter the circulation to form an embolism. Common sites of embolism are the arteries of the brain (*see* Stroke), the lungs (*see* Pulmonary Embolism below), and the legs.

Symptoms
Embolism in a major artery of the leg may result in acute limb ischaemia. Symptoms include pain and pallor of the affected limb. Claudication (limping) may be present. Chronic limb ischaemia is characterised by intermittent claudication (pain on exercise of the leg muscle which is relieved by rest). Pain on rest, however, may occur and ulceration and gangrene of the limb may develop.

Treatment
Emergency surgery may be required for embolism in a major artery to restore the circulation. In chronic ischaemia, patients should be advised to exercise, reduce weight, and avoid smoking. In order to avoid infection, great care must be taken when trimming nails, and attention to cleanliness of the affected limb is important. If symptoms are severe and persistent, treatment is by surgery (embolectomy). Amputation may occasionally be necessary.

Deep Vein Thrombosis

Definition and aetiology
Venous thrombosis is the formation of a blood clot (thrombus) within a vein and is usually accompanied by inflammation of the vein (thrombophlebitis). It is usually caused by venous stasis (e.g. during chronic ill-ness or after surgery), venous damage (e.g. in infection), or as a result of disruption of clotting mechanisms (e.g. in malignant disease or oral contraceptive administration). Venous thrombosis most commonly affects the veins of the legs.

Symptoms
In deep vein thrombosis no local symptoms may be produced, although warmth, aching, and swelling of the calf or thigh may occur, together with erythema. Severe pain may occur. The thrombus may become detached and be transported to the lung, resulting in pulmonary embolism (*see below*). This may be the presenting symptom.

Treatment
Treatment consists of the administration of anticoagulants (BNF 2.8.1 and 2.8.2), analgesics (BNF 4.7), and bed rest. Fibrinolytic drugs (BNF 2.10) may also be used in severe cases. Surgery may be required. Prophylactic measures include limb compression (e.g. with graduated compression hosiery) and elevation, and the use of anticoagulants.

Superficial Thrombophlebitis

Definition and aetiology
Superficial thrombophlebitis (phlebitis) is thrombosis of a superficial vein which occurs as a result of inflammation.

Symptoms
It is characterised by local pain and tenderness, erythema, oedema, and local warmth. The thrombosed vein may be felt as a hard 'cord'. It rarely results in embolism.

Treatment
Treatment consists of rest, limb elevation, and the administration of analgesics (BNF 4.7). The condition is usually self-limiting.

Pulmonary Embolism and Infarction

Definition and aetiology
Pulmonary embolism is the blockage of the pulmonary artery or one of its branches by an embolus, which leads to a reduction in pulmonary blood flow. It may be associated with necrosis of lung tissue (pulmonary infarction). It is almost always due to thrombi, which pass into the pulmonary circulation from a deep vein thrombosis. Rarely, the embolus consists of air, fat, or tumour cells.

Symptoms
The symptoms of pulmonary embolism depend on the extent and duration of the embolus. In minor disease,

patients may be asymptomatic, although sudden acute chest pain and haemoptysis are common and are associated with pulmonary infarction. In more severe cases, these symptoms are less likely, although right heart failure may develop and be associated with anginal pain. Other symptoms include acute dyspnoea, tachypnoea, and cyanosis. Syncope may occur as a result of a reduction in cardiac output, and may be fatal. Pulmonary hypertension and a rise in venous pressure may occur in subacute and chronic cases.

Treatment
Treatment is symptomatic in mild disease, although in severe cases emergency resuscitation may be necessary. In such cases, treatment may include oxygen therapy (BNF 3.6) and the administration of opioid analgesics (BNF 4.7.2) for chest pain, parenteral and oral anticoagulants (BNF 2.8.1 and **2.8.2**), and fibrinolytic drugs (BNF 2.10). Surgical embolectomy may be necessary if symptoms are life-threatening. Anticoagulant prophylaxis may be necessary for patients at risk.

Self-help organisation
Chest Heart and Stroke Association

Polycythaemia

Definition and aetiology
Polycythaemia is characterised by an increased mass of erythrocytes in the circulatory system. It may be of unknown aetiology (e.g. polycythaemia vera, *see below*), or be caused by a decreased total blood volume produced by severe dehydration or burns, diuretic therapy, or endocrine disorders (relative, pseudo-, or stress polycythaemia). Erythrocytosis (secondary polycythaemia) occurs as a physiological response to tissue hypoxia encountered in heart, pulmonary, or renal diseases. It may also occur in healthy individuals who live at high altitude.

Polycythaemia Vera

Definition and aetiology
Polycythaemia vera is a chronic myeloproliferative disorder characterised by proliferation of the bone marrow, resulting in an increased erythrocyte count and often accompanied by an increase in leucocytes, platelets, and total blood volume. It occurs most commonly between 50 and 60 years of age, but its exact cause is unknown.

Symptoms
The onset of polycythaemia vera may be insidious. Its presence may be initially diagnosed during an investigation of gout. Patients may have a ruddy complexion and initially suffer non-specific symptoms (e.g. fatigue, head-

ache, tinnitus, vertigo, and visual disturbances). Severe pruritus, especially after bathing, is common. Cardiovascular symptoms, due to increased blood viscosity, may develop and include angina pectoris and thromboses. Abnormal platelet function may result in haemorrhage, and abdominal pain may arise from peptic ulceration and splenomegaly. Death may follow haemorrhage or thrombosis, or the disease may progress to acute leukaemia.

Treatment
Treatment is controversial, but may include venesection and the administration of radioactive phosphorous-32 or certain cytotoxic drugs (BNF 8.1).

Splenomegaly and Hypersplenism

Definition and aetiology
Splenomegaly is enlargement of the spleen which may be accompanied by hypersplenism (*see below*). Splenomegaly occurs as a result of some other primary disorder. Common causes include infections (e.g. malaria and typhoid), inflammatory diseases (e.g. rheumatoid arthritis, sarcoidosis, and amyloidosis), chronic haemolytic anaemias (e.g. hereditary spherocytosis and thalassaemias), portal hypertension, malignant disease, or physical trauma.

Symptoms
In addition to palpable splenic enlargement, splenomegaly is often accompanied by abdominal pain, oesophageal varices, a feeling of satiety (due to pressure on the stomach), and purpura. Hypersplenism may occur and is characterised by a reduction in the number of circulating blood cells and a compensatory proliferation of bone marrow.

Treatment
Treatment is by the correction of the underlying primary disorder. Because of the inherent dangers (i.e. thrombosis and infection), splenectomy should only be performed in restricted circumstances (e.g. chronic haemolytic disorders and severe physical trauma).

9.1.2 ANAEMIAS

Anaemias

Definition and aetiology
Anaemia is a reduction in the concentration of erythrocytes or haemoglobin, or both, in the blood. In addition, the size and shape of erythrocytes may be altered. Anaemias may occur as a result of any condition in which there is defective production (e.g. iron, folic acid,

or vitamin B_{12} deficiency), or increased destruction (e.g. by drugs) or loss (e.g. haemorrhage) of erythrocytes.

Symptoms

The symptoms of anaemias are related to a reduction in the oxygen-carrying capacity of the blood and arise from tissue hypoxia. Mild anaemias may be asymptomatic, although fatigue, general weakness, and pallor may be evident. In more severe disease, a wide variety of additional symptoms are likely and may include angina pectoris, dyspnoea, heart failure with peripheral oedema, and tachycardia. Drowsiness, headache, irritability, tinnitus, and vertigo may also occur. Gastrointestinal symptoms include anorexia, constipation, diarrhoea, and nausea. Menstrual disturbances and loss of libido may develop.

Treatment

For treatment of the anaemias, see under the individual conditions.

Aplastic Anaemia

Definition and aetiology

Aplastic anaemia arises as a result of bone-marrow degeneration and is characterised by a failure to produce adequate numbers of erythrocytes, leucocytes, and platelets. Those erythrocytes which are produced are, however, normal in size and haemoglobin content. Aplastic anaemia may occur as a result of exposure to chemicals (e.g. benzene), drugs (e.g. chloramphenicol, chlorpromazine, cytotoxic drugs, phenylbutazone, or phenytoin), or to radiation. It may also follow a viral infection or be inherited (e.g. Fanconi's anaemia).

Symptoms

Symptoms include those stated under anaemias (see Anaemias above). In addition, the likelihood of infections is increased as a result of leucopenia, haemorrhage may occur due to thrombocytopenia, and these often prove fatal.

Treatment

Treatment comprises the avoidance of causative agents, reducing sources of infection, and the prompt administration of antimicrobial drugs (BNF 5.1) for any existing infection. Blood transfusion may be necessary, and anabolic steroids and corticosteroids (BNF 9.1.3) have been used. It may be necessary to administer a chelating compound and ascorbic acid (BNF 9.1.3) to treat iron overload arising from repeated transfusion. Bone-marrow transplantation is indicated in intractable disease.

Haemolytic Anaemias

Definition and aetiology

Haemolytic anaemias are characterised by an increased destruction of erythrocytes, although those that remain are of normal size and haemoglobin content. They may be caused by defective erythrocyte formation, they may be inherited (e.g. sickle-cell anaemia and beta thalassaemia), or may be due to the action of some other factor (e.g. blood transfusion, drug administration, infection or other systemic disease, or auto-immune mechanisms).

Symptoms

Symptoms are as stated under anaemias (see Anaemias above), but haemolytic anaemias may also be accompanied by hepatomegaly and splenomegaly, hyperbilirubinaemia, or jaundice. Haemoglobinuria and oliguria may occur.

Treatment

Treatment comprises the identification and withdrawal of the underlying cause. Anabolic steroids, corticosteroids, and pyridoxine (BNF 9.1.3) have been used.

Beta Thalassaemia

Definition and aetiology

Beta thalassaemia is an inherited, chronic, haemolytic anaemia occurring most commonly in Mediterranean and some Eastern races. There is a reduction in (beta thalassaemia minor), or complete absence of (beta thalassaemia major), production of beta chains, which are one type of polypeptide chain contributing to the structure of normal adult haemoglobin (haemoglobin A). The eventual result is ineffective erythropoiesis and failure of the red cells to mature.

Symptoms

Symptoms of beta thalassaemia major often occur in the first year of life, and include failure to thrive, short stature, bossed skull with prominent jaw, and a muddy complexion. There may be marked hepatomegaly with abdominal distension in addition to the symptoms stated under anaemias (see Anaemias above). Infection is a common complication. Iron overload is common as a result of repeated transfusion and heart failure may occur. Beta thalassaemia major is often fatal. The minor variant is usually asymptomatic, although intermediate forms of the disease do exist.

Treatment

Prevention in future generations may be achieved by genetic counselling or antenatal screening. Treatment is by repeated transfusion or more recently by bone-marrow transplantation. The maintenance of an adequate diet and the prophylactic administration of folic acid (BNF 9.1.2) may be beneficial. The administration of a chelating compound and ascorbic acid (BNF 9.1.3) may be required to treat iron overload.

Sickle-cell Anaemia

Definition and aetiology
Sickle-cell anaemia is a severe inherited haemolytic anaemia characterised by the presence of sickle-shaped erythrocytes. 'Sickling' occurs as a result of the formation of abnormal haemoglobin, and the disease occurs most commonly in negroes.

Symptoms
Mild forms of the disease may be asymptomatic, and only be discovered during hypoxic episodes (e.g. during anaesthesia). Symptoms may be mild or severe. All the symptoms stated under anaemias (see Anaemias above) may be present, but severe infection (e.g. bronchitis) and painful swelling of the hands and feet (hand and foot syndrome) may also occur, particularly during the first year of life. Thromboses may develop as a result of the abnormally shaped erythrocytes, and crises are likely, particularly in the presence of infection. Initial symptoms may include severe bone pain in the limbs and back. Dyspnoea with chest pain may occur, and there may be marked splenomegaly and hepatomegaly together with acute abdominal pain (which may occasionally be the major symptom). Complications include convulsions, jaundice, meningitis, and osteomyelitis. Sickle-cell anaemia is often fatal, commonly due to renal impairment.

Treatment
Prevention may be achieved by genetic counselling or antenatal screening. In the presence of the disease, prompt antibacterial therapy (BNF 5.1) is indicated for the treatment of concurrent infection. Patients should be hospitalised at the time of a crisis, and oxygen therapy (BNF 3.6) and opioid analgesics (BNF 4.7.2) may be required. Transfusion may be indicated. Folic acid (BNF 9.1.2) may be administered prophylactically.

Self-help organisation
Sickle Cell and Thalassaemia Information Centre

Haemolytic Disease of the Newborn

Definition and aetiology
Haemolytic disease of the newborn is caused by the passage of IgG antibodies from the mother across the placenta to the foetus. The antibodies can be derived from almost any source, but are most commonly caused by incompatability of rhesus factors in the maternal and foetal circulation. Haemolytic disease of the newborn caused by rhesus incompatability usually occurs in the second or subsequent pregnancies.

A second common, but less severe, cause of haemolytic disease is incompatibility between maternal and foetal ABO blood groups, which occurs predominantly when a foetus of blood group A or B is born to a mother of blood group O. Unlike rhesus incompatibility, ABO incompatibility can commonly produce symptoms in the first-born child.

Symptoms
In rhesus haemolytic disease, symptoms range from severe to mild. In severe cases, the foetus is usually prematurely delivered, has pronounced anaemia, and is usually born with *hydrops foetalis*. This syndrome consists of generalised oedema of the scalp, the lungs (pleurisy), and peritoneal cavity (ascites). The skin is extremely pale, the heart, liver, and spleen are grossly dilated, and heart failure may occur. Death often occurs rapidly. In less severe cases, many of these symptoms are still present, although physiological jaundice may develop from the continued breakdown of erythrocytes. Excess levels of bilirubin can lead to kernicterus. In mild cases, anaemia may be only mild and jaundice may be absent.

The symptoms of ABO haemolytic disease are considerably less severe than the rhesus form. Raised bilirubin levels and haemolysis infrequently occur, and it is thought that *hydrops foetalis* never arises from ABO incompatability.

Treatment
In cases of severe anaemia or where there is a risk of kernicterus, freshly donated rhesus-negative blood must be given to the neonate by exchange transfusion. Phototherapy may also be beneficial. In *hydrops foetalis*, diuretics (BNF 2.2), positive inotropic drugs (BNF 2.1), and fluid and electrolytes (BNF 9.2) are also vital.

Prevention in the mother by administration of anti-D (Rh$_o$) immunoglobulin in rhesus-negative women who have previously carried a rhesus-positive baby or had an abortion has significantly reduced the incidence.

Iron-deficiency Anaemias

Definition and aetiology
Iron-deficiency anaemias are due to inadequate iron intake (e.g. in dietary deficiency, malabsorption syndromes, or pregnancy) or to iron loss by haemorrhage (e.g. gastro-intestinal tumour, haemorrhoids, menorrhagia, or peptic ulceration). The erythrocytes are small (microcytic) and deficient in haemoglobin (hypochromic).

Symptoms
The symptoms of iron-deficiency anaemias are as described under anaemias (*see* Anaemias above).

Treatment
Treatment is by the administration of iron salts (BNF 9.1.1) and correction of any underlying pathology.

Megaloblastic Anaemias

Definition and aetiology
Megaloblastic anaemias are most commonly due to a deficiency of vitamin B_{12} or folic acid, or both, and are characterised by the failure of erythrocytes to mature. Despite a normal haemoglobin content (normochromic), the erythrocytes are fewer in number and larger (macrocytic) than usual. Vitamin B_{12} deficiency may occur in some vegetarians and vegans. If the intrinsic factor secreted by the gastric mucosa is absent, vitamin B_{12} is not absorbed. This is characteristic of pernicious anaemia and also occurs after total gastrectomy. Folic acid deficiency may occur in alcoholics, the elderly, during pregnancy, or in malabsorption syndromes. It may also arise as a side-effect of drugs (e.g. methotrexate and phenytoin).

Symptoms
The symptoms of megaloblastic anaemias are as described under anaemias (*see* Anaemias above), but in addition they are associated with glossitis, leucopenia, and thrombocytopenia. Vitamin B_{12} deficiency may also result in subacute combined degeneration of the spinal cord.

Treatment
Treatment comprises the identification of the specific deficiency and the administration of vitamin B_{12} or folic acid preparations (BNF 9.1.2), or both, as appropriate.

9.1.3 HAEMORRHAGIC DISORDERS

Haemophilia

Definition and aetiology
Haemophilia (classical haemophilia or haemophilia A) is an inherited haemorrhagic disorder occurring almost exclusively in males, and characterised by a tendency to excessive haemorrhage in response to trivial injury. It arises as a result of a deficiency of the antihaemophilic factor, factor VIII, in blood. Women may carry the disease, but do not normally suffer from it. Men inherit it from their carrier mothers (i.e. it is an X-chromosome-linked disease).

Symptoms
The extent of this inherited deficiency varies between families. Some symptoms of haemophilia may occur in an individual in whom the haemostatic capacity of factor VIII is reduced to about 25% to 50% of normal. In infancy, bleeding is characterised by the appearance of cutaneous ecchymoses or haematomata in the soft tissues. In severely affected children whose factor VIII level is 1% or less, joint haemorrhages (haemarthroses) are likely to occur as soon as crawling or walking begins. If untreated, these haemorrhages result in severe pain, limitation of movement, destruction of joints, and skeletal deformity. The knees, elbows, and ankles are most commonly affected. Bleeding into muscle and gastro-intestinal haemorrhage also occur. Excessive bleeding is also common after dental and surgical procedures, and major surgery or trauma may cause fatal haemorrhage.

Treatment
Prevention in future generations may be achieved by genetic counselling or antenatal screening. Haemorrhages may be treated by the intravenous administration of factor VIII, which may also be given as prophylaxis prior to dental or surgical procedures. Antifibrinolytic drugs (BNF 2.11) may be used as adjuncts. Drugs which may precipitate haemorrhage (e.g. aspirin and indomethacin) must be avoided.

Christmas Disease

Definition and aetiology
Christmas disease (haemophilia B), named after the patient first described with the condition, is an inherited haemorrhagic disorder characterised by a deficiency of factor IX. It is less common than haemophilia, and its inheritance and clinical presentation are identical to haemophilia A.

Symptoms and Treatment
Symptoms and treatment are similar to that of haemophilia (*see above*), with the exception that factor IX is administered.

Self-help organisation
Haemophilia Society

Purpuras

Definition and aetiology
Purpuras are a group of disorders characterised by purple-red skin discoloration, which occur, sometimes in the absence of physical trauma, as a result of leakage of blood from capillaries into the tissues.

Anaphylactoid Purpura

Definition and aetiology
Anaphylactoid purpura (Henoch-Schönlein purpura) is thought to occur as a result of an anaphylactic response to an infective allergen, predominantly caused by an upper respiratory-tract infection, although no specific allergen has been identified. It commonly occurs in children between 2 and 7 years of age, with a higher incidence in boys, although it can occur at any age.

Symptoms
The onset is usually sudden, with the appearance of characteristic symmetrical purpuras particularly on the lower limbs and buttocks. Somatic symptoms include abdominal pain with gastro-intestinal haemorrhage, arthralgia, fever and malaise, and myalgia. Renal complications (e.g. glomerulonephritis) may produce oedema, haematuria, and proteinuria. The disorder is usually self-limiting, although relapses are common, and death may infrequently occur as a result of gastro-intestinal haemorrhage or renal failure.

Treatment
Treatment is not normally required, although corticosteroids (BNF 6.3.4) have been given in the presence of severe symptoms.

Vascular Purpura due to Drugs or Infection

Definition and aetiology
Vasculitis (in the absence of thrombocytopenia) caused by blood-vessel wall damage may produce purpura during acute infections (e.g. meningitis), and following drug therapy (e.g. with penicillin, chlorothiazides, or sulphonamides) (Fig. 9.1).

Treatment
Exposure to known precipitating factors should be avoided.

Thrombotic Thrombocytopenic Purpura

Definition and aetiology
Thrombotic thrombocytopenic purpura is of unknown aetiology. It is characterised by histological and anatomical changes in small blood vessels and a decreased concentration of platelets, particularly in peripheral blood. It may be precipitated by an acute infection. The disorder may occur at any age and is more common in adult women.

Symptoms
The onset is sudden and common symptoms include anaemia, convulsions, fever, haemorrhage (particularly of the gastro-intestinal tract), psychiatric disturbances, and purpura. Symptoms may last for days or weeks, and acute relapses are common. Death may occur as a result of severe haemorrhage, renal failure, or stroke.

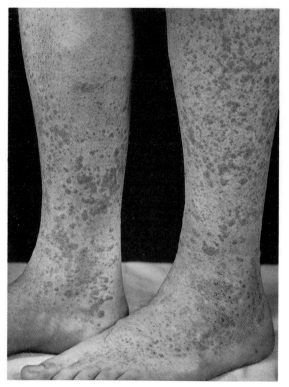

Fig. 9.1
Vasculitis caused by drug allergy. The blackened areas are points of necrosis, and are surrounded by erythema caused by leakage of blood into the regions around the vessels.

Treatment
Treatment is non-specific and symptomatic. Transfusion may be required for anaemia, and dialysis for renal failure. Other methods of treatment have included the administration of anticoagulant and antiplatelet drugs, splenectomy, and exchange transfusion.

Thrombocytopenia

Definition and aetiology
Thrombocytopenia is a deficiency of blood platelets which results in spontaneous haemorrhage. It may be caused by a decrease in the production of platelets or an increase in their rate of destruction. Thrombocytopenia caused by failure of platelet production may occur in aplastic anaemia, megaloblastic leukaemia, or malignant bone disease. Excessive platelet destruction may occur as a result of an auto-immune mechanism (idiopathic thrombocytopenic purpura) and may be acute or chronic. In addition, thrombocytopenia may be secondary to some other condition (e.g. hypersplenism or systemic lupus erythematosus). It may also follow

transfusion or an acute infection, or arise as a side-effect of drugs (e.g. quinidine). A transient thrombocytopenia may occur in infants born to mothers suffering from idiopathic thrombocytopenic purpura.

Symptoms
The acute idiopathic disease occurs most commonly in children, is usually of rapid onset and short duration, and is characterised by petechiae. Chronic disease is marked by bruising, scattered petechiae, and mucous membrane bleeding. Epistaxis, gastro-intestinal haemorrhage, and menorrhagia may occur. Relapses may be frequent and death is common.

Treatment
Idiopathic disease is treated by the administration of corticosteroids (BNF 9.1.4), and splenectomy may be indicated in the chronic form. Other drugs, including azathioprine, danazol, and vinca alkaloids (BNF 9.1.4), have been used. In drug-induced disease, the offending drug should be withdrawn. Any primary blood, or other systemic, disorder should be treated.

9.1.4 LYMPHATIC DISORDERS

Lymphangiectasia

Definition and aetiology
Lymphangiectasia is the dilatation of lymphatic vessels in the small intestine. It may be congenital or acquired, occurring secondary to malignant disease, pericarditis, or pancreatitis.

Symptoms
It is characterised by mild diarrhoea or steatorrhoea, or both, hypoproteinaemia, and oedema.

Treatment
Treatment consists of adoption of a low-fat diet (BNF 9.4.1). Surgical resection may be possible for localised disease.

9.2 NUTRITIONAL DISORDERS

9.2.1 GENERAL DISORDERS

Anorexia Nervosa

Definition and aetiology
Anorexia nervosa is characterised by a distorted perception of body image associated with marked anxiety regarding weight gain and physical appearance. It is a condition of unknown aetiology which predominantly affects females between 14 and 17 years of age, and may be chronic.

Symptoms
It results in weight loss of at least 25% of original body-weight caused by insufficient food intake, and may be accentuated by self-induced vomiting, purgation, or excessive exercise. There may also be evidence of emotional disturbance (e.g. bereavement or examinations) and family tensions. The patient may be withdrawn, depressed, and may suffer from insomnia and have difficulty in concentrating. There is usually denial of any illness. Physical signs include wasting of subcutaneous fat, resulting in hollow cheeks, stick-like limbs, shrunken breasts, flat abdomen, and wasted thighs and buttocks. The hands and feet are usually cold, and the skin is dry and covered with an excess of downy hair (lanugo) over the neck, cheeks, forearms, and legs. Bradycardia and hypotension are usually present and amenorrhoea, loss of libido, and impotence usually appear at an early stage due to endocrine disturbances.

Treatment
Severe cases should be treated in hospital, with psychological support aimed at gaining the patient's confidence, restoring body-weight, and reducing the duration of the condition. Intravenous (BNF 9.3) or enteral (BNF Appendix 3) nutrition may also be necessary. Long-term treatment with supportive psychotherapy is directed at preventing relapses.

Bulimia Nervosa

Definition and aetiology
Bulimia nervosa is associated with anorexia nervosa and is characterised by episodes of gross overeating, followed by a pathological fear of getting fat. This causes the patient to self-inflict vomiting or purgation, or both, often using fingers or a toothbrush to induce the gag reflex. The condition commonly arises in women who are slightly older than those presenting with anorexia nervosa alone.

Symptoms
Overeating and vomiting occur at least once daily, rising to an incidence of up to forty times in severe forms. Persistent vomiting causes depletion of body fluids and electrolytes, resulting in hypokalaemia, hyponatraemia, and alkalosis. Consequently, muscle weakness, tetany, and convulsions may occur, with urinary-tract infections, and renal failure resulting from loss of potassium.

There may be depressive symptoms of gloom, irritability, and occasionally suicidal contemplations. Body-weight may be normal, and menstruation and fertility are not impaired.

Treatment
Severe cases are treated in hospital, but most cases respond to counselling or group therapy. Treatment is directed towards the restoration of normal eating habits, and convincing the patient to accept a higher body-weight. Antidepressant drugs (BNF 4.3) may have a beneficial effect.

Obesity

Definition and aetiology
Obesity is characterised by an increase in body-weight in excess of physical requirements, and results from excessive accumulation of body fat. It is most commonly caused by a dietary intake which exceeds that required for physical activity, tissue repair, and vital functions. However, obesity may very occasionally arise from genetic disorders, often in association with hypogonadism. Endocrine causes of obesity are rare, but may include Cushing's syndrome or hypothyroidism. Obesity may also be drug induced (e.g. by corticosteroids, oral contraceptives, or phenothiazines). A family history of obesity is common in overweight individuals, and the condition is often considered to have an emotional or behavioural component.

Complications
Obesity is often responsible for a deterioration in health and, in severe cases, can lead to premature death. Obesity may be associated with an increased likelihood of cardiovascular disease (e.g. angina pectoris, heart failure, hypertension, and stroke), diabetes mellitus, and gastro-intestinal disease (particularly of the colon or gall bladder), some of which may be life-threatening. Obese women may suffer from menstrual disorders, and all overweight individuals are more susceptible to back pain, osteoarthritis, respiratory disorders, and varicose veins. Severely obese patients are also at greater risk during surgery involving general anaesthesia.

Treatment
Treatment is primarily by dietary management which is usually necessary on a permanent basis. A group approach (e.g. weight-watchers) is often beneficial. Behaviour modification may be tried in some patients and psychological support is often valuable. Appetite suppressants (BNF 4.5) are available and may be of some short-term value in selected patients. Surgical techniques (e.g. gastro-intestinal bypasses and jaw wiring) have been used in severe cases.

9.2.2 INTOLERANCE CONDITIONS

Lactose Intolerance

Definition and aetiology
Lactose intolerance is an inability to metabolise and absorb lactose. It arises as a result of a deficiency of the enzyme, lactase, which is responsible for converting lactose to galactose and glucose in the small intestine. As a result, lactose accumulates and is subject to fermentation. Lactase is synthesised by the intestinal mucosa and deficiency may arise from an intestinal disorder (e.g. coeliac disease, Crohn's disease, gastro-enteritis, and short-bowel syndrome).

Symptoms
The characteristic symptom is explosive, frothy diarrhoea associated with abdominal cramps and distension, and nausea and vomiting. Affected children fail to gain weight.

Treatment
Treatment is by the introduction of a lactose-free diet (BNF Appendix 3).

9.2.3 DEFICIENCY DISORDERS

Beri-beri

Definition and aetiology
Beri-beri is caused by dietary thiamine (vitamin B_1) deficiency. It occurs as a result of starvation (or high carbohydrate intake following starvation), and may occasionally occur in chronic alcoholism.

Symptoms
Early symptoms (e.g. general weakness) are vague. Subsequently, cardiovascular symptoms may predominate (wet beri-beri), and these include congestive heart failure with marked oedema and dyspnoea. Polyneuropathy may occur (dry beri-beri) and paraesthesia and cramps of the legs are common. Ataxia, confusion, nystagmus, and speech disorders may develop. In untreated cases, encephalopathy, coma, and death may result.

Treatment
Treatment is by the oral or parenteral administration of thiamine hydrochloride (BNF 9.6.2).

Pellagra

Definition and aetiology
Pellagra is caused by a deficiency of nicotinic acid, although other vitamin deficiencies are often present. It

commonly occurs as a result of poor diet, but may also arise as a result of malabsorption disorders or alcoholism.

Symptoms
It is characterised by a symmetrical erythematous rash (pellagra dermatitis) followed by hypertrophy and subsequently atrophy of the skin. Diarrhoea and dementia are common, but encephalopathy only rarely develops.

Treatment
Treatment is by the administration of nicotinamide (BNF 9.6.2). Accompanying nutritional deficiencies may also require treatment.

Rickets and Osteomalacia

Definition and aetiology
Vitamin D deficiency is characterised in growing infants and children by rickets, and in adults by osteomalacia. The deficiency is often of dietary origin, but it may also be caused by inadequate exposure to sunlight, particularly in the elderly and in Asians, or to the administration of antiepileptics. Occasionally a malabsorption disorder may be responsible, and rarely it may be caused by an inherited renal tubular disorder (i.e. hypophosphataemic vitamin D-resistant rickets). Vitamin D deficiency results in decreased gastro-intestinal absorption of calcium and phosphate, which leads to the defective mineralisation of bone. Osteomalacia is more common in women as a result of the additional nutritional demands exerted by pregnancy.

Symptoms
Rickets is characterised by a reduced growth-rate and skeletal deformities (e.g. bowing of the long bones, enlargement of epiphyses, and bossing of the skull). Chest and spinal deformities may also be evident, and muscle weakness may occur.

In osteomalacia, bone pain and tenderness are common, and fractures (e.g. of the neck of the femur) may occur. Muscle weakness may reduce the patient's mobility, causing a waddling gait, difficulty in climbing and descending stairs and in standing from low chairs.

Treatment
Treatment is similar for both rickets and osteomalacia. Vitamin D preparations (BNF 9.6.4) may be given in combination with calcium, and also as prophylaxis. A phosphate supplement (BNF 9.5.2.1) may be required in hypophosphataemic rickets. An appropriate diet should be maintained, and adequate exposure to sunlight is beneficial. Any underlying primary disorder should be treated.

Scurvy

Definition and aetiology
Scurvy is caused by a dietary deficiency of ascorbic acid (vitamin C) and is characterised by impaired collagen synthesis. It is most common in elderly or alcoholic patients, but may occur in artificially fed infants.

Symptoms
In adults, the onset is usually insidious and is marked by anorexia, fatigue, and general malaise. Other common symptoms include haemorrhage in, and inflammation of, the gums, gingival infection, and loose dentition. Haemorrhages may also occur in the gastro-intestinal or urinary tracts, the muscles, nose, and skin, and wound healing may be impaired. In infants, subperiosteal haemorrhage with pain and tenderness of the legs may occur, but gingival symptoms are less common.

Treatment
Treatment consists of the administration of ascorbic acid (BNF 9.6.3), which may also be given as prophylaxis.

Vitamin A Deficiency

Aetiology
Vitamin A deficiency is usually due to an inadequate diet and is often accompanied by protein deficiency. It may also result from a malabsorption syndrome or hepatic impairment.

Symptoms
Visual symptoms are characteristic of vitamin A deficiency. Dark adaptation is impaired and night blindness often follows. The cornea may become soft (i.e. keratomalacia) and dry. Blindness may occur if the deficiency is untreated. Other non-specific symptoms are anaemia, growth retardation, and increased susceptibility to infection.

Treatment
Treatment is by the administration of vitamin A (BNF 9.6.1), which may also be given as prophylaxis. An adequate diet should be introduced and any underlying disorder treated.

Vitamin B Deficiencies

(*See also* Beri-beri *and* Pellagra above.)

Riboflavine Deficiency

Aetiology
Riboflavine (vitamin B$_2$) deficiency is due to an inadequate diet.

Symptoms

Symptoms are usually mild, and include fissuring and scaling of the lips (cheilosis) and of the angles of the mouth (angular stomatitis). Glossitis and seborrhoeic dermatitis may also occur.

Treatment

Treatment is by the administration of riboflavine (BNF 9.6.2). An adequate diet should be introduced.

Pyridoxine Deficiency

Aetiology

Pyridoxine (vitamin B$_6$) deficiency may occasionally arise from an inadequate diet, but may also result from a malabsorption syndrome or may be drug-induced (e.g. by isoniazid).

Symptoms

Symptoms include anaemias, cheilosis, seborrhoeic dermatitis, glossitis, and peripheral neuropathy. Convulsions may occur in infants.

Treatment

Treatment is by the administration of pyridoxine hydrochloride (BNF 9.6.2), which may also be given as prophylaxis to prevent drug-induced deficiency. Any underlying cause should be treated.

Vitamin K Deficiency

Aetiology

Vitamin K deficiency may occur in underweight neonates through inadequate synthesis. Breast-fed infants may also suffer deficiency as breast milk is a poor source of vitamin K. Other causes include decreased absorption due to obstructive jaundice or malabsorption syndromes. Drugs may antagonise vitamin K (e.g. coumarin anticoagulants) or inhibit its synthesis (e.g. sulphonamides).

Symptoms

The most common symptom, which results from low prothrombin concentrations, is haemorrhage. Likely sites of bleeding include the gastro-intestinal tract, gums, nose, and wounds. Intracranial haemorrhage may occur at birth.

Treatment

Treatment is by the administration of vitamin K preparations (BNF 9.6.6), which may also be given routinely to all neonates or to mothers prior to delivery.

Zinc Deficiency

Aetiology

Zinc deficiency may occur as a result of inadequate dietary intake (e.g. in young children fed on milk products which are low in zinc). Zinc may be chelated by dietary fibre or phytate, and this may also lead to deficiency. Patients suffering from malabsorption syndromes, physical trauma, burns, and those fed intravenously are also susceptible to zinc deficiency. Acrodermatitis enteropathica, a previously fatal inherited disorder, is now known to be caused by zinc malabsorption.

Symptoms

Anorexia, growth retardation, hypogeusia, and hypogonadism may occur in children. Impaired dark adaptation and night blindness may also develop and wound healing may be impaired. Acrodermatitis enteropathica is characterised by alopecia, eczema, diarrhoea, growth retardation, and paronychia.

Treatment

Treatment is by the administration of zinc salts (BNF 9.5.4) and dietary management.

9.3   METABOLIC DISORDERS

9.3.1   GENERAL DISORDERS

Gout

Definition and aetiology

Gout is a disorder of purine metabolism characterised by hyperuricaemia, followed by deposition of urate crystals in joints and other tissues. Hyperuricaemia is caused by an increase in production, or decrease in renal excretion, or both, of uric acid. It may be idiopathic, inherited, secondary to some other disorder (e.g. polycythaemia vera or renal failure), or may be due to the administration of drugs (e.g. loop or thiazide diuretics). A diet high in purines (e.g. brain, game, kidney, liver, meat extracts, and sea foods) and alcohol consumption may be contributory factors.

Symptoms

Symptoms usually occur only after prolonged hyperuricaemia. The onset, however, is sudden and is characterised by severe pain and inflammation of a single joint, often the metatarsophalangeal joint of the great toe. This may be accompanied by fever and rigors. These initial symptoms commonly disappear within a few days or weeks. Recurrent attacks are likely, however, with the joints of all limbs eventually becoming chronically affected (Fig. 9.2). Urate deposits (tophi) may develop in other tissues (e.g. bursae, cartilage of the pinna, and tendon sheaths) and may also occur in the kidney, leading to renal impairment and even renal failure. Renal calculi are common.

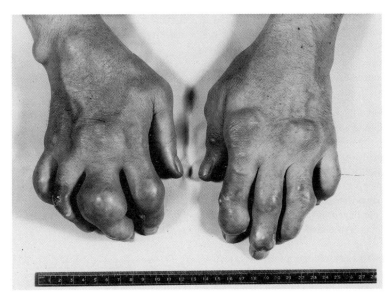

Fig. 9.2
Involvement of all joints of the hands in chronic gout.

Treatment
Acute gout attacks may be treated by the administration of non-steroidal anti-inflammatory drugs (BNF 10.1.1), although salicylates must not be used. Colchicine (BNF 10.1.4) may also be useful and corticotrophin (BNF 10.1.4.1) may be used in unresponsive cases.

Long-term management and prophylaxis comprises the administration of a xanthine-oxidase inhibitor or a uricosuric drug (BNF 10.1.4). These must not be given during, or just after, an acute attack. Patients should be encouraged to avoid excessive consumption of foods high in purines, and of alcohol.

Self-help organisations
Arthritis Care
Arthritis and Rheumatism Council

Hyperlipidaemias

Definition and aetiology
Hyperlipidaemias are a group of disorders characterised by increased plasma-lipid concentrations (i.e. cholesterol, triglycerides, or both). Disorders which may be inherited (primary hyperlipidaemias) include common hypercholesterolaemia, familial combined hyperlipidaemia, and familial hypercholesterolaemia. They may also be acquired (secondary hyperlipidaemias), commonly through excess alcohol consumption or hypothyroidism. Other causes include cholestasis, chronic renal failure, diabetes mellitus, and gout. The administration of drugs (e.g. oral contraceptives, thiazide diuretics, or chlorthalidone) may also precipitate hyperlipidaemia.

Symptoms
The most important implication of hyperlipidaemias is the consequent development of atherosclerosis with attendant ischaemic heart disease and stroke. The accumulation of yellowish lipid deposits under the skin (i.e. xanthomas) may occur in some types of hyperlipidaemia, and common sites include the eyelids (xanthelasma), elbows, and knees.

Treatment
The detection and treatment of hyperlipidaemia are important factors in the prevention of atherosclerosis and heart disease. Dietary intake of saturated fats should be restricted and body-weight controlled. The administration of lipid-lowering drugs (BNF 2.12) may be indicated.

9.3.2   CARBOHYDRATE METABOLIC DISORDERS

Galactosaemia

Definition and aetiology
Galactosaemia (galactose intolerance) is an autosomal inborn error of metabolism which may occur in two forms. It is most commonly due to a deficiency of the

enzyme galactose 1-phosphate uridyl transferase and a consequent inability to metabolise galactose. As a result, galactose 1-phosphate and galactose accumulate in the tissues. It may also be due to galactokinase deficiency, in which galactose accumulates in the blood and tissues.

Symptoms

In galactose 1-phosphate uridyl transferase deficiency, symptoms develop in the first few days of life. Diarrhoea is followed by dehydration and hypoglycaemia. Other symptoms include a failure to thrive, cataract formation, hepatomegaly, jaundice, and vomiting. Mental retardation may occur. The disorder may be fatal in the absence of treatment, and some degree of handicap may persist even in treated patients. Antenatal brain damage may occur.

Cataract formation is the only symptom of galactokinase deficiency.

Treatment

Early treatment is essential and comprises the adoption of a galactose-free lactose-free diet. Special foods and milk substitutes are available (BNF 9.4.1 and BNF Appendix 3). Prevention may be possible by prenatal diagnosis of the carrier state.

Glycogen Storage Diseases

Definition and aetiology

Glycogen storage diseases are a group of inherited metabolic disorders. Several types have been identified, and each type is characterised by deficiency of a different enzyme (e.g. glucose 6-phosphatase and glycogen synthetase) involved in glycogen metabolism. Almost all these deficiencies result in the accumulation of glycogen in body tissues.

Symptoms

Symptoms, which vary according to enzyme deficiency and body system affected, include heart failure, hepatomegaly, hypoglycaemia, physical and mental retardation, and muscle cramps and weakness.

Treatment

Some types of glycogen storage disease respond to frequent carbohydrate feeds, and special foods (BNF 9.4.1 and BNF Appendix 3) are available. Others, however, do not respond to any treatment and result in early death.

Hereditary Fructose Intolerance

Definition and aetiology

Hereditary frucose intolerance is an autosomal inborn error of metabolism caused by decreased activity of the enzyme fructose 1-phosphate aldolase, and a consequent inability to metabolise fructose.

Symptoms

Symptoms occur in infants soon after introducing fructose into the diet. Vomiting, anorexia, and a failure to thrive are common, and are accompanied by fructosaemia, fructosuria, and hypoglycaemia. Other symptoms include hepatomegaly, jaundice, proteinuria, and renal impairment, and untreated cases may result in death.

Treatment

Treatment consists of the adoption of a diet completely free of fructose, sorbitol, and sucrose.

9.3.3   ELECTROLYTE DISORDERS

Acidosis

Definition

Acidosis is a disturbance of acid-base balance characterised by an accumulation of acid or depletion of alkaline content of extracellular fluid. There is an increase in the hydrogen ion concentration (i.e. a fall in pH). Acidosis may be metabolic or respiratory (see below), although their aetiology and mechanisms of compensation may be closely interrelated.

Metabolic Acidosis

Definition and aetiology

Metabolic acidosis is caused by a metabolic disturbance in which acid accumulates in, or bicarbonate is lost from, the extracellular fluid. It may be due to shock or cardiac arrest, in which tissue hypoxia causes anaerobic metabolism and the production of lactic acid (i.e. lactic acidosis). Severe diarrhoea may also result in a metabolic acidosis through increased excretion of hydroxyl ions in the faeces. Uncontrolled diabetes mellitus and starvation may cause metabolic acidosis through increased production of organic acids (i.e. diabetic ketoacidosis). In chronic renal disease, the distal tubules may fail to excrete hydrogen ions and a metabolic acidosis develops (i.e. renal tubular acidosis). Other causes of metabolic acidosis include ingestion of acid and ethanol poisoning.

Symptoms

Mild metabolic acidosis may be asymptomatic, but it can be accompanied by fatigue, and nausea and vomiting. Rapid deep respiration (hyperpnoea) is characteristic, however, and severe acidosis may lead to the development of shock and be fatal.

Treatment

Any underlying disorder must be treated. Severe acidosis is treated by the administration of sodium bicarbonate (BNF 9.2.2) preceded by isotonic sodium chloride intravenous infusion.

Respiratory Acidosis

Definition and aetiology

Respiratory acidosis is an acidosis arising from the accumulation of carbon dioxide caused by hypoventilation. There is a rise in the partial pressure of carbon dioxide (i.e. an increase in PCO_2). It may be due to respiratory depression (e.g. by drugs), chronic obstructive airways disease (e.g. chronic bronchitis or emphysema), or obstruction of the larynx or trachea.

Symptoms

Respiratory acidosis produces vasodilatation leading to encephalopathy with headache and drowsiness. Stupor and coma may develop.

Treatment

Treatment is as for metabolic acidosis (*see above*). Assisted ventilation and oxygen therapy (BNF 3.6) may be required.

Alkalosis

Definition

Alkalosis is a disturbance of acid-base balance characterised by the accumulation of base or the depletion of acid in the extracellular fluid. There is a decrease in the hydrogen ion concentration (i.e. a rise in pH). Alkalosis may be metabolic or respiratory (*see below*), although their aetiology and mechanisms of compensation may be closely interrelated.

Metabolic Alkalosis

Definition and aetiology

Metabolic alkalosis is due to a metabolic disturbance in which bicarbonate accumulates in, or acid is lost from, the extracelluar fluid. It may arise through persistent vomiting (e.g. in pyloric stenosis) resulting in the loss of gastric acid, renal retention of bicarbonate, excessive ingestion of alkali, potassium depletion, or volume depletion (e.g. in burns or diuretic therapy).

Symptoms

Common symptoms include irritability and neuromuscular excitability. Tetany may develop.

Treatment

The underlying disorder should be corrected. In mild alkalosis, treatment may be unnecessary. In more severe cases, fluid replacement (BNF 9.2.2) may be undertaken and potassium and sodium depletion may require correction (BNF 9.2.2).

Respiratory Alkalosis

Definition and aetiology

Respiratory alkalosis is an alkalosis arising from excessive elimination of carbon dioxide in expired air. It occurs as a result of hyperventilation and is characterised by a fall in the partial pressure of carbon dioxide (i.e. a decrease in PCO_2). Hyperventilation may result from a central nervous system disorder (e.g. stroke or meningitis), anxiety, exertion at high temperature or altitude, or from excessive assisted ventilation (e.g. during anaesthesia). It may also be due to drug administration (e.g. salicylates).

Symptoms

Respiratory alkalosis is marked by tetany with spasm of the hand muscles and acroparaesthesia. Convulsions may occur and respiratory arrest may develop. Peripheral vasoconstriction is likely, resulting in pallor.

Treatment

Treatment may consist of rebreathing expired carbon dioxide. Any underlying disorder should be treated and anxiolytics (BNF 4.1.2) may be beneficial. Excessive assisted ventilation should be corrected by appropriate adjustment of the equipment.

Hypercalcaemia

Definition and aetiology

Hypercalcaemia is an increase in the plasma-calcium concentration above normal (i.e. >2.6 mmol/L). It usually occurs as a result of calcium reabsorption from bone into the bloodstream or a decrease in the renal excretion of calcium. The most common cause is primary hyperparathyroidism, although malignant diseases with bony metastases, vitamin D administration, or excessive calcium ingestion (e.g. milk-alkali syndrome) may be responsible. Other causes include Addison's disease, diuretic therapy, and sarcoidosis.

Symptoms

Mild hypercalcaemia may be asymptomatic, but if symptoms develop, they may include abdominal pain, anorexia, constipation, fatigue, nausea and vomiting, and polyuria with nocturia and thirst. Severe cases are characterised by confusion, delirium, and psychosis. Stupor and coma may also develop. Marked muscle weakness may occur, or renal impairment may develop as a result of calculi formation. This may progress to renal failure which may be fatal.

Treatment
The underlying cause should be identified and treated. Intravenous fluid replacement (BNF 9.2.2) and the restriction of dietary calcium may, however, be the only treatment required. The administration of binding or chelating agents (BNF 9.5.1.2) may be beneficial. In severe hypercalcaemia, a calcitonin preparation (BNF 6.6.1), plicamycin (BNF 8.1.2), or a corticosteroid (BNF 6.3.4) may be given to inhibit calcium reabsorption from bone.

Hyperkalaemia

Definition and aetiology
Hyperkalaemia is an increase in the plasma-potassium concentration above normal (i.e. >5 mmol/L). It usually occurs as a result of defective excretion arising from renal failure, although excessive potassium administration or potassium-sparing diuretic therapy may also be responsible.

Symptoms
Hyperkalaemia may be initially asymptomatic, although a flaccid paralysis occasionally occurs. Characteristic ECG changes may occur, and the development of asystole is often associated with sudden death.

Treatment
In mild cases, a reduction in potassium intake or the discontinuation of potassium-sparing diuretics may be sufficient, although an ion-exchange resin (BNF 9.2.1.1) may be beneficial. Marked hyperkalaemia (i.e. >6.5 mmol/L) constitutes a medical emergency and urgent treatment (*see* Acute Renal Failure) is essential.

Hypernatraemia

Definition and aetiology
Hypernatraemia is an increase in the plasma-sodium concentration above normal (i.e. >148 mmol/L). It usually occurs as a result of fluid loss in excess of sodium loss. This may arise as a result of diarrhoea or vomiting, excessive sweating, diabetes insipidus, or osmotic diuresis. In addition, hypernatraemia may be caused by inadequate fluid intake (particularly in infants, elderly, or unconscious patients) or to excessive intake of sodium (e.g. in inappropriate intravenous fluid therapy or dialysis).

Symptoms
Thirst is less marked than might be anticipated. Symptoms may include confusion, drowsiness and lethargy,

dry skin, hypotension, muscle twitching, and peripheral vasoconstriction. Coma may develop. Hypernatraemia is especially dangerous when it occurs suddenly, and thromboses may occur in infants. Brain cells may become dehydrated resulting in cerebral, subarachnoid, or subdural haemorrhage.

Treatment
Treatment is by the gradual correction of fluid balance and may comprise the intravenous (BNF 9.2.2) or oral (BNF 9.2.1) administration of fluid.

Hypocalcaemia

Definition and aetiology
Hypocalcaemia is a reduction in the plasma-calcium concentration below normal (i.e. <2.1 mmol/L). It is an infrequent occurrence, but may develop as a result of hypoparathyroidism, vitamin D deficiency, renal disease, magnesium depletion, acute pancreatitis, or hypoproteinaemia.

Symptoms
Hypocalcaemia is often asymptomatic. However, symptoms may develop depending on the severity, and include paraesthesia of the face, fingers, and toes, tetany, or prolonged tonic spasms of muscles due to neuromuscular instability. This may result in laryngeal spasm and stridor. Convulsions and psychosis may also occur.

Treatment
Treatment depends upon the underlying disorder. Intravenous infusion of calcium salts (BNF 9.5.1.1) or oral calcium, sometimes in combination with vitamin D, may be used in hypoparathyroidism. Dietary phosphorus restriction or phosphate-binding agents (BNF 9.5.2.2) may be beneficial in renal failure.

Hypokalaemia

Definition and aetiology
Hypokalaemia is a reduction in the plasma-potassium concentration below normal (i.e. <3.5 mmol/L). It may occur as a result of potassium loss in the urine, renal disease, or in diuretic therapy (e.g. with thiazide or loop diuretics). Excess potassium may also be lost in the faeces and may occur as a result of diarrhoea or laxative abuse. Other causes include Cushing's syndrome, corticosteroid therapy, diabetes mellitus, hyperaldosteronism (*see* Primary Aldosteronism), or vomiting. Dietary deficiency may occur in elderly patients.

Symptoms
Hypokalaemia may be characterised by neuromuscular disturbances, cramps, muscle weakness, and tetany. In severe cases, muscle weakness may progress to paralysis

and respiratory failure. Arrhythmias may also develop, particularly in patients receiving cardiac glycosides.

Treatment

Any underlying cause should be corrected. If diuretics are being given, a potassium-sparing drug (BNF 2.2.3 and 2.2.4) should be used, especially in those patients also receiving cardiac glycosides. The administration of oral potassium supplements (BNF 9.2.1.1) may be indicated, and intravenous therapy (BNF 9.2.2) may be necessary in severe hypokalaemia.

Hyponatraemia

Definition and aetiology

Hyponatraemia is a reduction in the plasma-sodium concentration below normal (i.e. <135 mmol/L), although it is more commonly associated with an excess of water in the absence of reduced plasma-sodium concentrations. Sodium depletion may be caused by loss via the gastrointestinal tract (e.g. diarrhoea or vomiting) or the kidney (e.g. in polycystic kidney disease or pyelonephritis), or as a result of excessive sweating. It may also arise from the administration of loop or thiazide diuretics. Water excess (i.e. water intoxication) may be caused by increased fluid ingestion, inappropriate postoperative intravenous fluid therapy, or acute renal failure.

Symptoms

Symptoms include orthostatic hypotension and reduced skin turgor. Confusion may occur, and convulsions may develop in severe cases. Water intoxication, however, is marked by anorexia, heart failure, hypertension, muscle weakness, and oedema.

Treatment

Hyponatraemia may be corrected by an increased dietary salt intake. Oral sodium supplements (BNF 9.2.1.2) may be indicated in some patients, although the administration of sodium chloride intravenous infusion (BNF 9.2.2) may be necessary.

Pseudohypoparathyroidism

Definition

Pseudohypoparathyroidism is a rare hereditary condition in which there is failure of the target tissues to respond to parathyroid hormone.

Symptoms

Clinically it resembles hypoparathyroidism, with symptoms produced through hypocalcaemia. However, pseudohypoparathyroidism is also associated with certain developmental abnormalities (e.g. round face, short stature, and shortening of the metacarpals and

metatarsals). Other associated disorders include amenorrhoea, diabetes mellitus, hypothyroidism, and Turner's syndrome.

Treatment

Treatment consists of correction of hypocalcaemia by administration of vitamin D preparations (BNF 9.6.4), initially with calcium supplements (BNF 9.5.1.1) if necessary.

9.3.4 INBORN ERRORS OF METABOLISM

Hepatolenticular Degeneration

Definition and aetiology

Hepatolenticular degeneration (Wilson's disease) is a rare, autosomal, inborn error of metabolism characterised by the accumulation of copper in the brain, kidneys, liver, and certain other tissues. It is a progressive disorder which is usually fatal in the absence of treatment.

Symptoms

The onset, which is insidious, usually occurs in childhood or adolescence, but it may not develop until the fifth decade. It is characterised by the development of neurological and hepatic symptoms. Common neurological symptoms include akinesia and rigidity, chorea, convulsions, drooling, dysphagia, speech disorders, muscle wasting and weakness, and tremor. The presence of a golden-brown ring around the outer edge of the cornea (Kayser-Fleischer ring) is a positive diagnostic feature. Behaviour and personality disorders are common and may be extreme, and untreated patients become immobile, demented, and mentally impaired. Cirrhosis, hepatitis, and jaundice are common hepatic symptoms, and ascites and hepatic coma may develop.

Treatment

Treatment, which comprises the long-term administration of a copper-chelating agent (BNF 9.8), must begin as soon as the disorder is diagnosed. Prompt treatment produces successful control and a correspondingly favourable prognosis. Patients should be advised to avoid foods rich in copper (e.g. shellfish and liver).

Maple-syrup Urine Disease

Definition and aetiology

Maple-syrup urine disease is a rare inborn error of amino-acid metabolism. It occurs as a result of a reduction in the activity of the enzyme, keto-acid decarboxylase, which is responsible for the metabolism of the keto acids formed from certain amino acids (e.g. isoleucine, leucine, and valine).

Symptoms

Symptoms vary according to the severity of the disorder. In the most severe (classical) form, symptoms develop soon after birth and include convulsions, feeding problems, lethargy, and metabolic acidosis. Patients have a characteristic maple-syrup odour caused by excretion of keto acids in sweat and urine. This form of the disorder is often fatal and those who survive may suffer severe brain damage. Other patients suffer from an intermittent form of the disorder and only experience episodic symptoms, which are usually precipitated by an acute infection. Such patients remain well between episodes, although they may suffer some psychomotor impairment. Milder forms of the disorder, with continuous but less marked symptoms, also exist.

Treatment

Treatment is by the dietary restriction of the relevant amino acids and, if begun immediately after birth, is usually successful. Special foods are available (BNF Appendix 3). One of the mild forms of the disorder responds to treatment with thiamine (BNF 9.6.2). Dialysis or exchange blood transfusion may be required during acute attacks and any infection should be treated immediately.

Phenylketonuria

Definition and aetiology

Phenylketonuria is an autosomal, recessive, inborn error of metabolism. It is characterised by deficiency of the enzyme phenylalanine hydroxylase and a consequent inability to convert phenylalanine to tyrosine. This results in the accumulation of phenylalanine in the blood and tissues.

Symptoms

Affected neonates may appear normal at birth, but phenylalanine accumulation gives rise to brain damage with mental retardation. The degree of retardation may vary, but is marked if the condition is not treated. Other symptoms include convulsions, eczema, hyperkinesia, microcephaly, light pigmentation, and a 'mousy' body odour.

Treatment

Early diagnosis is essential and is usually achieved soon after birth by routine screening using the Guthrie test. Genetic counselling may be beneficial as a means of prevention in future generations.

Treatment comprises the prompt introduction of a diet low in phenylalanine but adequate in other nutrients, and special foods are available (BNF Appendix 3).

Self-help organisation

National Society for Phenylketonuria and Allied Disorders

Porphyrias

Definition and aetiology

The porphyrias are a group of rare inherited disorders resulting from disturbed porphyrin metabolism, which under normal conditions contributes to the formation of the iron-containing complex, haem. Attacks may be spontaneous and sporadic, but may be precipitated by drug administration (e.g. barbiturates, oestrogens, and some antiepileptic drugs) or by alcohol consumption. Infection, menstruation, and pregnancy have also been implicated as contributory factors.

Symptoms

The passage of dark urine is the most usual common factor in the different forms of porphyria. Acute intermittent porphyria is the most serious of the acute forms and may be fatal. Common symptoms include acute abdominal pain with vomiting and constipation or diarrhoea, peripheral neuritis with limb pain and paralysis, psychiatric disturbances (e.g. anxiety and psychosis), and convulsions. Hypertension and tachycardia are common cardiovascular symptoms. Variegate porphyria and hereditary coproporphyria are other acute forms, and are characterised by photosensitivity in addition to the above symptoms. Porphyria cutanea tarda and erythropoietic porphyria are non-acute forms of the disorder, and are also characterised by skin photosensitivity.

Treatment

Precipitating factors must be identified and removed. A high-carbohydrate diet should be maintained during attacks to reduce excessive production of porphyrins. Treatment of acute attacks is symptomatic and the administration of analgesics (BNF 4.7), anti-emetics (BNF 4.6), antiepileptics (BNF 4.8), antipsychotic drugs (BNF 4.2), and beta-adrenoceptor blocking drugs (BNF 2.4) may be indicated. Care must be taken to avoid drugs contra-indicated in porphyrias. In addition, fluid and electrolytes (BNF 9.2) may be necessary and physiotherapy may be beneficial for paralysis. No specific treatment exists for skin symptoms, although betacarotene has been used in erythropoietic porphyria.

9.4 ANATOMY AND PHYSIOLOGY RELEVANT TO BLOOD AND LYMPH DISORDERS

Introduction

Each cell within the body is a discrete unit, carrying out

the functions for which it is genetically programmed. However, despite their apparent independence, cells are kept in continual contact with one another and with other parts of the body by the inward transmission of fluids containing nutrients, hormones, enzymes, and the outward flow of toxic and waste materials through the cell wall. The medium for the delivery and the removal of cellular components is the compartmentalised body fluid.

The largest compartment is the intracellular fluid in which the activities of the cell are carried out. The cell's intimate contact with the environment outside its walls is maintained by the presence of fluid around the cell wall, the interstitial (tissue) fluid. The third compartment of fluid is the blood plasma and lymph, which transports materials to and from the interstitial fluid. The interstitial fluid and the plasma are together referred to as the extracellular fluid.

It is vital that the plasma, lymph, and the interstitial fluid are maintained free of the potentially harmful elements introduced into the body (e.g. by absorption from the gastro-intestinal tract). The main circulatory defence mechanism within the body is the lymphatic system which collects material from the interstitial fluid.

Blood

Blood is a complex fluid, consisting of cellular components (approximately 45% of the total volume) suspended in a fluid environment, the plasma. An average adult male has about 5 to 6 litres of blood, whilst the blood volume in an average adult female is 4 to 5 litres.

Erythrocytes   The greater proportion of the cellular components of blood is erythrocytes (Fig. 9.3), numbering approximately five million per mm^3 (5 × 10^{12}/L). The process of formation of erythrocytes (erythropoiesis) is carried out in the red bone marrow (myeloid tissue) of the sternum, vertebrae, ribs, femur, humerus, and pelvis. Development within the bone marrow proceeds via erythroblasts (in which haemoglobin is synthesised) and reticulocytes. The reticulocytes become denucleated before they leave the bone marrow, and develop into erythrocytes within 1 to 2 days of entering the general circulation. Erythrocytes have a lifespan of approximately 120 days, at the end of which time they are destroyed by macrophage engulfment in the liver, spleen, and bone marrow.

Each erythrocyte is a biconcave disc about 8 μm in diameter, consisting of a lipoprotein membrane surrounding cytoplasm and a red pigment, haemoglobin. The role of haemoglobin is crucial. Each haemoglobin

ERYTHROCYTES

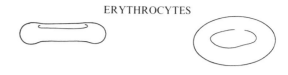

GRANULAR LEUCOCYTES

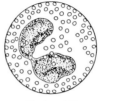   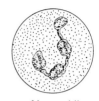

Eosinophil   Neutrophil

AGRANULAR LEUCOCYTES

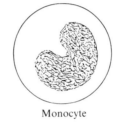   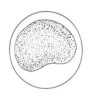

Monocyte   Lymphocyte

Fig. 9.3
Erythrocytes and leucocytes.

molecule contains four haem molecules which are structurally derived from the porphyrin ring. Each ring contains an iron atom and can bind reversibly to oxygen. Haem combines with inhaled oxygen in the ratio of one haem molecule to one oxygen molecule to form oxyhaemoglobin. Once haemoglobin has divested itself of oxygen, the proteinacious globin portion combines with waste carbon dioxide to form carbaminohaemoglobin, which is transported to the lungs for dissociation and exhalation.

At the end of the life of the erythrocyte, haemoglobin is broken down into haemosiderin (which may be stored and reused to make new haemoglobin), bilirubin (secreted by the liver in the bile), and globin.

Leucocytes   There are between 5000 and 7000 leucocytes per mm^3 of blood (5 to 7 × 10^9). They are classified into two main groups, the granular leucocytes (granulocytes) and the agranular leucocytes. Granular leucocytes are subdivided into neutrophils (polymorphs), eosinophils, and basophils (Fig. 9.3). Agranular leucocytes are subdivided into lymphocytes and monocytes.

The myeloid tissue of the red bone marrow is the origin of agranular and granular leucocytes. Agranular leucocoytes are also produced in lymphoid tissue. The three different types of granular leucocytes are produced from a common myeloblast, whereas monocytes and lymphocytes develop from monoblasts and lymphoblasts respectively. The proportion of each type of leucocyte is an important gauge of the state of health of the body. In health, the bulk of the elements are formed of neutrophils (60% to 70%) and lymphocytes (20% to 25%), but changes in the ratios may indicate allergic reactions, infection, or antigen-antibody reactions.

The principal function of the leucocytes is to counteract potentially pathogenic invasion of the body, and each leucocytic element is modified to provide a particular aspect of the defence mechanism.

Neutrophils (polymorphonuclear leucocytes) consist of a nucleus which is divided into 3 to 5 lobes linked by thin strands. They ingest bacteria by phagocytosis and secrete the bactericidal enzyme, lysozyme (see Section 15.4). They are also attracted by chemicals released at the site of tissue damage (chemotaxis).

Eosinophils are structurally similar to neutrophils, although the nucleus generally consists of only two linked lobes. Their functions, however, are different and may involve a role in the immune response. They may modulate the severity of the antigen-antibody reaction and counteract the release of histamine from mast cells in allergic reactions. They may also enhance the body's resistance to reinfection with helminths.

The granules in basophils contain a range of components (e.g. heparin, serotonin, and histamine) which play a role in the mediation of allergic reactions (see Section 15.6). Basophils may also be the precursors of the mast cells from which the basophilic granules are released.

Lymphocytes play a fundamental role in the immune response. They are functionally divided into T-cells (thymus-dependent cells) and B-cells.

The T-cells derive their immune competence within the thymus gland during foetal development. They are distributed throughout the body by the bloodstream and the lymphatic system. They are activated in response to a specific foreign agent (an antigen) to which they become attached and ultimately destroy. The response of T-cells is referred to as cell-mediated immunity as the antigen (e.g. a virus, cancer cell, or a transplanted tissue) is attacked within the cell. Several subdivisions of T-cells have been identified (e.g. killer, helper, and suppressor T-cells). The presence of T-helper cells is essential to

enable B-cells (see below) to divide and produce plasma cells. Conversely, T-suppressor cells prevent the production of antibodies possibly through an effect on the corresponding helper cells for that antibody. T-cytotoxic cells kill specific cells (e.g. those infected with a virus). Null cells are non-specific cytotoxic T-cells, which comprise natural killer cells, lymphokine-activated killers, and killer cells.

The B-cells (so-called because in birds they develop in the bursa of Fabricius) are thought to mature in the bone marrow, liver, and spleen and are transported to the lymphoid tissue for storage. These cells are the precursors of plasma cells which produce antibodies and provide humoral (circulating) immunity. The antibodies are produced from the plasma cell within the storage tissue and are specific for a particular antigen. Memory cells are also produced from the B-cells, and these may generate a more rapid and much greater antibody response should the antigen be identified on a subsequent occasion.

Monocytes, like neutrophils, are attracted to the site of infection by chemotaxis, and ingest bacteria and dead material by phagocytosis (see Section 15.4). As monocytes, these cells are short-lived but they enlarge to form highly efficient and long-lived phagocytic cells, the macrophages. The macrophages circulate widely throughout the body, but are also concentrated in certain tissues (e.g. bone marrow, liver, lungs, and spleen). These fixed macrophages are described as the cellular components of the reticulo-endothelial system, which plays an important role in clearing the blood of bacteria and particulate matter.

Platelets The sequence of platelet (thrombocyte) formation starts in the red bone marrow from megakaryoblasts, which mature into megakaryocytes. Multiple fragmentation of the cytoplasm of the megakaryocyte leads to the production of tiny packets which become enclosed within a cell membrane. Platelets of 2 to 4 μm diameter are formed in this way from each 40 μm megakaryocyte. There are between 150 000 and 400 000 platelets per mm^3 of blood (150 to 400 $\times$ 10^9/L). The lifespan of platelets is approximately 5 to 9 days, and they play an essential role in the processes of blood clotting. In trauma, they reduce the loss of erythrocytes from blood vessels by increasing in size and adhesiveness, resulting in the formation of plugs within arterioles, which also prevents fluid and cell loss. They also promote coagulation of blood through interaction with clotting proteins.

Blood Groups

Except under emergency circumstances, it is not possible to transfuse blood from one patient to another without a knowledge of the blood group of the patient. An individual's blood group is determined by the presence or absence of specific antigens (agglutinogens) on the surface of the erythrocyte and of corresponding antibodies (agglutinins) in the plasma. In the ABO system of blood groups, the erythrocyte antigens are polysaccharides; the antigenic character of the rhesus system is unknown. The antibodies to both sets of blood groups are primarily IgG or IgM, or both.

The ABO system   In the ABO system, the presence of two surface antigens, A and B, determines the presence of antibodies anti-A and anti-B, and these are summarised in Table 9.1. Subgroups to group A and group AB exist and are described as A_2 and A_2B. It is recommended that the terms 'universal donor' and 'universal recipient' are no longer used, partly because of the formerly unidentified presence of subgroups, and because other antigens, notably the rhesus factor, must also be considered in any proposed transfusion.

TABLE 9.1
The ABO system of blood groups

Group	Antigens	Antibodies	Frequency (%) in UK population
A_1	A_1	anti-B	34
A_2	A_2	anti-B and anti-A_1 in 10%	8
B	B	anti-A	9
A_1B	A_1 and B	neither anti-A nor anti-B	2.7
A_2B	A_2 and B	neither anti-A nor anti-B or, in 25%, anti-A_1	0.3
O	neither A nor B	anti-A and anti-B	46

The rhesus system   Rhesus factors (so called after their initial identification in rhesus monkeys) are present on the membranes of erythrocytes of about 85% of the population in the UK, who are described as rhesus-positive. The most common rhesus factor is the D antigen, but unlike the ABO system in which antibodies to absent factors are always present in the blood, anti-D antibodies are only produced when a rhesus-negative person comes into contact with rhesus-positive blood. This most commonly occurs when a rhesus-negative mother carries a rhesus-positive foetus. Anti-D rhesus antibodies can be produced in the maternal circulation, particularly at partruition, when the mother's blood may mix with that of the neonate. If a subsequent foetus has rhesus-positive blood, the transplacental transfer of anti-D antibodies can cause the potentially fatal haemolytic disease of the newborn.

Lymphatic System

The lymphatic system is a specialised form of circulatory system which consists of lymph vessels and the lymphatic organs (the bone marrow, thymus, spleen, and lymph nodes). Lymph nodes (which are 1 to 25 mm in size and limited within a capsule) are located along the lymph vessels, usually in groups. The connective tissue present in some mucous membranes (e.g. in the tonsils, the Peyer's patches of the ileum, the appendix, the respiratory system, and the reproductive system) also contains unencapsulated non-nodular lymphatic tissue.

Lymph capillaries originate in the spaces between cells and consist of walls which allow the one-way inward transfer of material from the blood capillaries. The movement of fluid is dependent upon contractions within the smooth muscle of the vessels and skeletal muscle, as there is no pump comparable to the heart. The lymphatic vessels eventually merge to form two major channels, the thoracic (left lymphatic) duct and the right lymphatic duct.

The lymphatic system serves several purposes. Excess fluid and the small amount of protein which leaks from blood capillaries into the interstitial fluid cannot return directly to the capillaries, but passes to the lymph capillaries as lymph fluid. The fluid is then passed through the lymphatic system and is returned to the blood at the right and left internal jugular and subclavian veins.

The lymphatic system assists in the absorption of fat from the small intestine. Complexes of bile salt and fat diffuse into intestinal epithelial cells and combine with lipids and proteins to form small particles (chylomicrons). These are too large to be absorbed directly into the circulation and so they pass into the lymph vessels for indirect transfer to the blood.

Lymph nodes participate in the defence mechanisms of the body. As lymph passes into the nodes, unwanted materials are filtered and destroyed by the action of macrophages, T-cells, and B-cells. Lymphocytes are also produced within the nodes and some are distributed to other parts of the body through the lymphatic and blood circulatory systems.

Spleen

The spleen is situated in the upper abdominal cavity and is the largest organ of the lymphatic system. It consists of red pulp, which occupies the venous sinuses and is filled with blood and splenic (Billroth's) cords, and white pulp which surrounds arteries and comprises white lymphatic tissue, consisting mainly of lymphocytes. Malpighian bodies, which are thickened lymphocytic nodules, are closely associated with the white pulp. Blood flows through the spleen in open and closed systems. The rate of blood flow through the closed system is fast and direct and this is the major route during health. Blood flows much more slowly through the open system as it has to negotiate a network of splenic cord spaces.

The spleen is responsible for the development of a small proportion of erythrocytes and lymphocytes in the foetus and newborn baby. This capacity is lost in early life but may be held in reserve in the event of haematological stress.

Splenic activity is responsible for reconditioning erythrocytes and destroying old erythrocytes and foreign material. As blood flows through the spleen, platelets and reticulocytes are temporarily removed for storage and maturation respectively. Blood is also stored in the spleen in the blood pool and this may be drawn on in the event of reduced blood volume (e.g. following haemorrhage).

The presence of the body's largest concentration of lymphocytes and stimulation of these cells by antigens results in antibody formation in the spleen.

The Control of Blood Clot Formation

Blood clotting (haemostasis), vasospasm, and platelet plug formation are the mechanisms by which blood loss is minimised in the event of breakage of a blood vessel. These mechanisms are delicately balanced so that they are rapidly effective in the event of haemorrhage, but not so effective under normal circumstances that clot formation occurs spontaneously.

The message that trauma has occurred is amplified through a complex cascade of enzyme systems, which comprise the mechanisms of blood clotting. The key to the formation of fibrin is the production of prothrombin activator by one of two pathways (known as the intrinsic and extrinsic pathways) and the release of various coagulation factors (which are commonly designated by Roman numerals). The extrinsic pathway, which is the more rapid of the two, may produce prothrombin activator within a few seconds in the event of severe trauma. It is initiated by tissue factor III, a factor present in cell walls, which leads to the release of a group of substances referred to as tissue thromboplastin. In the presence of calcium ions and factor VIII (the antihaemophilic factor), thromboplastin activates factor X to form prothrombin activator.

The intrinsic pathway, which is more complex than the extrinsic pathway, may take up to several minutes to produce prothrombin activator, and is initiated within the blood by interaction between the collagen fibres of damaged blood vessels and the blood. This activates factor XII and causes the release of phospholipids from platelets. Factor XII activates factor XI, which in turn activates factor IX. The presence of calcium ions, factor VIII, activated factor IX, and platelet phospholipids result in the activation of factor X. Prothrombin activator is finally formed in the presence of factor X, factor V, calcium ions, and platelet phospholipids.

The complete clotting process may be considered to comprise three stages. The initial stage is the formation of prothrombin activator (*see above*), which then converts prothrombin in the plasma to thrombin. Thirdly, thrombin converts fibrinogen into fibrin, which forms intermolecular links to produce the network of threads which comprise the clot.

The prevention of unwanted thrombosis is due to the action of an endogenous fibrinolytic compound, plasmin, which is formed from its precursor, plasminogen. The conversion of plasminogen to plasmin is catalysed by specific activators, plasminogen activators, which may be derived from the circulation, from local tissues, or by the action of drugs (e.g. streptokinase and urokinase).

Chapter 10

MUSCULOSKELETAL AND CONNECTIVE TISSUE DISORDERS

10.1 GENERAL DISORDERS

Back Pain

Definition and aetiology
Back pain becomes more common with advancing age, and occurs most frequently in the lumbar (i.e. lumbago) or sacro-iliac regions. The cause is often uncertain, but the upright nature of mans' posture results in shear strains which give rise to degenerative spinal joint disturbances. Back pain may also arise from inflammatory disease (e.g. ankylosing spondylitis), prolapsed (slipped) intervertebral discs, spinal nerve root compression (e.g. sciatica), osteoporosis, bony metastases, congenital spinal defects (e.g. spina bifida), fractures, infection, mechanical injury, and pelvic or retroperitoneal malignant disease. It may also be caused by strain arising from inappropriate lifting technique, obesity, poor posture, or pregnancy. Back pain may also be psychogenic.

Symptoms

Pain may be local or diffuse and may radiate or be referred. It is, however, usually characterised by limitation of movement. If pain is exacerbated by movement and improved by rest, the cause is usually mechanical strain or injury, whereas pain caused by inflammatory disease is usually worse after rest. Pain arising from nerve root compression may be exacerbated by coughing or sneezing. The onset of pain caused by disc, muscle, or ligament injury is usually sudden, whereas pain caused by inflammatory disease often has a gradual onset.

Treatment

Treatment depends on the cause. Common treatment includes the administration of non-steroidal anti-inflammatory drugs (BNF 10.1.1), bed rest, and physiotherapy. Patients should avoid lifting heavy weights, and be instructed in proper lifting techniques and maintaining an appropriate posture. Manipulation and traction may be beneficial in some patients and, very occasionally, laminectomy may be indicated.

Muscular Dystrophy

Definition and aetiology

The commonest degenerative myopathy is Duchenne muscular dystrophy which invariably affects only boys, although cases in girls with Turner's syndrome have been reported. Duchenne muscular dystrophy is primarily a genetically inherited disorder, although cases do occur in the absence of known familial history. It is thought to be caused by the absence of a muscular protein, dystrophin. The absence of this protein permits the influx of calcium into the muscle cell, resulting in the activation of proteases which digest muscle fibres. The gene to form dystrophin is located on the X-chromosome and is transmitted recessively to male offspring. Occasionally, gene mutation may give rise to the condition in the absence of familial history.

Symptoms

Early symptoms may be recognised with the late onset of walking at about 18 months of age, although other earlier developmental milestones (e.g. crawling) may also be delayed. Further disturbances of motor function (e.g. difficulty in climbing stairs, unsteadiness in walking, and failure to run) can develop after three years of age. The majority of boys are diagnosed between 4 and 6 years of age. Compensatory hypertrophy of unaffected muscles (e.g. of the calf) may occur early in the disease but disappears later. Obesity is common and mental retardation or impaired intellectual development can also occur. Contractures and scoliosis are common late symptoms. Continued development of muscular weak-

ness is relentless, resulting in confinement to a wheelchair between 10 and 12 years of age, and death from respiratory failure, respiratory-tract infection, or heart failure, often in the late teens or early 20s.

Treatment

There is no treatment for Duchenne muscular dystrophy. Palliative measures can be adopted to minimise the discomfort caused by contractures and scoliosis. Obesity should be treated with dietary control and physiotherapy may be helpful in the early stages. Carrier detection can be carried out in families with a history of the disease, followed by appropriate genetic counselling for affected females. Amniocentesis can detect affected males *in utero*.

Self-help organisation

Muscular Dystrophy Group of Great Britain and Northern Ireland

Sciatica

Definition and aetiology

Sciatica is a severe pain experienced along the course and distribution of the sciatic nerve in the buttocks, back of thigh and calf, and outer side of the calf and foot. It is usually caused by a prolapsed (slipped) lower lumbar intervertebral disc. The prolapsed disc causes irritation and compression of one or more nerve roots of the cauda equina which usually lasts several weeks. There is often a history of low back injury and pain from lifting weights or sudden movement. Sciatic pain may also be referred from other structures within the nerve distribution of the spinal segments from which the sciatic nerve arises (e.g. the hip or sacro-iliac joints).

Symptoms

The pain usually begins in the lumbar region (lumbago) and extends along the course of the sciatic nerve. It may be aggravated by stooping, coughing, or turning in bed.

Treatment

Treatment consists of bed rest and the administration of analgesics (BNF 4.7). To prevent relapse, the patient should be advised to avoid lifting objects with the back flexed. Chronic or recurrent sciatica may be treated surgically. Treatment of referred sciatic pain is directed towards the underlying cause.

Torticollis

Definition and aetiology

Torticollis (wry neck) is any condition in which rotating and tilting of the head to one side occurs. It may be spasmodic or permanent and although the cause is ill-defined, the most common form is due to spasm of the cervical muscles of the neck. It has been suggested that emotional disturbances may contribute. A history of an extrapyramidal disorder may be identified.

Symptoms
The onset commonly occurs between 30 and 60 years of age, is usually gradual, but may occasionally be acute. It is characterised by painful spasms of the muscles on one side of the neck and the adoption of an unnatural head posture. The condition may be intermittent and mild, but may become chronic and produce immobility and deformity.

Treatment
Drug treatment and surgery are usually ineffective. The application of slight pressure to the jaw with the hand may give short-term relief in spasmodic torticollis. If emotional disturbance is a factor, psychiatric treatment may be beneficial.

10.2   ARTHRITIS AND RELATED CONDITIONS

Ankylosing Spondylitis

Definition and aetiology
Ankylosing spondylitis is a progressive chronic arthritis of the spine which most often occurs in men between 20 and 40 years of age. The disease usually has a milder course in women. It is characterised by inflammation of the sacro-iliac and intervertebral joints. Calcification and ossification may result in immobility and fusion (i.e. ankylosis) of these spinal joints. The cause of the disease is unknown, although a family history is often present.

Symptoms
Early symptoms include low back pain and morning stiffness which gradually progress up the back, sometimes reaching the neck. Pain around the ribs may develop and be exacerbated by deep breathing and coughing. Marked rigidity and kyphosis of the spine may occur. Some patients experience severe heel pain, and hip and shoulder joints may also be affected. Systemic complications include amyloidosis, cardiovascular disease (e.g. arrhythmias and aortic valve disease), iritis (*see* Uveitis), and respiratory disease (e.g. cough, dyspnoea, and infection). The disease may interfere significantly with the quality of life, although only a minority of patients suffer total spinal immobility.

Treatment
Treatment comprises vigorous physiotherapy and the administration of non-steroidal anti-inflammatory drugs

(BNF 10.1.1). Pulse doses of corticosteroids (BNF 10.1.2.1) may be beneficial in unresponsive disease. Surgical straightening of the spine may be necessary in severe cases. Radiotherapy has been successfully used, but there is a high risk of leukaemia following treatment.

Self-help organisations
Arthritis Care
Arthritis and Rheumatism Council
National Ankylosing Spondylitis Society

Cervical Spondylosis

Definition and aetiology
Cervical spondylosis is a common disorder characterised by degeneration of the intervertebral joints of the neck (cervical vertebrae) and the associated cartilage (intervertebral discs). Bony projections (osteophytes) may form and result in compression of spinal nerve roots or even of the cord itself. The cause of cervical spondylosis is unknown, although it is associated with advancing age.

Symptoms
Pain, stiffness, and immobility of the neck are common. The pain may be mild or severe. Neurological symptoms, arising from spinal nerve root compression, may include severe pain in the arms and hands and sensory loss and weakness. In severe cases, the legs may become affected, paralysis can develop, and bladder function may be impaired.

Treatment
Treatment consists of providing a supportive collar and analgesics (BNF 4.7) when necessary. Surgery is indicated only in severe intractable cases.

Chondrocalcinosis

Definition and aetiology
Chondrocalcinosis (pyrophosphate arthropathy) is characterised by the deposition of calcium salts (e.g. calcium pyrophosphate dihydrate) in articular cartilage and by their appearance in synovial fluid.

The cause of the disease is unknown, although a family history may be present, and it can occur in association with diabetes mellitus, gout, haemochromatosis, and hyperparathyroidism.

Symptoms
Chondrocalcinosis may be asymptomatic, but the commonest symptom is osteoarthritis which may affect several joints simultaneously. Acute attacks of gout-like symptoms (pseudogout) may occur. Large joints, particularly the hip and knee, are most often affected. The periods between attacks are usually free of symptoms.

Treatment
Acute attacks may be treated by aspiration of the affected joint(s) and the administration of a non-steroidal anti-inflammatory drug (BNF 10.1.1). The intra-articular administration of a corticosteroid (BNF 10.1.2.2) may be beneficial.

Juvenile Chronic Arthritis

Definition and aetiology
Juvenile chronic arthritis (Still's disease) is a term used to describe a variety of conditions which are characterised by the development of inflammatory joint disease before 16 years of age. The cause of these diseases is unknown, but auto-immune mechanisms may be responsible.

Symptoms
Systemic juvenile chronic arthritis is characterised by a mild polyarthritis, irregular fever, lymphadenopathy, a rash, and respiratory symptoms.

Polyarticular juvenile chronic arthritis is more common in girls. It may affect any joint and mild systemic symptoms usually develop. Rheumatoid factor (*see* Rheumatoid Arthritis) is not detectable.

Pauci-articular juvenile chronic arthritis is characterised by the development of arthritis in a small number of joints, although only one joint may be affected. With the exception of iridocyclitis (*see* Uveitis), systemic symptoms are rare.

Juvenile rheumatoid arthritis is the childhood equivalent of rheumatoid arthritis. It has a poor prognosis.

Juvenile ankylosing spondylitis is the childhood equivalent of ankylosing spondylitis. It is characterised by a peripheral arthritis, affecting predominantly the joints of the lower limbs.

Treatment
Treatment comprises the measures described under Rheumatoid Arthritis.

Osteoarthritis

Definition and aetiology
Osteoarthritis (osteoarthrosis) is a non-inflammatory joint disease characterised by the degeneration of articular cartilage, the hardening (i.e. sclerosis) and refashioning of underlying bone, and the formation of bony projections (osteophytes) at the edges of the affected joint. Usually only 1 or 2 of the large weight-bearing joints are involved, most commonly those of the hip, knee, and spine. The smaller joints of the hands and feet may, however, also be involved. Osteoarthritis is very common, affecting more than 1 in 10 of the population, and is considered to be a normal sign of ageing (over half of those affected are over 60 years of age). Predisposing factors include joint disease or injury, a family history, occupation, obesity, and postural defects.

Symptoms
The onset of symptoms, which usually occurs at about 50 years of age, is characterised by joint pain, stiffness, and immobility. Transient stiffness after rest is common, although pain is exacerbated by movement and becomes more pronounced through the day. Affected joints may 'creak' on movement, and bony projections (Heberden's nodes) may be visible on the finger joints (Fig. 10.1).

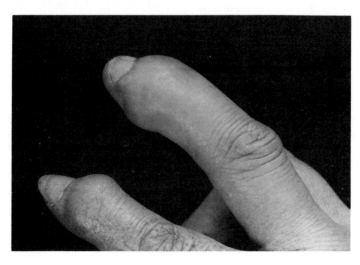

Fig. 10.1
Heberden's nodes, characteristic of osteoarthritis.

Effusions can occur and debilitating deformity may eventually develop.

Treatment
Treatment comprises the administration of non-opioid analgesics (BNF 4.7.1) or non-steroidal anti-inflammatory drugs (BNF 10.1.1) and gentle exercise, hydrotherapy, occupational therapy, physiotherapy, and weight reduction. Affected joints should be kept warm and local heat treatment may be used. Domestic aids (e.g. handrails and specially designed furniture) and walking frames or sticks are often beneficial. In severe cases, surgery may be required and osteotomy or total joint replacement may be indicated. The value of the intra-articular administration of corticosteroids (BNF 10.1.2.2) is controversial.

Psoriatic Arthritis

Definition and aetiology
Psoriatic arthritis is arthritis which develops in the presence of psoriasis. Very occasionally, arthritic symptoms precede the skin disorder. The cause is unknown, but psoriatic arthritis may be inherited and predisposing factors can include infection or trauma.

Symptoms
The interphalangeal joints are most commonly affected, and pitting and ridging of the nails often occurs (Fig. 10.2). Larger joints may also become involved and, in a minority of patients, ankylosis and marked deformity may develop. Ankylosing spondylitis may occur in association with psoriatic arthritis. Extra-articular symptoms are uncommon, although ocular complications (e.g. iritis and scleritis) may arise. Subcutaneous nodules do not develop. Although the erythrocyte sedimentation rate may be raised, rheumatoid factor is absent.

Treatment
The treatment for psoriatic arthritis is similar to that for rheumatoid arthritis, although antimalarials should not be given and penicillamine is ineffective. Immunosuppressants (BNF 10.1.3) may be given in unresponsive cases.

Rheumatoid Arthritis

Definition and aetiology
Rheumatoid arthritis is a chronic systemic disorder. It is characterised by inflammatory changes in the peripheral joints and associated connective tissues, by the atrophy and rarefaction of bone, and by a variety of extra-articular symptoms. The cause of the disease is unknown, but an auto-immune mechanism may be responsible and viral infection may be a predisposing factor.

Symptoms
Rheumatoid arthritis is more common in women and the onset, which may be acute or insidious, usually occurs

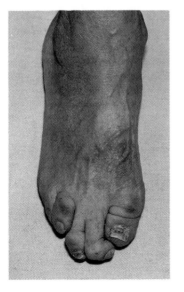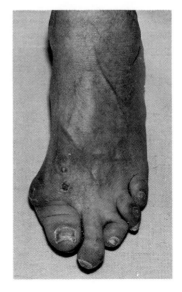

Fig. 10.2
Severe deformation of the toes in psoriatic arthritis. Psoriatic lesions are visible as pittings on the surface of the nails and on the upper toes.

between 35 and 60 years of age (for arthritis in younger age groups, *see* Juvenile Chronic Arthritis). The small synovial joints of the feet and ankles, hands and wrists, knees, and cervical spine are most commonly affected, although any synovial joint may become involved. Affected joints become acutely painful, swollen, and tender due to inflammation of the synovial membrane and the deposition of inflamed connective tissue (i.e. pannus) which destroys the articular cartilage. Ankylosis may occur and stiffness, particularly in the morning, is a common feature. As the disease progresses, partial joint dislocation may occur and marked deformity and disability may develop (Fig. 10.3). Subcutaneous nodules may occur, particularly over pressure points.

General extra-articular symptoms include anaemia, fever, malaise, and weight loss. Vasculitis may occur and respiratory symptoms (e.g. pulmonary effusion and fibrosis) may develop. Pericarditis is common. Ocular manifestations include keratoconjunctivitis sicca (*see* Dry Eye), which in conjunction with rheumatoid arthritis

or a connective tissue disorder (e.g. systemic lupus erythematosus) is referred to as Sjögren's syndrome. Scleritis, lymphadenopathy, peripheral neuropathy, and renal impairment may develop. The erythrocyte sedimentation rate in patients suffering from rheumatoid arthritis is raised and this, together with the presence in the blood of an immunoglobulin known as rheumatoid factor, is diagnostic of the disease. Amyloidosis is a potentially fatal complication.

Prognosis is variable. The disease is subject to remission and relapse with exacerbation, and a minority of patients suffer severe disability.

Treatment
Treatment is long term and comprises adequate rest and gentle exercise, although joint immobilisation (i.e. splinting) may be necessary to relieve pain. Physiotherapy and treatment with heat, ice packs, and ultrasound is beneficial. Occupational therapy and social support are often crucial, together with the provision of domestic and walking aids. Drug therapy is usually essential and includes the administration of non-steroidal anti-inflammatory drugs (BNF 10.1.1) and drugs which may affect the rheumatic disease process (BNF 10.1.3). Intra-articular injections of corticosteroids (BNF 10.1.2.2) are used but oral administration is usually avoided. Surgery may be indicated in severe cases, and procedures include joint fixation (arthrodesis), joint replacement (arthroplasty), and synovial membrane removal (synovectomy).

Self-help organisations
Arthritis Care
Arthritis and Rheumatism Council

10.3   BONE DISORDERS

Osteitis Deformans

Definition and aetiology
Osteitis deformans (Paget's disease of bone) is a chronic bone disease characterised by alternate periods of increased bone reabsorption and excessive and disorganised bone repair. This increased bone turnover leads to destruction of normal bone structure and consequent bone weakness and enlargement. The cause of osteitis deformans is unknown, although viral infection may be a factor. There is a marked geographical variation in the incidence of the disease.

Symptoms
The onset of the disease usually occurs after 40 years of age and its incidence generally increases with age.

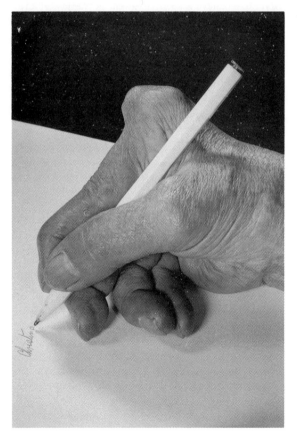

Fig. 10.3
The characteristic deformities of rheumatoid arthritis. The swollen joints can cause severe limitation of movement.

Characteristic symptoms include bone deformity, fracture, and pain. Common sites are the pelvis and spine and kyphosis is often seen. Bowing of the long bones (e.g. femur and tibia) may occur, and enlargement of the skull may be associated with nerve-compression deafness. Affected bones may become highly vascular and heart failure may result. Plasma-calcium and plasma-phosphate concentrations are usually normal, but there is marked elevation of plasma-alkaline phosphatase concentrations. Cancer of the bone (e.g. sarcoma) may develop in some patients.

Treatment
Often no treatment is necessary. Non-opioid analgesics (BNF 4.7.1) may, however, be required for pain. Calcitonin (BNF 6.6.1) or disodium etidronate (BNF 6.6.2) may be given in severe unresponsive cases. Plicamycin has also been used. Surgery may be required.

Osteopetrosis

Definition and aetiology
Osteopetrosis (Albers-Schönberg disease or marble bone disease) is a rare inherited disease characterised by increased bone formation and density. The bones become abnormally hard and easily fractured. Osteopetrosis may be mild (benign) or severe, and it is thought to be caused by disturbed bone reabsorption.

Symptoms
In both forms, fractures are common and may result in osteomyelitis. Severe osteopetrosis develops in childhood and produces anaemia by invasion of the bone marrow, and sensorineural deafness or blindness by cranial-nerve compression. Growth and mental retardation may occur, and early death is common, due to repeated fractures with haemorrhage and infection. The mild form of osteopetrosis does not develop until adolescence or adulthood and may be asymptomatic.

Treatment
Treatment comprises dietary calcium restriction with bone-marrow transplantation. Corticosteroids have been given and blood transfusion or antimicrobial therapy may be indicated.

Osteoporosis

Definition and aetiology
Osteoporosis is characterised by a reduced bone mass in the presence of normal bone composition. It is caused by changes in bone metabolism which may arise from alcoholism, endocrine disorders (e.g. Cushing's syndrome and primary hyperparathyroidism), nutritional deficiency or malabsorption, prolonged corticosteroid administration, or immobility. It is most commonly associated, however, with advancing age, particularly in postmenopausal women, although it may very occasionally occur during childhood, pregnancy, or in young adults.

Symptoms
Osteoporosis is characterised by brittle bones. Fractures, especially of the femoral neck, vertebrae, and wrist, are common and result in pain and deformity. Multiple crush fractures of the vertebrae result in vertebral collapse, which causes chronic back pain and kyphosis, with a consequent decrease in height.

Treatment
Treatment is aimed at preventing further reduction in bone mass and comprises the administration of calcium supplements (BNF 9.5.1.1). Vitamin D preparations (BNF 9.6.4) may also be given. The treatment of postmenopausal osteoporosis includes the administration of oestrogens (BNF 6.4.1), and anabolic steroids (BNF 6.4.3) have also been given. A variety of drug therapies have been tried including calcitonin, parathormone, and sodium fluoride. Calcium may be administered as prophylaxis.

Analgesics (BNF 4.7) are often necessary, particularly for back pain, and a spinal support may be beneficial. Orthopaedic treatment is required for fractures. Physical activity should, however, be maintained.

10.4 CONNECTIVE TISSUE DISORDERS

Bursitis

Definition and aetiology
Bursitis, which may be acute or chronic, is inflammation of a bursa. The cause is frequently uncertain, but physical injury, infection, or arthritic disease may be responsible.

Symptoms
Bursitis is characterised by local pain and tenderness, immobility, swelling, and erythema. It commonly affects the shoulder (subacromial bursitis) although the elbow (olecranon bursitis or miner's elbow) or the knee (prepatellar bursitis, Fig. 10.4, or housemaid's knee) may be affected. Bursitis may develop in association with deformity of the metatarsophalangeal joint of the great toe (i.e. a bunion). Popliteal bursitis (Baker's cyst) occurs when synovial fluid escapes from the knee-joint capsule and accumulates in the bursa in the popliteal space behind the knee joint.

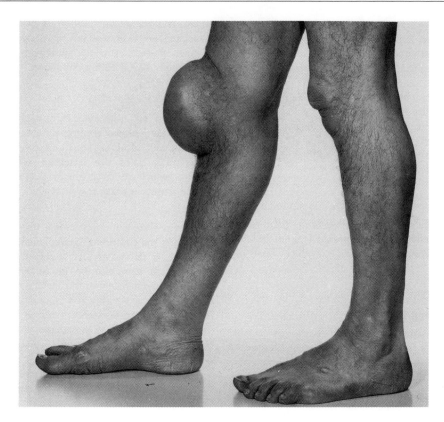

Fig. 10.4
An extreme case of prepatellar bursitis.

Treatment
Treatment consists of the administration of non-steroidal anti-inflammatory drugs (BNF 10.1.1) or local corticosteroid injections (BNF 10.1.2.2). Aspiration of accumulated fluid or surgical removal of the affected bursa may be necessary in chronic cases.

Fibrositis

Definition and aetiology
Fibrositis is a non-specific disorder of connective tissue characterised by generalised musculoskeletal pain and tenderness at certain clearly distinguished sites. It is often caused by physical injury, or exposure to cold or damp conditions. Other contributory factors include emotional disturbance and infection.

Symptoms
Symptoms may arise in almost any soft connective tissue, producing a variety of conditions (e.g. lumbago, torti-collis, and frozen shoulder). Onset may be sudden, and is marked by muscle pain with stiffness and tender-ness. Symptoms are commonly aggravated by move-ment, but are often self-limiting and disappear within a few days or weeks. Tension headache and irritable bowel syndrome may accompany fibrositis.

Treatment
Treatment includes rest and the application of heat and gentle massage. Non-steroidal anti-inflammatory drugs (BNF 10.1.1) may be indicated, and the application of a rubefacient (BNF 10.3.2) may be beneficial. Antidepres-sants and psychotherapy may be used for underlying psy-chological disturbances.

Frozen Shoulder

Definition and aetiology
Frozen shoulder (adhesive bursitis, adhesive capsulitis, or scapular arthritis) is characterised by an adhesive in-flammation of the shoulder-joint capsule and associated cartilage. It is almost always due to overuse or physical injury.

Symptoms

The onset is usually gradual and is marked by increasing pain in the shoulder, stiffness, and limitation of movement. Pain may be localised, but may also radiate into the neck (with muscle spasm) or the arm. Although the pain may be severe, it often resolves spontaneously. Joint mobility may, however, be permanently impaired.

Treatment

Treatment comprises adequate rest, physiotherapy, and the local application of heat or cold. Non-steroidal anti-inflammatory drugs (BNF 10.1.1) are often administered and local corticosteroid injections (BNF 10.1.2.2) may be indicated. Attempts should be made to recommence use of the shoulder once the initial pain, muscle spasm, and inflammation have been overcome. In severe cases, manipulation under anaesthesic may be necessary.

Giant Cell Arteritis

Definition and aetiology

Giant cell arteritis (cranial arteritis or temporal arteritis) is an inflammatory condition which may affect any of the larger arteries, especially the temporal and occipital arteries. The artery wall is damaged by granulomatous inflammation and, characteristically, giant cells are present which can cause thickening of the artery wall lining. Polymyalgia rheumatica frequently accompanies giant cell arteritis.

Symptoms

Giant cell arteritis rarely occurs under 50 years of age and may be preceded by a polymyalgic illness. Headache often occurs at a later stage and may be abrupt in onset with pain of great intensity and tenderness of the scalp, usually in the temporal region. The thickened temporal arteries may be tender and non-pulsatile, with erythema and oedema of the overlying skin. Up to 50% of patients have ocular disturbances which may result in irreversible blindness. Other symptoms are anaemia, fever, jaw pain (particularly on chewing), and weight loss.

Treatment

Early treatment with high-dose corticosteroids (BNF 10.1.2.1) is imperative to control inflammation and prevent blindness. Treatment should be continued for a minimum of 2 to 3 years at a reduced dose.

Polyarteritis Nodosa

Definition and aetiology

Polyarteritis nodosa may affect any organ and is characterised by marked inflammation and necrosis of small and medium arteries. These result in weakening of the artery walls with consequent aneurysm formation, thrombosis, and infarction. The cause is unknown, although it may be due to the formation of immune complexes, and hypersensitivity reactions (e.g. caused by penicillins or sulphonamides) have been implicated. The disorder is more common in men.

Symptoms

The onset of the disorder is characterised by non-specific symptoms (e.g. arthralgia, fever, malaise, myalgia, and weight loss). Thereafter, any body system may be affected. Skin symptoms include nodule formation (due to aneurysms), ulceration, and a wide variety of rashes. Renal complications characterised by hypertension are very common and are often fatal. Cardiac involvement frequently occurs and myocardial infarction, pericarditis, and tachycardia may lead to death. Confusion, peripheral neuropathy, and psychosis are symptoms of central nervous system involvement. Abdominal pain may arise as a result of gastro-intestinal haemorrhage or infarction. Respiratory symptoms do not usually occur, although asthma can develop.

Treatment

Although no specific treatment exists, the combination of corticosteroids (BNF 6.3.4 and 10.1.2.1) and immunosuppressants may retard the disease process and produce remission. Plasmapheresis has also been used.

Polymyalgia Rheumatica

Definition and aetiology

Polymyalgia rheumatica is characterised by muscle pain and stiffness. It usually develops after 50 years of age and may occur in association with giant cell arteritis. The cause of the disorder is unknown, although a family history may exist.

Symptoms

The onset may be acute or insidious and is often marked by non-specific symptoms (e.g. malaise, apathy, weight loss, and mild fever). Characteristic symptoms, however, include severe pain and early morning stiffness in the proximal muscles, particularly of the neck and shoulders. The disorder usually resolves spontaneously within 6 to 24 months, although it may persist for several years in a minority of patients.

Treatment

Treatment comprises the administration of corticosteroids (BNF 10.1.2.1) and non-steroidal anti-inflammatory drugs (BNF 10.1.1) may provide symptomatic relief.

Polymyositis and Dermatomyositis

Definition and aetiology

Polymyositis is characterised by inflammatory and degenerative changes in muscle tissue. When the non-suppurative inflammation also involves subcutaneous tissue and the skin, the condition is called dermatomyositis. The cause is unknown, but immunological mechanisms may be responsible and viral infection or a family history have also been implicated.

Symptoms

Onset usually occurs between 30 and 60 years of age and it may be acute or insidious. The most common initial symptom is progressive proximal muscle weakness, often affecting the thigh muscles, and resulting in difficulty in climbing stairs and arising. Muscle atrophy and contractures may eventually develop and dysphagia may be caused by disturbances of pharyngeal muscles. Respiratory muscles may also be affected, causing respiratory failure. In dermatomyositis, a characteristic scaly erythematous rash covers the face and exposed areas, often in association with oedema. This rash often fades but is replaced by brown pigmentation. Although most patients recover, symptoms may be persistent and death may occur.

Treatment

Treatment involves bed rest and the administration of corticosteroids (BNF 10.1.2.1) or immunosuppressants (BNF 10.1.3), or both. Physiotherapy may be beneficial.

Sarcoidosis

Definition and aetiology

Sarcoidosis is a non-caseating granulomatous disorder characterised by the formation of epithelioid cell tubercles (i.e. sarcoid) in almost any organ or tissue. Secondary fibrosis and necrosis may develop. The cause of sarcoidosis is unknown.

Symptoms

The onset of the disorder may be acute or insidious, and usually occurs between 20 and 35 years of age. The organs most commonly affected include the eyes, liver, lungs, lymph nodes, and skin but small bones, the central nervous system, heart, joints, muscle, or the spleen may also be involved. Common presenting symptoms are arthralgia, fever, and weight loss, but symptoms generally depend on the organ affected. Erythema nodosum and lymphadenopathy are frequent symptoms, and pulmonary involvement may be marked by cough, dyspnoea, and, eventually, pulmonary fibrosis and cor pulmonale. If the heart is affected, angina pectoris and heart failure may result. Spontaneous improvement and recovery is common, but sarcoidosis may become chronically progressive although death is uncommon.

Treatment

No specific treatment exists, although corticosteroids (BNF 6.3.4) may be useful in alleviating symptoms. Other drugs used include chlorambucil, chloroquine, and methotrexate.

Systemic Lupus Erythematosus

Definition and aetiology

Systemic lupus erythematosus (SLE) is a generalised connective tissue disorder of unknown aetiology. It is associated with a series of auto-immune mechanisms which result in auto-antibody formation. Antinuclear antibodies specific to DNA are formed, together with a variety of organ-specific auto-antibodies. These lead to necrosis and fibrosis of small blood vessels, collagen, and other connective tissues. The disorder occurs most commonly in Negroes and young women, and may be precipitated by drug administration (e.g. hydralazine), exposure to sunlight, or viral infection. A family history may be present.

Symptoms

The onset of symptoms, which can be mild or severe, may be acute or insidious. Non-specific symptoms (e.g. fever and malaise, alopecia, aphthous stomatitis, and an erythematous rash on exposed areas) are common. A butterfly rash covering the cheeks and nose is characteristic. Musculoskeletal symptoms are very common and include arthralgia and myalgia. Central nervous system involvement is often prominent and may be characterised by convulsions, depressive disorders, or psychosis. Renal impairment may occur and cause hypertension, oedema, and proteinuria, and can lead to renal failure and death. Other symptoms include anaemia, keratoconjunctivitis sicca (see Dry Eye), hepatosplenomegaly, lymphadenopathy, pericarditis, and pleurisy. The erythrocyte sedimentation rate is characteristically raised. The course of the disorder is often chronic with remissions and relapses, although the prognosis, even in the presence of renal involvement, is usually good.

Treatment

Exposure to precipitating factors should be avoided by susceptible patients. Sunscreening preparations (BNF 13.8.1) may be useful. Drug treatment includes the administration of corticosteroids (BNF 6.3.4 and 10.1.2.1) and antimalarials or immunosuppressants

(BNF 10.1.3). Non-steroidal anti-inflammatory drugs (BNF 10.1.1) are beneficial in treating musculoskeletal symptoms.

Self-help organisations
Arthritis Care
Arthritis and Rheumatism Council

Systemic Sclerosis

Definition and aetiology
Systemic sclerosis is a chronic disorder caused by increased collagen deposition and the obliteration of small blood vessels. The condition produces widespread fibrosis of internal organs (e.g. gastro-intestinal tract, heart, kidneys, and lungs). Involvement of skin is called scleroderma. The cause is unknown, although environmental factors (e.g. exposure to vinyl chloride) or a family history may be significant. The condition may arise at any age and is more common in women.

Symptoms
The initial symptom is often Raynaud's phenomenon (*see* Raynaud's Syndrome). Oedema of the hands and fingers is common and is followed by thickening and hardening (i.e. sclerosis) of the skin which becomes hyperpigmented, shiny, and tight. Cutaneous symptoms may spread to affect other areas (e.g. back, chest, and legs) and facial telangiectasia is common. Cutaneous calcification, particularly of the fingertips, may occur.

Symptoms may be restricted to the skin for several years, but progression to the visceral organs may develop and is associated with a poor prognosis. Dysphagia may occur as a result of disordered oesophageal motility. Pulmonary fibrosis may lead to dyspnoea and pulmonary hypertension, and fibrosis of cardiac muscle may give rise to arrhythmias and heart failure. Renal involvement may lead to progressive renal impairment and is a significant cause of death. Arthralgia and myalgia are common.

Treatment
Treatment is chiefly symptomatic. Cutaneous symptoms may be alleviated by providing protective clothing and local heat. Physiotherapy may promote mobility. Antihypertensive drugs (BNF 2.5) may be indicated and non-steroidal anti-inflammatory drugs (BNF 10.1.1) may relieve musculoskeletal symptoms. Dialysis or transplantation may be necessary in the event of severe renal disorder. A variety of systemic drug therapies have been tried (e.g. chlorambucil, colchicine, corticosteroids, and penicillamine) with variable success.

Tendinitis and Tenosynovitis

Definition and aetiology
Tendinitis is inflammation of a tendon and tenosynovitis is inflammation of the tendon sheath enclosing it. The cause of these conditions, which often occur together, is unknown although they may be due to a primary systemic disease (e.g. gout and rheumatoid arthritis) or to physical trauma or unaccustomed exercise.

Symptoms
Tendinitis and tenosynovitis are characterised by local inflammation, swelling, and tenderness. Pain, which may be severe, is usually exacerbated by movement. Common sites include the fingers and toes, hips, legs (e.g. hamstring or Achilles tendon), and shoulders.

Treatment
Treatment commonly includes rest, the application of heat or cold, gentle exercise, and physiotherapy. Non-steroidal anti-inflammatory drugs (BNF 10.1.1) may be indicated and local corticosteroid injections (BNF 10.1.2.2) may be beneficial.

10.5 ANATOMY AND PHYSIOLOGY RELEVANT TO MUSCULOSKELETAL AND CONNECTIVE TISSUE DISORDERS

Joints

A joint (articulation) is a junction between two bones or a bone and cartilage, and is classified according to its structure. If there is a space between the apposing surfaces and the structures are held together by a fibrous capsule, the joint is described as synovial. A joint with no space between the apposing surfaces may be held together by fibrous tissue (a fibrous joint) or by cartilage (a cartilaginous joint).

The most common type are the synovial joints (e.g. the knee, sacro-iliac, and elbow). They are characterised by a space, the synovial cavity, between the bones and a lining of hyaline cartilage on the apposing bone surfaces. The two bones are held together by a capsule formed of an outer layer of connective tissue (the fibrous capsule) lined internally by a secretory membrane, the synovial membrane. The fibrous capsule may be modified in some joints to form bundles of parallel fibres (the ligaments), which enhance the strength of the fibrous capsule. Synovial fluid, which lubricates the joint and nourishes the cartilage, is secreted by the inner synovial membrane. This alkaline fluid also contains macrophages, which remove debris produced during normal working of the joint.

A further layer of cartilage, the articular discs, may be present in synovial joints. The cartilage divides the synovial cavity and allows opposite bones of different shapes to form effective joints.

The potential for friction between moving bones and the overlying skin, tendons, ligaments, and muscles is reduced by the cushioning effect of sac-like fluid-filled cavities (the bursae).

Fibrous joints are characterised by irregular surfaces and are held together by a layer of fibrous connective tissue. The fibrous layer may be thin (e.g. the sutures between the bones of the skull) ensuring the complete absence of movement, or comparatively thick (e.g. the lower joint between the tibia and fibula) permitting small amounts of movement.

Cartilaginous joints are linked by a layer of hyaline cartilage or by fibrous tissue and cartilage. One example of a joint which is linked by hyaline cartilage, the joint between the first rib and the sternum, is immovable, and cartilage is gradually replaced by bone during adult life. The joints between the bodies of vertebrae are formed of discs of fibrocartilage and allow a minute degree of movement.

Bone and Skeleton

The skeletal system is the framework on which the organs and tissues of the body are supported. It provides protection for body systems, and acts as a lever for the action of muscles in the production of movement. It is also involved in homoeostatic mechanisms in the body in its role as a storage compartment for minerals and the production of blood cells.

Bone is a connective tissue in which bone cells (osteocytes) are separated by hardened intercellular collagenous material, rich in calcium salts. The strength and protection inherent in bones may be largely attributed to compact bone in which layers of osteocytes are arranged in concentric cylinders (Haversian canals) around a central channel which contains blood cells. Spongy bone contains a far less organised structure consisting of a network of thin plates of bone (trabeculae) interspersed in some bones by the marrow. In the mature skeleton, compact bone can be formed by the transformation of spongy bone (remodelling).

Although bone appears to be a permanent structure, it is continually being replaced throughout adult life, al-

lowing damaged bone to be replaced and bones to be refashioned. This is carried out by the deposition and reabsorption of calcium ions from the bone and the bloodstream. A balance exists in the formation of bone cells through the action of osteoblasts (ossification) and the reabsorption of calcium by osteoclasts. The homoeostatic balance is also controlled by the availability of vitamin D (which assists in the absorption of calcium from the gastro-intestinal tract and prevents the loss of calcium through the kidneys), an adequate dietary intake of calcium and phosphorus, and the presence of growth hormone, calcitonin, parathormone, and the sex hormones in balanced quantities.

The skeleton is a complex structure consisting of 206 bones, the majority of which may be classed as long (e.g. the thigh bone and the bones of the fingers), short (e.g. ankle and wrist bones), flat (e.g. scapula and cranium), or irregular (e.g. facial bones and the vertebrae).

The skeletal system may be divided into the axial and appendicular divisions. The axial skeleton consists predominantly of the bones of the trunk and head and includes the skull, sternum, ribs, and vertebral column. The appendicular skeleton is formed of the bones of the limbs and those which attach them to the axial skeleton.

The vertebral column (Fig. 10.5) is the central pivot on which the axial skeleton (and the musculature of the back) is supported. It also supports the head and protects the spinal cord. The column is made up of 33 vertebrae although the lower 9 vertebrae are fused into two chains. There are 7 cervical vertebrae in the neck region, 12 thoracic vertebrae at the rear of the thorax, 5 lumbar vertebrae in the lower back region, 5 sacral vertebrae which are fused to form the sacrum, and 4 fused coccygeal vertebrae which form the coccyx.

The junction between the top of the vertebral column and the head is formed at the atlas (C1) vertebra whose shape permits backward and forward movements, and the axis (C2) vertebra which allows rotation. Individual vertebrae are linked through the intervertebral discs of fibrocartilage, which are formed of a hard exterior surrounding an inner elastic structure. The discs strengthen the vertebral column whilst at the same time being capable of distension and absorbing pressure changes created from above and below.

The sacral and coccygeal portions of the vertebral column and the pelvic girdle form the pelvis. The pelvic girdle (Fig. 10.6) is formed of two hipbones and supports the abdominal contents. Although the hipbone is fused in the adult, in the neonate it is present as three separate bones, the ilium (which is the largest), the pubis, and the ischium. The sacrum is attached to the ilium at the sacroiliac joint.

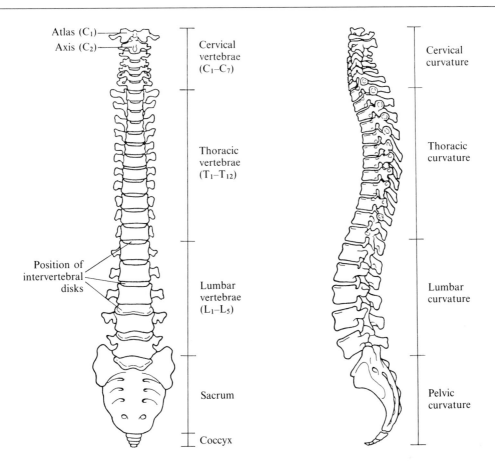

Atlas (C₁)
Axis (C₂)

Cervical
vertebrae
(C₁–C₇)

Thoracic
vertebrae
(T₁–T₁₂)

Position of
intervertebral
disks

Lumbar
vertebrae
(L₁–L₅)

Sacrum

Coccyx

Cervical
curvature

Thoracic
curvature

Lumbar
curvature

Pelvic
curvature

Fig. 10.5
Vertebral column (lateral view).

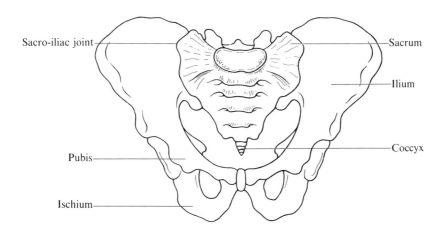

Sacro-iliac joint

Pubis

Ischium

Sacrum

Ilium

Coccyx

Fig. 10.6
Pelvic girdle, male (anterior view).

Muscle

There are three types of muscle tissue in the body of which the greatest proportion is skeletal (striated) muscle. Skeletal muscle is responsible for the movement of bones for which it may be attached directly to the bone. However, where the presence of muscle tracts would interfere with the free movement of the bone, attachments are made through tendons. Tendons may also link muscles, and may be enclosed in a sheath of fibrous connective tissue. The sheath is similar in structure to bursae (*see above*) and permits the smooth movement of the tendon when the attached muscle contracts.

The fibres of skeletal muscle are formed of parallel, elongated, multinucleated cells enveloped within a plasma membrane, the sarcolemma. The muscle fibres are themselves built up of thousands of myofibrils which are subdivided by areas of dense tissue into compartments, the sarcomeres. The myofibrils consist of thin myofilaments composed predominantly of actin, and thick myofilaments formed of myosin. Cross bridges link the actin and myosin proteins on the two filaments.

Skeletal muscle contractions are voluntary, are initiated within the central nervous system, and pass to the muscle via the anterior spinal nerve roots and motor nerves. A muscle contraction is generated by the arrival of an action potential from the axon of a motor neurone at the sarcolemma of the muscle (the neuromuscular junction, Fig. 10.7). The action potential within the nerve fibre causes the release of a neurotransmitter, acetylcholine, from the enlarged terminus of the axon, the synaptic bulb. This changes the permeability of the sarcolemma, causing a wave of excitation to pass through it which initiates muscle contraction.

Cardiac muscle is located exclusively in the heart wall and is structurally similar to skeletal muscle with the presence of actin and myosin, but only containing a single nucleus. The muscle fibres in cardiac muscle branch and are interconnected, permitting the rapid transmission of conduction from one filament to the next. The muscle also possesses an inherent ability to

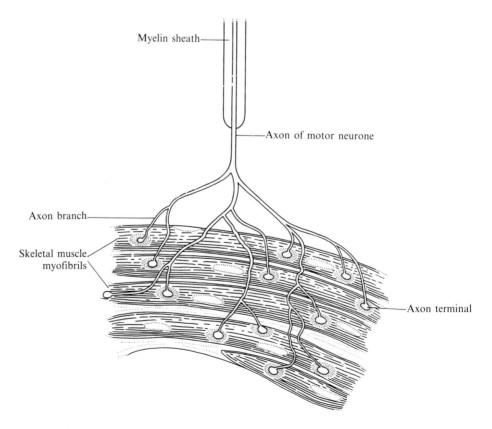

Fig. 10.7
Diagrammatic representation of a neuromuscular junction.

contract, and as a result requires a rich blood supply. The inherent rate of contraction may be modified by nervous stimulation.

Smooth (non-striated) muscle consists of sheets of spindle-shaped fibres each possessing a central oval nucleus. Smooth muscle found in the walls of small blood vessels and hollow organs (e.g. stomach, bladder, and uterus) is termed visceral (single-unit) muscle tissue. Contraction of one cell is quickly passed to adjacent cells, because the fibres are closely interwoven into a continuous network. Contraction is usually initiated by the autonomic nervous system (i.e. it is under involuntary control) and the cells can contract even when they have been considerably distended (e.g. in the bladder).

Other smooth muscle (e.g. the walls of the bronchi, the walls of the large arteries, and the intrinsic muscles of the eye) is formed of multi-unit tissues. These differ from single-unit fibres in that contraction of only one fibre can occur without spread to adjacent fibres.

Connective Tissue

Connective tissue 'connects' organs and supports the body's structures. It may be classified as loose (areolar) connective tissue, adipose tissue, dense (collagenous) connective tissue, elastic connective tissue, and reticular connective tissue. Cartilage is also classified as connective tissue.

Loose connective tissue consists of three types of fibres embedded within cells in a viscous intercellular substance, hyaluronic acid. Bundles of collagenous fibres, which impart strength and flexibility in the tissue, are formed from the protein collagen. Elastic fibres, formed of the protein elastin, provide strength and elasticity. Support within the fibril network is also provided by reticular fibres formed of collagen and glycoprotein. Cellular components of connective tissue include fibroblasts, macrophages, mast cells, and plasma cells (*see* Section 9.4).

Adipose connective tissue contains cells modified for fat storage, adipocytes, and is located wherever there is loose connective tissue. It is primarily distributed in subcutaneous tissue of the skin, over the surface of the heart, and as padding around joints. The cells help prevent heat loss, act as an energy store, and provide support.

Dense connective tissue fibres may be arranged irregularly or regularly. Irregularly orientated fibres contribute significantly to the fasciae and also occur in the protective fibrous capsules around organs. Fibres of dense connective tissue arranged in one direction impart strength but permit flexibility. These bundles form tendons and ligaments used to link muscles to bone, and bone to bone.

Elastic connective tissue has similar properties to regularly arranged dense tissue, but the frequent branching of the fibres renders them better suited to imparting strength and elasticity to organ and vessel walls. The tissue is found in laryngeal cartilage, arterial walls, and throughout the respiratory tree. It also links successive vertebrae and forms the vocal cords.

The liver, lymph nodes, and spleen are supported by a fine network of reticular connective tissue. The tissue also binds cells of other smooth muscle tissue.

Cartilage (consisting of hyaline cartilage, fibrocartilage, and elastic cartilage) is a resilient form of connective tissue characterised by the absence of blood vessels and nerve fibres. The cellular components are chondrocytes which are embedded within spaces (lacunae) and are surrounded by dense tissue, the perichondrium.

Chapter 11

EYE DISORDERS

11.1 DISORDERS OF THE EYE

Blepharitis

Definition and aetiology
Blepharitis is inflammation of the margins of the eyelids. The cause is often unknown, although it may be allergic or occur in association with seborrhoea of the face and scalp (i.e. squamous blepharitis). Bacterial infection may, however, be responsible (i.e. ulcerative blepharitis).

Symptoms
Squamous blepharitis is characterised by local inflammation, scaling, pruritus, and oedema. It is similar to seborrhoeic dermatitis of the scalp. In ulcerative blepharitis, yellow crusts form on the eyelashes, which may become stuck together. The eyelashes may be lost, lachrymation and photophobia may occur, and small ulcers can develop on the eyelid margins.

Both forms are subject to recurrence and may become chronic. Ulcerative blepharitis may be associated with the development of chronic conjunctivitis or corneal ulceration.

Treatment
The eyes should be cleansed with simple eye ointment or a suitably warmed eye lotion (BNF 11.8.2). In the presence of infection, an appropriate topical anti-infective preparation (BNF 11.3.1) should be used. Routine eye cleansing should be maintained and good hygiene encouraged. Rubbing or fingering the eyes must be avoided.

Cataract

Definition and aetiology
Cataract is any opacity of the lens of the eye or of its capsule. It may be inherited or may occur at, or soon after, birth (developmental cataract). It most commonly arises, however, as a result of degenerative changes associated with ageing (degenerative cataract). Other possible causes include diabetes mellitus, drug administration (e.g. corticosteroids), galactosaemia, ionising radiation, iritis (*see* Uveitis), and trauma.

Symptoms
Cataract is characterised by progressive visual impairment which varies according to the location and size of

the opacity. Vision may eventually be significantly reduced with the lens becoming visibly opaque. Cataract is usually painless, but pain may occur if the cataract swells and secondary glaucoma develops. Cataract formation is usually bilateral.

Treatment
No effective medical treatment exists. The provision of appropriate spectacles may be sufficient initially. If vision is markedly impaired, treatment is by the surgical removal of the affected lenses or their contents, and the insertion of a prosthetic lens. Corrective spectacles or contact lenses may also be worn.

Chalazion

Definition and aetiology
A chalazion (Meibomian cyst or tarsal cyst) is an inflammatory granulomatous swelling on the eyelid or its margin. It occurs as a result of the blockage of one of the Meibomian glands which lubricate the eyelid, and it is more common in adults than in children.

Symptoms
It is characterised by a painless slow-growing swelling (Fig. 11.1) which may be accompanied by conjunctival discoloration. Multiple swellings may appear but can disappear spontaneously. A chalazion may become so large, however, as to cause disfigurement, and secondary infection may occasionally develop.

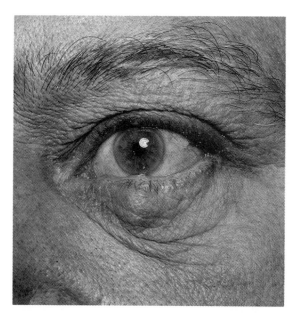

Fig. 11.1
A chalazion on the lower eyelid.

Treatment
Treatment is often by surgical removal under local anaesthetic (BNF 11.7). An appropriate topical anti-infective preparation (BNF 11.3.1) may be necessary if infection occurs.

Conjunctivitis

Definition and aetiology
Conjunctivitis is an inflammation of the membrane that lines the eyelids (i.e. the conjunctiva). It may be acute or chronic and is most commonly due to allergy or viral infection. Other causes include bacterial infection, which may accompany upper respiratory-tract infection, and irritation caused by dust, smoke, wind, or hand-to-eye contact (e.g. by contact-lens wearers).

Symptoms
Acute conjunctivitis is characterised by the production of a discharge which may be purulent, and by erythema and swelling of the eyelids. Local pruritus is a prominent feature if allergy is responsible. Chronic conjunctivitis is subject to remissions and relapses over a period of months or years. The symptoms are similar to those of the acute form, but less severe.

Treatment
The eyes should be kept clean and good hygiene should be encouraged. An appropriate topical anti-infective preparation (BNF 11.3) should be used if infection is responsible. In allergic conjunctivitis, a topical anti-inflammatory preparation (BNF 11.4) may be administered.

Corneal Ulceration

Definition and aetiology
Corneal ulceration may be described as the development of an area of necrosis in the tissue of the cornea. It is commonly caused by bacterial infection which occurs as a consequence of physical injury to the cornea. Viral infection may also be responsible, and dendritic ulcers are due to herpes simplex virus infection. Other possible causes include injury to, or defective closure of, the eyelids, or glaucoma.

Symptoms
Corneal ulceration is usually characterised by blinking, keratitis, lachrymation, pain, and photophobia. Ulceration may spread across the surface of the cornea and visual impairment may occur. In severe cases, corneal scarring or perforation may develop and destruction of the eye may eventually occur.

Treatment
Prompt treatment under specialist supervision is essential and usually comprises the topical (BNF 11.3.1), or systemic (BNF 11.3.2), administration of an appropriate anti-infective preparation. In severe cases, surgical repair or corneal transplantation may be necessary.

Dacryocystitis

Definition and aetiology
Dacryocystitis (dacrycystitis) is inflammation of the lachrymal sac usually caused by obstruction of the nasolachrymal duct. This obstruction may arise as a result of nasal polyps, nasal septum deviation, rhinitis, or trauma. In infants, it may be caused by congenital obstruction of the duct. Dacryocystitis is common and is often chronic.

Symptoms
The primary symptom is abnormal overflow of tears (i.e. epiphora), particularly on exposure to windy conditions. Local swelling and pain may occur. Chronic dacryocystitis is commonly progressive and may lead to the development of a lachrymal abscess.

Treatment
The condition usually resolves spontaneously in children. The application of hot compresses may be beneficial, and in the presence of an abscess, drainage and the administration of an appropriate anti-infective preparation (BNF 11.3) may be necessary. Dilatation of the nasolachrymal duct with a probe may be required in chronic cases. In unresponsive cases, surgical correction (i.e. dacryocystorhinostomy) is the only effective treatment.

Dry Eye

Definition and aetiology
Dry eye (keratoconjunctivitis sicca) is a chronic condition characterised by dryness of the conjunctiva, cornea, and sclera. It may be caused by a deficiency of conjunctival mucus (e.g. in Stevens-Johnson syndrome), corneal damage, eyelid disorders, or to tear deficiency arising from a systemic disease such as rheumatoid arthritis (i.e. Sjögren's syndrome).

Symptoms
Ocular irritation is the principal symptom, but photophobia and spasm of the eyelids (blepharospasm) may develop. Keratinisation of the cornea may eventually occur with ulceration, scarring, and visual impairment.

Treatment
Treatment is by the frequent administration of a preparation for tear deficiency (BNF 11.8.1).

Ectropion and Entropion

Definition and aetiology
Ectropion is the turning outward (i.e. eversion), and entropion is the turning inward (i.e. inversion), of the eyelid margins. Both conditions are usually associated with ageing, although they may arise as a result of scar formation on, or close to, the eyelid.

Symptoms
Ectropion is characterised by poor drainage of tears which consequently overflow (i.e. epiphora). The eye becomes irritated and the exposed cornea may become ulcerated.

Entropion is marked by irritation of the eye due to the inverted eyelashes. This may lead to conjunctivitis and corneal ulceration, and scarring.

Treatment
Surgery is the only effective treatment.

Exophthalmos

Definition and aetiology
Exophthalmos (proptosis) is the abnormal protrusion of one or both eyeballs. It arises as a result of swelling of the orbital tissues and is most commonly caused by hyperthyroidism. Other causes include orbital inflammation (e.g. orbital cellulitis), oedema, and malignant disease.

Symptoms
The surface of the eyeball becomes abnormally exposed. As a result, drying of the cornea may produce local infection or ulceration. Eye movement may be restricted and visual impairment may develop.

Treatment
The underlying cause should be treated. In some cases, exophthalmos may improve with the systemic administration of a corticosteroid, and surgery may be necessary.

Glaucoma

Definition and aetiology
Glaucoma is a group of ophthalmic disorders characterised by an increased intra-ocular pressure which results in damage to the optic disc and visual disturbances. Intra-ocular pressure increases through an imbalance between the production and drainage of aqueous

humour. The cause of glaucoma is unknown, but a family history and hyperopia may be predisposing factors. Glaucoma may also arise secondary to an existing disease (e.g. uveitis and cataracts).

Closed-angle Glaucoma

Definition and aetiology
Closed-angle glaucoma (acute congestive, narrow-angle, or obstructive glaucoma) is marked by a shallow anterior chamber and a narrow filtration angle which may be physically blocked by the iris. It may be acute or chronic.

Symptoms
The acute form of the disorder is characterised by a sudden rise in intra-ocular pressure, accompanied by severe eye pain, headache, nausea and vomiting, and prostration. Symptoms may be preceded by short periods of visual disturbance (e.g. haloes around lights) which are a consequence of corneal oedema and pupil dilatation. Usually only one eye is affected but, in the absence of treatment, blindness may follow. The chronic form is characterised by similar, but less severe, recurrent attacks.

Treatment
Early treatment of glaucoma (BNF 11.6) is essential and includes the topical administration of a miotic. A carbonic anhydrase inhibitor may also be given for its systemic effect and the osmotic effect of glycerol or mannitol may be useful. Surgery (e.g. iridectomy) may be necessary in severe or intractable cases.

Open-angle Glaucoma

Definition and aetiology
Open-angle glaucoma (simple, chronic simple, or wide-angle glaucoma) occurs in the absence of any abnormality in the structure of the anterior chamber or filtration angle. The drainage of aqueous humour gradually becomes impeded over a period of years, leading to a slow increase in the intra-ocular pressure. The cause is unknown.

Symptoms
Open-angle glaucoma may be asymptomatic in the early stages but is marked by a progressive loss of peripheral vision. Headache may occur, and central vision may deteriorate with blindness eventually developing. Usually both eyes are affected.

Treatment
Drug treatment (BNF 11.6) comprises the topical administration of miotics, adrenaline, or beta-adrenoceptor blocking drugs. A carbonic anhydrase inhibitor may also be given systemically. In severe cases, surgery may be required to facilitate drainage.

Self-help organisation
International Glaucoma Association

Macular Degeneration

Definition and aetiology
Macular degeneration is an important cause of visual impairment in the elderly. It is associated with ageing and arises as a result of interference with the blood supply to the macula lutea, a modified area of the retina responsible for detailed central vision. Both eyes are usually affected and a family history is often present.

Symptoms
The onset is often gradual and is painless. It is characterised by the progressive impairment of central vision. Although peripheral vision is unaffected, the entire central field may eventually be lost.

Treatment
No effective treatment exists.

Optic Neuropathies

Definition and aetiology
Optic neuropathy (optic neuritis) is inflammation of the optic nerve within the eyeball (i.e. papillitis) or behind it (i.e. retrobulbar neuritis). The cause is often unknown, but malignant disease, meningitis, multiple sclerosis, giant cell arteritis, chemical toxicity (e.g. caused by ethanol or lead), or viral infection may be responsible.

Symptoms
It is usually unilateral. Visual impairment may be slight or marked, and temporary blindness may develop and persist for many weeks. Movement of the eyeball may be painful. Although the condition usually remits spontaneously, relapses may occur, especially if multiple sclerosis is the cause.

Treatment
Any underlying cause should be treated. Systemic or retrobulbar and subconjunctival corticosteroid therapy may be beneficial.

Papilloedema

Definition and aetiology
Papilloedema (choked disc) is characterised by oedema of the optic disc. It is usually due to increased intracranial pressure (of which it is an important diagnostic sign) which may arise from intracranial tumours, cerebral haemorrhage, head injury, malignant hypertension, and meningitis.

Symptoms

Vision may not be impaired initially, although the 'blind spot' becomes enlarged. In the absence of treatment, however, atrophy of the optic nerve may occur, with the eventual development of blindness.

Treatment

Treatment is by the reduction of intracranial pressure, according to the underlying cause.

Ptosis

Definition and aetiology

Ptosis is drooping of the upper eyelid. It may be partial or complete and may affect one or both eyes. It is most commonly congenital and results from defective muscular development. It may, however, also be acquired (e.g. through malignant disease, myasthenia gravis, or physical injury).

Symptoms

Congenital ptosis is usually bilateral and acquired ptosis is usually unilateral. Visual impairment may occur, depending on the extent to which the pupil is obscured by the eyelid. As a result of trying to open the eyes, the head may be thrown back, the eyebrows raised, and the skin on the forehead may become wrinkled.

Treatment

Any underlying cause should be treated. Surgical correction may otherwise be necessary.

Retinal Detachment

Definition and aetiology

Retinal detachment is a rare disorder. It usually occurs as a result of the leakage of vitreous humour through a hole or tear in the retina, causing the retina to become separated from its underlying pigmented epithelium. The detachment is localised initially but may extend in the absence of treatment. The most common cause is retinal degeneration, which occurs in association with ageing. Other causes include the production of exudate, haemorrhage, injury, and malignant disease.

Symptoms

Retinal detachment is painless. Early symptoms include flashes of light and the appearance of 'floaters' in the field of vision. Central vision usually remains intact, but peripheral vision may become cloudy. As detachment progresses, the entire field of vision is lost and permanent blindness may follow through irreversible loss of retinal function. Retinal detachment usually affects only one eye at a time, but there is an increased likelihood of subsequent detachment in the other eye.

Treatment

Early diagnosis and location of offending retinal lesions is essential. Treatment is by surgery, and procedures used to repair retinal damage include cryosurgery, diathermy, and photocoagulation. Retinal re-attachment usually follows, but regular screening of both eyes is desirable.

Scleritis and Episcleritis

Definition and aetiology

Scleritis is deep-seated inflammation of the sclera. If the inflammation is superficial, the condition is known as episcleritis. These disorders are thought to develop as an allergic reaction in association with systemic diseases (e.g. rheumatoid arthritis).

Symptoms

Scleritis is marked by an intense purple discoloration of the sclera and discomfort or pain in the affected eye. Some visual impairment may develop and in severe cases perforation of the sclera may occur. The symptoms of episcleritis are similar, but milder.

Treatment

Treatment is by the administration of a topical corticosteroid or anti-inflammatory preparation (BNF 11.4), although a systemic preparation may be necessary in scleritis. Immunosuppressants have also been used in severe cases.

Strabismus

Definition and aetiology

Strabismus (cast, heterotropia, or squint) is a lack of co-ordination of the eyes so that the visual axes assume an abnormal position relative to each other. It may be caused by paralysis of an eye muscle (i.e. paralytic strabismus), in which the degree of deviation varies according to the position of the eyes. It may also arise through defective insertion of the eye muscles (i.e. concomitant strabismus), in which case the degree of deviation is constant. Strabismus may be present at birth, but also often develops in early infancy. Irregular strabismus is a normal occurence in the visual development of most babies and will normally resolve by three months of age. It is less common in adults in whom it is usually caused by a primary disease (e.g. brain injury, giant cell arteritis, and hypertension).

Symptoms

Strabismus may be convergent, in which the eyes turn inwards towards each other, or divergent, in which the eyes turn outwards. A common symptom is diplopia, although children often do not develop diplopia as the images from the divergent eye are 'ignored' by the brain.

Accordingly, this eye becomes 'lazy' and its vision impaired (i.e. amblyopia).

Treatment
Early investigation, diagnosis, and treatment are essential. Eye exercises with occlusion (i.e. patching) of the normal eye may be helpful. Corrective spectacles, with or without patching, may be appropriate. In severe cases, surgical correction is often necessary. If untreated, strabismus may result in complete visual loss in the affected eye.

Uveitis

Definition and aetiology
Uveitis is inflammation of the uvea (uveal tract) and may be anterior or posterior. Anterior uveitis is characterised by inflammation of the iris (iritis), the ciliary body (cyclitis), or, more commonly, of both (iridocyclitis). Posterior uveitis is characterised by inflammation of the choroid (choroiditis) or, more commonly, of the choroid and retina (chorioretinitis). Uveitis is often idiopathic, but it may occur secondary to systemic infections (e.g. syphilis, toxoplasmosis, and tuberculosis) or inflammatory disease (e.g. ankylosing spondylitis, rheumatoid arthritis, and sarcoidosis). A primary infection, or allergic or hypersensitivity reactions may also be responsible.

Symptoms
Anterior uveitis is characterised by inflammation, lachrymation, pain, and photophobia. The pupil becomes small, irregular, and unreactive. Visual impairment may develop and, if the disease becomes chronic, iris-lens adhesions (i.e. synechiae) may occur. Possible complications include cataract formation and glaucoma. In posterior uveitis, pain and lachrymation are less common, but visual shapes and sizes become distorted and 'floaters' may be seen. Retinal detachment is a possible complication.

Treatment
Local hot applications may be soothing, but treatment usually comprises the administration of a cycloplegic and mydriatic (BNF 11.5) to prevent adhesions, and of a topical or systemic corticosteroid, or both (BNF 11.4).

11.2 ANATOMY AND PHYSIOLOGY OF THE EYE

Introduction

The eye (Fig. 11.2) is a specialised visual structure into which light passes and within which it is focused onto a

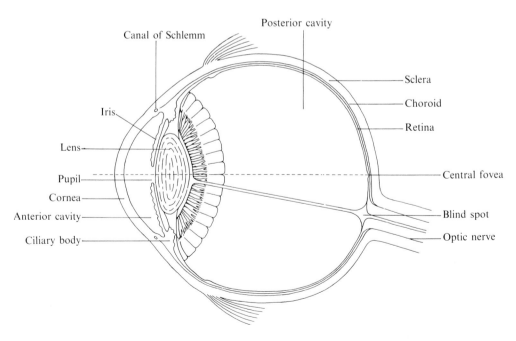

Fig. 11.2
Structure of the eye (horizontal section).

sensory surface. The image formed on the sensory surface is transmitted via the optic nerve to the visual cortex in the brain where the information received is interpreted by the surrounding occipital lobe of the cortex.

Internal Structure of the Eye

The eye, which is a fluid-filled sphere, measures about 2.5 cm in diameter. The bulk of the orb is contained within a bony orbit, with only approximately one-sixth visible externally. The orb is protected by pads of fat and by the muscles which control and initiate its movement. The wall of the eyeball is composed of three coats of which the fibrous tunic is the outermost. The white fibrous layer at the rear of the eyeball, the sclera, is continuous with the transparent window, the cornea, at the front through which light enters the eye. The junction of the sclera and cornea is marked by the canal of Schlemm, which lies deep within the sclera.

The central layer of the wall of the eyeball, the vascular tunic, is composed of choroid, the ciliary bodies, and the iris which are collectively known as the uvea. The choroid is a dark, non-reflecting membrane, which is highly vascularised. The choroid becomes modified immediately behind the scleral-corneal junction to form the ciliary bodies and the iris. The ciliary bodies are formed of the ciliary processes, which secrete aqueous humour, and the ciliary muscle, which on relaxation or contraction alters the shape of the lens for accommodation. The iris consists of pigmented radial and circular muscle at the centre of which is a hole, the pupil. The muscle of the iris relaxes and contracts to alter the amount of light which enters the eye.

The inner surface of the eye is formed of the nervous tunic, the retina. Unlike the outer two coats, the retina is only present in the rear portion of the eye. It is a highly complex multi-layered membrane, which may be broadly classified as nervous tissue with an outer pigmented layer. Blood vessels, forming a random pattern over its surface, may be readily seen in the retinal layer.

The nervous layer contains the morphologically descriptive rods and cones, which are the visual receptors. The rods, which number 70 to 140 million, operate in dim light and perceive different degrees of darkness and light. By comparison, there are only approximately 7 million cones, which are adapted for detecting colour and for the provision of visual acuity. The greatest concentration of cones occurs at a small depression, the central fovea, located in the middle of the yellow spot, the macula lutea. The central fovea is located at the visual axis of the eye and is the point of sharpest vision. The site at which the optic nerve leaves and at which the retinal blood vessels enter the eye is marked by the blind spot, optic disc. This lies close to the macula lutea and is marked by the absence of rods and cones.

The lens is a transparent proteinaceous body encapsulated in clear connective tissue. Its position forms the boundary between the anterior and posterior cavities of the eye. It is held in position and in a slightly stretched state by suspensory ligaments which arise in the ciliary bodies. The shape of the lens may be altered by the action of the ciliary muscles to allow light entering the eye to be sharply focused on the retina.

The shape of the anterior cavity, to the front of the lens, is maintained by the presence of a watery fluid, aqueous humour. Aqueous humour is continuously secreted by the ciliary body behind the iris and transported between the iris and lens through the pupil, and into the space between the lens and cornea. Normal pressure within the anterior cavity (about 16 mmHg) is maintained by the gradual drainage of aqueous humour through the canal of Schlemm into the blood.

The posterior cavity, behind the lens, is filled with a viscous fluid, the vitreous humour, which is formed *in utero* and, unlike the aqueous humour, is not recycled. It maintains the shape of the eyeball and helps to prevent distortion of the retinal membrane.

External Structure of the Eye

The eye is an extremely sensitive organ and requires protection from the external environment. The external surface of the eye and the inner lining of the eyelid are protected by a thin vascularised membrane, the conjunctiva, which in the space between the eyelid and the eyeball forms the conjunctival sac. Tears are secreted by the lachrymal glands (*see below*) into the upper conjunctival sac. The eyelids are formed of folds of muscle and skin above and below the eyeball. The movement of the eyelids assists in the lubrication of the surface of the eyeball by tears, although the lower eyelid is more firmly fixed than the upper.

The eyelids are strengthened by the presence of a tarsal plate in which are embedded the sebaceous Meibomian (tarsal) glands. The glandular secretions reduce the loss of tears by evaporation and prevent the upper and lower eyelids from sticking to each other. The border of each eyelid is lined with short hairs, the eyelashes, at the base of which are sebaceous glands, glands of Zeis.

The controlled secretion and drainage of tears (lachrymation) is essential for lubrication and the maintenance of a healthy eye. Tears are produced by the lachrymal glands located in the upper outer (i.e. furthest from the nose) portion of each eye orbit and contain an antibacterial enzyme, lysozyme. From the lachrymal gland, the tears are secreted through 6 to 12 lachrymal ducts onto the surface of the upper conjunctival membrane. Tears drain from the surface of the conjunctiva via the inner corner of each eye into the lachrymal sac, which is located along the side of the nose. The fluid drains into the nasolachrymal duct from the lachrymal sac and subsequently into the nasal cavity. Hence, eye-drops instilled into the conjunctival sac may end up in the nasal cavity to eventually be swallowed and absorbed.

Chapter 12

DISORDERS OF THE EAR, NOSE, AND OROPHARYNX

12.1   DISORDERS OF THE EAR

Deafness

Definition and aetiology
Conductive deafness is hearing loss which arises as a result of disturbance of the sound conduction mechanisms in the external auditory canal or the middle ear. Causes include physical obstruction (e.g. by ear wax), disease of the external or middle ear, perforation of the eardrum, or otosclerosis.

Sensorineural deafness is hearing loss characterised by disturbance of the inner ear or of the acoustic (eighth) nerve. It may be caused by neural or brain damage, loud noise (e.g. occupational deafness), or to the administration of drugs (e.g. aminoglycosides). Maternal rubella may produce congenital sensorineural deafness in neonates.

Treatment

Any underlying disorder must be identified and treated. Provision of a hearing aid may be beneficial.

Self-help organisations

British Association for the Hard of Hearing

National Deaf Children's Society

Royal National Institute for the Deaf

Labyrinthitis

Definition and aetiology

Labyrinthitis (otitis interna) is an uncommon disorder characterised by inflammation of the labyrinth which disturbs its function. It usually occurs as a complication of otitis media, in which the infection spreads from the middle ear. Viral labyrinthitis may occur as an epidemic.

Symptoms

The chief symptom is vertigo, which may be accompanied by severe nausea and vomiting. Nystagmus may occur and deafness may develop.

Treatment

Treatment comprises the administration of an antiemetic (BNF 4.6). In severe cases, surgery (i.e. labyrinthectomy) may be necessary and antibacterial drugs (BNF 5.1) may be indicated in the presence of bacterial infection.

Mastoiditis

Definition and aetiology

Mastoiditis is inflammation of the bony mastoid process which lies behind the ear. It occurs as a serious complication of otitis media, with bacterial infection spreading to the mastoid air cells from the middle ear. It has become less common because of effective antibiotic therapy of otitis media.

Symptoms

Common symptoms include inflammation, pain, and swelling over the mastoid process, and fever and malaise. The production of a profuse purulent discharge is also common and increasing conductive deafness may develop. Abscess formation may occur in severe cases.

Treatment

Treatment is by the oral or parenteral administration of an appropriate antibacterial drug (BNF 5.1). In severe cases, surgery (i.e. mastoidectomy) may be indicated in order to remove infected bone, and this may be followed by local topical treatment (BNF 12.1.2).

Ménière's Disease

Definition and aetiology

Ménière's disease is a labyrinthine disorder associated with vertigo. It usually develops in middle or old age and may be mild or severe. It is due to the damage of the receptor cells of the cochlea and vestibular system.

Symptoms

It is characterised by progressive deafness and tinnitus, eventually followed by recurrent attacks of vertigo. Deafness may become total. The vertigo is exacerbated by movement and may be accompanied by nausea and vomiting, and nystagmus. Attacks may last from several minutes to several hours.

Treatment

Treatment comprises the administration of drugs such as prochlorperazine, betahistine, and cinnarizine (BNF 4.6), or ultrasonic irradiation. In extreme cases, it may be necessary to destroy the labyrinth by surgery, but deafness will result.

Otitis Externa

Definition and aetiology

Otitis externa is characterised by inflammation of the external auditory canal. The acute form is usually caused by bacterial infection, although fungal infection may be responsible. The entire canal may be involved or infection may be localised in the form of a furuncle. The chronic form of otitis externa is most often eczematous and is commonly associated with eczema occurring at other body sites. Contributory factors include mechanical trauma, chemical irritants (e.g. hair products), and dampness (e.g. after swimming).

Symptoms

Eczematous otitis externa is marked by itching of the auditory canal which is often dry and scaly. Severe pain is characteristic of acute otitis externa and is often exacerbated by manipulation of the pinna. An offensive purulent discharge may be evident and the canal may become blocked as a result of local swelling and accumulated purulent debris. Accordingly, hearing may be impaired.

Treatment

The affected ear should be gently but thoroughly cleaned. The local application of warmth may be helpful and contributory factors should be avoided. A topical astringent or corticosteroid (BNF 12.1.1) may be administered in the presence of an eczematous reaction. If infection is responsible, however, an appropriate topical anti-infective preparation (BNF 12.1.1) should be used and an analgesic (BNF 4.7) may be required if pain is severe. In the presence of localised or unresponsive infections, a systemic anti-infective preparation (BNF 12.1.1) may be indicated.

Otitis Media

Definition

Otitis media (tympanitis) is inflammation of the middle ear. It may be classified as acute, chronic, or sero-mucinous otitis media.

Acute Otitis Media

Definition and aetiology
Acute otitis media is usually due to bacterial infection (e.g. *Haemophilus influenzae*, *Staphylococcus aureus*, or *Streptococcus pyogenes*), although viral infection may be responsible. It is most common in young children and is often preceded by an upper respiratory-tract infection. Physical injury to the eardrum, however, may be a precipitating factor.

Symptoms
Acute otitis media is characterised by severe pain and a degree of conductive deafness. Fever, and nausea and vomiting are also common. A purulent exudate is produced and may accumulate in the middle ear. This may cause bulging, or even perforation, of the eardrum.

Treatment
The treatment of acute disease may include the administration of a non-opioid analgesic (BNF 4.7.1) and, in the presence of bacterial infection, an appropriate antibacterial drug (BNF 5.1, Table 1). Antibacterial prophylaxis (BNF 12.1.2) may be considered. Surgical incision of the eardrum (i.e. myringotomy) may be necessary to drain accumulated exudate.

Chronic Otitis Media

Definition and aetiology
Chronic disease may follow an acute attack although its development may be insidious. It may also be associated with obstruction of the Eustachian tube or physical injury to the eardrum.

Symptoms
Chronic otitis media is marked by permanent painless inflammation of the middle ear and the production of a purulent discharge and perforation of the eardrum. Hearing impairment may be the presenting symptom.

Treatment
In the presence of chronic disease, the affected ear must be thoroughly cleaned. Topical treatment similar to that for otitis externa may be beneficial. A systemic antibacterial (BNF 12.1.2) may be indicated in severe cases. Surgical repair may be necessary.

Sero-mucinous Otitis Media

Definition and aetiology
Sero-mucinous otitis media ('glue ear' or secretory otitis media) is characterised by the accumulation of a viscous mucinous fluid in the middle ear. It is most common in children and often follows repeated attacks of acute otitis media arising from upper respiratory-tract infections. It may also be associated with obstruction of the Eustachian tube, allergic reactions, or inflammation of the adenoids or sinuses.

Symptoms
Sero-mucinous otitis media is characterised by varying degrees of conductive deafness. Deafness may become permanent in the absence of treatment and can cause learning difficulties and speech disorders in children. Pain and discharge are often absent, although discharge will become evident if perforation of the eardrum (myringotomy) is carried out.

Treatment
Expert supervision is essential. If an infection is thought to be responsible, an appropriate antibacterial drug (BNF 5.1) may be administered. A systemic nasal decongestant (BNF 3.10) or an antihistamine (BNF 3.4.1) may be beneficial in relieving Eustachian tube obstruction or allergy. Surgical incision of the eardrum may be necessary to drain off accumulated fluid, and a small drainage tube (i.e. a grommet or stopple) may be inserted in the eardrum. Any primary disorder of the nasopharynx should be corrected. Mucolytics have been used with varying success.

Otosclerosis

Definition and aetiology
Otosclerosis is characterised by the immobilisation of the stapes in the middle ear and is caused by abnormal formation of new bone around the stapes and the oval window. Its aetiology is unknown, although a family history is often present. It is a common cause of deafness, occurs more frequently in women, and is exacerbated by pregnancy.

Symptoms
Otosclerosis is marked by the progressive development of conductive deafness and may be accompanied by tinnitus and vertigo. Both ears are usually affected and total deafness may occur in the absence of treatment.

Treatment
Treatment consists of the surgical removal of the stapes (i.e. stapedectomy) followed by replacement with a prosthesis. The provision of a hearing aid may be helpful.

12.2   DISORDERS OF THE NOSE

Rhinitis

Definition and aetiology
Rhinitis is inflammation of the nasal mucosa which may be of allergic, infective (*see* Common Cold), or vasomotor origin.

Allergic Rhinitis

Definition and aetiology
Allergic rhinitis may be seasonal (i.e. hay fever) and occur at specific times of year as a result of allergy to plant pollens (e.g. trees or grasses). Alternatively, it may be perennial (i.e. nonseasonal) and arise from exposure to other allergens (e.g. animal danders, feathers, fungal spores, or house-dust mite).

Symptoms
Hay fever is characterised by the sudden onset of symptoms which include lachrymation, rhinorrhoea, and sneezing with itching of the eyes, ears, nose, and palate. Coughing, wheezing, and nasal congestion are also common. The symptoms of perennial allergic rhinitis are similar to those of hay fever. In addition, nasal congestion and obstruction are likely to become chronic, and may lead to blockage of the Eustachian tubes and hearing difficulties.

Treatment
Both forms of allergic rhinitis benefit from identification and avoidance of specific allergens. Corticosteroids or sodium cromoglycate (BNF 12.2.1) may be administered as both prophylaxis or treatment. Symptoms may be treated with an oral antihistamine (BNF 3.4.1) or a systemic nasal decongestant (BNF 3.10). Topical nasal decongestants (BNF 12.2.2) may be used on a short-term basis, but may cause rebound nasal congestion and obstruction (rhinitis medicamentosa).

Vasomotor Rhinitis

Definition and aetiology
Vasomotor rhinitis (non-allergic non-infective rhinitis) is caused by the dilatation of the blood vessels of the nasal mucosa, which may be due to sympathetic nervous system underactivity or parasympathetic nervous system overactivity. Common precipitating factors include emotional disturbances (e.g. anger, anxiety, and fatigue), low humidity (e.g. caused by central heating), and sudden changes in temperature (e.g. mild chilling).

Symptoms
Symptoms of vasomotor rhinitis are similar to those of allergic rhinitis, although nasal itching and sneezing are less common. In addition, the nasal mucosa may appear highly coloured, varying from bright red to purplish. Nasal polyposis, asthma, and an intolerance to aspirin may also occur.

Treatment
Treatment is similar to that of allergic rhinitis. Intranasal corticosteroids (BNF 12.2.1) may be beneficial in the treatment of nasal polyposis. Humidification of the atmosphere may provide general symptomatic relief. Severe cases may benefit from surgery (e.g. submucosal diathermy) and removal of polyps.

Self-help organisation
Action Against Allergy

Sinusitis

Definition and aetiology
Sinusitis is inflammation of the paranasal sinuses, affecting primarily the frontal and maxillary sinuses (Fig. 12.1). It is usually caused by viral or bacterial infection and often follows an attack of the common cold. It may also arise, however, as a result of an underlying dental

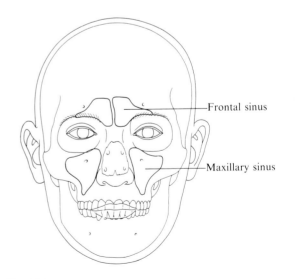

Fig. 12.1
Position of the frontal and maxillary sinuses.

infection or some anatomical defect (e.g. deviated nasal septum). Sinusitis may be acute or chronic.

Symptoms
Common symptoms include nasal obstruction with purulent rhinorrhoea. Fever may occur, and facial pain over the affected sinus is common and can be exacerbated by bending forwards or coughing. If the frontal sinuses are affected, pain occurs over the eyes as a frontal headache. If the maxillary sinuses are involved, pain occurs under the eyes and may extend into the jaw so as to resemble toothache.

Treatment
Steam inhalations and non-opioid analgesics (BNF 4.7.1) are often helpful. Any primary infection or defect should be treated. Symptoms may be relieved by the administration of a systemic nasal decongestant (BNF 3.10) or by the short-term use of a topical nasal decongestant (BNF 12.2.2). In the presence of bacterial infection, an appropriate antibacterial drug (BNF 5.1, Table 1) should be given. In unresponsive cases, surgery may be necessary to facilitate drainage of the sinus, which should also be washed out to remove any purulent debris.

12.3   DISORDERS OF THE OROPHARYNX

Aphthous Stomatitis

Definition and aetiology
Aphthous stomatitis (aphthous ulceration) is a common disorder characterised by the development of small ulcers (i.e. aphthae) on the oral mucosa. The cause is unknown, but a local immune mechanism may be responsible. Contributory factors may include folic acid, iron, or vitamin B_{12} deficiencies. Emotional disturbances or physical illnesses may also contribute.

Symptoms
The chief symptom is the appearance of shallow yellow or white ulcers on the tongue or the mucosal surfaces of the cheeks and lips. The ulcers are acutely painful, may occur singly or in groups, and are commonly surrounded by an area of erythema. Although they usually heal spontaneously after about 14 days, recurrence is common. In some severe cases, they may be persistent and can be accompanied by fever and malaise.

Treatment
The use of an antiseptic mouth-wash (BNF 12.3.4) may be beneficial in the prevention of secondary bacterial infection. Treatment (BNF 12.3.1) comprises the topical administration of a local anaesthetic or analgesic. A topical protective paste may also be useful and the administration of a corticosteroid lozenge or paste is often effective. A tetracycline mouth-wash may be used to treat recurrent ulceration.

Gingivitis

Definition and aetiology
Gingivitis is inflammation of the gums. It is almost always caused by poor oral hygiene, which is characterised by the accumulation of food debris and the formation of dental plaque and calculus. Other causes include dental defects, primary systemic diseases (e.g. diabetes mellitus and leukaemia), and mouth breathing. The administration of phenytoin may result in the development of gingivitis.

Symptoms
The gums become inflamed and swollen and bleed easily, particularly after brushing the teeth or eating. Periodontal disease may develop in the absence of treatment and may result in dental decay or loss. Vincent's infection is a further possible complication.

Treatment
Any underlying dental defect or systemic disease should be corrected. Prophylaxis involves the removal of plaque with dental floss, especially in high-risk individuals. Treatment consists of introducing and maintaining good oral hygiene and regular dental therapy.

Glossitis

Definition and aetiology
Glossitis is a common disorder characterised by inflammation of the tongue. It may be due to infection, mechanical trauma, or irritation (e.g. by alcohol, foods, and smoking). It may also occur as a result of primary systemic disorders (e.g. anaemia and vitamin deficiencies).

Symptoms
The tongue may become red, swollen, and ulcerated. In severe cases, pain may occur and swelling may be such that the tongue protrudes. Subsequent difficulties in eating and speaking may arise.

Treatment
Irritants should be avoided and good oral hygiene encouraged. Any underlying primary disorder should be treated. Treatment of glossitis may include the use of a topical anaesthetic or antiseptic preparation (BNF 12.3.3 and 12.3.4). An appropriate antibacterial drug (BNF 5.1) may be indicated in the presence of infection.

Halitosis

Definition and aetiology

Halitosis (bad breath) is characterised by an offensive unpleasant breath odour. It may be due to dental or gingival disease (e.g. Vincent's infection), respiratory disease or infection, nasopharyngeal disease (e.g. chronic tonsillitis), or simply to the retention of food debris in the mouth. Gastro-intestinal disease is not generally thought to be responsible. Although halitosis is often real, it may also be imagined (i.e. psychogenic) and can indicate the presence of anxiety or underlying personality disorders.

Treatment

Any underlying cause should be corrected and good oral hygiene should be encouraged. Reassurance may be beneficial in imagined halitosis.

Laryngitis

Definition and aetiology

Laryngitis is inflammation of the larynx. It is usually caused by viral or bacterial infection and often follows an attack of the common cold. It may also arise, in the absence of infection, as a result of exposure to irritants (e.g. tobacco smoke or alcohol), from excessive use of the voice, or in association with an allergic reaction or respiratory-tract disorders (e.g. bronchitis and influenza). It may be acute or chronic.

Symptoms

The most common symptom is hoarseness which may progress to complete voice loss. This may be accompanied by a sore, dry throat, local oedema, dysphagia, and an irritating cough. Fever is uncommon.

Treatment

The voice should be rested and irritants avoided. Steam inhalations are usually beneficial. Although no specific treatment exists for viral laryngitis, an appropriate antibacterial drug (BNF 5.1) may be indicated for the less common bacterial infection.

Oral Leucoplakia

Definition and aetiology

Oral leucoplakia is characterised by the development of white thickened patches on the mucosa of the cheeks, tongue, and occasionally, of the gums. It may be due to irritation (e.g. by friction or smoking), infection (e.g. candidiasis or tertiary syphilis), or it may be inherited. In most patients, however, the cause is unknown.

Symptoms

The white patches usually develop over a period of weeks. They may be soft or hard and cover large or small areas of mucosa. The patches cannot be rubbed off. Ulceration may occasionally occur. Recurrence is common; in a small number of patients, malignant changes may develop.

Treatment

Patients should avoid smoking and any sources of friction must be removed, which usually involves dental treatment. In the presence of infection, an appropriate antimicrobial (BNF 5.1 and 5.2) may be indicated. Treatment is often ineffective, and follow-up is essential in order to detect the development of any malignant disease.

Pharyngitis

Definition and aetiology

Pharyngitis (acute sore throat) is an acute inflammation of the pharynx. It is most commonly caused by viral infection, although Group A β-haemolytic streptococcal infections may produce bacterial pharyngitis, particularly in young children which, if untreated, can develop into acute rheumatic fever. In young adults, the causative agent appears to be predominantly *Corynebacterium haemolyticum*. It may also arise as a result of pharyngeal irritation (e.g. by alcohol or smoking).

Symptoms

Pharyngitis is characterised by sore throat, with pain on swallowing and hoarseness. In the presence of infection, fever may occur and the pharynx may develop a membranous covering. A purulent exudate may also be produced. Patients with *C. haemolyticum* infection commonly present with a scarlet fever-like rash.

Treatment

Patients should be encouraged to avoid pharyngeal irritation and to maintain a high-fluid intake. Symptomatic treatment includes the use of antiseptic or anaesthetic gargles, or both, lozenges, or mouth-washes (BNF 12.3.3 and 12.3.4). Non-opioid analgesics (BNF 4.7.1) may be required and, in the presence of bacterial infection, an appropriate antibacterial drug (BNF 5.1) may be indicated.

Sialadenitis

Definition and aetiology

Sialadenitis is inflammation of a salivary gland. It is most often caused by viral (e.g. mumps) or bacterial infection, although it may occasionally arise as a result of an allergic reaction. The obstruction of a salivary duct (*see* Sialolithiasis) may be a contributory factor. Alcoholism and sarcoidosis may also be implicated.

Symptoms

The parotid or submandibular salivary glands may be affected and common symptoms include pain which may be acute, and swelling. Local oedema may occur and a purulent discharge may arise from the duct of the affected gland. Fever and malaise may develop. Sialadenitis may be acute, chronic, or recurrent.

Treatment

Good oral hygiene must be encouraged. An appropriate antibacterial drug (BNF 5.1) should be administered in the presence of bacterial infection. Any salivary duct obstruction should be removed, and in chronic or recurrent cases surgical removal of the affected gland may be indicated.

Sialolithiasis

Definition and aetiology

Sialolithiasis is characterised by the formation of salivary stones (i.e. calculi) in the salivary ducts or, less commonly, in the salivary glands. The ducts of the submandibular glands are most often affected. Stones are formed by deposition of calcium carbonate and phosphate from saliva.

Symptoms

Sialolithiasis is most common in adults. It is marked by obstruction of the affected duct or gland, which leads to accumulation of saliva within the gland, particularly in association with eating. The salivary gland becomes swollen and pain may be experienced. Swelling may persist for several hours.

Treatment

Treatment comprises the removal of the offending stone, usually under local anaesthetic. In recurrent cases, corrective surgery may be necessary.

12.4 ANATOMY AND PHYSIOLOGY OF THE EAR, NOSE, AND OROPHARYNX

The Ear

The ear (Fig. 12.2) is the organ of hearing and balance whose primary centres are located deep within the temporal bone of the skull in fluid-filled chambers. The outer structures are used mainly as a means of channelling sound inward to the hearing receptors. Anatomically, the ear is divided into three distinct, but interconnected, zones.

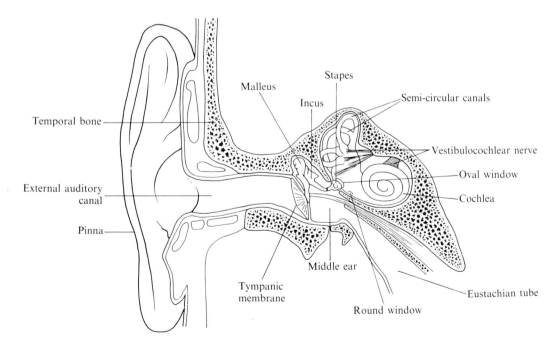

Fig. 12.2
The ear in section.

The outer ear consists of the pinna, the external auditory canal (meatus), and the tympanic membrane (eardrum). The pinna is the external portion of the outer ear, and is of variable size and thickness. It consists of a flap of fixed cartilage contained within thickened skin, and receives and directs sound waves from the environment into the ear. The external auditory canal leads from the pinna to the tympanic membrane. The surface of its outer end is lined with small hairs and ceruminous cells, which secrete cerumen (wax) and serve to minimise the entry of foreign materials into the canal. Sound entering the ear is transmitted along the external auditory canal to the tympanic membrane, which forms the boundary between the outer and middle ear. It is attached by a ring of cartilage to the temporal bone, and is lined by a membrane of thickened skin on its outer surface and a mucous membrane on its inner surface.

The middle ear (tympanic cavity) lies immediately behind the tympanic membrane, and is in an air-filled cavity within the temporal bone. The temporal bone lining the rear of the middle-ear compartment is lined by air cells of the mastoid process. The opening to the Eustachian tube is located in the opposite wall of the cavity and connects the middle ear to the nasopharynx. It acts to equalise pressure within the middle ear with that of the external environment, and prevent rupture of the tympanic membrane. The entrance to the Eustachian tube is normally closed except on swallowing, chewing, and yawning.

Sound which impinges on the tympanic membrane is transmitted and amplified within the middle ear by the action of the ossicles. These consist of three delicate bones, the malleus (hammer), incus (anvil), and stapes (stirrup). The vibrations created by the action of sound on the tympanic membrane generate an oscillating movement of the tiny bones which subsequently reaches the oval window (fenestra vestibuli). Amplification of sound is produced by the lever-like movement of the ossicles and the concentration of the vibrations at a single focus, the oval window. A second opening to the inner ear is formed by the round window (fenestra cochlea), which lies immediately below the oval window.

The inner ear is the primary centre of hearing and balance. It consists of a fluid-filled membranous labyrinth immersed in a watery fluid, the perilymph, which is itself contained by a bony labyrinth. The inner ear may be divided into the cochlea, the vestibule, and the semicircular canals. The cochlea, a spirally arranged bony tube, consists of three compartments, an upper and lower compartment containing perilymph and a central compartment containing endolymph. Vibrations which reach the oval window set up motions within the perilymph, and are transmitted to fine hairs lining the membrane of the central compartment. The movement

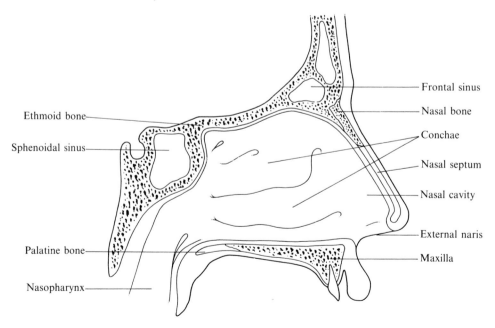

Fig. 12.3
Nasal cavity and sinuses.

of these fine hairs generates a nervous potential which is picked up and transmitted to the brain via the vestibulocochlear nerve (the acoustic eighth cranial nerve).

The vestibule is the central portion of the bony labyrinth, within which the membranous labyrinth is divided into the utricle and the saccule. In conjunction with the three semi-circular canals (arranged at right angles to each other), the vestibule is concerned with maintaining an awareness of orientation of the head and of body position during movements (e.g. rotation).

The Nose

The nose is the organ of smell, and the uppermost part of the respiratory tract. The external portion of the nose is formed of bone and cartilage, and contains two openings, the external nares (nostrils). The internal nasal cavity is bordered on its upper surface by the underside of the cranium, and is separated from the oral cavity at its base by the palate (Fig. 12.3). The palate is divided into a hard portion at the front of the nasal cavity and a soft portion at the rear. The nasal cavity is divided vertically by a cartilaginous membrane, the nasal septum. The rear of the nasal cavity is marked by two internal nares and the openings of the Eustachian tube from each ear. Pairs of air cavities, which comprise the paranasal sinuses (ethmoidal, frontal, maxillary, and sphenoidal sinuses), surround and are linked to the nasal cavity.

The nasal cavity and its internal structures warm and filter the air entering through the nostrils. The internal

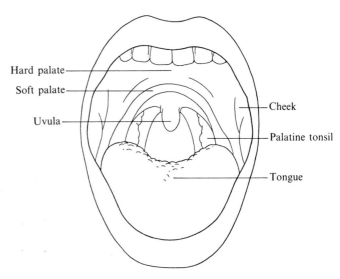

Fig. 12.4
The oral cavity.

cavity is divided by bony plates, the conchae, into passages (meatuses), which are lined by hairs contained within a mucous membrane. Olfactory functions are located in cells that lie immediately above the uppermost concha, and are stimulated by the presence of volatile agents in turbulent currents generated by inspired air.

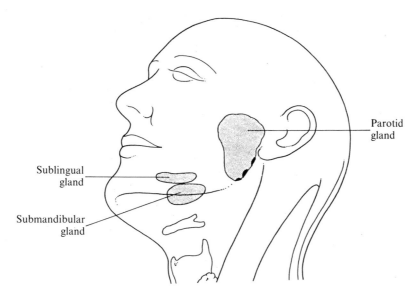

Fig. 12.5
Position of the salivary glands.

The Oropharynx

A detailed description of the structures of the upper respiratory tree may be found in Section 3.4. Only those structures within the oropharynx that have not been previously described will be discussed here.

The oral cavity (Fig. 12.4) consists of the cheeks, the hard and soft palates (*see above*), and the tongue. The sides of the mouth are marked by cheeks, which are muscular structures internally lined with squamous epithelium. Movement of the cheeks assists in the mastication of food and in keeping the bolus between the teeth.

The tongue is a highly flexible organ formed of skeletal muscle and covered with a mucous membrane. It plays a fundamental role in the sensation of taste, and assists in mastication, swallowing, and the articulation of sounds. The upper surface of the tongue is rough due to the presence of papillae. There are approximately 2000 taste buds found in certain papillae. Additional taste buds are located on the soft palate and in the throat. Particular sensations of taste are highly localised on the surface of the tongue, and may be broadly classified as sour, sweet, salt, and bitter.

Three pairs of salivary glands (Fig. 12.5) continuously secrete saliva into the oral cavity to keep the mucous membranes moist. The amount secreted increases considerably when food enters the mouth or in anticipation of food. The largest of the salivary glands, the parotid gland, is located immediately in front of each ear. The other two glands are situated below the floor of the oral cavity. The submandibular gland is found near the base of the tongue and immediately behind the sublingual gland, the smallest of the three pairs. The glands secrete fluids of varying composition to constitute saliva which enters the mouth near its roof (parotid duct) and on its floor (submandibular ducts).

Chapter 13

SKIN DISORDERS

13.1 DISORDERS OF THE SKIN

(The diagrammatic representation of a range of common skin lesions is illustrated in Fig. 13.1.)

Acne Vulgaris

Definition and aetiology
Acne vulgaris (common acne) is an inflammatory condition of the hair follicle and sebaceous gland (i.e. of the pilosebaceous unit). It commonly occurs at puberty and generally resolves by 30 years of age. It may be caused by increased plasma-androgen concentrations or by increased sensitivity of the sebaceous glands to androgens. This results in excessive sebum production and hyperkeratosis. The hair follicles subsequently become blocked with keratin and inflamed, and the sebaceous glands may become infected, often by *Propionibacterium acnes*. Acne may also be precipitated by the administration of drugs (e.g. corticosteroids, oral contraceptives, or antiepileptic drugs) or by the use of oily cosmetics. Other contributory factors include emotional disturbance and menstruation. Diet or sexual activity are not thought to play any part in the development of acne.

Symptoms
Acne is characterised by the formation of comedones which may be open (blackheads) or closed (whiteheads). They are usually distributed over the face, neck, chest, shoulders, and back. In more severe cases, inflamed papules and cysts may develop. Conglobate and cystic acne are characterised by the formation of inflamed purulent cysts deep in the tissues. Scarring may occur subsequent to healing, particularly after the more severe forms.

Treatment
Patients should be encouraged to wash regularly with water and detergent solutions and avoid picking or squeezing lesions. The value of reassurance and psychological support should not be underestimated. Treatment (BNF 13.6) comprises the topical administration of antiseptic and keratolytic preparations. The prolonged administration of an appropriate antibacterial drug (BNF 5.1, Table 1) may be beneficial particularly in more severe cases. An anti-androgen may be suitable for the treatment of women suffering intractable symptoms. In the presence of severe cystic or conglobate acne, the systemic administration of isotretinoin may be considered, but only under expert supervision. Plastic surgery may be indicated in patients who suffer severe scarring. Ultraviolet radiation can give positive improvement.

Albinism

Definition and aetiology
Albinism is an autosomal recessive genetic disorder in which there is an absence or malfunction of tyrosinase, an enzyme involved in melanin production. The severity of the condition, which may occur in all races, varies according to the extent of the enzymatic loss.

Symptoms
Albinism is characterised by lack of pigment in the skin, hair, and eyes. It may be accompanied by astigmatism, nystagmus, strabismus, and photophobia. There is a tendency to sunburn easily and develop malignant skin disease.

Treatment
There is no treatment available to correct the deficiency. Patients should be encouraged to wear tinted glasses, avoid exposure to sunlight when possible, and regularly apply sunscreening preparations (BNF 13.8.1) to exposed parts. Routine skin examination should be performed to allow early detection of malignant disease.

Alopecia

Definition and aetiology
Alopecia is the absence or loss of hair, and may be partial or complete. Causes are varied and include physical damage (e.g. excessive traction employed in some hairdressing techniques, vigorous use of stiff hairbrushes, and trichotillomania). Toxic alopecia is very often temporary and may be precipitated by chemical hair preparations, systemic disease (e.g. myxoedema, severe febrile illness, or early syphilis), and drugs (e.g. propranolol, carbimazole, cytotoxic agents, anticoagulants, or excessive doses of vitamin A). Injuries to the scalp or diseases resulting in inflammation and tissue damage (e.g. tinea capitis) may lead to permanent alopecia. Alopecia areata is a sudden, and often reversible, patchy hair loss with no apparent cause. Male-pattern alopecia (androgenetic alopecia) occurs as a result of genetically predisposed hair follicles in the scalp responding to stimulation by circulating androgens.

Symptoms
The hair loss due to physical or chemical trauma is generally confined to the areas of damage. Alopecia areata (Fig. 13.2) may involve any hairy part of the body and re-growth is characterised by hairs resembling exclamation marks. Male-pattern alopecia usually starts as recession of the hairline in the lateral frontal regions and may be associated with hair loss on the crown. These two areas may, in time, become confluent. The long coarse pigmented terminal hairs are progressively replaced by

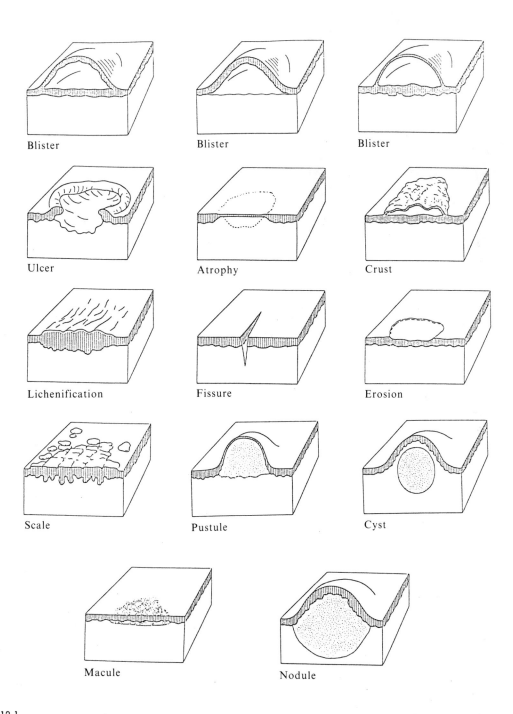

Fig. 13.1
Diagrammatic representation of common skin lesions.

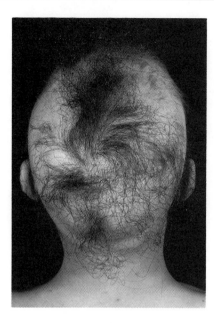

Fig. 13.2
The patchy hair loss characteristic of alopecia areata.

short fine colourless vellus hairs. The hair follicles themselves gradually shrink, resulting in a decrease, and eventual cessation, in hair production.

Treatment
Treatment comprises removing the cause where appropriate. Systemic or topical corticosteroids may be beneficial in treating some cases of alopecia areata. Minoxidil lotion (BNF 13.9) may be applied to reverse male-pattern alopecia, but treatment must be maintained indefinitely.

Angioedema

Definition and aetiology
Angioedema (which should be distinguished from hereditary angioedema, *see below*) is a form of urticaria characterised by large oedematous lesions, involving the dermis and subcutaneous tissues. The causes are as for urticaria.

Symptoms
The sites most commonly affected are the lips, eyelids, and genitalia. Other sites include the tongue, and the dorsal surfaces of the hands and feet. The onset is often sudden, marked by single or multiple lesions lasting for 1 to 2 hours, although occasionally persisting for up to three days. Oedema occurring in the upper respiratory tract may result in potentially fatal respiratory distress.

Treatment
The treatment of angioedema is as for urticaria. Injections of adrenaline (BNF 3.1.1.2), corticosteroids (BNF 6.3.4), antihistamines (BNF 3.4.1), and tracheal intubation may be indicated in severe cases.

Callosities and Corns

Definition and aetiology
A callosity (callus) is a hard circumscribed thickened area of hyperkeratosis. It is produced by repeated friction or pressure, usually over a bony prominence. It may be caused by a variety of factors (e.g. badly-fitting shoes or occupational activities).

A corn is a small circumscribed area of hyperkeratosis with a central core, always found on the feet. It is produced by repeated pressure or friction over a bony prominence, usually due to badly-fitting shoes. Hard corns are usually found on the upper surfaces of toes, while those found between the toes are termed soft corns.

Symptoms
Callosities are commonly found on the toes and soles of feet, and the fingers and palms of hands. They are generally of uniform thickness and colour, with a rough surface, and may cause discomfort, especially on application of pressure.

The point of the corn lies in the dermis, and causes pain by pressure on the nerve endings.

Treatment
Treatment of both callosities and corns comprises relieving the pressure where possible using self-adhesive pads. The application of keratolytics (BNF 13.7) may be beneficial in aiding removal of the hard skin. Careful paring of the hard skin with a file or pumice stone (dermabrasion) may also be helpful.

Decubitus Ulcer

Definition and aetiology
A decubitus ulcer (bedsore or pressure sore) is an area of ulceration caused by ischaemia and subsequent necrosis of tissues exposed to prolonged pressure. It is commonly seen in patients immobilised for a variety of reasons, especially the bedridden and elderly. Other precipitating factors include friction (e.g. due to wrinkled bedding or rough clothing), skin maceration (e.g. due to perspiration, and urine and faecal matter in the incontinent), and dulled or absent perception of sensation. Anaemia, malnutrition, secondary infection, decreased peripheral circulation, and any existing cachectic state may accelerate the process.

Symptoms

The initial stages of formation of a bedsore are characterised by erythema, oedema, and blister formation. Necrosis follows and may extend through the fatty tissues to muscles and even bone in severe cases (Fig. 13.3).

Treatment

Bedsore formation may be arrested in the early stages by the adoption of preventive measures. These include frequently changing the patient's position, relieving pressure on sensitive areas, regularly inspecting the skin to note any changes, efficient skin cleansing and drying regimes, and encouraging the patient in active movement when possible. Any underlying disorder should be treated and a regular high-protein diet maintained. The treatment of advanced stages consists of debridement using skin disinfecting and cleansing agents or desloughing agents and enzyme preparations (BNF 13.11). Dextranomer beads and gel and colloid dressings (BNF 13.13.8) may be beneficial. In severe cases, surgical excision of necrotic tissue and wound closure may be necessary.

Eczema

Definition and aetiology

Eczema (dermatitis) is an inflammatory condition of the skin. It is caused by endogenous factors (e.g. atopic dermatitis) or exogenous factors (e.g. external irritants) as in contact dermatitis and napkin rash.

Symptoms

The acute stage of eczema is characterised by the appearance of vesicles on the skin, formed by the spread of oedema from the dermis into the epidermis. The vesicles may rupture releasing a clear exudate which dries and forms crusts. Pruritus is a major feature of the condition and is usually accompanied by inflammation and tenderness. During the latter stages, the oedema subsides and the epidermis dries and thickens. Scales may be produced by a fast turnover of cells. Scratching and rubbing of the skin may contribute to the secondary stages and may also cause infection.

Treatment

Any underlying cause should be removed, if possible, and patients should be discouraged from scratching or using topical sensitising agents. Soap substitutes (BNF 13.1), and emollient and barrier preparations (BNF 13.2) may be beneficial for dry lesions. Keratolytics (BNF 13.5) may be required to soften and loosen scales. In some cases, an appropriate topical corticosteroid (BNF 13.4) may be indicated. Wet dressings (BNF 13.11) and anti-infective skin preparations (BNF 13.10) may be necessary for weeping or infected eczemas. Oral antihistamines (BNF 3.4.1) may be of value in reducing pruritus. Systemic corticosteroids (BNF 6.3.4) may be necessary in severe cases.

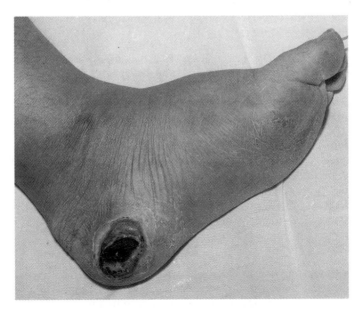

Fig. 13.3
A bedsore in which erosion has revealed the muscular tendons of the heel.

Atopic Dermatitis

Definition and aetiology
Atopic dermatitis (atopic eczema) is a chronic fluctuating inflammatory condition of the skin. The cause is unknown, although a family history of allergy (e.g. asthma or allergic rhinitis) is common. The age of onset is generally 2 to 6 months and it usually resolves spontaneously by 30 years of age. The skin may, however, remain sensitive to physical or chemical irritants.

Symptoms
Atopic dermatitis starts on the face and is characterised by red, weeping, crusted lesions. It spreads to the hands, flexures of the knees, elbows, wrists, ankles, and sides of the neck. Pruritus is a major feature and scratching may cause secondary infection. In older children and adults, erythema and lichenification predominate, and the condition is characterised by dry, itching, cracked skin. Contact allergens, emotional disturbances, and changes in temperature or humidity may exacerbate the condition.

Treatment
The treatment of atopic dermatitis is as described under eczema.

Contact Dermatitis

Definition and aetiology
Contact dermatitis (contact eczema) is an inflammatory skin condition (Fig. 13.4a) caused by exposure to physical or chemical irritants (i.e. irritant contact dermatitis) or allergens (i.e. allergic contact dermatitis). It may be acute or chronic.

Primary irritants (e.g. acids, alkalis, or organic solvents) damage the epidermis, allowing penetration and subsequent inflammation. Atopic dermatitis may predispose an individual to develop irritant dermatitis. Allergens that may cause dermatitis include organic dyes (e.g. hair colorants), topical medicaments (e.g. local anaesthetics and antihistamines), and metal (e.g. nickel fasteners in clothing). Allergic sensitisation may take days, months, or years to develop. Photoallergic and phototoxic contact dermatitis occur on exposure of the skin to light subsequent to the topical application of sensitising substances (e.g. after-shave lotions and sun-screening agents).

Symptoms
The symptoms of contact dermatitis are as described under eczema. In the acute phase, the site of the lesions caused by primary irritants usually coincides with the point of contact. Chronic cases and allergic reactions may show a more generalised spread.

Treatment
The treatment of contact dermatitis is as described under eczema. The resistance of the skin is lowered for several months after apparently healing, and patients should be encouraged to continue using emollients and barrier creams (BNF 13.2.1) and to avoid sensitising agents.

Exfoliative Dermatitis

Definition and aetiology
Exfoliative dermatitis is a severe inflammatory condition of the skin affecting a large proportion of the body surface. The cause is unknown, although it may be precipitated by other skin conditions (e.g. psoriasis and other forms of dermatitis) or drugs (e.g. penicillin, barbiturates, or phenytoin).

Symptoms
The onset of exfoliative dermatitis may be sudden, and initial symptoms include widespread erythema, fever, shivering, malaise, and sometimes pruritus. Scaling occurs as the condition progresses, and the skin becomes dry and thickened (Fig. 13.4b). After some weeks, body and scalp hair, and nails may be shed. Serious metabolic disturbances in chronic cases may be caused by increased blood flow through the skin and the loss of large amounts of exfoliated scale. These include hypothermia, fluid loss, peripheral circulatory failure, hypoproteinaemia, and in susceptible individuals, congestive heart failure. Skin and respiratory-tract infections may occur. The condition may be fatal if not treated promptly.

Treatment
Hospitalisation is usually necessary to monitor protein and electrolyte balance and regulate the environmental temperature. Other measures include the administration of oral corticosteroids (BNF 6.3.4) and the withdrawal of all non-essential medication. Oral antibacterial drugs (BNF 5.1) may be required to treat secondary infection. The application of soothing emollients (BNF 13.2) after bathing may be beneficial.

Napkin Rash

Definition and aetiology
Napkin rash (napkin dermatitis) is an inflammatory condition of the skin confined to the area in contact with the napkin (i.e. the pubic area, buttocks, genitalia, and thighs). Damage to the stratum corneum, resulting from prolonged skin contact with occluded moist napkins, appears to be a precipitating factor. The condition may be further aggravated by ammonia (formed by bacterial degradation of urea), *Candida albicans*, faeces, or

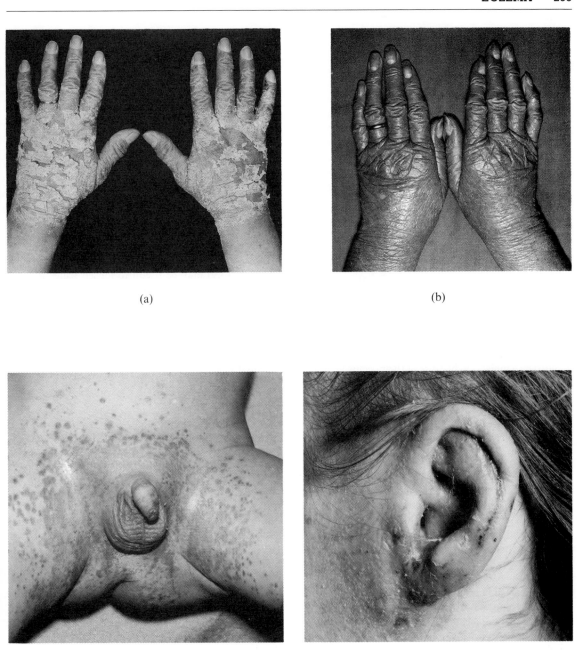

(a)

(b)

(c)

(d)

Fig. 13.4
Types of eczema: a) Contact dermatitis. The flaking crust has
been produced by the fluid from ruptured vesicles; b) The dried,
hardened, and non-elastic skin characteristic of exfoliative dermatitis; c) Widespread erythema and dried vesicles of napkin
rash; d) Greasy scales, inflammation, and erythema in
seborrhoeic dermatitis. (Compare with contact and exfoliative
dermatitis.)

residual detergents and antiseptics present in inadequately rinsed napkins.

Symptoms

The onset of napkin rash is rarely seen before the third week of life and resolves spontaneously on discontinuing napkin use. The condition is characterised by erythema (Fig. 13.4c) in the napkin area, and may be followed by skin peeling. Fine scaling may be apparent in chronic cases. Vesicles and ulcers may be present in severe cases, and dysuria may occur if the genitalia are affected. In some infants, napkin rash can be the first sign of a predisposition to chronic skin disorders (e.g. atopic dermatitis).

Treatment

Treatment comprises drying the skin surface and reducing the contact time with irritants. Parents should be encouraged to change napkins frequently and be instructed in correct laundering procedures. Exposing the skin to the air for as long as is practical may be beneficial. Mild topical corticosteroids (BNF 13.4) and an appropriate topical antifungal preparation (BNF 13.10.2) may be indicated. Ointment bases should be avoided on a moist skin because of their occlusive action, but may be useful for prophylaxis on unaffected skin. Emollients and barrier creams (BNF 13.2.1) may also help to prevent further outbreaks after healing.

Seborrhoeic Dermatitis

Definition and aetiology

Seborrhoeic dermatitis is an inflammatory condition of the skin of unknown cause. It affects areas of the body supplied by sebaceous glands, although the composition and flow of sebum is usually unaltered. Emotional disturbances, fatigue, or infection may precipitate the condition in predisposed adults, and a fungal infection has been implicated. It generally occurs between 18 and 40 years of age and is more common in men.

Cradle cap (infantile seborrhoeic dermatitis) is an inflammatory condition of the scalp in infants. It commonly occurs in association with napkin rash, although the cause is unknown. It is often seen in children with a predisposition to develop allergic disorders. The onset of cradle cap occurs during the first three months of life and generally resolves spontaneously within a year.

Symptoms

Seborrhoeic dermatitis is characterised by dry or greasy scales, mild erythema, and pruritus (Fig. 13.4d). Affected sites include the scalp, hair line, eyebrows, bridge of nose, sternum, external ear canal, and the area behind the ears. In severe cases, yellowish-red papules may be present. The distribution may extend to the axillae and inguinal and anal regions, and blepharitis may occur. In some cases, there is an increased susceptibility to infection.

Cradle cap is marked by thick yellow scales on the scalp, extending in some cases to the eyebrows and behind the ears. Other symptoms may include erythema. Small red papules may appear on the face, neck, and occasionally the trunk. Secondary infection may occur in severe cases.

Treatment

Treatment consists of medicated shampoos (BNF 13.9), topical corticosteroid preparations (BNF 13.4), and appropriate anti-infective skin preparations (BNF 13.10) for infected lesions. Keratolytics (BNF 13.5) may be indicated in severe cases.

In cradle cap, the application of olive oil or arachis oil (BNF 13.9) may be useful to loosen scales prior to cleansing with a mild shampoo. The use of potentially sensitising medicated shampoos should be avoided. Mild topical corticosteroids (BNF 13.4) may be indicated in severe cases.

Self-help organisation

National Eczema Society

Erythema Multiforme

Definition and aetiology

Erythema multiforme is an acute hypersensitivity reaction occurring in the skin and mucous membranes. It may be precipitated by drugs (e.g. barbiturates, penicillin, or sulphonamides), vaccines (e.g. BCG), viral infections (e.g. herpes simplex), and ionising radiation. In many cases, the cause is unknown.

Symptoms

The onset is generally sudden and marked by erythematous lesions, often with a purple centre (Fig. 13.5). They are symmetrically distributed over the extremities and, less often, the trunk and face. The lesions may be macules or slightly raised papules, gradually fading in 1 to 2 weeks. Vesicles may occur in similar sites and on the mucous membranes. The condition is often recurrent. The Stevens-Johnson syndrome is a very severe form characterised by bulla formation involving the eyes, genitalia, oral mucosa, and skin. Accompanying symptoms may include arthralgia, fever, and malaise. If left untreated, it may prove fatal.

Treatment

The causative agent should be identified and avoided where possible. Milder forms resolve spontaneously and may only need symptomatic treatment such as antipruritic preparations (BNF 13.3). Oral corticosteroids

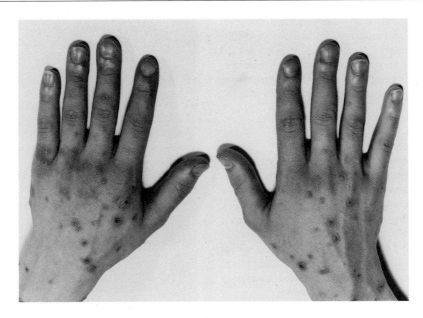

Fig. 13.5
Erythema multiforme. The circular lesions have a central purple area, and the similar distribution on both hands is characteristic.

(BNF 6.3.4) may be indicated in severe cases, and anti-bacterial drugs (BNF 5.1) may be necessary to treat or prevent secondary infection.

Erythema Nodosum

Definition and aetiology
Erythema nodosum is an acute inflammatory skin re-action characterised by erythematous nodules. It is most commonly caused by underlying streptococcal infec-tions or sarcoidosis. Other causes include mycotic and viral infections, tuberculosis, leprosy, psittacosis, and ulcerative colitis. Some drugs (e.g. sulphonamides, iodides, and oral contraceptives) may also precipitate this condition. The incidence of erythema nodosum is greater in females and is most frequently seen between 20 and 45 years of age.

Symptoms
The onset of erythema nodosum is often sudden and is characterised by red, painful, tender nodules appearing on the lower legs. Occasionally, the thighs, arms, or face may be affected. Characteristic nodular colour changes occur, from bluish-purple to yellowish-green, finally resembling a bruise. It is generally accompanied by arthralgia, fever, and malaise. Spontaneous resolution usually occurs in about 3 to 6 weeks. The condition may be recurrent on subsequent challenge by an offending agent or infection.

Treatment
Treatment of the underlying disorder and bed rest may be all that is required. In some cases, administration of aspirin or other non-steroidal anti-inflammatory drugs (BNF 10.1.1) may also be helpful. Ambulant patients should be encouraged to wear support bandages or stockings.

Folliculitis

Definition and aetiology
Folliculitis is a superficial inflammation of the upper part of the hair follicle, often caused by infection with *Staphylococcus aureus*. Folliculitis of a non-infective origin may arise as a result of chemical or physical trauma (e.g. contact with mineral oils, tar products, or adhesive dressings). Re-penetration of the skin by sharp shaved hairs results in the inflammatory condition pseudofolliculitis.

Symptoms
Folliculitis commonly occurs on the face and is marked by small papules or pustules at the point of emergence of the hairs. The condition may become chronic (*see* Sycosis Barbae).

Treatment
Suspected irritants should be avoided where possible. The use of a suitable skin disinfecting and cleansing

agent (BNF 13.11) may be of value and the application of an appropriate anti-infective skin preparation (BNF 13.10) may be necessary in severe cases. In many instances, however, no treatment is required. Pseudofolliculitis may be prevented by altering shaving technique to leave hairs a little longer, or by not shaving at all.

Haemangiomas

Definition and aetiology
Haemangiomas are benign, vascular tumours arising as a result of hyperplasia of blood vessels. Most are congenital or develop shortly after birth, and may be due to part of the angioderm remaining isolated as the vascular system develops. They may be superficial, subcutaneous, or a combination of the two. Superficial haemangiomas are more likely to be of the capillary type in which localised hyperplasia of the angioderm has taken place. Subcutaneous lesions are generally of the cavernous type which consist of irregular vascular spaces.

Strawberry Naevus

Definition and aetiology
A strawberry naevus is a superficial capillary haemangioma, which may develop subcutaneous components as it enlarges. It is usually not present at birth, but develops shortly afterwards.

Symptoms
Growth commences shortly after birth and progresses rapidly for a few weeks. The lesion then continues to enlarge slowly, generally reaching maximum size within 6 months. It appears as a soft, scarlet, well-defined swelling with a lobulated surface of variable size (Fig. 13.6). Any part of the body may be affected, but it occurs most frequently on the head and neck. Other sites include the trunk and anogenital region. The lesion may ulcerate, especially if near the mouth or in the nappy area. Bleeding may also occur although this is not usually serious. Lesions close to the eye may result in visual impairment. Spontaneous and complete regression occurs in most cases after 2 to 5 years, although some individuals may be left with a brown pigmentation, telangiectases, wrinkling, or scarring in the affected area.

Treatment
Reassurance is all that is required for most patients. Treatment is necessary only if there are complications or a poor cosmetic appearance is predicted subsequent to regression (i.e. ulcerative lesions or those with a deep subcutaneous component). Intralesional injections of corticosteroids or oral corticosteroids may facilitate shrinkage. Local injections of sclerosants may be necessary in those cases where regression is incomplete, or

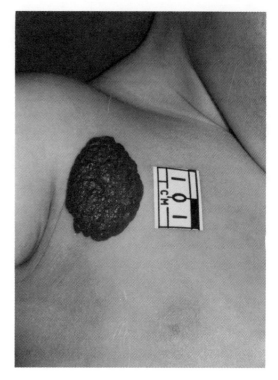

Fig. 13.6
Strawberry naevus in a young baby. The lobulated surface stands proud of the skin.

surgical excision may be required to remove any excess skin folds remaining.

Cavernous Haemangioma

Definition and aetiology
A cavernous haemangioma is subcutaneous but may be overlaid in some cases by a strawberry naevus.

Symptoms
It may be seen as a soft, bluish, ill-defined swelling beneath the skin, generally present at birth. It may occur at any site and regresses less readily than superficial haemangiomas.

Treatment
Treatment is as for a strawberry naevus, although it may be less successful.

Port Wine Stain

Definition and aetiology
This is a capillary haemangioma present in most cases at birth.

Symptoms

It occurs as a pink, red, or purple lesion of variable size, generally unilateral and appearing most commonly on the head. It is initially flat, but may gradually become raised and of a deeper colour. Most cases persist for life.

Treatment

Camouflaging preparations (BNF 13.8.2 and BNF Appendix 3) may be of value in cases where the cosmetic appearance causes the patient psychological distress. Laser therapy has been used with success in some cases.

Hereditary Angioedema

Definition and aetiology

Hereditary angioedema (which should be distinguished from angioedema, *see above*) is the result of an auto-somally dominant inherited deficiency or, in some cases, malfunction of C1 esterase inhibitor. The result is the continuous activation of C1, the first component of complement (*see also* Section 15.6). Attacks may be precipitated by emotional disturbances, viral infection, or trauma.

Symptoms

The condition is characterised by recurrent, hardened, painful swellings of the skin and mucous membranes. If the gastro-intestinal tract is affected, accompanying symptoms may include nausea and vomiting, colic, and occasionally obstruction. Common symptoms of urticaria are not present. Obstruction in the upper respiratory tract causes the death of about 20% of all cases before middle-age.

Treatment

Hereditary angioedema does not readily respond to the treatment used for urticaria. Fresh frozen plasma administered in the early stages of a severe attack may be beneficial in temporarily replacing the deficient enzyme inhibitor. Tranexamic acid and danazol (BNF 6.7.3) are of value in long-term management, and stanozolol (BNF 6.4.3) may be used for preventing attacks.

Hyperhidrosis

Definition and aetiology

Hyperhidrosis is characterised by overactivity of the sweat glands, resulting in excessive perspiration. It may be precipitated by an underlying systemic disorder (e.g. febrile illness, hyperthyroidism, an infection, malignant disease, or the menopause). Other causes include alcoholic intoxication, lesions in the sympathetic nervous system, obesity, and psychogenic factors.

Symptoms

Hyperhidrosis may be generalised or localised, common sites being the axillae, palms, and soles. The skin often appears pink and in severe cases may become macerated, fissured, or scaly. Decomposition of the sweat by bacteria and yeasts may result in an unpleasant odour (bromhidrosis).

Treatment

Any underlying systemic disorder should be treated, where possible. Sweat production in the feet may be reduced by soaking them in solutions of formaldehyde or glutaraldehyde. The local application of aluminium chloride salts (BNF 13.12) to the axillae may be beneficial. In severe cases, sympathectomy or excision of portions of axillary skin may be necessary.

Ichthyosis

Definition and aetiology

Ichthyosis is a generalised non-inflammatory skin disorder, characterised by abnormal scalings. This may be caused by overproduction of keratin or abnormalities in desquamation. It is inherited (e.g. ichthyosis vulgaris) or acquired following systemic diseases (e.g. carcinoma, Hodgkin's disease, hypothyroidism, and leprosy).

Symptoms

Ichthyosis is characterised by a rough and scaly skin surface which affects all parts of the body, although it is usually most severe on the lower legs (Fig. 13.7). There is often reduced secretion from the sebaceous and sweat glands, which exacerbates the condition. The symptoms may worsen during the winter months.

Treatment

Treatment is palliative and consists of the topical administration of emollients (BNF 13.2.1). Patients should be discouraged from excessive bathing and use of degreasing agents (e.g. soap). Removal of scale in severe cases may be assisted by the use of keratolytics (BNF 13.5). Etretinate (BNF 13.5) may be indicated in severe cases under hospital supervision.

Keloid

Definition and aetiology

A keloid is a raised nodule formed in the skin as a result of excessive amounts of collagen laid down during repair of connective tissue (e.g. after trauma). It may also arise spontaneously. The cause is unknown, although precipitating factors include burns, infections, surgical incisions (Fig. 13.8), tension on a wound, and the presence of foreign bodies (e.g. surgical sutures). Keloid formation is rare in infancy and the elderly, occurring

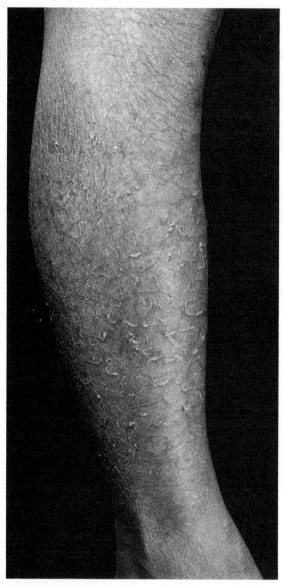

Fig. 13.7
Ichthyosis on the lower leg. This non-inflammatory condition can be readily distinguished from the forms of eczema illustrated in Fig. 13.4.

most commonly between puberty and 30 years of age. There is a genetic tendency and keloids occur more frequently in Negroes and women; pregnancy appears to increase the incidence.

Symptoms
Commonest sites of keloids include the chest, ear lobes, neck, and shoulders. A keloid is generally shiny, smooth, firm, and pink or red.

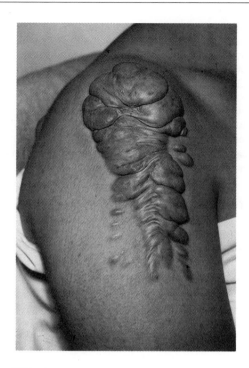

Fig. 13.8
A keloid occurring along the length of an incision on the shoulder.

Treatment
Local corticosteroid injections (BNF 10.1.2.2), radiotherapy, and compression therapy may each be of value alone, or as an adjuvant to surgical excision, to prevent reformation. Keloid formation may be prevented by avoiding all non-essential surgery in predisposed individuals. Where surgery is necessary, measures should be taken to prevent secondary infection and reduce the tension on wounds.

Lichen Planus

Definition and aetiology
Lichen planus is an inflammatory skin disorder characterised by collections of papules (lichen) which are small, shiny, and violet-coloured with angular borders. It appears to be idiopathic, although it may be associated with an altered state of immunity. It often occurs in conjunction with myasthenia gravis, thymoma, ulcerative colitis, and vitiligo. Drugs (e.g. antimalarials or gold) and chemicals (e.g. dyes used as developers in colour photography) may cause similar lichenoid eruptions. The onset of lichen planus is often insidious and generally occurs between 30 and 60 years of age, affecting more women than men. It is usually self-limiting and

will regress spontaneously within 6 to 18 months, although it may recur.

Symptoms

The condition may be acute or chronic, the acute form showing a sudden onset, a more generalised distribution of lesions over the whole body, and a shorter course. The characteristic lesions are often distributed symmetrically and may occur at any site. They appear most commonly on the wrists, ankles, and trunk. They may be separate or confluent, linear or annular, and may exhibit white lines (Wickham's striae) on the surface of the papule. The area may show increased pigmentation subsequent to healing. Hypertrophic lesions may form, usually on the lower legs, if the papules increase in size and thickness, and these may result in atrophy and scarring. Papules are rarely seen on the scalp, but an associated complication for some patients is permanent patchy hair loss. Pruritus of varying degree occurs in most cases of lichen planus. Some patients have bluish-white linear lesions on mucosal surfaces, especially the mouth, but also arising in the anogenital region, the larynx, and nails. Oral lesions may become eroded and painful.

Treatment

Treatment is symptomatic and may include the application of topical fluorinated corticosteroid preparations (BNF 13.4) and oral antihistamines (BNF 3.4.1) to relieve pruritus. Corticosteroids in lozenges or in dental paste (BNF 12.3.1) may be indicated in cases of erosive oral lesions. Systemic corticosteroids (BNF 6.3.4) may be necessary in severe cases.

Mole

Definition and aetiology

A mole (melanocytic naevus or naevocytic naevus) is a benign pigmented circumscribed growth of the skin. It is idiopathic and formed by proliferation of melanocytes at the junction between the dermis and epidermis. Moles are common and occur in all races. Their development is greatest in children and adolescents, decreasing with advancing age.

Symptoms

There are several different forms which are classified histologically. Most are small (<15 mm diameter) and may vary in colour from flesh-tinted to yellow or light brown through to dark brownish-black. They may be flat, raised, or pedunculated, and with a smooth or rough surface. They can arise at any site on the body and may be hairy (Fig. 13.9). Occasionally, melanomas may arise from the melanocytes in a mole.

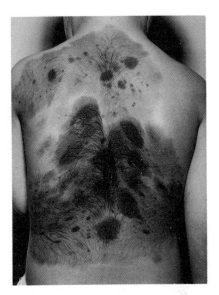

Fig. 13.9
Widespread distribution of pigmented and hairy moles on the back of a young girl.

Treatment

Excision and biopsy may be necessary in cases where a mole has shown a sudden increase in size, changed in colour, become inflamed, painful, or pruritic, or started to bleed or ulcerate. In most cases, however, treatment is unnecessary and the patient should be reassured that moles are generally quite harmless.

Pemphigus

Definition and aetiology

Pemphigus is a group of skin diseases characterised by severe and chronic blistering. It is thought to be due to an auto-immune reaction. It is often associated with myasthenia gravis and thymoma, and may be precipitated by drugs (e.g. captopril, penicillamine, or rifampicin). Pemphigus tends to occur in middle or old age and is rarely seen in children. The incidence is greater in specific populations (e.g. the Brazilian, Indian, and Jewish races).

Symptoms

The initial stage is characterised by bullae on the oral mucosa, formed as a result of the destruction of intercellular bonds between epidermal cells (acantholysis). The lesions are painful and slow to heal. Other mucous membranes may be affected, including the conjunctiva, upper oesophagus, and vulva. Similar eruptions occur on the skin (Fig. 13.10) several months later, and commonly affect the face, trunk, groin, and axillae. Second-

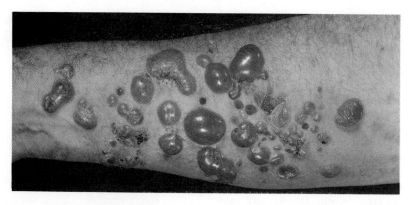

Fig. 13.10
The severe multiple blisters characteristic of pemphigus.

ary skin infection and septicaemia may be further complications. The condition may be fatal if left untreated.

Treatment
Treatment consists of the oral administration of very high doses of corticosteroids (BNF 6.3.4). Immunosuppressants (BNF 8.2) may be indicated in cases where a reduced corticosteroid dose is necessary. An appropriate antibacterial drug (BNF 5.1) may be necessary to treat secondary infection.

Photosensitivity

Definition and aetiology
Photosensitivity is an abnormal reaction of the skin to ultraviolet radiation. Sunburn is caused by excessive exposure to UVB light (wavelength 290 to 320nm). It should be distinguished from phototoxicity, which can develop from exposure to normal amounts of sunlight in sensitive or sensitised individuals. Precipitating factors of photosensitivity caused by phototoxicity include contact with perfumes, plants, and preparations containing coal tar, or ingestion of drugs (e.g. griseofulvin, nalidixic acid, sulphonamides, tetracyclines, or thiazides). It may be caused or aggravated by disease (e.g. porphyria or systemic lupus erythematosus).

Symptoms
Symptoms are of varying intensity and include erythema, oedema, urticaria, eruptions of vesicles or bullae, and in chronic cases, thickened scales. Herpes labialis often results from exposure of the latent herpes simplex virus to strong sunlight.

Treatment
Treatment of any underlying disorder or the removal of precipitating substances will be effective in many cases.

Where this is not possible, preventive measures include avoiding exposure to sunlight or covering exposed areas. The application of sunscreening preparations (BNF 13.8.1) may be of value, particularly the reflectant barrier-type such as titanium dioxide paste (BNF 13.2.1). Topical corticosteroids (BNF 13.4) may be beneficial in treating severe reactions.

Pilonidal Disease

Definition and aetiology
Pilonidal disease is characterised by the formation of a cyst or sinus in the midline of the sacrococcygeal area. This condition occurs most commonly in young hirsute males.

Symptoms
The lesion may be pigmented and contain hair, and is asymptomatic unless infected, in which case abscesses may form.

Treatment
Acute abscesses may be treated by incision and drainage. Chronic sinuses must be completely removed by surgical excision followed by closure.

Pityriasis

Definition
Pityriasis is a term applied to disorders of the skin in which fine branny scales are formed.

Pityriasis Alba

Definition and aetiology
Pityriasis alba is a common non-specific eczema of unknown cause, although impetigo, exposure to sunlight, and soap have been suggested as aggravating factors.

Symptoms

The condition generally occurs in children and adolescents. It most commonly affects the face, particularly the cheeks and chin, but other sites include the neck, shoulders, and upper arms. The lesions are well-defined, round, or oval; they may be skin-coloured (and barely visible), or erythematous. They may become depigmented with persistent fine scaling. It may last for a year or more and is often recurrent, although it usually clears completely by puberty.

Treatment

There is little effective treatment. Application of emollient creams (BNF 13.2.1) may facilitate removal of scales and prevent dryness.

Pityriasis Capitis

Definition and aetiology

Pityriasis capitis (dandruff) is a chronic non-inflammatory condition of the scalp characterised by the excessive production of scales. The cause is unknown, although it may arise as a result of increased sebaceous activity and hormonal changes occurring at puberty. The incidence of dandruff peaks between 10 and 20 years of age and is rarely seen in children.

Symptoms

The condition is marked by greyish-white scales which may be dry or greasy. They can occur in small patches or involve the entire scalp.

Treatment

The frequent use of mild shampoos may be beneficial in removing scales. Shampoos containing cytostatic agents (BNF 13.9) may help to slow down the rate of production of epidermal cells. Keratolytic agents (BNF 13.6) may be useful, and topical corticosteroids (BNF 13.4) may be indicated in severe cases.

Pityriasis Lichenoides

Definition and aetiology

Pityriasis lichenoides resembles psoriasis in some of its features, and occurs mainly in adolescents and young adults. The cause is unknown.

Symptoms

The chronic form is characterised by small reddish-brown papules, each with an adherent but detachable scale, distributed over the trunk and limbs. Individual lesions generally disappear in 3 to 4 weeks, but new crops continually form and the condition may persist for years before completely resolving. An acute form exists and has a shorter course, often resolving within 6 months. It may be preceded or accompanied by mild symptoms of fever, headache, and malaise. The lesions are oedematous and may become haemorrhagic, resulting in scarring on healing. Transient depigmented areas may be a consequence of both acute and chronic forms.

Treatment

There is little effective treatment, although psoralens and ultraviolet A (PUVA) (BNF 13.5) has been beneficial in some cases.

Pityriasis Rosea

Definition and aetiology

Pityriasis rosea is an acute, self-limiting, common skin disorder, possibly of viral origin. It occurs mainly between 10 and 30 years of age, and is less common during the summer months.

Symptoms

It is characterised by a single, red, scaly, round or oval macule (the herald patch, Fig. 13.11) appearing on the trunk or upper limbs. Smaller red papules and pink oval macules covered with silvery grey scales appear a few days later. The macules lose their pink colour, wrinkle in the centre, and peel outwards to form a collarette of scale around the margins. Pruritus may be present, but constitutional symptoms are usually absent and the condition generally resolves in 6 to 8 weeks without further recurrence.

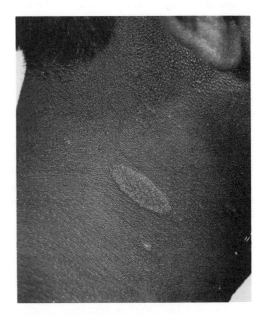

Fig. 13.11
The single oval macule (herald patch) of pityriasis rosea.

Treatment

Most cases require no treatment. Soap, water, and wool may irritate the lesions and contact should be minimised. Application of calamine cream or lotion (BNF 13.3) or topical corticosteroid preparations (BNF 13.4) may be beneficial in relieving irritation.

Pruritus

Definition and aetiology

Pruritus (itching) is a cutaneous sensation from which relief is sought by scratching or rubbing the skin. Localised pruritus may arise as a result of an allergic reaction or may be caused by eczema, insect bites, or infections (e.g. intestinal worms, which cause pruritus ani). Factors contributing to generalised pruritus include dry skin, atopic and contact dermatitis, lichen planus, urticaria, and psoriasis. Systemic disorders (e.g. diabetes mellitus), hepatic, renal, or malignant disease, and polycythaemia may also be responsible. Many drugs (e.g. antidepressants, barbiturates, chloroquine, and opioid analgesics) produce pruritus. Emotional disturbances may precipitate or exacerbate the condition. In some individuals, essential pruritus occurs without any apparent cause.

Symptoms

The symptoms are due to self-inflicted skin damage and include varying degrees of erythema, urticarial eruptions, excoriation, fissures, and crusting. Lichenification and changes in pigmentation may occur after prolonged scratching and rubbing.

Treatment

The cause should be identified and avoided where possible, and any underlying disorder treated. Patients should be encouraged to avoid dry atmospheres, the intake of vasodilators (e.g. alcohol), wearing rough or irritating clothing, and becoming overheated. Oral antihistamines (BNF 3.4.1) may be beneficial, especially the sedative type if pruritus at night is a problem. Local applications containing calamine or crotamiton (BNF 13.3), and emollients (BNF 13.2.1) may also be of value. Local corticosteroid preparations (BNF 13.4) may provide relief in some cases, but should not be used indiscriminately.

Psoriasis

Definition and aetiology

Psoriasis is a common chronic recurrent skin disorder of unknown cause. There is a genetic predisposition to develop the condition, although individual attacks may be precipitated by a variety of factors. These include emotional disturbances, hormonal changes, strong sunlight, streptococcal infection of the throat, local trauma, topical irritants, and drugs (e.g. chloroquine or lithium). A resistant form of psoriasis often develops following withdrawal of systemic corticosteroids.

Symptoms

The onset is gradual and usually occurs in young adults. An increase in the rate of proliferation of epidermal cells results in well-defined, slightly raised, dry, vivid-red lesions covered with silvery scales (Fig. 13.12). Common sites include the scalp, elbows, knees, and lower back, and less commonly the axillae, anogenital region, eyebrows, and nails. There may be remissions and relapses throughout life. It rarely affects the patient's general health, although psoriatic arthritis and generalised exfoliation are serious complications which may occasionally arise.

Treatment

In many cases, the removal of any precipitating factors, reassurance, and simple remedies such as emollients

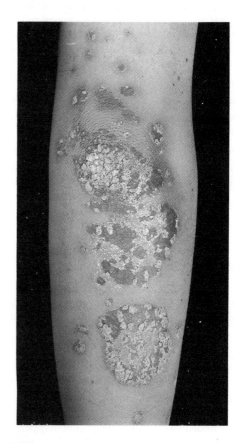

Fig. 13.12
Psoriasis on the elbow and lower arm. Silvery scales have been shed, revealing erythema and thickened underlying epithelium.

(BNF 13.2.1) are all that is required. Topical preparations containing keratolytics (BNF 13.5) to facilitate scale removal may be of value. Psoralens and ultraviolet A (PUVA) (BNF 13.5) in controlled doses may be beneficial in severe cases. Antimetabolites (BNF 8.1.3) and etretinate (BNF 13.5) may be used under expert supervision to treat resistant lesions.

Self-help organisation
Psoriasis Association

Pyoderma Gangrenosum

Definition and aetiology
Pyoderma gangrenosum is a non-infective necrosis of the cutaneous tissues. The exact cause is unknown, although it may be caused by a disorder of the immune system. It is often associated with Crohn's disease, rheumatoid arthritis, and ulcerative colitis. Lesions may also arise in the presence of existing skin disease (e.g. acne) or at a site of trauma.

Symptoms
The condition is characterised by two different types of lesion, which may be present simultaneously or sequentially. Both are painful and rapidly ulcerate. Tender erythematous nodules, which become blue in the centre before ulcerating, may develop on any part of the body, but most commonly occur on the face, calves, thighs, and buttocks. A scar often remains after healing. Pustular vesicles can also occur at any of the above sites and on the eyelids, lips, and oral mucosa. Haemorrhagic bullae may occur in the presence of leukaemia.

Treatment
Treatment consists of the oral administration of very high doses of corticosteroids (BNF 6.3.4). In addition, any underlying disorder should be treated.

Sebaceous Cyst

Definition and aetiology
Cysts, commonly referred to as sebaceous cysts, are more correctly termed epidermoid cysts. The contents consist primarily of keratin and its breakdown products, although follicular and sebaceous materials may also be present. They arise in damaged or blocked pilosebaceous follicles. Cysts containing sebum as their main component are called steatocystoma multiplex and are relatively uncommon.

Symptoms
Sebaceous cysts are common in adults, and frequently occur on the face, ears, scalp, neck, upper trunk, and scrotum. They are pale, firm, globular swellings of variable size, and may be single (Fig. 13.13) or multiple. They enlarge slowly, and are usually painless and harmless unless they become infected and result in abscess formation and suppuration.

Treatment
Removal is unnecessary unless a cyst is infected or cosmetically unacceptable. Infections may be treated

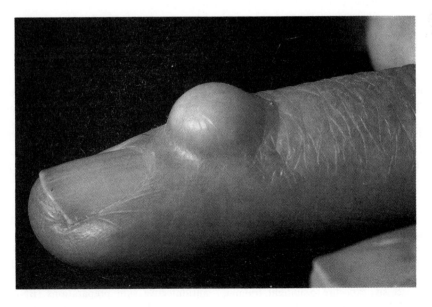

Fig. 13.13
A sebaceous cyst on a finger.

using an appropriate oral antibacterial drug (BNF 5.1), and the cyst drained through an incision. Larger cysts may require surgical excision. The cyst wall must be removed to prevent recurrence.

Sunburn

Definition and aetiology
Sunburn is an inflammatory skin condition resulting from excessive exposure to ultraviolet radiation, in particular to the shorter wavelengths of 290 nm to 320 nm (i.e. UVB).

Symptoms
The extent of the reaction varies between individuals, the most susceptible being pale-skinned people. Erythema usually appears 2 to 8 hours after exposure and fades within 36 hours. Symptoms of heavier doses include bullae, oedema, pain, and tenderness, which generally reach a peak on the second day. Extensive areas of sunburnt skin may result in constitutional symptoms (e.g. fever, malaise, and headache). Hyperpigmentation and epidermal thickening occur in varying degrees a few days later, and constitute an attempt to protect the skin against further doses of radiation. Prolonged and repeated exposure may in time cause premature ageing of the skin and the development of malignant disease (e.g. melanoma and rodent ulcer).

Treatment
Further exposure should be avoided until successful treatment has been completed. The skin should be cooled by cold-water compresses or sponging. Topical corticosteroid preparations (BNF 13.4) may be prescribed to reduce minor inflammation, and non-opioid analgesics (BNF 4.7.1) may be indicated for pain. Systemic corticosteroids (BNF 6.3.4) may be necessary in severe cases. The patient should be counselled on preventive measures, which include using sunscreening preparations (BNF 13.8.1) and gradual suntanning to allow the skin to acclimatise.

Telangiectasia

Definition and aetiology
A telangiectasia is a lesion on the skin or mucous membranes formed by a group of permanently dilated, superficial blood vessels. Contributory factors include the prolonged topical administration of fluorinated corticosteroids, prolonged vasodilatation (e.g. in rosacea and varicose veins), or atrophy of local supporting tissue caused by ageing, excessive exposure to sunlight, trauma, or X-ray therapy. Telangiectases may also accompany systemic diseases (e.g. dermatomyositis, systemic lupus erythematosus, and systemic sclerosis). Some forms may be genetically inherited, although in many cases the cause is unknown.

Symptoms
Lesions may be linear, punctate, spider-like, or stellate and can be accompanied by increased melanin pigmentation. They are generally small and dull-red in colour, and blanch temporarily on the application of pressure.

Treatment
In many cases no treatment is required, although camouflaging preparations (BNF 13.8.2 and BNF Appendix 3) may be used to conceal cosmetically unacceptable lesions. Where appropriate, small telangiectases may be destroyed by cauterisation, cryotherapy, or electrolysis.

Toxic Epidermal Necrolysis

Definition and aetiology
Toxic epidermal necrolysis (scalded skin syndrome or Ritter-Lyell syndrome) is a serious skin disorder characterised by exfoliation of extensive areas of necrotic epidermis. The cause is unknown, although it may arise as a reaction to drugs (e.g. barbiturates, ethambutol, phenolphthalein, phenytoin, or sulphonamides). It may also be associated with viral infections, leukaemia, and radiotherapy. In infants, it usually occurs as a result of staphylococcal infection.

Symptoms
The onset is rapid and initial symptoms include erythema and tenderness, often accompanied by anorexia, fever, and malaise. In addition, flaccid bullae may be present. Desquamation of the skin, which may be localised or extensive, occurs after 36 to 48 hours and leaves raw, painful areas. The prognosis in adults is poor due to possible complications (e.g. secondary infection, and fluid and electrolyte imbalance). Scarring, and loss of hair and nails may follow healing. The prognosis is more favourable in the staphylococcal-induced form because the damage to the epidermis does not extend to as great a depth.

Treatment
Any underlying infection or disorder should be treated and causative agents withdrawn or changed. Other measures include hospitalisation, correction of fluid and electrolyte imbalance, and minimal physical handling to reduce the degree of skin loss. Careful application of anti-infective skin preparations (BNF 13.10) may be necessary. Infants may require isolation to prevent contagion.

Ulcers

Definition and aetiology
The formation of an ulcer in the skin is caused by local destruction of the epidermis and part of the underlying dermis. It may be simple and without further complications, or chronic and unresponsive to treatment.

Varicose (venous) ulcers are caused by venous stasis, which may be a consequence of deep vein thrombosis, varicose veins, or peripheral vascular disease (e.g. in diabetes mellitus). Ischaemic (arterial) ulcers are caused by a diminished arterial blood supply to the skin, which may be a consequence of atherosclerosis, hypertension, or scar tissue. Decubitus ulcers occur at sites exposed to prolonged pressure. Infections, malnutrition, or trauma may precipitate ulceration in predisposed individuals, or complicate existing ulcers.

Symptoms
Venous ulcers occur most commonly in the elderly, particularly in women. They generally occur on the lower leg and are of variable size, encircling the whole leg in severe cases. There is an initial erythema which progresses to a bluish-red discoloration and finally to necrosis (Fig. 13.14). The edge is often irregular in outline and may be indurated. The skin around the ulcer may show deposits of haemosiderin. Ischaemic ulcers are more painful than venous ulcers, have less pigmentation in the surrounding skin, and have well-defined margins. They frequently occur on the front of the tibia. There is little exudate and healing is generally slow.

Treatment
Any underlying disorder should be treated. Patients should also be encouraged to exercise when possible to improve the circulation. Successful treatment of venous ulcers may be promoted by improving venous drainage by the use of compression bandages and support stockings. Non-ambulant patients should spend part of each day with their legs in an elevated position. Treatment of the ulcer itself consists of debridement using various skin cleansing or desloughing agents and enzyme preparations (BNF 13.11). Dextranomer beads and gel and colloid dressings (BNF 13.13.8) may be beneficial. The use of anti-infective skin preparations should be avoided unless absolutely necessary, as these can be sensitising.

Urticaria

Definition and aetiology
Urticaria is characterised by transient erythema and wheals in the dermis. It is the result of localised oedema caused by increased permeability of the small blood vessel walls due to the release of mediators (e.g.

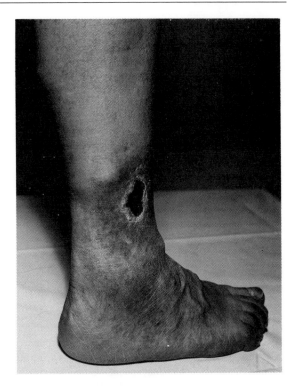

Fig. 13.14
A varicose ulcer. The central area of necrosis is delineated by an irregular border and surrounded by pigmentation caused by deposition of haemosiderin.

histamine, kinins, or prostaglandins). Acute urticaria may be precipitated by a variety of stimulants (e.g. drugs, foods or food additives, and underlying systemic infections or disorders). The cause is unknown in 50% of chronic cases, but psychogenic or physical factors (e.g. heat, cold, or sunlight) may be important.

Symptoms
The first common symptom is pruritus. It is followed by large or small wheals, which may occur at any site (Fig. 13.15), and disappear after a few hours. The larger wheals characteristically show a white centre surrounded by a ring of erythema. In some cases, erythema occurs without wheals, and occasionally bullae may be present. Larger swellings occur more diffusely and may be characteristic of angioedema. The condition is often self-limiting. Acute urticaria generally disappears within 1 to 7 days, while chronic cases may take up to two years to regress.

Treatment
Where possible, the cause should be identified and avoided, and any underlying disorder treated. The

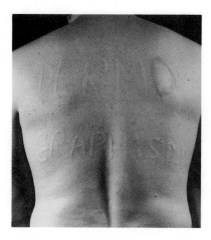

Fig. 13.15
The localised oedema of urticaria can be illustrated by dermatographism.

patient should be counselled to avoid potentially
sensitising agents (e.g. azo colouring agents and benzo-
ates used as food additives, and salicylates). Oral antihistamines (BNF 3.4.1) may be of value in relieving
symptoms, and oral corticosteroids (BNF 6.3.4) may be
indicated in severe cases. Adrenaline (BNF 3.4.3) may be
required in severe acute attacks).

Vitiligo

Definition and aetiology
Vitiligo is an acquired condition characterised by lesions
devoid of pigment, possibly caused by a toxin or an auto-
immune reaction which destroys melanocytes. It often
arises in association with Addison's disease, diabetes
mellitus, melanoma, myasthenia gravis, pernicious
anaemia, and thyroid disorders. It may be idiopathic or
inherited.

Symptoms
The condition affects all races and generally develops
before 20 years of age. Common sites initially affected
include the face and neck, and areas exposed to trauma
(e.g. knuckles, hands, elbows, knees, ankles, and feet). It
spreads gradually, and in rare cases may affect the entire
skin surface. The lesions, which generally show a symmetrical distribution, have well-defined and often
hyperpigmented margins (Fig. 13.16). The melanocytes
of the hair follicles are usually unaffected, although
hairs in older lesions may become white. Spontaneous
repigmentation, commencing at the hair follicles, occurs
in a small proportion of cases but is rarely complete.
The condition does not affect general health, although

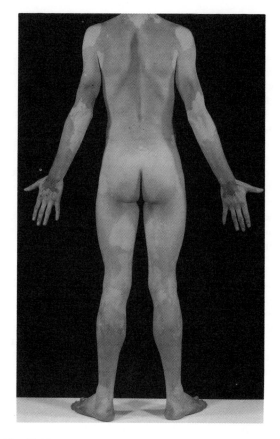

Fig. 13.16
Widespread vitiligo in a young man. The symmetrical distribution of the areas of depigmentation (e.g. around the elbows,
shoulders, hands, and buttocks) is clearly visible.

there is an increased tendency to sunburn in the depigmented areas.

Treatment
Cosmetic camouflage preparations (BNF 13.8.2 and
BNF Appendix 3) may be of value, and sunscreening
preparations (BNF 13.8.1) should be applied to exposed
lesions. Skin bleaching agents may be used to remove the
few remaining pigmented areas in cases of extensive
vitiligo.

13.2   ANATOMY AND PHYSIOLOGY OF THE SKIN

The Skin
The skin is one component of the integumentary
system, which also includes the nails, hair, sebaceous

and sudoriferous glands, and ceruminous glands. It is the single largest system in the body, and provides one of the major routes through which the external environment is monitored and experienced. It is an organ which is being continuously replenished to replace cells lost or damaged.

The skin may be considered to consist of a layer of dermis supporting an outer layer of epidermis and padded from within by a layer of fat (Fig. 13.17). The microscopic structure, however, is considerably more complex reflecting the diverse roles that the skin plays.

The outermost layer of the skin is composed of the epidermis. It consists of four types of cells of which the bulk are the keratinocytes. Keratinocytes are formed from the deepest layer of the epidermis, the stratum basale (stratum germinativum), and migrate upwards to the surface. In their passage towards the surface, the cells are responsible for the formation of a protein, keratin. The waterproof keratin resides in the outermost layer of the epidermis, the stratum corneum, within denucleated dead keratinocytes. The cells of the stratum corneum also provide a barrier to other potentially harmful agents (e.g. bacteria, heat, and light waves). Dead cells are eventually sloughed off the surface of the epidermis and continually replaced by new cells from below. The period between their formation in the basal layer and their loss is approximately 2 to 4 weeks.

The epidermis also contains melanocytes, Langerhans cells, and Granstein cells. Melanocytes synthesise the pigment melanin from the amino acid tyrosine, and the rate of melanin synthesis, rather than the number of melanocytes, determines the darkness of the skin. Increased production is induced by exposure to ultraviolet radiation. As a result, the degree of skin tanning is increased, and the underlying dermis is protected from the harmful effects of further irradiation. The rate of synthesis and distribution of melanin is also affected by an anterior pituitary hormone, melanocyte-stimulating hormone. The Langerhans cells are similar to melanocytes but are derived from the bone marrow. Both the Langerhans cells and the Granstein cells play an active role in the immune system. They are responsible for rendering T-cells aware of the presence of antigens that penetrate the upper layers of the epidermis.

Immediately below the epidermis is the dermis. This layer of the skin is highly vascularised and innervated, and contains hair follicles and sebaceous glands. The bulk of the dermis comprises a network of elastic and collagen fibres throughout a bed of connective tissue,

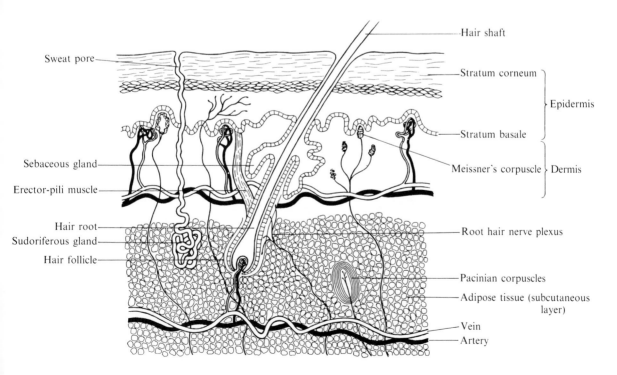

Fig. 13.17
Skin section.

which imparts extensibility, elasticity, and strength to the skin.

The sensation of touch is provided by the presence of Meissner's corpuscles in dermal projections into the epidermis, and by epidermal tactile discs. Root hair nerve plexuses, which surround hair follicles, transmit sensations induced by the movement of the hair. Naked nerve endings are also widely distributed over the surface of the skin. Pressure on the surface is monitored by Pacinian (lamellated) corpuscles located within the dermal projections into the subcutaneous fat layer.

The sensation of pain is monitored by pain receptors (nociceptors) distributed throughout the skin. An awareness of pain in the skin is described as superficial somatic pain, whilst pain arising in deeper structural tissues (e.g. tendons and muscles) is described as deep somatic pain. The nerve impulse generated by stimulation of the nociceptors is transmitted to the central nervous system via the spinal and cranial nerves.

Hair

One of the most distinctive features of the skin is the presence of hair. Each hair consists of a shaft, the majority of which lies above the surface of the skin, and a root, which lies within the dermis. In dark hair, the central layer of the shaft contains pigmented cells, whereas the same cells in white hair are filled with air. The root of the hair is contained within a follicle whose base is enlarged to form a bulbar structure. This swelling contains the blood supply to nourish the hair, and the germinal cells to produce a new hair when the old one is shed.

The primary function of hair is protection (e.g. prevention of the effects of harmful radiation on the scalp and entry of objects into cavities). Hair grows at the rate of approximately 1 cm per month and has an average life of three years. Although the numbers vary considerably, there may be about 300 000 hairs on the scalp, and of these about 50 to 100 are shed each day.

Glands of the Skin

The majority of the sebaceous glands, which secrete sebum, are closely associated with the hair follicles (forming the pilosebaceous unit). Sebaceous glands are widely distributed over most of the body with the exception of the soles of the feet and the palms of the hands. Glands not associated with hair follicles, and which secrete sebum directly onto the surface of the skin, may be found in the tarsal glands of the eyelid, the lips, and in genital regions. The activity of these glands is stimulated by androgens and inhibited by oestrogens. Sebum is an oily fluid containing wax esters, triglycerides, squalene, and sterol esters and serves to moisturise the skin and hair, limit the evaporation of water from the surface of the skin; it is bacteriostatic.

Sudoriferous (sweat) glands, which may be classified as apocrine or eccrine, occur all over the body. Apocrine glands are localised to the pigmented areas of the breast, the axillae, and the pubic area, and only become active at puberty. Body odour is produced by the bacterial decomposition of the sweat from apocrine glands. Eccrine glands are more widely distributed than apocrine glands. About 500 mL of sweat may be normally produced by the 3 or 4 million eccrine glands each day. Sweat comprises a mixture of components (e.g. inorganic salts, urea, ammonia, and lactic acid), but eccrine sweat is less viscous than apocrine sweat. The production of sweat is a major component of thermoregulation, and only a minor contributor to the excretion of body waste.

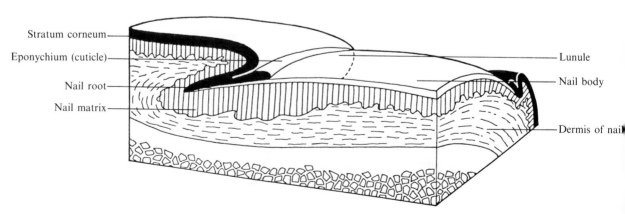

Fig. 13.18
Longitudinal section showing the structure of a nail.

The activity of the glands is regulated by cholinergic neurones, which are controlled by the hypothalamus. Increased activity, particularly of glands of the hands and feet, may occur in response to anxiety and stress.

Nails

A nail is a plate of flattened, keratinised, epithelial scales located on the upper portion of the end of each digit (Fig. 13.18). The fingernails are used primarily to assist in picking up small objects and for scratching. Growth of a nail occurs by the conversion of epithelial cells in the nail matrix (nail bed) into nail cells at the root of the nail. The growth of the nail from its root forces the nail body forward to the tip of the digit. Toenails grow at a slower rate (approximately 1 cm in 9 to 24 months) than fingernails (1 cm in 3 months).

Chapter 14

MEDICAL MICROBIOLOGY

14.1 INTRODUCTION

Micro-organisms are living entities that are visible only with the aid of a microscope. They are of importance to pharmacists for a number of reasons:

- They are the causative agents of infections.
- Some of them, particularly the actinomycetes, are the source of antibacterials used in the control of these diseases.
- Their products can be used in the form of vaccines or antisera to immunise man against infection.
- Chemical and physical methods of sterilisation have to be applied to many pharmaceutical preparations (e.g. injections, eye-drops, and surgical dressings), and the efficiency of these processes has to be checked. Tests for sterility must be carried out on the final products as routine controls.
- Disinfectants have to be formulated which will kill micro-organisms without affecting the materials treated, and the suitability of these disinfectants has to be assessed.
- Many pharmaceutical preparations will support the growth of bacteria and moulds on storage and must be preserved.

- The quality control of pharmaceutical products requires regular inspection for microbial count at all stages of manufacture.

It is amongst the micro-organisms that the most powerful poisons known and the most resistant forms of life are found. Pharmacists must therefore be armed with a sound knowledge of their characteristics to fulfil their role in combating disease.

Relationships between Groups of Organisms

All organisms may be classified in 1 of 3 kingdoms, animals, plants, or protists. Protists are further subdivided into algae, bacteria, fungi, and protozoa, and thus include photosynthetic and non-photosynthetic micro-organisms. They are differentiated from animals and plants by their low level of organisation, and many micro-organisms in this group are unicellular or coenocytic.

A further classification of organisms is based on the cell type making up their structure. The eukaryotic cell is the basic structural unit of animals, plants, fungi, protozoa, and most algae. It possesses an external, semipermeable, cytoplasmic membrane and contains discrete membrane-bound organelles. These include a nucleus, Golgi body, mitochondria, chloroplasts (in photosynthetic organisms), lysosomes, and vacuoles. There is an endoplasmic reticulum which ramifies throughout the cytoplasm, is continuous with the cytoplasmic and nuclear membranes, and has ribosomes attached to its surface.

Bacteria and bluish-green algae are made up of prokaryotic cells. These are much less complex, possessing a poorly defined nucleus and ribosomes within the protoplasm, and are bound by a cytoplasmic membrane.

The cells of plants and some micro-organisms also have a protective outer cell wall.

Viruses form a separate class altogether and are sharply differentiated from any cellular organism. They could be regarded as a link between complex macromolecules (e.g. DNA, RNA, and proteins) and the simplest form of prokaryotic cell.

Although helminths cannot be strictly classed as micro-organisms, they are included in this Chapter to complete the discussion of organisms that can cause disease.

14.2   BACTERIA

Bacteria are small, unicellular, prokaryotic protists which possess a relatively simple morphological structure compared with fungi or protozoa. They are, however, micro-organisms of highly complex enzymatic behaviour which enables them to adapt to a wide variety of environments. They are universally distributed in nature, being found in soil, in fresh and sea water, at all levels of the atmosphere, and on and in animals and vegetation. The infections caused by bacteria are described in Section 5.2.

Morphology

Bacteria exist in three basic shapes which can be described as spherical or ovoid (coccus), cylindrical or rod-shaped (bacillus), or helical (spirillum). The cocci range in size from $0.75\,\mu m$ to $1.25\,\mu m$ in diameter, and the bacilli from $0.7\,\mu m$ to $8.0\,\mu m$ in length. The spirillar forms are very variable, from the smallest vibrio of $1\,\mu m$ in length to multiple coiled types $18\,\mu m$ to $20\,\mu m$ long. Individual bacterial cells may remain attached to each other after cell division and form typical aggregates. The cocci can thus form chains (e.g. streptococci) or grape-like clusters (e.g. staphylococci). Bacilli may also produce chains, although this is only typical of certain

groups. 'Higher' bacteria (e.g. *Actinomyces* and *Streptomyces*) are filamentous and form mycelia in a similar way to fungi.

When growing in a mass on solid media, colonies are produced whose shape may be typical for that bacterium.

The three main parts of most bacterial cells are:

- the exterior cell wall

  This is a rigid, relatively permeable structure of considerable strength, defining the shape and maintaining the integrity of the cell. It contains mucopeptide which is responsible for strength, and other components which differ in Gram-negative and Gram-positive bacteria (*see* Classification below).

- the inner cytoplasmic membrane

  This area of intense enzymatic activity lies immediately beneath the cell wall, and is composed of lipids and lipoproteins. It is semipermeable, controls the passage of substances into and out of the cell, and is responsible for the cell's energy supply.

The cell wall and the cytoplasmic membrane are collectively known as the cell envelope.

- the protoplast

  This comprises the interior cytoplasm of the cell and nuclear material. The chromosome exists as a closed circle of double-stranded DNA, without a nuclear membrane. Further DNA is contained in circular plasmids present in the cytoplasm. The cytoplasm also contains ribosomes which are composed of RNA and other proteins, and are the sites of protein synthesis. Some bacteria may also contain transient granules of cellular reserve materials (e.g. volutin granules, polysaccharide granules, fat droplets, and elemental sulphur in sulphur bacteria).

Some bacteria secrete complex polymers which form an external glycocalyx capsule (*see also* Section 15.5). These polymers are generally polysaccharides, although some species secrete polypeptides. The capsule may contain toxins which can be responsible for the virulence of the micro-organism. Bacteria capable of producing capsules only do so in the correct environment.

Some species are motile by means of flagella. These are very fine, hair-like processes of a wavy form composed of a specific protein, flagellin. They are often longer than the micro-organism and may be arranged at the poles of the cell or all over its surface (peritrichous types). The flagella rotate rapidly about their long axis, thus driving the cell through fluids.

The surface of many bacteria (especially Gram-negative species) is covered with numerous, fine, shorter threads called fimbriae or pili. They are composed of a single protein, fibrilin, and in some species facilitate adhesion of the cell to surfaces.

Metabolism

All bacteria require a source of water, nitrogen, and carbon in relatively large quantities, and phosphorus and sulphur in smaller amounts. In addition, many inorganic ions (e.g. K, Ca, Mg, and Fe) and heavy metal trace elements (e.g. Co and Cu) may be needed. Bacteria with complex enzyme systems are able to use the simplest substrates (e.g. carbon dioxide and inorganic salts) for synthesis and as energy sources and are called autotrophs; they are generally non-parasitic. Many bacteria of clinical importance, however, are heterotrophs and require organic compounds as substrates for free energy production.

Metabolism is also affected by temperature and pH. Most animal pathogens have an optimum temperature range of about 35°C to 38°C and an optimum pH range of 7.2 to 7.6 for growth.

Most bacteria are unaffected by relatively large changes in osmotic pressure owing to the strength of their cell walls. In hypertonic solutions, partial dehydration of the substrate may occur and this may inhibit growth, but very high pressures are needed before plasmolysis is seen.

Bacteria can be divided into four classes on the basis of their behaviour towards molecular oxygen:

- Obligate (strict) aerobes (e.g. *Mycobacterium tuberculosis*) require a high oxygen tension for growth or even survival, and cannot grow anaerobically.
- Obligate (strict) anaerobes (e.g. *Clostridium* spp.) require a complete absence of oxygen for growth. Even small quantities may prove toxic.
- Facultative anaerobes (e.g. *Staphylococcus* and *Escherichia* spp.) constitute the majority of bacteria which can use either aerobic respiration or anaerobic fermentation as a means of obtaining energy. As respiration is a more efficient method, these micro-organisms usually grow more rapidly in oxidative conditions.
- Microaerophiles (e.g. *Actinomyces* spp.) are obligate aerobes which are sensitive to the very high oxygen tensions found in normal air. They can only be cultivated at much reduced oxygen concentrations.

Apart from its role as a main carbon source for autotrophic bacteria, carbon dioxide has a stimulatory action on the growth or toxin production of many heterotrophic micro-organisms (e.g. growth of *Escherichia coli* and toxin production in *Corynebacterium diphtheriae*). In some cases it appears to be an essential nutrient for the growth of a number of bacteria, including anaerobes.

Reproduction

The true bacteria reproduce asexually by simple binary fission. The cell first enlarges to about twice its normal size with an increase in cytoplasmic contents, and DNA replicates to form two daughter chromosomes. A transverse septum is formed by the ingrowth of the cytoplasmic membrane and cell wall, separating the cytoplasm into two equal parts each containing nuclear material. The daughter cells may eventually part or can remain attached through several succeeding generations, giving aggregates.

Conjugation can occur in bacteria, resulting in the transfer of genetic information from a donor ('male') cell to a recipient ('female') cell. The ability to donate DNA is determined by the presence of F (fertility) plasmids (F factors). R plasmids (R factors) are responsible for transferring antimicrobial resistance between cells (e.g. *Salmonella*, *Shigella*, *Staphylococcus*, *Streptococcus*, and *Clostridium* spp.). This is not true sexual reproduction.

The genera *Bacillus* and *Clostridium* produce endospores, possibly in response to the development of unfavourable conditions for vegetative growth. Spore shape, which may be elongated, ovoid, or spherical, is characteristic of a species. They form within the vegetative cell and have a thick, tough, impermeable outer layer, a high calcium and dipicolinic acid content, and a low water content. DNA, RNA, and protein are present within the protoplast, although enzymatic and metabolic activity is reduced. Spores are highly resistant to heat, chemical disinfectants, and radiation, and may remain viable for years.

Spores germinate under favourable conditions of optimum moisture and nutrients. They become less resistant, lose calcium and dipicolinic acid, and the tough outer layer is shed and becomes more permeable. The net result of sporulation and germination is a single vegetative cell from each spore.

'Higher' bacteria (e.g. *Actinomyces* spp.) have a transitory mycelial type of growth resembling fungi. Vegetative growth is by elongation of the filaments and lateral branches, which are formed from budding cells within the chain. Multiplication is by transverse fission, fragmenting the filaments to produce cocci and bacilli. *Streptomyces* spp. produce conidia (exospores) which are formed extracellularly from aerial hyphae. Although a resting state, conidia are not highly resistant but serve as a means of dissemination.

Classification

There is at present no single internationally accepted method of classification of bacteria. Systems are constantly changing, which reflects the extreme diversity of the bacterial kingdom and the continual acquisition of fresh information. In structurally complex organisms (e.g. plants and animals), the differences between types are fairly clear-cut, relatively stable, and often visible to the naked eye. In addition, fossil evidence of common ancestry is available. With bacteria, the reverse is true. They are generally better defined by their physiological features, which provide a better estimate of their genetic relationships, rather than by relying solely on morphological characteristics. Micropalaeontological studies do point to the existence of fossil micro-organisms, although the currently available data are insufficient to assist in presenting an evolutionary scheme. In the absence of any completely satisfactory system, two main types of classification are in use:

- the natural classification

  This is based on a combination of morphological and physiological characters (e.g. shape, motility, distribution of flagella, and formation of spores). Some characteristics are given more weight than others in grouping the bacteria into classes, orders, families, genera, and species. The inclusion of a bacterium in any of these depends on the presence or absence of certain key characters which are considered of major importance. The taxonomic unit of this system is the species and it is essentially a modified form of the classical botanical and zoological classification method.

  The best known classification is that set out in *Bergey's Manual of Determinative Bacteriology*, which has been considerably modified since it was first published in 1923. The 8th edition of 1974 was followed by an abbreviated version in 1977, *The Shorter Bergey's Manual of Determinative Bacteriology*. This in turn was followed in 1984 by a book of much wider scope, *Bergey's Manual of Systematic Bacteriology*, which is an extremely useful and complete reference work for the identification of all bacteria.

- the numerical classification (Adansonian classification or taxometrics)

  This is based on the phenetic relationships between strains. As many characteristics as possible are determined for each strain, but no weighting is applied to any of them. Similarities are expressed as percentages, 100% representing identical characteristics, through to 0% which indicates no similarity at all. Bacteria are then grouped into phenons according to the extent to which they share characteristics. This system lends itself to computer analysis and, in the cases where it has been used, has shown some unexpected relationships between micro-organisms, hitherto unsuspected.

Staining techniques, particularly Gram's stain, are important aids in the identification and classification of bacteria. The first stage of Gram's stain involves treatment with ammonium oxalate-crystal violet solution and Lugol's iodine which colours bacterial cells purple. Subsequent washing with an iodine-acetone solution decolorises Gram-negative bacteria which may then be counterstained cherry-red using dilute carbol-fuchsin. Gram-positive bacteria retain the initial purple colour, a property determined by the composition and structure of the cell wall which is thicker and stronger than the cell wall of Gram-negative bacteria and appears to be less permeable to the strength of the iodine-acetone solution employed in the reaction.

A few species (e.g. *Mycobacterium* spp.) take up carbol-fuchsin only after prolonged exposure or treatment with heat. They do not decolorise or counterstain blue on subsequent treatment with dilute sulphuric acid and methylene blue, and are thus termed acid-fast.

Reliable results from such methods are dependent on the integrity of the cell wall and age of the culture. Older Gram-positive cells may give a false Gram-negative result due to physical and chemical changes in the cell wall. Treatment with isoniazid renders tubercle bacilli non-acid-fast.

Other methods of classification include genetic studies using DNA homology which is used to establish new species. Chemotaxonomy utilises chemical and physical data to build up a precise picture of the molecular structure of individual bacteria, and is proving an extremely effective means of classification.

Nomenclature

Bacterial nomenclature, in contrast to classification, is governed internationally by a set of rules contained in the Bacteriological Code (current edition: Lapage *et al.*, 1975). The Linnaean binomial system with latinised names is used, with the name of the genus given first and always capitalised and the species name second with a lower-case initial letter, and both names printed in italics (e.g. *Clostridium perfringens*). Higher taxa also have an initial capital but are usually, by convention, printed in Roman type (e.g. Enterobacteriaceae). There are many accepted colloquial terms in common use which are not regulated by the Code, and these are usually printed in Roman type (e.g. it is acceptable to refer to rod-shaped bacteria as bacilli even though they may not belong to the genus *Bacillus*; members of the genus *Streptococcus* may be called streptococci; and

Mycobacterium tuberculosis is commonly referred to as the tubercle bacillus).

Many variations can occur within a species, and these may be characterised by the following terms. These terms do not have any official standing, but are useful practical descriptions. They are often used in conjunction with the name of the bacterium to define it more precisely:

Biotype	displays different physiological characteristics, although the genetic constitution (genotype) remains the same
Form	a suffix denoting a subdivision of a species
Morphotype	displays similarities in form or structure
Pathotype	displays similarities in pathogenicity
Phagotype	displays similarities in sensitivity towards bacteriophages
Phase	alternative immunological states in a species
Serotype	displays similarities in antigenic properties
Strain	micro-organisms that possess different inherited properties from other micro-organisms, although some features may be common in strains within the same species
Var.	*see* Variety
Variant	a micro-organism that shows some variation from the parent culture
Variety	a subdivision of a species

The Bacteriological Code recommends use of the suffix -var instead of -type, although this is not mandatory and indeed meets with a lot of opposition from some bacteriologists.

Transmission of Bacterial Infections

Transmission of bacterial diseases to man occurs in a variety of different ways. Some diseases exist as a zoonosis where man may be an incidental host as a result of some particular occupation (e.g. anthrax and brucellosis), while other diseases are transmitted directly from person-to-person (e.g. pertussis and tuberculosis). In some instances, disease occurs when a micro-organism present as part of the normal flora invades and becomes pathogenic (e.g. *Actinomyces* spp. causing actinomycosis, and *Clostridium difficile* causing pseudomembranous colitis in the presence of some antibacterials).

There are many mechanisms whereby a micro-organism is introduced to the host, and several possible portals of entry. Bacteria may be inhaled in airborne water droplets expelled from an infected individual (e.g. *Corynebacterium diphtheriae*) or from air-conditioning cooling towers (e.g. *Legionella pneumophila*), or in dried infected excreta (e.g. *Chlamydia psittaci*). Ingestion is a common mode of infection, particularly ingestion of faecal-contaminated food or water (e.g. *Vibrio cholerae*, and *Salmonella* and *Shigella* spp.). Unpasteurised milk from infected cows was a source of *Mycobacterium bovis* or *Brucella* spp. prior to routine heat-treatment of milk and stringent controls governing livestock. Infections may also be acquired by contact with urine from infected animals (e.g. *Leptospira interrogans*), blood and secretions (e.g. *Brucella* spp.), nasal secretions from infected patients, or from infected fomites (e.g. *Chlamydia trachomatis*).

Sexually-transmitted micro-organisms include *Treponema pallidum* and *Neisseria gonorrhoeae*, and infants may become infected with *Chlamydia oculogenitalis* during passage along the birth canal. Soil-contaminated wounds may become infected due to germination of spores (e.g. *Clostridium tetani, C. perfringens*, and *Bacillus anthracis*). Arthropods which may act as vectors for micro-organisms (e.g. *Borrelia burgdorferi, Yersinia pestis*, and *Rickettsia* spp.) include ticks, rat fleas, and lice respectively. Accidental inoculation of laboratory personnel is also a possible route of transmission for many infections.

Pathogenic bacteria may damage host cells directly by multiplication or use of cellular nutrients, or indirectly by production of potent toxins which disseminate to sites removed from the initial infection (e.g. *Corynebacterium diphtheriae*). In some cases, disease is caused by ingestion of toxin which has been produced by micro-organisms multiplying in another medium (e.g. *Clostridium botulinum* in canned foods). For a more detailed account of toxin production and the pathology of infections, *see* Section 15.5.

14.3 VIRUSES

Viruses are very small structures, ranging in size from approximately 20 nm to 300 nm, which means that the majority of them may only be seen with the aid of an electron microscope. All but the very largest are smaller than bacteria.

They are obligate intracellular parasites and utilise the metabolic pathways of living cells for their own replication. They infect all forms of life, displaying specificity for the different groups (i.e. animals, bacteria, fungi, invertebrates, and plants). There are, however, examples of vertebrate and plant viruses also multiplying in insects which in some cases act as vectors (e.g. yellow fever virus in mosquitoes). Viruses also exhibit a degree of specificity for species within a group, often causing a milder illness in their usual host compared to serious disease if they cross the host barrier (e.g. Lassa virus).

Viruses are capable of producing a diverse range of neoplasms in animals. Almost all those identified to date are DNA viruses, with the singular exception of the retrovirus family which are RNA viruses. Examples of oncogenic viruses include human T-cell leukaemia virus, human papillomavirus (causing warts), Epstein-Barr virus (causing Burkitt's lymphoma), and hepatitis B virus (causing hepatocellular carcinoma). The infections caused by viruses are described in Section 5.3.

Morphology

Viruses are clearly differentiated from other forms of cellular life. In their simplest form (naked viruses), they are made up of nucleic acid surrounded by a protective protein coat (the capsid) which together are referred to as the nucleocapsid. The nucleic acid may be DNA or RNA, but not both, and in either case may be single- or double-stranded. Many animal viruses are more complex, possessing a lipoprotein layer surrounding the nucleocapsid and are thus termed enveloped viruses. An additional component of the envelope is glycoprotein which may project from the surface as spikes. Surface proteins may play a role in binding to the host cell during the initial stages of infection and they also have antigenic properties.

The capsid is composed of blocks of protein (capsomeres), conferring in most cases either a cubical (usually icosahedral) or helical shape. In some cases, the outer coat is not so obviously symmetrical and spherical, brick-shaped, or pleomorphic structures have been observed. Many bacterial viruses (bacteriophages) are shaped like spermatozoa, possessing a protein tail attached to a polyhedral head. Some viruses are illustrated diagramatically in Fig. 14.1.

Most viruses are sensitive to heating at 50°C to 60°C for 30 minutes but are not inactivated by freezing. They are also sensitive to extremes of pH, preferring a range of 5 to 9. The lipid membranes of enveloped viruses are destroyed by ether and mild detergents, whereas naked viruses remain quite stable and require harsher treatment for disruption. Viruses are insensitive to antimicrobials.

Reproduction

A virion is the term applied to the complete viral particle as it exists extracellularly prior to infection of a cell. The infective unit of the virion is the nucleic acid, which is protected from the external environment by the capsid. The first stage of infection is random contact between the virion and host cell. Surface proteins may bind with specific receptor sites on the host cell, or there may be fusion between the host cytoplasmic membrane and viral lipid envelope.

In order to replicate, the nucleic acid must be uncoated which may take place extra- or intracellularly. The precise way in which the nucleic acid penetrates the cell wall is not understood in many cases, although endocytosis may be the means for some animal viruses. Bacteriophages use their protein tails to inject nucleic acid into bacterial cells, while plant viruses are often injected by an insect vector (e.g. aphids).

The viral nucleic acid must be delivered to the replication sites which may be in the nucleus (e.g. DNA viruses, except poxviruses) or within the cytoplasm (e.g. poliovirus). Synthesis of viral proteins takes place within the cytoplasm. The pathways of replication vary depending on the type and form of nucleic acid present. In some RNA viruses where RNA is present as a single strand, it may act as its own messenger RNA (mRNA) and thus protein synthesis may commence directly with translation of the genome. In DNA viruses and other RNA viruses, transcription must first take place to produce mRNA, and is followed by translation. The enzymes required for these processes may be present within the virus (e.g. poxvirus transcriptase, or reverse transcriptase of retroviruses) or derived from the host cell. The proteins produced have differing roles. They may be enzymes which catalyse replication of the viral nucleic acid or inhibit host cellular functions, or they may be the proteins which will form the new capsids.

The final stage in reproduction involves the addition of the capsid to the nucleic acid to form a new virion, which is released into the extracellular environment. This may be by budding through the cytoplasmic membrane or by other as yet unknown mechanisms, and may or may not involve destruction of the host cell. Enveloped viruses acquire their outer membranes at this stage using virally-modified components of the host cytoplasmic membrane.

Viruses can vary their genetic structure by spontaneous mutation, producing variants of known strains. This may increase or decrease the virulence of virus infections (e.g. influenza type A) and is in part responsible for cyclic pandemics of this type of infection. Recombination of genetic material from different viruses may also occur to produce new viral types.

Classification and Nomenclature

Classification and nomenclature of viruses is regulated by the International Committee for the Taxonomy of Viruses which has drawn up a set of rules for this purpose. The code of bacterial nomenclature is not to be

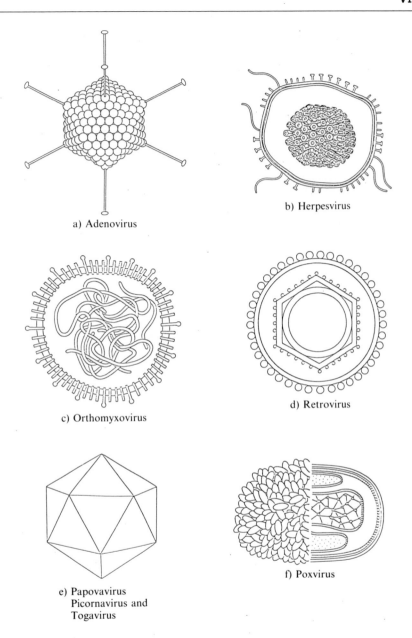

a) Adenovirus

b) Herpesvirus

c) Orthomyxovirus

d) Retrovirus

e) Papovavirus
   Picornavirus and
   Togavirus

f) Poxvirus

Fig. 14.1
Diagrammatic representation of viruses.

followed, although an effort is to be made towards latinisation of names. The name of a viral genus should end in '...virus' and that of a family in '...viridae'. The family name is often printed in italic type with a capital initial letter, the genus name in Roman type also with a capital initial letter, and the species name in Roman type with lower case initials. However, this is not necessarily standard throughout the different texts on the subject.

The classification is based on various criteria, including host type (e.g. animal, bacteria, or plant), morphology, and nucleic acid structure. Similarity between viruses does not necessarily produce similar diseases in their hosts, even amongst those viruses possessing common antigens (e.g. parainfluenza and mumps viruses). The classification of certain animal viruses is listed in Table 14.1.

TABLE 14.1
Classification of some important animal viruses causing disease in man.

	Viruses	Characteristics
RNA viruses		
Family: Genus: Species:	*Arenaviridae* Arenavirus group Lassa virus	pleomorphic (approximating to spherical), enveloped, single-stranded RNA
Family: Genus:	*Orthomyxoviridae* Influenza virus	helical, enveloped, single-stranded RNA
Family: Genus: Species: Genus: Species:	*Paramyxoviridae* Morbillivirus measles virus Paramyxovirus mumps virus, parainfluenza virus	helical, enveloped, single-stranded RNA
Family: Genus: Species: Genus: Species:	*Picornaviridae* Enterovirus poliovirus Rhinovirus rhinovirus	cubic, naked, single-stranded RNA
Family: Genus: Species:	*Rhabdoviridae* Lyssavirus rabies virus	helical, enveloped, single-stranded RNA
Family: Subfamily: Species: Subfamily: Species:	*Retroviridae* Lentivirinae human immunodeficiency virus Oncovirinae human T-cell leukaemia virus	pleomorphic, enveloped, single-stranded RNA
Family: Genus: Species: Genus: Species:	*Togaviridae* Flavivirus yellow fever virus Rubivirus rubella virus	pleomorphic (approximating to spherical), enveloped, single-stranded RNA
DNA viruses		
Family:	*Adenoviridae*	icosahedral, naked, double-stranded DNA
Family: Subfamily: Species: Subfamily: Species: Subfamily: Species:	*Herpesviridae* (herpesviruses) Alphaherpesvirinae herpes simplex virus, varicella-zoster virus Betaherpesvirinae human cytomegalovirus Gammaherpesvirinae Epstein-Barr virus	icosahedral, enveloped, double-stranded DNA
Family: Genus: Species:	*Papovaviridae* Papillomavirus human papillomavirus	icosahedral, naked, double-stranded DNA
Family: Genus: Species:	*Poxviridae* Orthopoxvirus variola virus, vaccinia virus (used to produce smallpox vaccine)	brick-shaped, enveloped, double-stranded DNA

Transmission of Viral Infections

Viral infections are transmitted in a variety of ways. A common route is via airborne droplets (e.g. common cold, chickenpox, influenza, measles, mumps, rubella, and poliomyelitis). Rabies is transmitted primarily in saliva, usually as the result of an attack by a rabid animal, and oral and genital secretions carry herpes simplex viruses. Contact with body fluids from infected hosts is responsible for transmitting Lassa fever, Marburg disease, Ebola fever, and cytomegalovirus infections. Insects can act as the vector (e.g. yellow fever) and such viruses have been given the general name arboviruses. Other means of transmission include the faecal-oral route (e.g. poliomyelitis), contact with active lesions (e.g. herpes simplex and chickenpox lesions), and hand-to-face contact (now believed to be an important route for transmission of the common cold).

For an account of the pathology of viral infections, *see* Section 15.5.

14.4   FUNGI

Fungi are non-photosynthetic, coenocytic, eukaryotic protists, which are larger than bacteria and possess a more complex structure.

They are saprophytic or parasitic in nature. The saprophytic fungi utilise dead organic matter as a nutrient source. Spoilage of stored grain or other food may be commercially detrimental to man while mycotoxins released by some saprophytic species may be directly harmful (e.g. alfatoxin produced by *Aspergillus flavus* on maize and legumes). Some species are pathogenic and cause disease in man, animals, and plants. Other species may be of benefit to man and are employed in food processing (e.g. *Saccharomyces cerevisiae* in bread making and alcohol fermentation) or in the production of antimicrobials (e.g. penicillins, cephalosporins, or griseofulvin). The infections caused by fungi are described in Section 5.4.

Morphology

There are two forms of fungi, the moulds and yeasts, which differ in their morphology and methods of reproduction.

The basic unit of vegetative growth of moulds is the hypha, which is a branched tubular structure with a characteristic rigid cell wall composed of chitin, cellulose, and mannans. Hyphae contain membrane-bound nuclei and mitochondria. Perforated cross-walls (septa) may divide the hyphae up into separate cells containing one or more nuclei (septate hyphae); non-septate hyphae have no cross-walls. Growth proceeds only from the tips of hyphae which form a tangled meshwork of interlacing filaments called the mycelium, a dry colony visible to the naked eye. The mycelium in non-aquatic species is composed of two parts: the vegetative mycelium which is usually located below the surface of the substrate and takes in nutrients, and an aerial portion above the surface responsible for the formation and dissemination of spores into the external environment. Examples of moulds include dermatophytes (*see* Tinea Infections), *Aspergillus* and *Penicillium* spp.

Yeasts (e.g. *Cryptococcus neoformans* and *Saccharomyces* spp.) are unicellular and ovoid, spherical, or ellipsoidal in shape. They generally form moist colonies but do not form a mycelium. In some cases, however, there may be incomplete separation of cells following reproduction giving an appearance of filaments (i.e. a pseudomycelium). Such species are referred to as yeast-like fungi (e.g. *Candida albicans*). Dimorphic fungi (e.g. *Sporothrix schenkii*) exist as both moulds and yeasts, depending on the environment. Many pathogens are moulds in the saprophytic state, but become yeasts or yeast-like in animal tissues.

Generally, fungi are non-motile, although spores and gametes of some aquatic species do possess flagella.

Metabolism

Fungi are heterotrophic, relying on an organic substrate as a nutrient source. They can only absorb soluble nutrients and thus excrete extracellular enzymes from the hyphal tips to break down the organic material. They are aerobes and can tolerate a wide range of temperatures, although the optimum is around 28°C. They are also more resistant to acidic environments than bacteria.

Reproduction

The unit of reproduction is the spore, which may be produced asexually or sexually. When the right conditions prevail, spores germinate and produce new mycelia.

The asexual spores of mycelial fungi are produced by abscission of the tips of the hyphae which are often specialised spore-bearing structures distinguishable from the basic hyphae. In some cases, these structures may be large and complex (e.g. mushrooms).

Sexual spores are formed by the fusion of two specialised cells from different hyphae and the transference of nuclear material.

Yeasts multiply vegetatively by budding, usually from the narrowest end of the cell. They may also produce spores sexually.

Classification

Taxonomically, fungi can be divided into three main classes according to the septation of their hyphae and type of spore formation:

- *Phycomycetes* have non-septate hyphae and produce endogenous asexual spores (sporangiospores) within a sac called a sporangium at the tip of an aerial hypha (the sporangiophore). Their sexually produced spores may be oospores or zygospores, giving rise to two subdivisions within this class, *Oomycetes* (*Oomycotina*) and *Zygomycetes* (*Zygomycotina*). *Rhizopus*, the common bread mould, and *Mucor* (genera within *Zygomycetes*) are frequently found as aerial contaminants.
- *Ascomycetes* (*Ascomycotina*) possess septate hyphae although the cytoplasm is continuous through the perforated cross-walls. Their asexual spores (conidia) are exogenous and produced by a specialised cell borne on a conidiophore (often an aerial hypha) which has a variety of different shapes. The sexual spores (ascospores) are produced endogenously in a sac called an ascus. This group contains edible morels and truffles, plus the genus *Saccharomyces* and many plant pathogens.
- *Basidiomycetes* (*Basidiomycotina*) like the *Ascomycetes*, possess septate hyphae and occasionally produce conidia. Asexual reproduction is not common in this group. They differ, however, in the mode of formation of the sexual spores (basidiospores) which are formed on a characteristic club-shaped structure, the basidium. This group includes mushrooms (e.g. *Amanita* and *Psilocybe* spp.).

Fungi can only be assigned to one of these classes where the form of sexual reproduction (referred to as the perfect form) has been observed. The *Deuteromycetes* (*Deuteromycotina*) or *Fungi Imperfecti* is a provisional taxonomic group which includes those fungi known only to reproduce asexually. This group includes the dermatophytes (ringworm fungi) such as *Microsporum*, *Trichophyton*, and *Epidermophyton* spp; also *Candida*, *Aspergillus*, and *Sporothrix* spp. It has become common practice to retain in this group those fungi which are known to exhibit a sexual phase in special conditions but which normally reproduce asexually in laboratory culture, even though many of them are strictly *Ascomycetes*.

Transmission of Fungal Infections

Many fungal infections are transmitted to man from the environment by inhalation or direct inoculation. Spores may be present in soil, vegetation, grain, pigeon excreta, building materials, or skin flakes shed from animals or man. Only dermatophytes (*see* Tinea Infections) and *Candida* spp. (*see* Candidiasis) are transmitted from person-to-person. *Malassezia furfur* and *Candida* spp. are the only two fungi with a commensal relationship with man under normal conditions and thus may give rise to opportunistic infections (*see* Pityriasis Versicolor and Candidiasis) if those conditions change.

Mycoses is the collective name given to infections caused by fungi; mycoallergosis refers to allergic reactions precipitated by fungal allergens (e.g. allergic bronchopulmonary aspergillosis). Mycoses may be further subdivided into superficial, cutaneous, subcutaneous, and systemic infections.

Pityriasis versicolor is an example of a superficial mycosis which arises endogenously and involves only the stratum corneum.

Tinea infections are cutaneous mycoses in which the micro-organisms attack keratin in tissues (e.g. hair, nails, and skin).

Sporotrichosis is an example of a subcutaneous fungal infection in which the dimorphic micro-organism *Sporothrix schenkii* exists as a saprophytic mould in the environment (in soil or vegetation), but reverts to a yeast in animal tissues. It must be inoculated into the subcutaneous tissues, often via an abrasion.

Systemic mycoses may involve any organ of the body, although the primary site is often the lungs as a result of spore inhalation. True pathogens (e.g. *Cryptococcus neoformans*) may cause disease in any individual receiving a sufficient dose. Opportunistic pathogens produce disease only in susceptible hosts (e.g. *Aspergillus* spp. in the presence of underlying lung disorders or *Candida* spp. in immunocompromised hosts).

14.5   PROTOZOA

Protozoa are relatively large, non-photosynthetic, unicellular eukaryotic protists, possessing an outer membrane of varying rigidity. Many species are parasitic.

They are motile by means of flagella, cilia, or amoeboid movement (protrusion of pseudopodia). In some species nutrition is derived by the uptake of soluble nutrients, while other species engulf and internally digest particulate matter (phagotrophic nutrition). Excretion may be by discharge of waste products through the outer membrane or the release of products at cell division. Reproduction is asexual by means of binary fission or multiple fission (schizogony). Some species include sexual phases (sporogony) in their life-cycle. Resistant cysts capable of surviving unfavourable conditions may also be formed and facilitate spread of the micro-organism.

Transmission of diseases caused by parasitic protozoa occurs in a variety of ways. There may be direct contact between hosts (e.g. *Trichomonas vaginalis* transmitted sexually) or faecal contamination of food and water with resistant cysts (e.g. *Entamoeba histolytica*, *Giardia lamblia*, and *Toxoplasma gondii*). *T. gondii* may also be ingested by prey animals (including man) as tissue cysts. Vectors, in the form of blood-sucking arthropods, are required to transfer *Leishmania*, *Plasmodium*, and *Trypanosoma* spp. between hosts. Some free-living amoebae are pathogenic to man and invade the host directly from the environment (e.g. *Naegleria fowleri* in freshwater pools and *Acanthamoeba* spp. as windborne cysts). Many protozoal infections are transmitted as a zoonosis, involving man and wild or domestic animals in the same cycle (e.g. leishmaniasis). The infections caused by protozoa are described in Section 5.5.

14.6   HELMINTHS

Helminths are well developed multicellular organisms belonging to the animal kingdom. Some species of helminth live within the gastro-intestinal tract or tissues of a definitive host during the adult phase of their life-cycle, but most are unable to multiply within the host. Eggs or larvae passed into the external environment must rely on an intermediate host to continue the life-cycle, or they must incubate in appropriate soil conditions before developing into infective forms. This is in contrast to other infectious agents (e.g. bacteria, fungi, protozoa, and viruses, *see above*) in which a small inoculum can build up sufficient numbers to cause disease.

Light helminthic infections, particularly of gastro-intestinal parasites, are often asymptomatic and further exposure is necessary to produce a worm load of sufficient size to cause symptomatic disease. Conditions for reinfection exist in endemic areas and measures must be taken to break the cycle of transmission. These include improving sanitation and farming methods; health education with respect to eating habits, food handling, and general hygiene; steps to avoid bites from infected arthropods; and in some cases, mass chemotherapy to reduce the reservoir of human infection.

The maturation phase and life span of some species is very long (e.g. *Taenia* spp. may survive for 20 years or more), and symptoms may not be apparent until some time after infection. This can be particularly important in the case of returning travellers or immigrants from endemic areas who may develop symptoms after a prolonged period in a non-endemic area.

Helminthic infections are prevalent in many tropical and subtropical regions, but are by no means confined to those areas. Enterobiasis and toxocariasis are examples of infections commonly occurring in urban areas of temperate zones. The infections caused by helminths are described in Section 5.6.

The three classes of medical importance to man are Cestoda, Trematoda, and Nematoda.

Cestoda and Trematoda

Cestoda and Trematoda belong to the phylum Platyhelminthes (flatworms). Platyhelminthes are characterised by the absence of a body cavity (coelom). They are bilaterally symmetrical, flattened in dorsoventral section, and protected by an outer protective cuticle. There is a head, which may incorporate a rudimentary brain, but there are no sense organs or blood circulation. Most are hermaphroditic with well developed reproductive organs.

Adult cestodes (tapeworms) inhabit the gastro-intestinal tract of definitive hosts, and are protected from the action of host digestive juices by the outer cuticle. They do not possess a digestive tract, but absorb nutrients through microvilli on their body surfaces. The length of a mature cestode varies between species from 2 mm to 10 m. Hooks and suckers attach the head (scolex) to the host gastro-intestinal wall. Proglottides emerge behind the head and develop an excretory canal, nerve trunks, and reproductive organs as they mature. The most distal proglottides (containing eggs) are shed in the host's faeces; or in some species, the eggs are shed into the gastro-intestinal tract before passing to the external environment. If these eggs are ingested by an intermediate host, they develop into larval forms (cysticerci) in the host body tissues. Raw or undercooked contaminated meat eaten by a definitive host allows the development in the gastro-intestinal tract of the larval forms into adult helminths.

Adult trematodes (flukes) inhabit specific organs of the definitive host, depending on the fluke species. They are unsegmented, and possess suckers for attachment, a well developed nervous system, and a mouth leading to a branched alimentary tract. The life-cycle invariably involves more than one host. All but *Schistosoma* spp. are leaf-like in shape, range in size from a few millimetres to several centimetres, and are hermaphroditic. If eggs passed from a definitive host reach fresh water, they hatch into miracidia, which penetrate particular species of snail. Further development produces cercariae and these are released back into the water. They may attach to, or penetrate, a second intermediate host (e.g. fish, frogs, or aquatic plants), which may be ingested by a definitive host. Development into adult flukes takes place followed by migration to the final target organ (e.g. liver, biliary tract, gastro-intestinal tract, or lung), and eggs are subsequently passed from the definitive host in bile, faeces, or sputum.

Schistosomes (blood flukes) are elongated and worm-like, ranging in length from 2 mm to 4 mm (males) or 1 mm to 2 mm (females). The female is held along a groove in the ventral surface of the male, and together they inhabit the vascular system of specific organs of the definitive host. The life-cycle of schistosomes is similar to that of hermaphroditic flukes (*see above*), except in their requirement for only one intermediate host. The cercariae released back into the water from snails attach themselves by their suckers to the skin of mammalian definitive hosts. They burrow through the skin and form schistosomula, which migrate to the liver to complete their development. Adult schistosomes migrate to the target organ and produce eggs. The eggs penetrate venous capillaries and migrate to the bladder or gastro-intestinal tract in an attempt to reach the external environment. Some become trapped in tissues and cause inflammatory reactions.

Nematoda

Authorities disagree on the classification of Nematoda, which has been separately considered a class in each of the phyla Aschelminthes and Nemathelminthes, and has also been classified as a separate phylum.

Adult nematodes (roundworms) may be free-living, or some species may inhabit the gastro-intestinal tract or tissues of a definitive host. They are unsegmented motile roundworms, varying in length from a few millimetres up to 120 cm. They possess a body cavity, and a well developed alimentary tract with two openings, one to serve as a mouth and the other as an anus. The body is covered by a cuticle but is devoid of cilia. Sexes are separate in all species, but individual life-cycles may vary. In many cases, no intermediate host is required, and eggs or larvae are transferred between definitive hosts directly or indirectly.

In certain species (e.g. *Ascaris lumbricoides* and *Trichuris trichiuria*), eggs passed in the faeces of a host may remain viable in soil for some time before ingestion in contaminated food or water. Alternatively, in other species (e.g. *Ancylostoma duodenale*, *Necator americanus*, and *Strongyloides stercoralis*) eggs passed in the host's faeces hatch in appropriate soil conditions and larvae penetrate the skin, usually the feet, of another host. Eggs of *Enterobius vermicularis* cause intense pruritus ani, and scratching allows the eggs to be transmitted on the fingers directly to others, to food, or to oneself (auto-infection). Encysted larvae of *Trichinella spiralis* present in raw or undercooked meat in one host may be consumed by another host. The ingested larvae mature into adult forms and produce more larvae, which migrate to striated muscle.

Some species do, however, require intermediate hosts. *Dracunculus medinensis* relies on an aquatic crustacean. Filarial larvae are transmitted by arthropods.

Man is an incidental host to *Toxocara* spp., which mature to the adult form in cats and dogs. Eggs passed in the faeces of a definitive host may be ingested by humans. They hatch into larvae, which migrate to body tissues but are unable to undergo further development.

Chapter 15

GENERAL PATHOLOGY

15.1 GENERAL AND SYSTEMIC EFFECTS OF DISEASE

Introduction

Pathology is the science concerned with the study of disease, and is one of the most fundamental of the medical disciplines. Its scope covers the causes, mechanisms, manifestations, and functional consequences of disease. It is not a study which readily stands alone, as its proper understanding depends primarily upon knowledge of the normal conditions and functions of the body. Hence, anatomy, physiology, biochemistry, and psychology are complementary. Similarly, additional contributions must be sought from specialist disciplines, including microbiology, parasitology, toxicology, and radiobiology (concerning disease causation), or endocrinology, immunology, and haematology (concerning mechanisms or manifestations).

For the pharmacist, pathology is not a traditional field of knowledge. Despite the inclusion of physiology, aspects of biochemistry, microbiology, histology, and the rudiments of anatomy in pharmaceutical curricula of the past, the logical progression from the study of the normal to the abnormal did not always follow. Undeniably, the requirement for pathology as a basis for diagnosis, surgery, or therapeutics is much more the natural prerogative of the medical profession. However, in relation to the pharmacist's developing role, which includes a deeper involvement in the applications of drug therapy, it follows that there is greater necessity for disease processes to be understood. In particular, knowledge of pathology would be the basis for understanding the rationale of therapy and appreciating the inherent limitations of its effectiveness. The acquisition of sufficient knowledge for the anticipated purposes of the pharmacist is not an insurmountable problem. For anyone capable of mastering the other pharmaceutical sciences, pathology presents no intellectual problem. What is required is the appropriate mastery of the principles, in conjunction with the intelligent application of this knowledge when confronted by the need to understand a particular case.

Disease manifestations may be structural or functional, or both. Functional abnormality may involve biochemistry or performance. An individual defect may in general be called a lesion and may be single or multiple. If several different types of lesion are involved as a feature of a disease, the condition is known as a syndrome. In every case, the severity or extent of the lesion may vary from minor to major and the condition may be stable, exacerbating, or remitting. Given that there may be defects of structure and function in any one or all of the possible range of tissues, organs, or systems, the range of recognisably different diseases becomes immense. It must be accepted that the coverage achieved in this Chapter and Chapter 16 is not comprehensive. However, they aim to provide a useful working knowledge.

At this stage, it is important to emphasise not only the great diversity of diseases, but also the considerable degree of common ground featured in disease processes. To state the point simply, there are limits to the range of ways in which a tissue or organ can go wrong. Furthermore, the consequences may be even more limited. An organ may malfunction only in quantitative terms (i.e. working either more or less effectively, or not at all). Generally, qualitative changes in function are rare. Muscles, nerves, or gland cells, even if radically changed, do not generally perform any function apart from that of which they are normally capable. Thus, the greatest diversity exists in relation to causation and mechanistic detail. Immense numbers of different toxic agents, allergens, pathogenic micro-organisms, and genetic mutations cause bewildering varieties of lesions at the molecular or cellular ultrastructural levels. These are ultimately revealed in terms of the tissue or organ responses, and in which the possible range is more limited. It is upon these limited manifestations of the disease processes that the subject material of these first sections will concentrate.

For the purposes of precise diagnosis, attention must be given to the diverse detail which distinguishes one disease from another. Thus, most specific diseases are described in terms of the individual features, taking account of lesions in target structures and giving rise to local malfunctions. On the other hand, for the purposes of rational therapy, the essential features of the pathology are sought and attention is given to common properties linking diseases. At a more general level, there are a number of less specific effects which apply to the whole body. These will form the subject of the rest of this introductory section. They range in severity from life-threatening major system malfunctions to the more superficial discomforts, which provide the common awareness of feeling unwell.

Cardiovascular and other Systemic Effects of Disease and Injury

The general well-being of all tissues and organs depends, above all else, on the optimal supply of oxygen and nutrients and the removal of waste material by the blood supply. Thus, proper functioning of the cardiovascular system is vital, in close association with the homoeostatic and control mechanisms provided by the nervous and endocrine systems. Blood component production must be maintained. Input of nutrients (e.g. from the gastro-intestinal tract, liver, and adipose tissues), an adequate supply of water, and effective control of fluid and electrolyte balance are essential. Respiratory function must also be effective, and must be controlled and integrated with circulatory functions. This therefore represents a complex system of fundamental importance. Numerous specific disorders of components of the system will be dealt with in later Sections. In addition, general malfunction of the circulation may represent the less specific consequences of a wide range of disease states, thus extending adverse influences throughout the body.

Many of the effects of disease and injury are reflected by pressure changes that alter blood flow and volume distribution throughout the system. One consequence, which may be local or widespread, is congestion. The volume of blood located in vessels at any one time is increased to an abnormal extent (hyperaemia). Congested vessels are engorged with blood and the affected tissues become noticeably altered in colour. The tissues range from bright red, if the blood is arterial and well-oxygenated (erythema), to bluish if it is venous and very poorly oxygenated (cyanosis). Congestion may be passive or reactive. In passive congestion, blood may accumulate in a part of the vascular network through pressure changes elsewhere (e.g. by increased upstream pressures or impeded downstream flow). Thus, the actual congestion is most likely to occur in relatively low

pressure (venous) parts of the system. Important examples of such systemic congestion are the involvement of the entire venous system due to right side heart failure (see Section 16.1) or parts of the system (e.g. mesenteric veins engorged from portal venous occlusion, see Section 16.4). Left ventricular failure results in similar pooling of blood in the lower-pressure pulmonary vascular bed (see Section 2.6). More localised congestion may be due to blockage of drainage veins (e.g. by thrombus, embolus, or compression by tumour).

Reactive congestion is a feature of inflammation (see Section 15.4), one of the most fundamental of disease processes. Blood volume increases in the affected vascular network as a result of arteriolar vasodilatation. Rates of flow may be increased (contrasting with impeded flow in passive congestion), or small-vessel vasodilatation may result in reduced flow or cessation (stasis) when pressures have dropped markedly. Other reactive hyperaemia may occur physiologically (e.g. in exercised skeletal muscles or due to the blushing reflex).

The accumulation of fluid in the interstitial spaces between tissues (i.e. extravascular) is called oedema and may often be associated with vascular congestion. It results in swelling of the affected part. There may be a reactive mechanism, as in acute inflammation, whereby changes in the permeability of capillary walls allow the exudation of plasma; this may also be influenced by local vascular pressure changes. Alternatively, changes may occur in the physiological balance of forces controlling relative distribution of fluid between blood vessels and tissues (Fig. 15.1). Normally, the higher

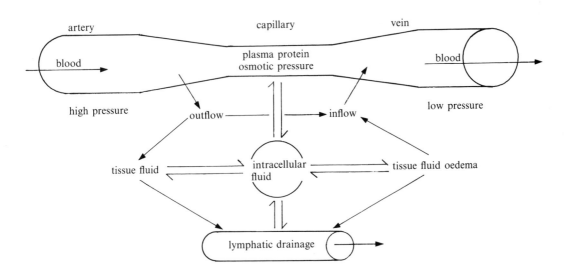

Fig. 15.1
Blood plasma fluid-tissue balances determined by pressures and osmosis. Net increase of outflow over inflow causes oedema.

pressure at the arterial end of the capillary bed results in outflow of fluid. Osmotic pressure produced by plasma proteins causes a return flow from the tissue fluid compartment into the vessels at the lower pressure (venous) end of the system. Back-pressure in the veins or decreased osmotic pressure from the plasma proteins may result in net outflow (transudation) from blood vessels. If the venous drainage is due to hydrostatic back-pressure, as in the lower limbs, the condition is known as dependent oedema. Tissue fluid also drains away via lymphatic vessels, and any obstruction of such drainage will cause fluid accumulation (lymphoedema). Accumulated fluid may not always be retained in the tissues. If escape is possible into cavities, free-standing fluid may collect (e.g. ascites).

Another general circulatory malfunction associated with a variety of pathological states is shock. This takes the form of an acute general circulatory failure in which blood flow through tissues becomes inadequate to meet their requirements. Obvious symptoms result from low pressure which produces markedly reduced blood flow. The skin becomes typically cold and clammy, depressed oxygenation of tissues gives a cyanosed appearance, kidney function is curtailed, and urine production is reduced.

Disorders which radically reduce cardiac output (e.g. heart failure) produce cardiogenic shock (see Section 16.1). Loss of blood volume (oligaemic shock) will have similar consequences. This occurs in severe haemorrhage, extensive burning or bruising, and loss of fluid as a result of vomiting or diarrhoea. Other varieties of shock are due to a marked inability to maintain peripheral vasomotor tone, so that blood pools and pressure cannot be maintained. Toxic shock may result from a wide range of agents, especially endogenous toxins generated by infectious micro-organisms. Neurogenic shock is due to widespread vasodilatation secondary to loss of sympathetic nerve activity. This occurs as a result of nervous system damage (e.g. of the spinal cord). More rarely, anaphylactic shock involves vasodilatation and plasma-volume loss due to systemic histamine release by allergic mechanisms (see Section 15.6).

The most profound consequence of shock is death. This represents radical failure on a systemic scale, involving total loss of cardiovascular and nervous functions. Death may occur almost immediately if a very severe state of shock develops, or it may be delayed. Unless the circulation is speedily restored, some degree of damage may occur in any tissue with impaired perfusion. The damage or death of cells in particular organs or systems, and the possibilities for reversal of such damage, are explored in subsequent sections. At this stage, it is sufficient to note the particular susceptibility of nervous and cardiac tissues to hypoxia resulting from poor blood supply. Thus, shock from any cause may give rise to progressive disorder of these and other vulnerable systems. A vicious cycle results (refractory shock) in which cardiogenic and neurogenic failures exacerbate the situation until there is a total cessation of all functions.

Endocrine and Metabolic Responses to Disease and Trauma

Certain disease mechanisms (e.g. inflammation and wound healing) constitute local responses with protective and reparative functions. In addition, particularly in response to severe or widespread disease, changes occur in the biochemical systems of the body as a whole. Such changes are manifestations of pathology and are also protective or restorative, aimed at ultimate reversion to normality. The most important mechanisms affect metabolism and the fluid and electrolyte balance of the body; changes in these systems occur in parallel and the mechanisms are interrelated. The metabolic response has two phases. The first phase, which is catabolic, involves the progressive mobilisation of energy resources. Commencing with carbohydrate reserves, stores are made available for tissue consumption, elevating blood levels and depleting the stores. Glycogen, fat, and protein are affected, producing supplies of glucose, free fatty acids, and amino acids respectively. The latter may be used for the formation of new protein or converted to carbohydrate. The overall effect is a reduction in muscle mass and a negative nitrogen balance. This phase may only be brief in minor injury, but can last for 1 to 2 weeks after surgical injury and may extend to months in severe chronic infection. Recovery is accompanied by an anabolic phase, in which nutrient stores are restored and muscle tissue rebuilt.

The accompanying biphasic changes in fluid and electrolyte balance occur over similar periods. Initially, there is fluid retention plus decreased urinary excretion of sodium and chloride ions. At the same time, potassium excretion is increased. In the second phase, the processes are reversed and the normal balance eventually restored. These changes have implications for normal functioning of cells (e.g. nerves and muscle fibres) and also affect the fluid requirements of those people who are ill.

The metabolic and the fluid and electrolyte changes are influenced by changes in hormonal control, and in particular by secretions from the pituitary and adrenal glands. An early response to a wide variety of disease states is the release of adrenaline from the adrenal medulla, and this contributes to the rapid provision of additional glucose supplies in the blood. This may be associated with an extension of the alarm reaction. The longer-term catabolic phase of the metabolic response is attributable to secretion of corticosteroids (hydrocortisone). Again, the effect is to provide extra nutrient supplies, even though fat and protein are lost. This hormonally mediated response is a general response to states of stress (almost any severely adverse condition), providing a degree of protection and constituting the general adaptation syndrome. The corticosteroid effects also partially explain the ionic changes, especially the sodium and water retention, in which aldosterone and vasopressin are also involved.

Nervous System Involvement in Disease

A variety of disorders arise as a result of nervous activity or malfunction, and the combination of these effects produces the state of feeling unwell. The general response is adaptation to the pathological circumstances, but this may actually impede normal functions. The outcome for the patient is, at the least, discomfort.

Activation of the sympathetic system accounts for some of the discomfort, particularly from physical injury, and may feature restlessness and agitation accompanying a racing pulse, and cutaneous discomfort. Similar sensations may be provoked by the fear of impending unpleasant events (e.g. forthcomimg surgery). Another aspect of sympathetic activity may occur in mental disease (e.g. during attacks of agitation in anxiety neurosis, in which feelings of fear are matched by palpitations, hypertension, deep breathing, flushing, sweating, piloerection, and dry mouth).

Pain or pruritus are the principal results of sensory nerve stimulation, and a major feature of local and whole-body disease. The mental state of the patient is also important, because the perception and tolerance of these sensations are worsened by fear or other mental distress. Sensations of bodily discomfort result from the circulation of toxic materials or alterations in blood content (e.g. pruritus associated with jaundice, or nausea from gastro-intestinal infection). Shivering and pyrexia are the results of altered nervous function. These appear with other effects and sensations in various combinations, typifying specific diseases. In most cases, there will also be a general sensation of malaise.

Abnormal mental activity is a major component of illness and may even be responsible for physical disease. Psychosomatic influence on physiological controls may disturb general body functions, or may cause specific diseases (e.g. essential hypertension or gastric ulcer-

ation). Such manifestations complicate the presentation of other disease states, possibly obscuring or misleading diagnosis. Alternatively, mental disorder may lead to the presentation of spurious or imaginary illness (hypochondriasis). In the worst cases, this may lead the patient to self-inflicted injury in order to sustain the illusion of illness.

15.2 MODES OF ACTION OF INFLUENCES CAUSING CELLULAR DAMAGE OR DEATH

Introduction

There are many more ways in which damage may be inflicted on living cells or tissues than there are ways for the cells to respond to the damage. The minute mechanistic details of all possible causes of damage are diverse, and may even differ between cell types or in the tissues of individuals. Nevertheless, there are important features in common and some general principles which may be explained, particularly by offering categorisation of effects and quoting key examples. Above all, it is essential to attempt an explanation of how the diversity of actions may all link up with the very limited range of subsequent cellular changes.

Modes of action of pathogens, immune mechanisms, irritants, and genetic errors will be explained in other sections with the appropriate topics. This section is concerned with physical and chemical actions, toxic mechanisms, and resulting biochemical defects.

Hypoxic Mechanisms

Most of the cells of the body derive essential energy by oxidative (aerobic) metabolism of nutrients. Metabolism is oxygen-dependent and therefore impaired if the supply is deficient (hypoxia) or absent (anoxia). Hypoxic cells deprived of energy resources may have impaired function and suffer structural damage; severe hypoxia may kill the cell and possibly the whole body. The duration of oxygen lack may be as important as its degree of severity. Cell types vary considerably in their dependence on oxidative metabolism. Some cells can, at least temporarily, produce energy by alternative anaerobic metabolism. Cells therefore differ in their relative vulnerability.

The energy-supplying metabolism normally utilises

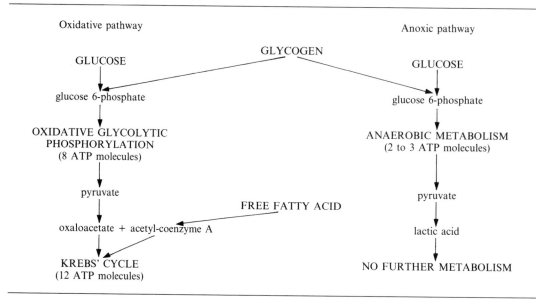

Fig. 15.2
Outline pathways of oxidative (aerobic) and anoxic (anaerobic) metabolism of nutrient materials supplying utilisable cellular energy. Utilisable energy is indicated in terms of the numbers of ATP molecules produced per molecule of respective nutrient.

both glucose and free fatty acid (FFA)(Fig. 15.2). Glucose is oxidised by oxidative glycolytic phosphorylation to pyruvate and thence to the oxygen-dependent Krebs' cycle. Fatty acid is oxidised to acetyl-coenzyme A (active acetate) which also enters the Krebs' cycle. In the absence of oxygen, glucose may be used anaerobically, but there is no anaerobic counterpart for fat metabolism.

This distinction is important. For cells performing continually and having large energy requirements, FFA is a very substantial nutrient energy source. Cardiac muscle is the principal example, but the same applies to other tissues during more intense activity. Hypoxia will deny these cells this source of energy and they will then attempt to use glucose anaerobically. However, this will be much less efficient because the pyruvate produced as a result of anaerobic metabolism cannot progress into the oxygen-dependent Krebs' cycle. Instead, pyruvate is converted to lactic acid and no further metabolism occurs. Much less energy is produced by anaerobic glycolysis (2 molecules of ATP as opposed to 8 per original glycogen unit); cellular ATP levels will fall when there is continued usage in the absence of Krebs' cycle energy. The situation will be even worse if the supply of glucose is also impaired. Neurones and myocardial cells are particularly vulnerable as they have little stored

glycogen, and high rates of metabolism ensure that this is speedily depleted. Skeletal muscle may have a reasonable temporary supply of glycogen and may therefore incur oxygen debt, whereas cardiac muscle may not.

Other cells, particularly some connective tissue cells, are less affected by hypoxia and can subsist entirely on anaerobic metabolism. Macrophage monocytes, especially the non-motile epithelioid or giant-cell forms (*see* Section 15.4), thrive in anoxic sites where specialist functional cells will die. Fibroblasts proliferate and produce collagen fibres under similar conditions. Microglia and astrocytes, the counterparts of these cell types in the central nervous system, are similarly able to survive and proliferate where hypoxic neurones have rapidly perished.

Hypoxia may be a condition affecting whole systems, particularly when due to deficient oxygenation of the blood. This may arise as a result of asphyxia, suffocation, respiratory failure, broncho-occlusion, or pulmonary alveolar damage. Oxygen transport by the blood is reduced by impaired pulmonary blood-flow, anaemia, or carbon monoxide-denatured haemoglobin. A major cause of hypoxia is the failure of blood supply perfusing the tissues (*see* Ischaemia, below, *and* Section 16.1).

Ischaemia

Insufficient blood supply to a tissue will cause both hypoxia and deficiency of nutrient supplies (e.g. FFA, glucose, and amino acids). Tissues will also lack other essential materials (e.g. insulin, thyroxine, trace elements, electrolytes, and vitamins). The most devastating effects, however, are from combined hypoxia and glucose-lack. Systemic abnormalities (e.g. heart failure, vasomotor failure, shock, haemorrhage, pulmonary circulation occlusion, or very low blood volume) may cause widespread ischaemia, producing reduction or cessation of blood flow in various organs or tissues. More localised ischaemia results from individual blood vessel blockage (e.g. embolus or thrombus, *see* Section 16.1), occlusion (e.g. due to pressure, atherosclerotic plaques, or other vascular wall damage), or constriction (e.g. arteriosclerosis). Stasis due to severe inflammation or very viscous blood may also impair local blood flow. Anatomical factors are prime determinants of ischaemic effects. Apart from differing sensitivities of tissues to deprivation of blood-borne materials, the possibilities of alternative blood supplies (by collateral or anastomosing vessels) may alleviate the full consequences of ischaemia or allow restoration of an effective supply. Combinations of systemic and local ischaemia are likely to be serious and, when severe, the result is necrosis.

Areas of necrotic tissue caused by local cessation of blood flow (infarcts) tend to be cone- or wedge-shaped, because the distribution of downstream vascular tributaries from the point of cessation generally spreads out in such shapes. Cross-flow from adjacent normal vessels may, however, alter the pattern. Ischaemic necrosis develops distal to any impediment to flow, and therefore remote areas (e.g. limb extremities or inner layers of cardiac muscle) are common sites of infarction.

Local ischaemia is rare in the liver. The lobules of this organ have a dual blood supply, consisting of oxygen-rich arterial blood mixed with nutrient-rich hepatic portal blood from the intestine. However, the organ as a whole is more vulnerable to the systemic effects of congestive heart failure. The liver is a reservoir for a large volume of low-pressure venous blood, and its drainage is particularly impaired when the main veins of the body become engorged. This adversely affects flow though the whole organ, and tissue necrosis may result.

Cardiac muscle is especially vulnerable to ischaemia, not only through hypoxia but also as a result of the marked extent to which it may respond to increased work demands. It may be impossible to match increased energy demands with the prevailing coronary blood supply, especially when coronary arteries are narrowed by atherosclerosis. Hypoxia of atherosclerosis is therefore aggravated (e.g. by exercise).

Even greater vulnerability is displayed by cerebral neurones (*see* Section 16.5), the most sensitive of all cells to ischaemia and hypoxia. Equally, anterior horn cells of the spinal cord, the Purkinje cells of the cerebellum, and pyramidal cells of the hippocampus are almost as sensitive. Neurones generally have high metabolic activity and very little capacity to respire anaerobically; they are also almost totally dependent on glucose. Retinal cells, also neural in origin, are highly dependent upon adequate glucose and oxygen supplies. Deprivation of circulation in all these cells can stop function within a very short time (5 to 20 seconds for cerebral neurones). Damage may be reversible up to about three minutes only. Destruction of the cortex and basal ganglia occurs after 8 minutes, the entire brainstem at 10 minutes, and spinal cord by 15 minutes. The grey matter is much more severely affected than the white. Systemic ischaemia produces more severe effects than local ischaemia. Some local ischaemia may be negated by an alternative blood supply via the circle of Willis (*see* Section 4.6).

Other tissues subject to ischaemic damage are the parenchymatous epithelial tissues of the kidney, and endocrine and exocrine glands. These commonly have single track blood supplies and, at times, may have high metabolic energy requirements and hence high vascular dependence. Surface or lining epithelial cells (e.g. of the skin, respiratory tract, and cornea) are less energy demanding. Some surface cells have access to atmospheric oxygen (e.g. in the lungs) so that their survival is prolonged, even after body death. Pressure and occlusion of surface cells may cancel this advantage (e.g. as seen in the development of necrotic decubitus ulcers in skin).

Physical Forms of Damage

Traumatic damage is caused by mechanical forces disrupting tissue and cellular structures. Energy imparting damage may occur from forces of compression, laceration, piercing, cutting, shear forces, deceleration, and impact. Certain structures (e.g. nerve fibres) are especially vulnerable. The main effect is the separation of cells or the rupture of blood vessels, or both. Haemorrhage and ischaemia from blood-vessel severance are important causes of secondary and possibly remote damage. Local haemorrhages are revealed as contusions or bruising. Blood accumulation from haemorrhage may cause damage due to pressure (e.g. in the cranium) or by causing further ischaemia.

Thermal injury caused by excessive heat denatures

tissues by burning or scalding. Dry heat may be less damaging than heat combined with hydrolytic effects (e.g. steam). Denaturing and coagulation of cellular protein affects intracellular organelles, membranes, and enzymes; nuclear contents are also affected with the destruction of DNA. Fatty materials (i.e. stored triglyceride fat and the lipid of membranes) are also degraded. A heating effect, observed especially in skin, is the separation of cells and tissue layers together with fluid accumulation, causing blistering (vesiculation). This is a combination of inflammatory exudation from blood vessels and transudation from damaged cells. Body hyperpyrexia (hyperthermia) also produces adverse effects but at lower temperatures. Neurones, especially cerebrocortical, pyramidal, and cerebellar Purkinje cells, have special sensitivity and become necrotic from temperatures as low as 41°C, with fatal effects ensuing within a few hours.

Reduced temperatures lower cellular metabolism and reduce functional activity. Actual cellular damage requires freezing (or near-freezing) temperatures and results mainly from ice-crystal formation. Rapid freezing is more damaging than slow, because it results in intracellular crystallisation and disruption. Slower freezing gives larger, mainly extracellular, crystals. Membrane damage (cell or organelle) may be caused by ice penetration or distortion. Injuries are also caused by abnormal osmotic gradients that develop in freezing or thawing. Cold temperatures cause physical changes in lipoprotein and DNA. An additional cause of cell death is ischaemia, resulting from vasoconstriction, thrombosis, and blood-cell damage. Frozen necrotic tissue becomes blackened by the presence of haemoglobin breakdown products.

Damage caused by Ionising Radiation and Nuclear Particles

Radiation effects in tissues are the result of energy transfer to component matter. Chemical changes follow from molecular activation. Three physical processes which operate at different energy levels account for energy transfer: photo-electric absorption, Compton recoil absorption, and ionic pair production. Radiation from different sources may thus differ in its physical actions and this may give a different quality to the effect on tissues. This is taken into account in relation to the physical units used to define radiation dosage. The energy dose absorbed by tissues is expressed according to the International System of Units (SI) as the gray (1 joule of energy per kg). Dose-effect relationships are further refined by application of a Quality Factor for particular types of radiation, expressing the relative biological

TABLE 15.1
Relative biological effectiveness of different types of radiation: absorbed energy dosage producing equivalent effects in tissues

Radiation	Quality factor (QF)
X-rays	1
γ-radiation	1
β-particles	1
neutrons	2 to 10
α-particles	20

effectiveness. The SI unit arising from the use of the Quality Factor is the Sievert (Table 15.1). Energy levels and qualities determine the ability to penetrate tissues and the ways in which cellular structures are attacked.

Energy transferred to matter results in ionisation of component atoms or, at least, elevation of the atom to a higher excitation state, both effects increasing chemical reactivity. Excited atoms give rise to molecular changes and the major consideration is the absorption of sufficient energy to form free radicals. In tissues, the main component affected is water; ionic pairs are formed and give rise to various ions plus free radicals. Ionised and free radical products (particularly hydroxyl free radicals) are chemically highly reactive. Hydrogen peroxide and peroxy free radicals are also formed. These free radicals attack enzymes, membrane lipoprotein, or proteins, denaturing vital cellular components and causing the toxigenic effects of irradiation. Cellular results will be degeneration, leading to necrosis (*see* Section 15.3). These effects are energy-dose dependent and therefore predictable on a dose-related basis (non-stochastic effects).

Other effects in cells are believed to depend upon target interactions of radiation with molecules of particular character or importance, especially macro-molecules (e.g. DNA). The high susceptibility of lymphocytes to irradiation is explained on the basis that the relatively very large mass of nuclear material in these cells exposes a vulnerable target. Target damage is called a stochastic effect, frequency rather than severity being dose-related. Genetic abnormalities (*see* Section 15.8) and neoplastic changes (*see* Section 15.7) result from such effects.

Tissues respond to irradiation with markedly different susceptibilities. The response may be explained by the Law of Bergonie and Tribondeau (1904), which states that 'radiosensitivity of cells is related directly to their ability to divide and inversely to their degree of differentiation'. Tissues may therefore be assigned categories ranging from radiosensitive, through radioresponsive, to radioresistant:

- Proliferating cells are most radiosensitive (e.g. blood-forming stem cells, gastro-intestinal basal epithelia, epidermal basal cell layer, and gonadal germinal cells).
- Differentiating cells (e.g. intermediate forms in development of blood cells, spermatozoa, and ova).
- Intermediate sensitivity is displayed by sporadically dividing cells for repair or maintenance in blood vessels and connective tissues (e.g. endothelial cells and fibroblasts).
- Regenerating, differentiated functional post-mitotic cells (e.g. in liver, glands, and kidneys).
- End cells, highly differentiated with little or no ability to divide (e.g. neurones, and skeletal and cardiac muscle) are quite radioresistant.

Systemic effects range from minor acute discomfort to death (Table 15.2), depending upon dosage, frequency of exposure, and form of radiation. Local effects include focused irradiation, sunburn, or effects of low penetration particles (β-burns). Interrupted dosage is less severe than the same dose received all at once. This is because some repair or recovery may take place in the interval between exposures. Repair mechanisms can reverse some effects, even potentially mutagenic or carcinogenic changes in DNA. In the case of ultraviolet exposure, skin prepared by previous low level exposure is less susceptible to otherwise harmful doses.

Chemical and Toxic Damage

It is not possible to deal with the entire range of toxic effects; some forms of toxicity are more pertinent to other sections of Chapters 15 and 16, so that irritants (*see* Section 15.4), sensitising agents (*see* Section 16.7), carcinogens (*see* Section 15.7), and teratogens (*see* Section 15.8) are dealt with elsewhere. Another major, but very diverse, category of harmful substances is comprised of agents which modify function rather than cause overt structural damage. These often specific interactions are covered in more detailed texts of pharmacology or toxicology.

TABLE 15.2
Acute radiation syndrome

Whole body effects of relatively short exposures to ionising radiation. Dosage is expressed in terms of absorbed radiation (100 rad = 1 gray), as typified by X-ray or γ-radiation, low Linear Energy Transfer radiation (Quality Factor 1). Other forms of energy require application of the appropriate Quality Factor, giving dosage in rem (100 rem = 1 Sievert)

Dosage (rad or cgray)	Time		
0 to 20	No detectable effect at any time		
20 to 70	Slight fall in lymphocytes and sperm counts. Chromosomal abberations. No vomiting.		
70 to 150	Prodromal symptoms: anorexia, nausea, vomiting, fatigue. Effects minor and recovery rapid.		
	Week 1	Week 2	Week 3 (plus)
150 to 300	Prodromal symptoms 2 to 24 hours. Lymphocytes fall to <1200/mm³ at 48 hours.	100% recovery.	—
300 to 500	Prodromal symptoms with diarrhoea 1 to 48 hours. Lymphocytes fall to 500/mm³ at 48 hours.	Latent period. Erythema 7 to 10 days, hair loss in 10 to 14 days.	Anaemia, purpura, haemorrhages 50% mortality in 10 to 40 days. Male/female sterility in 2 to 3 years.
500 to 800	Severe prodromal symptoms, very rapid with fever and headaches. Lymphocytes 200/mm³ at 48 hours.	Fall in platelets, leucocytes, and erythrocytes. Bleeding, abdominal pains, fever. Immunosuppression.	100% mortality from 8 to 21 days. Combined effects on haemopoietic and gastro-intestinal systems.
1000 to 2500	Prodromal symptoms and incapacitation within minutes.	Nausea and vomiting, diarrhoea, fever, weakness, weight loss, DEATH.	
Up to 20 000	Cardiovascular and cerebral effects. Very rapid onset of prodromal symptoms, with headache, disorientation, ataxia, coma, convulsions, shock, and DEATH in 1 day.		

Many substances produce damaging effects or even cell death by direct chemical action. Obvious examples are strong acids or alkalis whose effects on tissues are directly corrosive, denaturing protein, lipid, and other tissue constituents very readily. Many other chemically highly-reactive substances (e.g. oxidising agents, heavy metal salts, aldehydes, alcohols, and nitro ($-NO_2$) groups) will do likewise. Severe chemical action may completely destroy tissue or denature its protein to the extent of coagulating it (tanning action). Under many circumstances, however, the action will be less intense, and selective damage will occur. Three types of effect warrant attention. Firstly, numerous compounds act largely by oxidative or free radical mechanisms, affecting intracellular structures (e.g. those involved in cell energy production and utilisation). Secondly, the materials with cytoplasmic membrane structures (enzyme or receptor bearing) are especially vulnerable and subject to lipoperoxidation. Thirdly, some important groups of compounds react selectively with vital enzymes, notably those involved in energy generating metabolism. Such toxicity will involve the same structures in the cell as those affected by hypoxia (*see* Hypoxic Mechanisms above) and which are also vulnerable to the toxigenic actions of radiation (i.e. the common theme is attack on energy production).

Many other compounds are intrinsically less chemically reactive and would not directly interact with tissue components under physiological conditions. They may, however, exhibit secondary toxicity by being converted *in vivo* to chemically more reactive derivatives. Many drugs display such covert activity. This is usually the result of chemical biotransformations by Phase I metabolism, which occurs mainly in the liver but is also possible in lung, skin, and other tissues. This produces transient, unstable, reactive, intermediate products which cause toxic damage. The second phase of metabolism completes a process of detoxification.

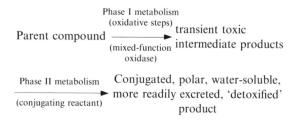

Damage is caused when toxic intermediates gain access to locally available vulnerable material in the cell (e.g. enzymes or membranes) rather than proceeding to Phase II metabolism.

The mechanism primarily responsible for production of the offending materials, the mixed-function oxidase (MFO) system, is a versatile multi-enzyme combination capable of processing a very wide range of compounds. Its great range is all the more remarkable because specific enzymes are required for particular compounds (or groups). Phase I metabolism does not invariably cause toxicity; the main reasons why it will do so are if the MFO activity is enhanced (induction), if high dosage leads to the activity of an abnormal metabolic pathway, or if repeated dosage leads to inadequacy of the system available for Phase II detoxification (e.g. glutathione depletion).

In many cases, the product of MFO activity will be unstable or will exist temporarily as a reactive free radical or even as an ionised reactive molecule. For many compounds, series of metabolic steps may give several reactive and harmful products (e.g. different stages of the oxidising pathways for phenacetin, *see below*, or paracetamol produce epoxide or quinoneimine derivatives).

Numerous other compounds produce such epoxides or quinonoid structures (Table 15.3). Others (e.g. carbon tetrachloride) give rise to free radicals. Thus, a wide range of energised molecules, large or small, may be generated within cells.

Complementary to the oxidising reactions are reduced

TABLE 15.3
Toxic products resulting from activating biotransformation of drugs or chemical agents

Compound	Transformation	Toxic product (transient or intermediate)
Benzene	epoxidation	benzene 1,2 oxide (epoxide)
Carbon tetrachloride	reductive dehalogenation	carbon trichloride free radical
Chloroform	oxygen insertion with dehydrohalogenation	carbonyl chloride
Frusemide	oxidation of furan ring	epoxide
Halothane	reductive dehalogenation	free radical
Isoniazid	acetylation and oxidation	acetylating carbonium free radical
Paraquat	reduction	methyl viologen, free radical, and superoxide

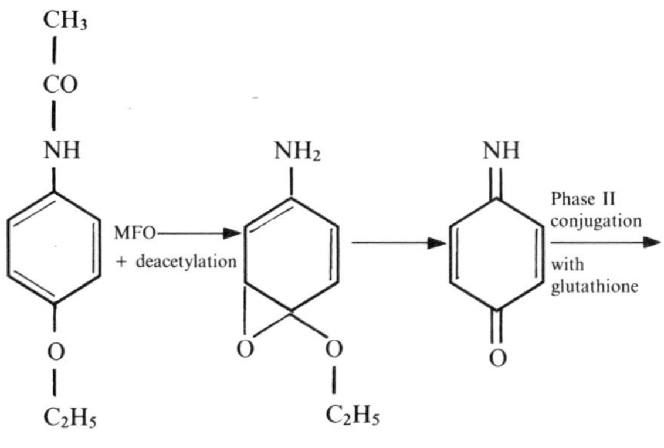

Phenacetin Epoxide Quinoneimine

coenzymes (the hydrogen acceptors) or the cytochrome system. These in turn give rise to reduced products acting upon suitable substrates. A reduced substrate of particular interest is oxygen. While many reducing reactions will culminate in the production of H_2O or CO_2, in some there may be intermediate activated products. Single oxygen atoms and reduced oxygen free radicals (superoxide, $O_2^{\bullet-}$) are generated from molecular oxygen. These chemically highly reactive species are normally well controlled. Nevertheless, like the other activated molecules, they are potentially harmful. Protective reactant systems in the cytoplasm or organelles of cells normally prevent significant damage due to such reactive agents. Antoxidants and free-radical scavengers provide physiological buffers to mop up the excess. In many cases, this function is performed by the Phase II metabolising enzymes (e.g. the glutathione-glutathione transferase system). More specifically, the oxygen radicals are eliminated by the superoxide dismutase, catalase, peroxidase combination. However, deficiencies or overload of these buffering systems may allow the offending products to accumulate or leak into adjacent sites, thus leading to damage. Production of superoxide to this extent may result particularly from autoxidation of chemicals, which is mediated by xanthine oxidase, aldehyde oxidases, dehydrogenases, or by abnormal loads causing electron transport leakage. It is noteworthy that as a consequence of superoxide interactions, hydroxyl free radicals and peroxides may also be formed, analogous to the products generated by irradiation. Paraquat is a potent toxigen which generates superoxide.

Target substrates for the chemically highly reactive products of these mechanisms are generally the enzymes and cellular organelle components. Various interactions are possible, but lipoperoxidation is of particular interest because it may partially explain the intracellular structural derangement which occurs in toxic events (it has its counterpart also in radiation damage). Lipoperoxidation results from oxidative attack on the lipid component of the membranes providing the cell structures (including mitochondria, endoplasmic reticulum, and nuclear membranes).

Lipoperoxidation damage is sustained by the input of both oxidising agents and molecular oxygen, and is impeded by the natural antoxidants in tissues. Radiochemical or photochemical radical-producing actions will trigger or exacerbate it. It may also occur directly as a result of hyperoxic toxicity. As an insidious change with time, it may account for some ageing deterioration in tissues (*see* Section 15.9 *and* Chapter 18).

One of the main targets within the cell is the mitochondrial membrane and its associated enzyme systems. The importance of hypoxia and ischaemia is once more apparent, because mitochondrial destruction must preclude effective energy generation. The same effects may, however, occur rather more specifically without structural mitochondrial damage. Some very important toxic agents inhibit energy-generating metabolism (especially the aerobic function) as a result of selective inhibition of key components of the system. Cyanides and hydrogen sulphide poison the oxidative chain by interacting with iron in the cytochrome-system molecules, thus preventing electron transfer. Nitro compounds uncouple the chain from the nutrient metabolism processes. Arsenic and other heavy metals bind covalently with sulphydryl (-SH) groups in organic molecules, particularly interacting with sulphydryl-rich proteins. Among such proteins are some vital enzymes (e.g. pyruvate oxidase), which will be altered and inactivated. Such an effect, blocking an essential stage in glucose oxidation, inhibits cellular metabolism. Other heavy metals have similar effects.

Overall, it is possible to show a great variety of toxic and other pathological influences interfering with the fundamental energy-producing mechanisms in cells. Likewise, other intracellular structures and mechanisms may be similarly or separately affected (e.g. endoplasmic reticulum and protein synthesis). Although there is great diversity of damage-causing action, some common themes may be discerned. As explained in Section 15.3, the ways in which the cell as a whole can respond to the damage are quite limited. Thus, many varied chains of adverse effects may lead to the same general consequences.

15.3 CELL AND TISSUE RESPONSES TO DAMAGE

Introduction

This section concerns only the effects on the established cellular components of a tissue (e.g. hepatocytes or cardiomyocytes) provoked by mechanisms discussed in Section 15.2. Additionally, a damaging influence is likely to affect the vascular and connective tissue components that produce inflammation, and this is considered in Section 15.4. Typical cellular responses to damage are restricted in variety, in direct contrast to the great diversity of causes. Another aspect of cellular injury is the impairment or cessation of functional activity, although the cell may remain alive. Characteristic structural changes may also indicate the injury in a still-viable cell; such changes are termed degenerations. If the damage is severe, viability may not be sustained and the cell may die. Cell death resulting from injury is termed necrosis. Degenerative changes may be reversible; necrosis is, of course, irreversible.

The damaged cell that suffers a biochemical or substructural lesion will attempt compensatory or reparative changes. The success of these measures may depend on the availability of alternative or reserve energy supplies, or the provision of an advantageous environment; cells may survive and recover from some degree of damage without major overt structural or even functional change. Recovery is promoted by the removal of the damaging influence. More severe or persistent injury causes the observable degenerative processes described below. Even more serious damage may change the cell into a stage beyond recovery, involving cessation of useful function but leaving the cell alive. Ultimately the cell's mechanisms fail totally, and death ensues (Fig. 15.3) rapidly or after delay, depending on the severity of the insult. Whatever the case, it is still impossible to determine precisely the event or change which actually denotes the point of death and necrosis is largely defined by observation of changes which follows its occurrence.

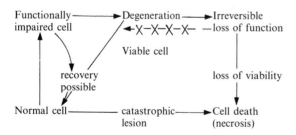

Fig. 15.3
Progression of cellular changes resulting from damage.

Not all cell death is explained in such terms, nor is it only caused by damaging influences. Another normal process appears to operate largely on a predetermined or programmed basis, and accounts for much of the massive cellular loss involved in foetal development and organ modelling. This process (apoptosis) is understood to continue throughout life, accounting particularly for the natural ageing deterioration of the body (see Section 15.9).

Degenerations

Observable changes in damaged cells, described as degenerations, are largely attributable to some continued activity within the cell. Such changes have also been described as cellular agony, representing a response to damage. One feature of this may be a change in motile activity (e.g. observable in cells in culture which display abnormal contractile or rounding-up activity), while a more generally observable characteristic of all degenerations is cell swelling. Three main degenerations are recognised (Fig. 15.4).

Damage to energy production or utilising mechanisms results in hydropic degeneration (cloudy swelling or aqueous swelling). This involves the influx of water from surrounding extracellular fluid due to changes in internal osmotic pressure. The main factor causing this is impairment of the energy-requiring sodium pump in the cell membrane. The sodium pump normally extrudes sodium ions (with chloride ions), and accounts for the normally polarised state of the membrane in the cell at rest. As the pump energy fails or the membrane is otherwise damaged, the ions re-enter the cell, also drawing in water to increase cell volume. Not only does the damaged cell function imperfectly, but it loses its responsiveness to stimulus or excitation because the membrane becomes depolarised. Cytoplasmic changes are also seen as some of the water causes swelling of organelles (e.g. mitochondria or endoplasmic reticulum) and appears in enlarged vacuoles. Perinuclear spaces (haloes) distended with fluid also occur. Distortion or disruption of organelles results from damaged membranes, or denatured protein and redistribution of calcium (which appears in abnormal deposits associated with damaged protein).

Toxic or hypoxic damage to intracellular structures may particularly result in accumulation of denatured protein. Alternatively, impaired functioning or reabsorbed protein from adjacent areas may lead to internal accumulation of proteinaceous secretions, enzymes, antibodies, or hormones. The deposits are observable microscopically as globules or droplets of protein in the cells, and the defect is termed hyaline degeneration. Hyaline material is thus indicative of, or associated with, malfunction. It occurs in alcohol-damaged liver cells and dying cardiac muscle.

In some tissues, cell damage features accumulation of

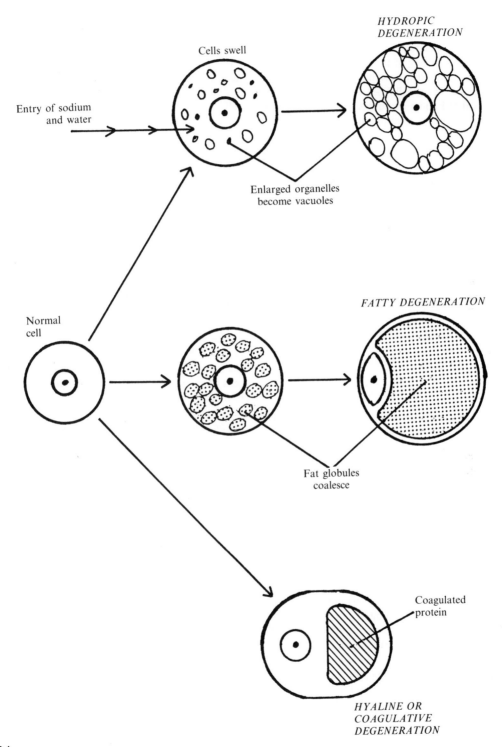

HYDROPIC DEGENERATION

Cells swell

Entry of sodium and water

Enlarged organelles become vacuoles

Normal cell

FATTY DEGENERATION

Fat globules coalesce

Coagulated protein

HYALINE OR COAGULATIVE DEGENERATION

Fig. 15.4
Degenerative changes in cells.

fat as globular deposits and is termed fatty degeneration. This may occur in otherwise normal tissues as a result of excessive supply of fatty material (e.g. in obesity), in which case the cells merely function as stores. However, cell damage, particularly of the endoplasmic reticulum and its protein-synthesising mechanisms, can also cause fat accumulation. Many cell types, which have absorbed free fatty acid (FFA) as an energy-providing nutrient, dispose of the excess by excreting it in the form of lipoprotein. However, if protein synthesis generally and hence lipoprotein synthesis in particular is impaired, the fatty acid cannot be excreted (Fig. 15.5). Instead, it is stored in the cell as triglyceride fat. Large accumulations distend the cell, which may remain viable but with severely curtailed functioning. Fatty accumulations may also occur in conjunction with hydropic degeneration in energy-damaged cells (e.g. in hypoxia) when nutrient fatty acid cannot be properly utilised.

Cellular utilisation or elimination of free fatty acid (FFA) involving energy production, storage, or elimination. If elimination is prevented, excess FFA accumulates and is retained as triglyceride fat.

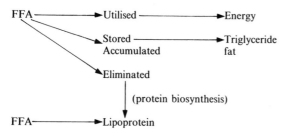

Fig. 15.5
Fatty degeneration mechanism.

Necrosis

Severe deficiency of usable energy within the cell, disruption of mechanisms sustaining life, or destruction of vital membranes, organelles, or nuclear structure beyond a certain degree, all result in cell death. Because of the interrelationships with usable energy, necrosis may generally be associated with hydropic degeneration. If death occurs rapidly, the full manifestation of degeneration may not have time to develop. If death is delayed, as in severe degeneration with a dying period, the cellular disruption will continue past the indefinable point of death.

Post-necrotic changes involve abnormal behaviour of the nucleus and progressive deterioration of cellular structure. If the process is slow or conditions after death are not extreme, the nucleus may go through a sequence of changes: pyknosis, karyorrhexis, and karyolysis (Fig. 15.6), leading to its disintegration. This sequence is not invariable, and catastrophic death may involve rapid and radical disorganisation. Depending upon the type of cell and the prevailing conditions, one general consequence is that the tissue may become a mass of coagulated protein (coagulation necrosis or dry gangrene). Such a change is typical of an ischaemic/anoxic necrosis in muscle. Other types of dead cells will, however, liquefy (e.g. those which contain lysosomes or secrete proteolytic enzymes, as in gastro-intestinal mucosal glands). Such cells are subject to autolysis, or self-digestion, and the tissue undergoes liquefaction necrosis.

Areas of dead tissue existing in living bodies may persist unchanged as infarcts or gangrene. In most cases, however, further destruction will be performed by action of cells from surrounding tissue or residual blood supply. Such lysis and phagocytosis of necrotic tissue by polymorphonuclear leucocytes and monocyte macrophages constitute very important features of the repair processes of damaged tissues. Such removal of dead cells is a necessary preliminary to their replacement by living cells or connective tissue, or both. Dead cells may also be destroyed in living or dead bodies by microbial action (e.g. gas gangrene infection in live tissues, and saprophytic or putrefactive action of bacteria and fungi in dead bodies). The latter actions are, of course, the usual postmortem putrefaction initiated by intestinal flora.

The other major process for cellular removal, apoptosis, also involves the ultimate removal of cellular fragments by phagocytosis. However, the process leading up to cell death is the opposite to that which occurs in degenerative swelling. In apoptosis, the cells shrink. Whereas necrosis occurs as a cessation of energy-using function, apoptosis appears to be an energy-requiring process in which the shrivelled cells break up into membrane-bound fragments (Fig. 15.6). It is these fragments which are ingested by macrophages or even adjacent tissue cells such as hepatocytes (e.g. in yellow fever). Apart from embryonic and geriatric cell death, other extensive atrophy of tissues (e.g. some virus effects, cytotoxic actions, regression of malignant tissues, and the involution of lymphoid tissue caused by corticosteroids) may take place by apoptosis.

Regeneration

In living tissues, one possible sequel to the loss of cells after death and phagocytosis is regeneration, replenish-

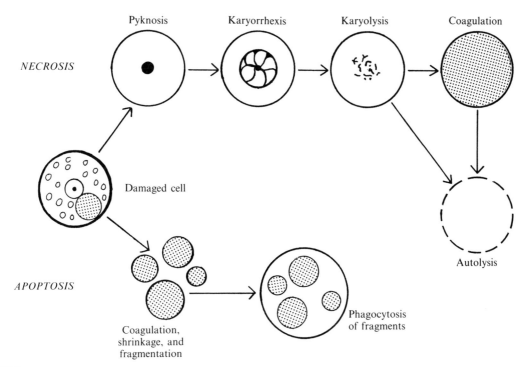

Fig. 15.6
Cell death: necrosis and apoptosis and subsequent destructive changes.

ment by cell-division. This is a desirable effect as it would lead to restoration of the functional-cell stock of the tissue. Unfortunately, not all of the body's tissues have effective regenerative capacity. Relative abilities of tissues to regenerate are shown in Table 15.4.

Generally, cellular regeneration occurs at varying rates in relation to tissue wear and tear. After substantial cell death (e.g. ischaemic infarct), full replacement of functional tissue may depend upon the restoration of ideal conditions (e.g. regrowth of effective blood supply) or may require an appropriate connective tissue framework (e.g. Schwann cells for axonal regrowth, or reticulin network for liver cells).

When damaged tissue does not have appropriate regenerative ability or when a pathological influence is persistent (e.g. toxic effect or hypoxia), the tissue replacement may instead be achieved by formation of connective tissue (*see* Section 15.4). In these circumstances, mechanical tissue repair may be achieved, although the tissue formed is scar tissue and functional-cell capacity is diminished.

TABLE 15.4
Regenerative capacities of tissues

Very effective regeneration
    bone marrow haemopoietic cells and connective
        tissue cells (e.g. bone and fibroblasts)

Generally effective in optimal conditions
    parenchymal epithelial tissues (e.g. liver lobules,
        renal tubules, endocrine gland cells such as
        adrenal cortex and thyroid, and other glands)

Intermediate effectiveness
    surface epithelia (e.g. skin, gastro-intestinal mucosa,
        and respiratory tract)

Limited regeneration
    axonal processes of neurones

Little or no regenerative activity
    muscle cells and central neurones

15.4 INFLAMMATION: DAMAGE, PROTECTION, AND REPAIR

Introduction

Inflammation is an important component of many forms of disease, particularly those in which tissue damage occurs (e.g. toxic and necrotic lesions, hypersensitivities or auto-immune conditions, and traumas). It may account for much of the discomfort and disability which results, and in some conditions, the inflammation itself may be aggressive and tissue damaging. Thus, inflammation may be a response to disease processes, but it may also be instrumental in causing further damage (e.g. fibrosis). In the main, however, the mechanisms are essentially protective and reparative, so that inflammation plays a part in healing processes and in the control of most infections.

Inflammatory processes involve the blood vessels and interstitial connective tissue of the affected area. Pathological changes in the functional cells of a tissue constitute a separate aspect (*see* Section 15.3). The cardinal signs of inflammation are erythema, oedema, heat, pain or pruritus, and often impairment of function. These signs indicate the acute aspects of inflammation. Further developments involving cellular accumulation, structural breakdown, and ultimate fibrous changes constitute more chronic changes in tissues.

These processes are non-specific responses to damage (i.e. essentially the same process is activated whatever the cause). Common causes include trauma, burning, corrosive action of chemicals, toxic damage, cell death, infections, hypersensitivities, and plant, animal or microbial venoms and toxins. Agents causing inflammation without necessarily resulting in any other damage are called irritants, although irritancy is usually closely associated with other toxic or pathological influence. Although there are few major qualitative differences in the inflammation from diverse causes, there are very strong quantitative relationships. The severity and extent of inflammation are clearly dependent upon intensity of the irritant or damaging effect. Similarly, inflammation normally persists only for as long as the process is needed (Fig. 15.7). However, in pathological inflammation (e.g. hypersensitivities, rheumatoid, and auto-immune diseases), the severity and persistence of inflammation are abnormal, harmful, and not apparently protective or reparative.

Acute Inflammation

Following provocation, the first signs of inflammation develop very rapidly. In most sites, the immediate response is due to the activation of mast cells which release stored secretory granules (*see also* Section 9.4). The granules contain various materials, including the potent vasoactive agent histamine which dissolves in tissue fluid and diffuses throughout adjacent connective tissue. Sufficiently high local concentrations stimulate receptors of sensory nerves and smooth muscle. These stimuli cause vasodilatation, commencing with capillaries in the immediate vicinity. Local nerve (axon) reflexes extend the blood-vessel dilatation to arterioles (Fig. 15.8). Blood flow is thus increased, resulting in local reddening and often a temperature rise. Increased blood flow is potentially beneficial, improving oxygenation and nutrition and transporting haemostatic and protective components of plasma.

Another effect of histamine is the increase in permeability of capillary walls, permitting passage of plasma fluid into the tissue spaces of the affected area. This causes oedema, a dynamic phenomenon which results in an increased flow of fluid through the interstitial space of the tissue, with ultimate drainage usually via lymphatic vessels. This may help to dilute and flush away foreign material. Furthermore, it spreads plasma proteins with protective functions (e.g. fibrinogen, antibodies, and complement) through the tissues.

These early responses may not persist. If histamine is washed away or metabolised, the blood vessels could revert to normal and the inflammation subside. How-

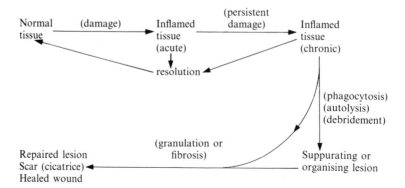

Fig. 15.7
Stages and reversibility (resolution) of inflammation.

Vascular dilatation

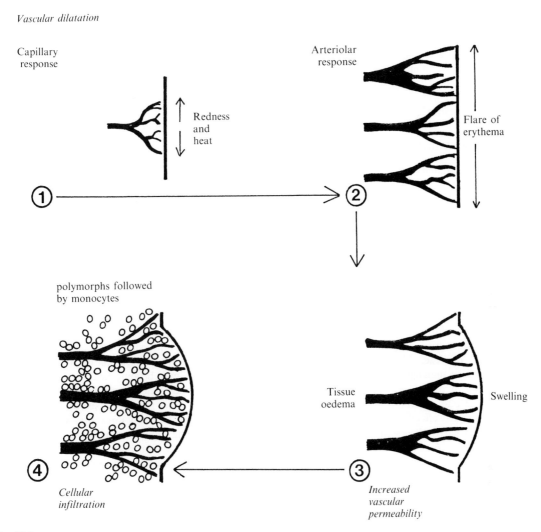

Fig. 15.8
Acute inflammation.

ever, continued causative action is matched by continued vasodilatation and fluid exudation. The role of histamine is taken over by other inflammatory mediators (*see below*) derived from plasma (e.g. kinins or complement components) or from adjacent damaged tissue (e.g. prostaglandins, leukotrienes, or lysosomal enzymes). Such mediators also give rise to further changes involving cellular infiltration (Fig. 15.8).

Cellular infiltration occurs from the blood. Leucocytes are initially influenced to adhere to blood-vessel walls, then to move through pores or channels in or between the cells of the walls, and finally to migrate through the accumulated exudate in the inflamed tissue. These actions are determined by the mediator effects,

partly on the blood vessels and partly chemotactic influence, to attract cell migration. Once attracted, the cells are then activated. Initially, the main inflammatory cell type is the polymorphonuclear neutrophil. This may in time be supplemented or replaced by others (e.g. monocytes), but the infiltration of neutrophils may continue for long periods with the accumulation of astronomical numbers. If required, bone-marrow production of these cells is stimulated.

The function of neutrophils is mainly the secretion of destructive enzymes which are capable of attacking micro-organisms or digesting tissues. To a lesser extent, neutrophils have phagocytic capabilities and can also kill cells by a cytotoxic action known as oxygen burst (*see* Section 15.5). Neutrophils themselves are killed in the course of their actions, and the accumulation of living and dead cells forms pus (pyogenesis).

Pus forms in cavities which develop within inflamed tissue (abscesses). Even though this is destructive, the process is potentially beneficial as it promotes the elimination of infection, debridement of dead tissue, or the removal of foreign matter.

Chronic Inflammation

Pyogenesis may be initiated early in inflammation, but it may also be persistent, thus constituting a feature of both acute and chronic inflammation. Two outcomes are possible in chronic inflammation. The total elimination of the cause may proceed to tissue repair or, in the case of intractable causes (e.g. foreign bodies, resistant infection, or persisting immune reactions), the reaction continues to isolate and repair the lesion as far as is possible.

Both the repair or the prolongation of chronic inflammation depend upon two additional cell populations. Following, or in addition to, polymorphonuclear activity, monocytes infiltrate the lesion, again mainly from the blood. Bone-marrow production may be increased for this purpose. Monocytes also perform phagocytosis, more so than neutrophils, but they are less effective in killing or digesting some material. Monocytes may mature into macrophages (scavenger cells) and may be particularly effective at the final elimination of material already partly processed by the neutrophils. Alternatively, monocytes may be very active as phagocytes in even very early phases of inflammation, especially if particles of foreign material are present. Accumulation of macrophages in nodular masses in response to substantial quantities of material, especially if very persistent, may develop, and they remain in tissues for long periods. Nodular masses of monocytes form granulomas (*see* Section 15.5). Cells in these structures cease aggressive phagocytosis and accumulate in layers (epithelioid cells). Epithelioid masses form around large or irremoveable foreign objects, and numbers of very heavily laden macrophages often coalesce to form multinucleate giant-cells. These mechanisms appear to provide long-term containment of persistent material. Chronic infection is similarly contained.

In and around inflammatory lesions, the proliferation and activation of fibroblast cells is provoked. Masses of these cells accumulate and form an enclosing layer. The fibroblasts are also activated to promote the synthesis and deposition of fibrillar protein (collagen). Commonly, fibroblasts will migrate into an area of coagulated, denatured, or digested protein, pus, thrombus, or macrophage nodule. The fibroblasts are also capable of digestive enzyme secretion, particularly proteolytic enzymes, and make use of the breakdown products as nutrient, with amino acids contributing to collagen biosynthesis. Thus, encroaching masses of fibroblasts are involved in the removal of lesion components and their replacement by collagen fibre deposits. Collagen fibre deposition may be followed by the formation of new capillary blood vessels (Fig. 15.9). Layers of collagen fibres permeated by a capillary network have a characteristic appearance (granulation tissue). This term is not to be confused with granuloma, although the two often occur together (*see* Fig. 15.10).

A layer of granulation tissue forms a barrier between normal and pathological tissue, and may be especially valuable for the containment of invasive cells. It forms around abscesses (pyogenic membrane) and commonly around infected granulomas (e.g. tubercle, *see* Section 15.5). Restraining barriers also surround some tumours, persistent foreign bodies, or necrotic tissues.

If fibroblasts are able to continue to penetrate abnormal material, an advancing front of granulation tissue will progressively replace pus, thrombus, or dead cells with vascular fibrous connective tissue (*see* Section 10.5). In this way, a necrotic or pyogenic cavity may be filled or, with advancing granulation from either side, surgical wounds may become healed. Such fibrous replacement performs a mechanical repair but the result is a scar (this term is not to be confused with eschar, which is necrotic tissue). This may not represent full healing if the fibrous tissue replaces the specialist functional tissue. In some cases, fibroblast activity may be particularly aggressive, attacking and replacing normal tissue; this effect is fibrosis (e.g. in silicosis, asbestosis, or fibrosing alveolitis in the lungs).

Ideally, tissue repair also involves the regeneration of functional cells, and some tissues (e.g. bone-marrow haemopoietic tissue) can perform this particularly well (*see* Table 15.4). Epidermal or gastro-intestinal epithelia also regenerate well, as do some tubular or glandular epithelia (e.g. kidney tubules, liver cells, and endocrine glands). However, regeneration may be ineffectual in other tissues (e.g. muscles). Thus, necrotic cardiac muscle can only be repaired by collagen fibre scar tissue. Even when regeneration is possible, its effectiveness may be impaired (e.g. by chronic toxicity continually killing newly-formed tissue). In such circumstances, the associated and more resilient granulation tissue growth may be favoured, again resulting in collagen fibre replacement of specialist cells. Conflict of this sort accounts for the fibrotic changes in liver damaged by chronic alcohol intake or other toxicity (cirrhosis). Chronic infection, immune damage, or trauma may produce a similar result (e.g. in rheumatoid arthritis).

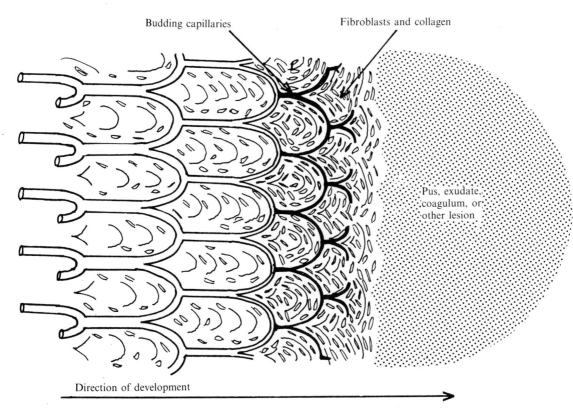

Budding capillaries

Fibroblasts and collagen

Pus, exudate, coagulum, or other lesion

Direction of development

Fig. 15.9
Granulation tissue.

The process of acute or chronic inflammation, up to and including fibrosis, may occur in all body tissues except the central nervous system. In the latter, equivalent changes occur but specialist cellular activities of a protective or reparative nature take place involving astrocytes and glial cells. Neurones of the central nervous system cannot regenerate and are replaced by gliosis, a scarring mechanical repair. Other forms of specialist repair by inflammation occur in damaged connective tissues (e.g. the cicatrisation of bone). These processes are, however, closely analogous to granulation tissue formation originating in areolar tissue.

Inflammatory Mediators

The complex series of interacting vascular and cellular changes in inflammation are explicable on the basis of the combined actions of mediator substances released or formed *in situ* in the area of the lesion. Numerous agents that participate in the various stages are now partially understood (Table 15.5). They cause vascular changes or influence cellular behaviour, or both; there is also considerable overlap in mediator properties.

The initial effects are caused by histamine, which is stored ready-formed in tissue mast cells and is available for action almost immediately. As these effects wear off, supplementary mediators are brought into play. Generally, they are derived from inert precursor substances which have been activated, usually by enzyme action. For precursor activation to occur, the enzyme itself needs to be activated and often the process requires a chain or cascade of successive enzyme activations. Good examples of such cascades are the kallikrein-kinin system and the complement system, both originating in plasma proteins passing into inflammatory exudate. The polypeptide kinins, bradykinin and kallidin, derived from the kallikrein-kinin system appear to be brought into operation at an early stage to replace histamine. Complement components provide a much wider, general purpose combination of mediators, accounting for a wide variety of inflammatory mechanisms. A common initiating mechanism for several of the mediator systems is clotting factor XII.

TABLE 15.5
Inflammatory mediators

Histamine	vasodilator, increases vascular permeability, sensory stimulant (pruritus)
Bradykinin and kallidin (polypeptides)	potent vasodilators, exudate promoters, chemotactic agents for leucocyte infiltration, pain-producing
Complement components	various fractions causing histamine release, inflammatory exudation, leucocyte chemotaxis, macrophage phagocytosis and enzyme secretion, tissue lysis, and cytoplasmic-membrane breakdown
Fibrin deposition	haemostasis, protective barrier formation, lesion limitation; involved in vascular damage (associated with hyaline degeneration, collagen degradation, and fibrinoid necrosis)
Mediators derived from arachidonic acid	
• cyclo-oxygenase	produce prostaglandins, thromboxanes, prostacyclin, and endoperoxides; alter blood vessels (dilatation, constriction, or increased permeability)
• lipoxygenase action	produce leukotrienes; vascular responses and exudation, chemotaxis, and activation of secretion by polymorphs and macrophages
Lysosomal enzymes	acid hydrolase, protease, polysaccharidase, lipase, nuclease, and collagenase activities; lyse all components of tissues
Lymphokines	provoke infiltration and activity of inflammatory cells and promote immune and hypersensitivity reactions (cell-mediated)
Acute phase proteins	produced by synthesis in hepatocytes due to humoral stimulation by interleukin-1; include fibrinogen, complement precursors, and other mediator materials; also inhibitory and reaction restraining mediators

Products derived from enzyme action on arachidonic acid, a common component in the phospholipids of cytoplasmic membranes, also appear to account for several aspects of acute reactions. In inflammation, phospholipase-A released from damaged cells converts phospholipids to arachidonic acid. The action of further enzymes gives leukotrienes (lipoxygenase enzyme system) or prostaglandins, thromboxanes, and prostacyclin (cyclo-oxygenase system), which together are capable of causing vasodilatation, exudation, smooth muscle contraction, and cell migration.

The cellular mechanisms in late acute or chronic stages are similarly mediated. Cell migration into the lesion and activation of phagocytosis may be caused by leukotaxin (a kinin mixture), complement components, prostaglandins, and leukotrienes. Secretory products of other cells have an important role in the later stages, especially of immune-controlled reactions. Lymphokines or monokines, from lymphocytes and monocytes respectively, cause mutual activation or chemotaxis, or both. Lymphokines are particularly important in immune-initiated inflammation. Interleukin-1, a monokine, provokes neutrophil secretion and fibroblast proliferation.

Breakdown of tissue components (i.e. cells, fibres, or connective tissue matrix) is effected by various enzymes, some of which may be produced by mediator activation cascades, particularly as a final result of complement activation. Others are secreted by activated inflammatory cells (e.g. lysosomal enzymes from eosinophils or neutrophils have a wide range of actions, and macrophages secrete neutral proteinases that include elastase and collagenase). All of these are responsible for inflammatory tissue degradation which may be a feature of pathological inflammation (e.g. abscess formation or cartilage erosion in inflamed joints). In some cases (e.g. removal of necrotic tissue prior to repair), it may be beneficial. Enzymatic digestion is also an important part of attack on pathogens (e.g. phagocytosed bacteria, multicellular parasites, or virus-containing cells). Similarly, aberrant (e.g. malignant or senile cells) or incompatible tissues (e.g. rejected allografts) may be subject to such attack.

Fibrin in Inflammation

The combined entry of plasma protein and fluid exudate into inflamed tissue provides fibrinogen and a source of the coagulating enzyme system (prothrombin-thrombin) responsible for converting it into fibrin (*see* Section 9.4). This is another of the cascade activation mechanisms and is closely related to the kinin and complement activations, especially with respect to initiation by the Hageman factor. Thus, in addition to the action of mediating agents, fibrin coagulation occurs in acute inflammatory lesions. This may be essential for haemostasis in damaged tissues, or may be seen as beneficial in forming a coagulated protein layer at the periphery of lesions. The fibrin barrier may limit potential spread of toxins or infection. It probably serves also to limit the extent of the influence of inflammatory mediators and hence controls the size of the affected area. However, the presence of excess fibrin in tissues may contribute to the mechanism of chronic inflammation. A further plasma-enzyme activation mechanism (plasminogen-plasmin) provides a fibrinolytic action, dissolving clotted fibrin. This results in the liquefaction of inflammatory exudate, allowing drainage, and is one of the main ways in which inflammation resolves.

Deposition of fibrin in the walls of inflamed blood vessels, associated with deterioration of normal structure (fibrinoid necrosis), is a feature associated with pathology of various kinds (e.g. immune-complex lesions, atherosclerosis, arteriosclerosis, and rheumatoid lesions). Fibrin deposits are often associated with degradation of collagen (e.g. in rheumatoid nodules or in senile atrophy of tissues). Platelets are particularly involved with fibrin deposition in haemostasis, thrombus formation, and in other vascular lesions. Amyloid formation, another deposition of fibrillar protein similar to fibrin or degraded collagen, is also a feature of inflammation, especially in chronic lesions.

15.5 PARASITES, PATHOGENS, AND INFECTION

Introduction

This section is concerned with the mechanisms and effects of infection and of consequent disease processes. The causative infectious micro-organisms are also important, and these have been described in the individual disease monographs (*see* Chapter 5). A brief outline of the general characteristics of pathogens is given in Chapter 14 and appropriate texts on microbiology or parasitology should be consulted for further information. This account will be limited to micro-organisms, although much of the general nature of infection may also apply to the higher organised pathogens (e.g. helminths).

Parasites and Pathogenicity

The relationship that exists when one organism lives on or in a different type of organism is termed symbiosis, and each party to the relationship is called a symbiont. The essential feature to be considered here is parasitism, in which one organism benefits from but adversely affects another, although other types of relationship may exist. Commensalism benefits the dependent symbiont without harmful effects to the host, while in some cases, each symbiont may derive mutual benefit.

From birth we are rapidly and effectively parasitised, although the parasite advantage is usually not so unbalanced that it is detrimental to the host; when this happens, the parasite becomes a pathogen. The resident population, which is usually microbial, is not pathogenic and may protect the host from those micro-organisms that are. Some of the microbial activity will be saprophytic, in which the micro-organisms utilise dead material (intestinal or cutaneous debris) as a substrate. Generally, however, the relationship is saprophytic only after death of the whole body, when the cadaver is partially consumed by the microbial flora. Overall, whatever the relationship, the usual residence is external (cutaneous) or limited to externally connected internal surfaces (e.g. gastro-intestinal, genito-urinary, or respiratory tracts); internal tissues are normally sterile.

There are few, special, disease-producing features possessed by most resident parasites, although many of these are potentially infectious and pathogenic given a change in circumstances. The main requirements are access to host tissues and impairment of host defences. Thus, infection mainly amounts to a newly acquired opportunity for commensals to extend their environment beyond their normal location (e.g. spread of upper respiratory-tract micro-organisms into sinuses or lower respiratory spaces, usually free of such occupation). Penetration into cells or tissues (e.g. from skin or gastro-intestinal populations) may result especially from mechanical or other tissue damage.

Features enabling micro-organisms to become pathogens are readiness of transmission to the host (which may depend on survival during passage between different environments), invasiveness, and resistance to host defences. The additional liability of the micro-organism to give rise to disease is an attribute called virulence, and depends on the micro-organism's multiplication and specific metabolic activities. Specialised means of transmission may be required by some parasites (e.g. the bite of an insect vector or the provision of an intermediate host).

All of these features are set to counteract body defences, giving rise to a number of categories of pathogenicity:

- opportunistic pathogenicity

    Normally commensal micro-organisms with little ability to penetrate defensive barriers or to survive in normally defended tissues (e.g. skin bacteria or fungi gaining access via wounds or weeping eczema). Other opportunists become pathogens only when host immunity is impaired (e.g. *Pneumocystis carinii*), or secondary to major debilitating diseases (e.g. cancer).

- extracellular pathogenicity

Micro-organisms able to survive and multiply on or in tissues but outside cells. Interstitial fluid, blood, or even cell surfaces provide suitable environments for numerous bacteria and fungi. Micro-organisms in this category are particularly vulnerable to phagocytic activity, although some of the most effective pathogens have the ability to prevent or survive phagocytosis by various means such as possession of protective capsules (e.g. pneumococci).

- facultative intracellular parasites

These micro-organisms survive when phagocytosed into cells, as they are resistant to the intracellular killing mechanisms of neutrophils or macrophage cells.

- obligate intracellular parasites

These live almost entirely in cells. Cell residence is essential to ensure long-term survival and multiplication of all viruses and rickettsia, and some fungi and bacteria. Protozoa (e.g. *Plasmodium* spp., *Leishmania* spp., and *Toxoplasma* spp.) have periods of obligate intracellular multiplication in their complex life cycles, gaining extra benefit from host-cell nutrition and energy.

Multiplication is necessary for establishment and perpetuation of an infection on or within tissues. This ability depends on the type of micro-organism and the host tissue conditions. Only small numbers of virus particles may suffice to cause an infection, whereas millions of bacteria may be essential. Bacterial growth by binary fission may take so long to reach effective numbers from an initially small population that the host has time to develop more effective defences. The more pathogenic strains of micro-organisms may feature more rapid rates of multiplication.

Virus multiplication utilises the internal synthetic mechanisms in the infected host-cell to produce masses of new virion particles in proportion to a relatively small infection. It does this by introducing its own nucleic acids into the control of the production of the cell's protein and nucleic acids, diverting the process to the replication of viral DNA or RNA and provoking biosynthesis of viral protein. Such synthesis or release of new virions, or both, may injure or kill the cell. Alternatively, there may be slow sustained virus production over prolonged periods without cell damage. These effects have considerable bearing on the relative pathogenicity and virulence of the infection. Again, host susceptibility is a determinant factor.

Pathogenicity also depends upon suitable locations for penetration and multiplication. These often require cell-surface attachment as a preliminary, involving interactions with receptor sites (e.g. on epithelial cells). Various kinds of micro-organisms, and in particular viruses and bacteria, adhere to cell surfaces in a manner that indicates the existence of specific receptor sites. The non-pathogenic microbial residents of mucous membranes are attached to the surfaces by virtue of such receptors. Access by potential pathogens to the receptors is therefore denied unless, as with some aggressive bacteria, there is strong competition for the sites. Otherwise, opportunist infections may only succeed if normal micro-organisms are displaced, and this may arise as a consequence of virus action. Attachment of viral particles to host cells, an essential preliminary to penetration, again requires specific receptors.

Pathogenic Damage

Harmful effects of infections occur by a variety of mechanisms and are often multifactorial. Invasiveness, multiplication, toxigenicity, depletion of nutrition, and host defensive action are among the most important damaging activities, alone or in combination.

Direct cellular damage is a common result of intracellular multiplication, as typified by virus growth. Internal disorganisation and diversion of cellular resources causes general metabolic depression and lack of functional enzymes. Membranes are weakened or broken down, giving mitochondrial malfunction; and lysosomal membrane destabilisation allows enzyme leakage, giving rise to even more internal disruption. The combined effects lead to cell death and lysis, with infected cells typically becoming shrunken and spheroidal in the course of dying. Cells involved in the replication of viral particles swell and vacuolate before lysing. An alternative result is the coalescence of several cells to form multinucleate giant-cells (*see also* Section 15.4). However, not every infected cell displays pathological change; the infection may be dormant for very long periods or, in some cases, the cells are not harmed by the parasites.

Consequences of intracellular growth depend considerably upon the type of host cell, with viruses showing great selectivity for specific cells. For example, poliovirus lives harmlessly in lymphoid or gastrointestinal epithelial cells, but causes severe damage if the infection spreads into the central nervous system where the virus replicates in spinal motor neurones;

nerve cell-bodies degenerate, lose granular constituents, and suffer necrosis and lysis. Vigorous functional activity in these neurones, associated with muscular exertion, exacerbates the virally-induced damage. Other examples of specific cellular attacks include nasal epithelium (rhinovirus), bronchial epithelium (influenza virus), and hepatocytes (hepatitis A or B virus). Protozoa also use particular cells for multiplication, and several types of cells may be attacked in different phases of a life-cycle (e.g. malarial parasites). Overall, the major sites for intracellular pathogen residence and multiplication are the phagocytic cells, neutrophils, and macrophages.

Toxin production is the other major cause of direct infection-induced disorders. Toxins are high molecular weight, very potent, tissue poisons (usually proteins) secreted by micro-organisms (exotoxins) or existing as a structural component (endotoxins).

Exotoxins are primarily bacterial products. Their effects may be exerted locally in or around infection sites, but there may often be systemic circulation, causing major disease. Some exotoxin effects are specific (e.g. toxins of *Clostridium botulinum* or *C. tetani*, which seriously impair nervous function and in particular inhibit secretion of neurotransmitters). Lethal effects of severe infections may be the result of exotoxins on vital organs (e.g. cardiotoxin effects of diphtheria toxin). Others exert more general cell-damaging actions (e.g. *C. perfringens* and *Pseudomonas aeruginosa*), causing necrosis in exposed tissues.

Certain exotoxic products of intestinal pathogens are secreted in the intestinal lumen and affect the surrounding mucosal wall with only superficial penetration, thereby causing only local effects. Such secretions are termed enterotoxins. *Vibrio cholera* enterotoxin causes gastro-intestinal epithelial cells to secrete copious quantities of fluid, causing severe general dehydration. Enterotoxins of *Escherichia coli* have similar effects while the inflammatory enteritis caused by various species of *Campylobacter* may also be due to enterotoxins.

Endotoxins are produced when components of bacteria are shed or released by cell disruption. These are generally less potent than exotoxins and effects may result only from disintegration of large numbers of micro-organisms (e.g. when bacteria spread systemically in septicaemia). Typical endotoxin material comes from the glycosaminoglycan or glycolipid layers of the glycocalyx capsules surrounding the cytoplasmic membranes of *Salmonella* spp. and other Gram-negative micro-organisms. Effects of such endotoxins include necrosis of lymphoid, reticulo-endothelial, and haemopoietic tissues, liver and gastro-intestinal damage, neuronal toxicity, and fever with loss of consciousness.

Endotoxins thus account for the widespread and varied pathology of typhoid fever.

A feature of endotoxin release, met especially in septicaemia or severe infection, is a general syndrome of fever, rigors, and hypotension, amounting to severe shock (*see* Section 15.1). This is termed septic (bacteriogenic or endotoxin) shock. Some pyrogenic and endotoxin-like effects are also due to products released from damaged neutrophils or macrophages. Immune complexes may also be pyrogenic and shock-inducing, directly or via neutrophil damage. Disintegration of micro-organisms in foci of infection due to antibiotic action (e.g. penicillin effects on the bacteria causing syphilis) may give endotoxin-like effects, probably as a result of released products. This produces the Jarisch-Herxheimer reaction, which features a combination of fever, sweating, malaise, rigors, headache, and skin rash.

Inflammation, local or generalised, is a very common aspect of most kinds of infections. Not only is it the result of tissue-damaging actions exerted by the pathogens, but it may also be the protective measure deployed to combat, contain, or eliminate the micro-organisms. Inflammation and the functions of the immune system are dealt with in detail in Sections 15.4 and 15.6. It is only necessary to emphasise here the harmful as well as the beneficial roles of inflammation. When determined by the immune system, inflammatory damage may exceed the potential for harm of many parasitic micro-organisms. In particular, systemic manifestations of disease or long-term pathology may be aspects of damage well beyond the direct influence of what might be a localised or relatively short-term infection (e.g. skin rashes from gastro-intestinal infections or long-term effects of syphilis).

Infective Lesions: Acute Infection

Despite the various combinations of pathogenic influence at work in different infections, the range of tissue reactions possible is relatively limited and certain forms of lesion may be considered to be typical of infection sites. Specialised differentiated cells will be subject to degeneration, necrosis or, more rarely, proliferative changes. The connective tissue and blood vessel components of the tissue will respond with inflammatory changes.

In general, the active development of a focus of infection will be associated with the earlier manifestations of inflammation. A degree of erythema (due to vasodilatation), swelling (inflammatory exudation), and pruritus or pain are typical of even very minor infections. These effects are readily reversible when the provocation has subsided, or they may be sustained and extended.

Further development of the inflammatory process, involving the infiltration of neutrophils from the blood, provides a very important antimicrobial defence, especially against bacteria and fungi. Very large numbers of these cells rapidly accumulate at sites of infection, forming pus (*see* Section 15.4). These cells have some capacity for phagocytosis of microbial pathogens, and this is coupled with the secretion of antimicrobial substances (e.g. lysozyme and lactoferrin) or lysosomal enzymes capable of digesting the micro-organisms. They also have the capability for oxygen-dependent killing (Table 15.6). Ingested micro-organisms are exposed to chemically reactive products of oxidative metabolism: superoxide and hydroxyl free-radicals produced by an oxygen burst are powerfully microbicidal. Hydrogen peroxide, linked with iodination or chlorination reactions intracellularly, is particularly effective against catalase-negative bacteria and some fungi. Catalase-positive pathogens are much less affected and are thus more resistant to neutrophil attack.

Micro-organisms with some resistance to uptake or microbicidal attack may provoke massive formation of pus in an effort to eradicate the infection. This process is known as suppuration and micro-organisms causing this are termed pyogenic (Table 15.7). Pus accumulates in cavities in the tissues forming abscesses, carbuncles, or furuncles (boils). The cavities are caused by cellular necrosis, tissue digestion, and pressure; the pus itself, releasing lysosomal enzymes and toxic products, is

TABLE 15.6
Antimicrobial oxygen-burst mechanisms through which phagocytic cells attempt to destroy ingested micro-organisms

Sequence of intracellular actions

1. Metabolic oxidation mechanisms activated (oxygen-burst, with increased oxygen uptake).

2. Oxidative phosphorylation of glucose by the hexose monophosphate shunt involves reduction of elemental oxygen and produces toxic superoxide anion ($O_2^{\cdot}$).

3. Superoxide dismutase enzyme action
$$O_2^{\cdot} + O_2^{\cdot} + 2H^+ \rightarrow O_2 + H_2O_2$$
and
$$H_2O_2 + O_2^{\cdot} \rightarrow O_2 + HO^- + HO^{\cdot}$$
Hydrogen peroxide and hydroxyl free radicals are chemically reactive, toxic, and microbicidal.

4. Action of hydrogen peroxide and halogenation
$$H_2O_2 + I^- \text{ or } Cl^- \rightarrow \text{attack on bacterial components}$$
dependent on the enzyme myeloperoxidase (mainly in neutrophils).

TABLE 15.7
Pyogenic micro-organisms: pathogens typically associated with accumulation of pus in infected lesions

Bacteroides species	*Proteus* species
Escherichia coli	*Pseudomonas aeruginosa*
Gonococcus species	*Staphylococcus aureus*
Meningococcus species	*Staphylococcus pyogenes*
Pneumococcus species	*Streptococcus pyogenes*

tissue-eroding. Pus-filled cavities are usually lined by a layer of granulation tissue, the pyogenic membrane, serving as a protective barrier and the means for ultimate tissue repair. Pus is not readily eliminated unless the cavity should rupture (spontaneously or through surgical intervention), with the opening forming a sinus or fistula through which drainage may occur.

In some areas, infected pus may be less readily confined and thus spreads through adjacent air spaces (e.g. as in bronchopneumonia). Aggressive infections may not be confined in pyogenic lesions and may spread progressively.

Infective lesions: Chronic Infection

Pyogenic infections may become chronic when the antimicrobial functions of neutrophils are defective. In particular, cells may fail to phagocytose the micro-organisms or, having done so, may fail to kill them, possibly due to ineffective production of oxygen-burst agents (*see* Table 15.6). The majority of persistent lesions, however, are due to resistant micro-organisms. In abscesses, infections may persist because the micro-organisms are inaccessible in necrotic tissue, in the walls, or sloughed off into the cavity.

A number of severe and chronic infections (Table 15.8) involve granuloma formation (Fig. 15.10), a further extension of inflammatory defences. As with suppuration, certain infections lead to massive cellular infiltrations, but in this case by macrophage cells. These form nodular masses, sometimes with other cells (e.g. lymphocytes

TABLE 15.8
Chronic infections associated with intracellular pathogens, typically causing formation of granulomatous lesions

Actinomycosis	Schistosomiasis
Aspergillosis	Strongyloidiasis
Brucellosis	Syphilis
Filariasis	Toxocariasis
Leishmaniasis	Trypanosomiasis
Leprosy	Tuberculosis
Onchocerciasis	*Yersinia* infections

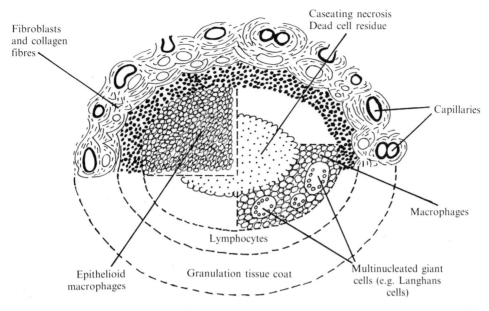

Fibroblasts
and collagen
fibres

Caseating necrosis
Dead cell residue

Capillaries

Macrophages

Lymphocytes

Epithelioid
macrophages

Granulation tissue coat

Multinucleated giant
cells (e.g. Langhans
cells)

Fig. 15.10
Granuloma.

and plasma cells, indicating immune activity), and are generally avascular. Such granulomas are typified by the tubercle lesions of tuberculosis. Macrophages are generally more effective at phagocytosis than neutrophils and again deploy microbicidal internal secretions (lysosomal enzymes and oxygen-burst products). Macrophage activities augment neutrophil functions and the combination may well eliminate many severe infections. However, micro-organisms listed in Table 15.8 are facultative intracellular parasites and have the ability to survive within cells for long periods. Macrophages themselves are long-lived, often even when laden with viable pathogens, and hence accumulate in nodular masses.

Most of the macrophages in a granuloma are single cells packed in an epithelioid mass. Their initial activity is phagocytosis, but when laden with micro-organisms this ceases and the microbicidal activities commence. Although they produce oxygen-burst products, macrophages lack the enzyme myeloperoxidase and cannot perform the hydrogen peroxide-halogenation function. This may be why they are less effective than neutrophils in certain cases. Some macrophages undergo fusion to form large multinucleate giant-cells (e.g. the Langhans cells in tuberculosis) and these are features of many forms of granuloma. Giant-cells may function to remove cellular debris rather than eliminate pathogens. The lymphocytes, which accumulate in granulomas (often in an outer layer) as a manifestation of cell-mediated immunity, stimulate enhanced antimicrobial activity in macrophages.

Old or large lesions may enclose masses of caseous material which is made up of coagulated protein residues of dead macrophage cells. Alternatively, the contents may liquefy, especially when containing active micro-organisms, giving rise to a cold abscess. Infection may spread readily from such a site if the contents are released. In most cases, however, granulomatous lesions are encapsulated by granulation tissue (separate mechanisms despite the similarity of the names). As with the occurrence around pyogenic abscesses, the granulation layer forms a protective barrier and acts to repair the lesion when the infection may ultimately become inactive. Subsided lesions become fibrous scars and may eventually calcify.

Survival of micro-organisms and persistence of lesions may be prolonged despite active immune function. However, immunity may at least hold an infection in check (e.g. in tuberculoid leprosy, as opposed to the more flourishing lepromatous form of the disease when immunity is poor). Immune reactions may give rise to much of the tissue damage associated with the chronic infections, as the reactivity may be directed against residues of dead, as well as living, pathogens. Later phases of these diseases may thus be sustained by hypersensitivity to residues of dead bacteria, as occurs in the tertiary stages of syphilis.

Chronic infections may occur when an otherwise acute

or treatable infection is neglected. It may also represent a failure of early therapy, and therefore microbial resistance (e.g. to antimicrobials) is another factor predisposing to chronicity. Relative inaccessibility of micro-organisms in suppurating or granulomatous lesions may further add to the intractability of chronic infections against immune or therapeutic attack.

15.6 IMMUNITY AND IMMUNOPATHOLOGY

Introduction

The immune system functions to detect the presence of alien material in the body or the occurrence of aberrations in the substance of the body. Having detected such material, the system is activated in an attempt to eliminate it. These functions serve to guard against abnormal cell development and to protect the body against parasitic micro-organisms or some toxic materials. Nevertheless, the process is neither totally effective nor totally beneficial. In the performance even of beneficial immune functions, a degree of tissue damage may be sustained so that some harmful features (e.g. of infections) are often the result. Furthermore, a number of important disease states are largely caused by activity of the immune system without any apparent significant element of protective function (e.g. allergies and auto-immune diseases).

Any material to which the system will react is called an antigen. To have antigenic reactivity the material has to be organic, have a very large molecular structure, and be polymeric. Typically, such materials are proteins but other macromolecules (e.g. polypeptides, polysaccharides, and polylipids) may also be antigenic. The ability of antigens to activate and react with the immune system is determined by surface features of these structures: chemical configurations that the system can recognise as being alien (i.e. differing from the surface patterns of normal molecules). These key abnormal configurations are referred to as antigen determinant groups. Antigenic material may have its origin outside the body (e.g. pathogens, incompatible blood or tissue transplants, and vaccines). Alternatively, it may be the body's own material which has become altered (e.g. mutated or diseased cells and chemically denatured protein).

A substantial number of low molecular weight, non-polymeric substances also activate the immune system, but they are not antigens and do so indirectly. These chemicals (Table 15.9) are effective only because they

TABLE 15.9
Hapten-forming chemicals which may act as skin-contact sensitising agents or photosensitisers

Chemical haptens	
• Aniline group	
p-aminophenol	procaine
aniline	quinoneimine
butesin	quinonediimine
hydroxybenzoates (parabens)	saccharin
p-phenylenediamine	sulphonamides
• Antibacterial agents	
acriflavine	nitrofurazone
cetrimide	phenols
chloroxylenol	propamidine
halogenated hydroxyquinolines	thiomersal
• Antibiotics	
cephalosporins	penicillins
neomycin	streptomycin
• Antihistamines	
chlorocyclizine	mepyramine
crotamiton	phenothiazines
diphenhydramine	tripelenamine
• Dyestuffs	
aniline black	eosin
azo compounds	
• Local anaesthetics	
amethocaine	benzocaine
amylocaine	cinchocaine
• Metals and salts	
beryllium	mercury
chromium	nickel
cobalt	platinum
• Plastics	
(sensitising species are generally monomers or additives, not polymers)	
acrylic or epoxy monomers	phthalic anyhydride
butyl maleate	thiuram accelerators
formaldehyde	tolylene diisocyanate
methyl methacrylate	
Photosensitisers	
chlorodiazepoxide	oral hypoglycaemics
griseofulvin	phenothiazines
halogenated salicylanilides	sulphonamides
hexachlorophane	tetracyclines
nalidixic acid	thiazide diuretics

possess the ability to interact with, and thus alter, material more capable of being antigenic (e.g. protein or other polymers). The latter material is referred to as the carrier; it may be part of the body's normal protein or it may itself be of foreign origin. In either case, the essential requirement is that the denatured or altered carrier becomes abnormal or alien. The denaturing chemical reagent (a hapten) provides determinant groups, altering the configuration of the carrier and giving specificity to the newly-formed antigen. Thus, a hapten-carrier complex becomes an antigen. Many highly-reactive chemicals readily act as haptens. Others (including numerous drugs) are initially chemically inert and require preliminary activation by metabolic transformation in the body or by ultraviolet irradiation (photosensitisers, see Table 15.9).

The response to an antigen depends upon the combined functions of the cells of the lymphoid tissues, with one or more types of lymphocyte performing the main activities. Accessory or subsidiary functions are provided by cells of the reticulo-endothelial system. Interaction with each antigen type is a separate and specific phenomenon, giving rise to a state of immunity to that antigen. Alternatively, the state may be harmful, in which case it is called hypersensitivity or allergy. These activations require a sequence of events (Table 15.10); the complete manifestation of the reactivity actually involves two separate series. Once the system has responded to the preliminary antigenic stimulus, further antigen exposure interacts with the products from the cells, mediating the states of immunity or hypersensitivity. Such products take the form of circulating lymphocytes (e.g. effector T-cells) or of plasma-protein antibody (Fig. 15.11). As these products are specifically directed against the antigen which provoked their formation, there will be many different species of antibody and lymphocytes in the circulation at the same time. Other types of lymphocytic cells may be recruited by further influences to aid immune-cell functions (e.g. to act as T-killer cells, Fig. 15.11). Production of lymphocytes for both effector-cell function and also for accessory purposes (T-helper cells or T-suppressor cells) involves division of precursor cells, the lymphoblasts. Antibody production occurs after the specialised secretory cells (plasma cells) have been produced by division of plasmablast precursors. At the same time, memory cells are produced that extend and perpetuate this antibody response, spreading and persisting throughout the immune system; these are responsible for long-term responsiveness to the antigen.

Cell-mediated Immunity

This is the most important form of immune response; it is involved in most reactivity to abnormal tissues and many forms of infection, particularly those in which pathogens reside within cells. The cellular response is provoked by tissue antigens and particulate or fibrillar material. It plays a prominent role in transplant rejection, reacting to incompatible cell-surface antigens.

Initially, the presence of appropriate antigen, plus the action of antigen-presenting macrophages, leads to the proliferation of T-cells in the lymphoid tissue of that

TABLE 15.10
The immune state or hypersensitive (allergic) reactivity: sequence of events involved in the activation of the immune system

Primary exposure (sensitisation phase)	Stage one Exposure to antigen (e.g. incompatible protein, aberrant tissue, or pathogen)
	Stage two Antigen processing or presentation – influence on immune system (macrophage/lymphocyte interactions)
	Stage three Lymphoid cell proliferation (precursos cells transformed into blast cells and development of specific populations (clones) of lymphocyctes or plasma cells)
	Stage four (i) Antibody production (ii) Activated lymphocyte production – effector T-cells (specifically directed against antigen)
	Stage five Products in circulation or in target tissues
Subsequent exposure (challenge phase)	Stage one (i) Antigen-antibody interaction (ii) Antigenic provocation of activity in effector cells
	Stage two Consequences • beneficial: immunity or immunosurveillance – cell-mediated, humoral, or both (neutralisation, destruction, detoxification, or elimination of antigenic material) • harmful: hypersensitivity, allergy, or auto-immune disease state (tissue damage; release of inflammatory mediators)

Immunisation Sequences

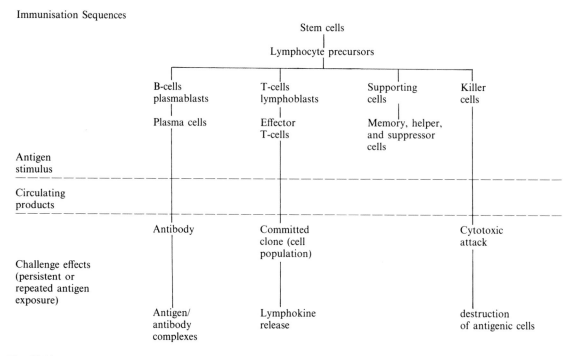

Fig. 15.11
Origins and production of cells or products involved in immune functions or immunopathological actions.

area (usually the drainage lymph-nodes). Effector T-cells pass from the node into efferent lymph channels and thence via the blood to the tissues. After a short latent period of 5 to 7 days, increasing numbers appear in the circulation. When contact is made between specifically programmed effector cells and the appropriate antigen (the original source or a further entry or occurrence of that type), these cells are stimulated to release lymphokines (Table 15.11). These are systemically and locally acting hormones which influence a variety of other cell populations to react to the antigenic material. This response attracts inflammatory and phagocytic cells into the tissues containing the anti-genic material, the lymphokines having appropriate chemotactic properties for neutrophils or monocytes. The infiltrating cells are further provoked into functional actions (e.g. secretion of tissue-lysing lysosomal enzymes or the activation of phagocytosis). Lymphokine release has another purpose, cellular recruitment, which augments the active cellular population. In particular, T-cell numbers are increased by non-specific stimulation of release and attraction of additional cells from lymphoid tissues. The required role of the combined infiltrating cell populations is the elimination of the antigenic material. However, the process commonly also involves the destruction of adjacent normal tissue and a severe inflammatory state may be produced. The ability to attack cellular structures is, however, generally desirable, as it provides the means for attacking intracellular parasites. Thus, cell-mediated immunity is the most effective control for viral, fungal, and many bacterial or protozoal infections. It obviously has a role to play in the digestion of damaged or aberrant (mutated) cells. It may, in the process, cause necrosis or chronic inflammation (e.g. eczema or granuloma formation). Some auto-immune diseases (see Section 16.10) may be explained in terms of this activity.

TABLE 15.11
Lymphokines (products from antigen-stimulated effector T-cells)

Interferon (antiviral)
Lymphotoxin (local cell damage)
Macrophage migration inhibition factor
Mitogenic factor (immunoblast stimulating)
Monocyte and neutrophil chemotactic factors
Skin reactive factor
Transfer factor (recruits other lymphocytes)

Humoral Immunity

This function may be associated with cell-mediated immunity, or either form may occur independently. It results from the secretion and circulation of antibody proteins. These are carried in the blood and are also able to penetrate into tissues, especially when inflammation renders blood vessels more permeable. Antibody production is primarily provoked by soluble protein (e.g. toxins), by polysaccharide antigens, or by small-particle antigens (e.g. virions or bacteria). If the provoking stimulus is by larger multicellular structures, humoral immunity is more likely to be accompanied or surpassed by cell-mediated immunity. Antibody mediated effects more commonly operate in relation to material accessible in blood or tissue fluid, whereas reactions with tissues are mainly restricted to cell-surface attack. Antibodies play a part in graft rejection but are less important in immunosurveillance.

Antibodies are referred to as immunoglobulins, designated Ig. All immunoglobulin molecules are composed of at least four polypeptide chains arranged as mirror image pairs, each pair consisting of a light chain and a heavy chain. Human immunoglobulins are formed from five main varieties of heavy chain (each of the paired chains being identical), thus giving five classes of immunoglobulin: IgA, IgD, IgE, IgG, and IgM. Other lesser variants of light and heavy chain are known, giving immunoglobulin subdivisions. IgM molecules differ in structure, being formed from five of the mirror image units. This provides many more antigen-binding valencies (10), contrasting with the divalency of most other immunoglobulin types.

Following administration of antigen, the system first synthesises IgM antibody. Prolonged antibody production subsequently generates IgA and IgG, depending on the maturing plasma cells. Secondary responses to antigen, sometime after an initial stimulus, are mediated predominantly by the production of IgG by memory cells and plasma cells previously evoked by that antigen. Production of IgE, the type involved in various allergic conditions, is particularly associated with the genetically-determined atopic predisposition of individuals.

Most antibody immunoglobulin is divalent, whereas antigens are multivalent. This allows for a wide variation in interactions of antigen and antibody, from the formation of small soluble complexes to large multimolecular lattice aggregates; the exact combination is determined by the relative concentrations. Simple combination in small complexes may suffice to neutralise toxin molecules, while larger combinations may form insoluble precipitates, leading to phagocytosis of the antigen by macrophages. The simpler divalent antibodies (IgG) may form monomolecular layers on bacterial cells or other antigen particles, again facilitating phagocytosis. The larger multivalent IgM antibody forms cross-linkages and brings about agglutination or aggregation of bacteria or other cells, once again leading to destruction by macrophages. Many examples of humoral immune function may be explained by such complex formation.

Portions of the immunoglobulin molecule may also bind to non-antigen sites. One of the most important of such combinations is complement fixation and activation. Complement is found in plasma protein as a mixture of interrelated enzyme substrates and precursors. These enzymes are activated in a sequence following the formation of an appropriate antigen-antibody complex. The sequential activation gives rise to subsidiary products which become available to evoke various immune or inflammatory mechanisms (e.g. anaphylatoxins provoke histamine release from mast cells). Opsonising components stimulate phagocytic activity (e.g. of bacteria) by macrophages. Various chemotactic components influence inflammatory cell infiltration. The completion of the complement sequence produces cell-lysing enzyme action. This effect may be exerted on pathogens, although blood-cell or normal tissue lysis may also result, as occurs in hypersensitivity.

Immune-mediated Disease: Hypersensitivity or Allergy

The terms hypersensitivity and allergy are virtually synonymous when applied to harmful effects ensuing from activities of the immune system. Generally, allergy denotes the state of specific reactivity acquired by unintentional or natural exposure to a provoking antigen (allergen). The use of hypersensitivity has slightly broader connotations and includes deliberate, experimental, or less natural causes. Either term may be applied to adverse results of immune attack directed at a pathogen. This may involve direct cell damage (e.g. on cells containing viruses or fungi), although numerous infections result in additional damage from the system, quite unconnected with any beneficial or protective function. Pathology of a similar kind also arises from reactivity to apparently normal tissue components, for which the term auto-immune disease is used.

In relation to all of these, it is worth reiterating the essential immune mediation. This is to differentiate the conditions clearly from a range of non-immune but apparently similar conditions, which usually involve inflammation due to some other but often obscure cause (e.g. intrinsic asthma or idiopathic skin eruptions). The immune aetiology requires a period of time for the state to develop, and manifestations of the condition require either persistence of, or renewed exposure to, the causative material. These simple criteria are often clearly inapplicable to the pseudo-allergic conditions.

A hypersensitive state should be possible in any individual, providing a sufficiently intense stimulus is applied to provoke it. In contrast, susceptibility to allergy is extremely variable between individuals and is largely determined by genetic factors. Thus, 25% to 30% of the population are especially prone to allergic disease. These subjects are given to persistent production of IgE antibodies, often in response to relatively minute allergen exposures. They easily acquire allergies to numerous materials; the earlier the first appearance of the allergy, the wider the potential range of allergens. Such susceptibility is said to be atopic. Typically, atopic allergies commence as eczema at an early stage and develop into asthma later in life (which may only slowly fade). An additional general susceptibility to allergic rhinitis features in youth and early adulthood, but this decreases with age.

A useful classification of allergic/hypersensitive conditions was compiled by Coombs and Gell in 1968, who defined four main types of reaction. Types I, II, and III are mediated by antibody, while type IV is cell-mediated. Antibody-evoked reactions are relatively rapid in onset (immediate hypersensitivity), whereas cell-mediated type IV reactivity requires periods of 12 hours or more before becoming apparent (delayed hypersensitivity).

Type I or anaphylactic hypersensitivity is exemplified by urticaria (skin), rhinitis (nasal mucosa), angioedema (loose subcutaneous tissues of the face), allergic conjunctivitis (eyes), extrinsic allergic asthma (bronchioles), and anaphylactic shock (cardiovascular system). These are all essentially similar acute inflammatory reactions of the specified parts and depend on mediators (e.g. histamine, leukotrienes, prostaglandins, and kinins). The underlying states of hypersensitivity are established by cell-bound IgE antibody fixed to mast cells or blood basophils. The affected site is largely determined by the point of access of causative allergen.

Reactions of type II hypersensitivity are also termed cytotoxic, because they involve damage exerted on particular cells or tissues. The prime targets are often blood cells or their precursors. The cells have or acquire antigenic characteristics, possibly by chemical change, and are then attacked by cytotoxic antibody plus complement. Such attack may be directed against incompatible blood transfusion.

Type III hypersensitivity depends upon immune complex formation in blood vessels. The nature of the condition depends upon the circulating antibody levels and the form of the complex. A combination of soluble complexes and excess antigen gives whole body reactions of the serum sickness type. Complexes formed by localised antigen with excess antibody give restricted lesions (localised necrosis) called Arthus reactions. The formed complexes of antigen and antibody activate complement and may provoke kinin and prostaglandin formation. Platelet disruption (leading to intravascular blood clotting) and Arthus reactions (leading to fibrous scarring) are features of a variety of pulmonary allergic conditions produced by inhaled particulate antigens (e.g. farmer's lung and bird-fancier's lung caused by inhaled mould spores) which result in extrinsic allergic alveolitis. Infection with *Streptococcus pyogenes* (type 12) or *Plasmodium malariae* may provoke remote tissue damage (e.g. glomerulonephritis) due to immune complexes.

Delayed hypersensitivity (type IV) occurs in a number of bacterial infections, especially to those intracellular micro-organisms causing chronic infections. Fungal and virus infections also generally evoke this type, in association with cell-mediated immunity. Delayed hypersensitivity also plays a role in the rejection of incompatible tissue transplants and in chemical-hapten induced eczema (contact sensitisation). The reactions take the form of cellular inflammation with necrotic tissue damage. Effector T-cells infiltrate tissues and subsequently provoke accumulation and activity of macrophages (and sometimes neutrophils), resulting in granuloma formation, tissue destruction, and fibrous scarring.

15.7 PROLIFERATIVE AND NEOPLASTIC DISORDERS

Normal Growth, Adaptive Growth, and Regeneration

During the embryonic period, the activity of cells comprising the developing body is devoted almost solely to division and orientation as required for tissue organisation. Current understanding suggests that cells require little or no direct stimulus to proliferate and that they continue to divide until some influence inhibits this activity. The major influences appropriate to the normal formation of tissues appear to be either that the cells have divided a certain number of times or that the cell has arrived in an optimal position within a tissue (e.g. an epithelial cell is surrounded by similar cells and has one face exposed on the tissue surface). Cessation of proliferation at the correct time appears to be a genetically programmed influence; in most cases the cessation of division is a necessary precondition for the subsequent differentiation and maturation into a specialised functional cell. Ultimately, most of the cells of the adult body are transformed into such a state and many of them may not be called upon to divide ever again. This enduring cessation is called repression. However, in some tissues, continued cellular proliferation proceeds throughout life (e.g. in bone marrow and the basal cells of the gastro-intestinal or cutaneous epithelia). Even so, the products of these divisions (blood cells or epithelia) mature, acquire functional characteristics, and are repressed. These essential proliferations are subjected to further control, again mainly by inhibitory influences. For the majority of remaining tissues, cell division is only occasionally required for renewal of cells lost by wear and tear; for this purpose, a limited de-repression is possible. Only when it is necessary for the replenishment of substantial masses of tissue (e.g. lost by necrotic damage) is there de-repression and cell division on a large scale. This proliferative activity is called regeneration.

Another cause for renewed cell division, usually more insidious, is the enlargement of tissues required by continual elevated functional demands or by continual adverse insult. Tissue growth in this way (compensatory or adaptive hyperplasia) results from controlled de-repression. This type of tissue growth involving in-creased cell numbers must be distinguished from enlargement due to increase in cell size (e.g. the hypertrophy of vigorously exercised muscles). Relative abilities of various tissues to regenerate or undergo hyperplasia are shown in Table 15.12. Some cells, notably central neurones, become permanently repressed. Although much of this activity, or lack of it, is determined by genetic programming supplemented by other inhibitory influences (e.g. chalones), special growth-stimulating influences also play a part. Growth stimulation may be local (e.g. prostaglandins) or systemic (e.g. pituitary trophic hormones).

Abnormal Growth and Neoplasia

Some influences, usually prolonged states of abnormality or harmful insult, result not only in changes in size of tissues but also in transformation of the tissue character (metaplasia). An example is the change of epithelial structure from simple single layers to the compound squamous type in the surface tissues of the respiratory airways exposed chronically to irritant pollutants (e.g. cigarette smoke). The thickening is hyperplastic, but it involves loss of cilia from the cell surfaces and hence impaired function. Furthermore, mucus-producing cells also proliferate on the metaplastic surface. Metaplasia may also involve connective tissues (e.g. in an extensively calcified area, osteoblasts may develop and a dis-

TABLE 15.12

Normal proliferative activities in organs and tissues: relative ability to regenerate

Controlled cellular production, also associated with hyperplasia when necessary.	
a) Continuous activity	bone marrow epidermis gastro-intestinal mucosa
b) Facultative regeneration	
	glandular epithelia: • innervation dependent growth (exocrine tissues) • trophic hormone effects on endocrine tissue
	kidney (nephron epithelium) liver peripheral nervous system axons
Proliferation necessary to maintain or replace tissue structure, required by cellular turnover, loss by wear and tear, or damage. Adaptive hyperplasia as required for increased functional demand.	
c) Epithelial (surface or lining) repair	
• very effective	bladder transitional epithelium vascular epithelium
• effective but liable to lead to metaplasia	pulmonary alveolar epithelium respiratory-tract airways lining
d) Only partially effective	central nervous system axons myocardium skeletal muscle (innervation dependent)
e) Ineffective	peripheral and central neurones

tinctively osseous structure be constructed, even to the extent that marrow with haemopoietic cells may be present). Apart from the loss or change in function, metaplasia is of significance in view of the association with further development into neoplasia. This association appears to be strongest when the metaplastic tissue is particularly disorganised, with irregularities of cell sizes and structures (cell dysplasia). In particular, nuclear abnormalities, increasingly irregular mitoses, and loss of cell orientations are regarded as premalignant changes, forewarning neoplasia.

Neoplastic change produces a tissue in which the cells proliferate in an uncontrolled manner, presumably due to a loss of repression of division. They do not necessarily divide at an abnormal rate but division occurs when it should not and continues to do so. This produces an abnormally increased number of cells with resultant disorganisation of the tissue structure. The reversion to a proliferative state often results in a partial or total loss of the specialised functions of the affected cells. The change may take place in one or more cells of a tissue, but the result is the persistent development of a population of permanently altered cells to replace the normal tissue. This forms a colony or tumour of neoplastic cells. Alternatively, neoplastic change in a mobile cell population (e.g. blood cells) results simply in the production of strikingly excessive cell numbers in the circulation (e.g. forms of leukaemia).

When neoplastic cells develop as coherent tissues (i.e. as tumours), two different characteristics in behaviour have a very important bearing on the general consequences for the body, the prognosis for the disease, and the requirements of treatment. When the cellular proliferation is limited to its site of origin and simply produces an expanding mass of cells, the tumour is classed as benign. Such tumours are usually distinctly demarcated from surrounding normal tissue by a capsule of fibrous connective tissue. This capsule may originate partly from the residual compressed framework of the tissue, but in many cases there are indications of an active inflammatory reaction, probably determined by immune activity. The resultant fibrous layer (granulation tissues, *see* Section 15.4) appears to act as a restraining barrier.

The alternative form, malignant growth, is not restricted to one site and such tumours frequently show no distinct demarcating barrier of fibrous tissue. These neoplastic cells invade surrounding tissue by vigorous outgrowths of strands, projections, or sheets, spreading particularly along lines of weakness in normal tissues. In many cases, spreading also occurs by detachment of small clumps of cells from the tumour, which are carried to other sites by blood or lymph metastasis. These cells, if deposited in suitable locations, establish secondary colonies. In turn, extensive invasion or further metastasis is possible from these colonies.

Principal features contrasting benign and malignant growths are shown in Table 15.13. In general, benign tumour growth is slow and cell division is less frequent. Malignant growth is often more rapid, although the lack of restriction of the extent of this growth is the characteristic feature of this type. Current understanding of neoplastic cell production, irrespective of whether malignant or benign, is based upon the concept of cycles applied to normal cell division (Fig. 15.12). Cell populations are composed of quiescent (Q) cells plus variable numbers of cells ready for regular proliferative activity (P-cells). Q-cells in a mature population include end-cells, which are the final product (i.e. fully-

TABLE 15.13
Comparison of the characteristics of benign and malignant neoplastic growth

	Benign	Malignant
Growth	expansion at one site, slow and erratic, may cease	invasive, rapid, and rarely ceases
Spread	restricted to site of origin, not invasive, no metastasis	not restricted, invasive, and often metastatic
Structure	well differentiated, regular, resemblance to origin, retention of function to some extent	less well differentiated, irregularly distributed and misshapen, function rudimentary
	few mitoses	more frequent mitoses, aberrant
	well formed capsule	not encapsulated effectively
	well formed stroma of blood vessels and connective tissues	stroma and blood supply irregular, haemorrhage and cell-necrosis common
Clinical features	compression or obstruction of other tissues causing severe effects depending on site, quantitatively inappropriate malfunctions	much more extensive tissue replacement, local and systemic compression or obstruction causes serious malfunctions of vital organs, poor prognosis, ultimately fatal in most cases

differentiated functional structures), plus dormant and dying cells. Normally, only a few cells at any one time are in a P-state, whereas neoplastic populations have much larger proportions of such cells. The cyclic behaviour of P-cells takes them through sequences of changes involving the preparation of new chromosomal material, the separation of the genetic material between two new nuclei, and the final cell division (mitosis). Once embarked upon mitosis, the processes proceed at controlled and characteristic rates, so that sequences S, G_2, and M are completed within periods of about 12 hours for most cell types. However, considerable differences occur in the times taken for the post-mitotic growth phases (G_1). As with normal cells, in which G_1 may differ from 12 hours to months or even years, many neoplastic cells may have prolonged G_1 phases. These

differences may have important consequences, both with regard to tumour development and its response to therapy. While frequent cycling may imply rapid neoplastic growth, it also means that at any one time, a higher proportion of cells will be in the non-resting (S, G_2, or M) states which are much more vulnerable to some forms of cytotoxic chemotherapy or irradiation. Thus, acute leukaemia and Burkitt's lymphoma, with short generation times, have markedly different characters from pulmonary or gastric carcinomas which are much more insidious.

Note is taken of the characteristics of development and behaviour for classification of neoplastic disease, in particular the distinctions between benign and malignant forms (Table 15.14). Particular attention is also paid to the originating tissue (where such determination is

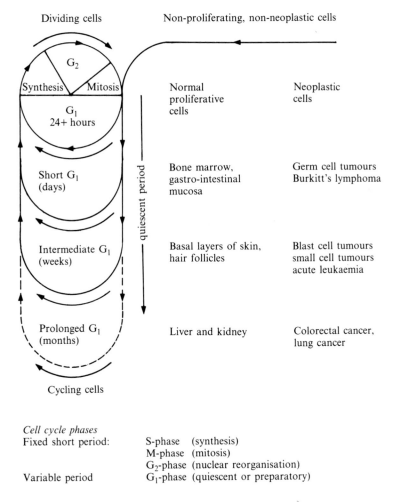

Cell cycle phases
Fixed short period: S-phase (synthesis)
                        M-phase (mitosis)
                        G_2-phase (nuclear reorganisation)
Variable period G_1-phase (quiescent or preparatory)

Fig. 15.12
Cell-division cycles and quiescent or non-proliferative periods in normal and neoplastic cells.

TABLE 15.14
Nomenclature and classification of neoplastic diseases based upon tissue of origin or other usage

Tissue	Benign	Malignant
Connective tissues or muscle		
blood vessels	angioma	angiosarcoma
bone	osteoma	osteosarcoma
cartilage	chondroma	chondrosarcoma
fibrous	fibroma	fibrosarcoma
lymphatic vessels	lymphangioma	lymphangiosarcoma
skeletal muscle	rhabdomyoma	rhabdomyosarcoma
smooth muscle	leiomyoma	leiomyosarcoma
Epithelia		
glandular/parenchymal	adenoma	adenocarcinoma
surface or lining	papilloma	carcinoma
Further characterised in terms of the form of epithelium (e.g. squamous or basal cell) or else the form of glandular structure (e.g. cystadenoma)		
Haemopoietic tissues		
lymphoreticular tissues	benign lymphoma	lymphosarcoma, reticulum-cell sarcoma, Hodgkin's disease
myeloproliferative tissues (bone marrow)		leukaemia, multiple myeloma, polycythaemia
Neural tissues		
neuroglia and ependymal cells		glioma
peripheral nerve sheaths	neuroma	neurofibrosarcoma
Embryonic origin		
foetal trophoblast (placental)	hydatidiform mole	choriocarcinoma
multipotential cells	benign teratoma	malignant teratoma
Eponymous diseases (complex, mixed-cell, or other unusual characteristics)		
Burkitt's lymphoma		lymphocytic lymphoma
Hodgkin's disease		lymphoreticular sarcomas
Kaposi's sarcoma		sarcoma
Paget's disease		dermato-fibrosarcoma
Hamartomas (tumour-like tissue malformations in which neoplastic change is common)		
melanocytes	naevus-melanoma	melanoma
nerve sheaths	neurofibromatosis	neurogenic sarcoma

possible). The identity of the tissue is indicated by an abbreviated term (e.g. fibro-, osteo-, or neuro-), often accompanied by the name of the organ if appropriate. These terms prefix a description of the nature of the neoplasia, important distinctions being made between tumours of epithelial and connective tissues. Thus, benign connective tissue tumours are designated simply by -oma, whereas malignancy is denoted by -sarcoma (e.g. osteoma or osteosarcoma for bone tumours). Benign epithelial tumours are called papillomas if they develop on surface tissues, whereas those in glandular epithelia are called adenomas. Malignant forms are carcinomas. Neoplasia of blood and lymphoid tissues is also described on the basis of the cell type which is affected. White-cell neoplasia (leukaemia) is qualified by the type of cell produced (e.g. myelocytic, affecting the polymorphonuclear cell lines) or the precursor (blast) cells affected (myeloblastic). Tumours of neural, embryonic,

or primitive tissues are rather less systematically classified. There is also another miscellaneous group (eponymous) named after an associated medical authority (e.g. Hodgkin's disease and Kaposi's sarcoma). Generally, these do not fit easily into the other systems because they involve multiple cell types or may originate in several different types of tissue.

In benign tumours, the cellular formations often clearly resemble the tissue of origin. The cells are usually well differentiated (i.e. distinctively organised) as in the mature, specialised tissue. Often, the specialised function of the differentiated tissue is retained, at least to some extent. Thus, thyroid adenoma cells may secrete the appropriate hormones. However, such aberrant tissue may secrete excessive quantities, due to the larger mass performing the function or because of the lack of normal constraints regulating the function (e.g. as in hyperthyroidism and hyperinsulinism).

Cells of malignant tissue are usually less well differentiated and may show a much greater diversity of size and shape. Cellular abnormalities are also much more common, to the extent that often large numbers of them fail to survive for long. As in benign tissue, some vestige of function may be retained, but abnormality is often greater (e.g. a malignant thyroid adenocarcinoma may be unable to secrete hormones yet display some capacity for concentrating iodide).

Tumour Structures

Tumour development in surface epithelia usually starts as a sheet but the build-up of new cells leads to protrusion, giving outgrowths, warts, or papillae. As typified by most early warts, surface tumours may have a wide base. Further growth may continue without extension of this base, leading to the formation of a polyp structure (Fig. 15.13), a large tumour mass attached by a peduncle or stalk. A core of connective tissue carrying blood vessels and lymphatics runs through the stalk to nourish the tumour. Should it be impossible for a surface

tumour to protrude, the growth, less commonly, will be inward. Inward growth in the absence of such a constraint is an indication of invasiveness and malignancy. Alternatively, when polyps occur on gastro-intestinal epithelia, the continual passage of bolus material past the tumour may exert a drag, causing marked extension of the peduncle.

Tumours of involuted glandular epithelia at a distance from a surface take the form of roughly spherical nodules; invasive or spreading malignant forms (adenocarcinomas) may be more diffuse or irregular. Neoplasia in a gland nearer a tissue surface may give outward growth (fungating tumour), developing into papillae or polyp structures. If the neoplastic origin is a secretory cell type and benign or well-differentiated, the tumour will retain a glandular structure and may form secretions. In an exocrine gland the neoplastic duct structures may be inadequate, causing accumulation of secretions. In such cases the tumours display large, fluid-filled, cystic spaces (cystadenoma) containing serous or mucinous secretions.

Connective tissue commonly develops at the same

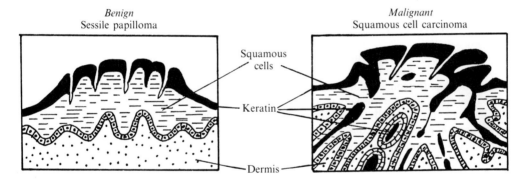

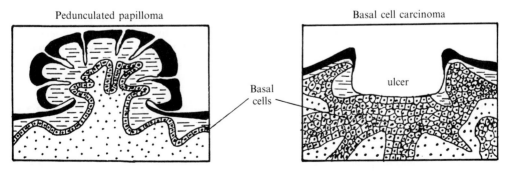

Fig. 15.13
Varieties in forms of epithelial tumours (benign and malignant).

time as benign and malignant tumours. It may surround both forms but usually does not succeed in encapsulating malignant tissue. Connective tissue growth within the tumour is usually also associated with the growth of blood vessels that provide support necessary for the survival of the tumour tissue; their development is known as the stromal reaction. Either component may grow profusely, sometimes to such an extent that suggests neoplastic change also in the blood vessel or fibrous growth. In this case the tumour may be described as a mixed type (e.g. fibroadenoma). A very profuse fibrous growth produces a hard tumour (scirrhous). Collagen fibres in the stroma of tumours tend to contract with time (as they do in scar tissue) and considerable tissue distortion may result. Contraction in the fibrous tumours of the breast may result in nipple retraction (see Breast Cancer). Encircling tumours of the gut may similarly contract, causing blocking stricture (e.g. in colorectal cancer).

Tumours of connective tissue are generally less common and less complex than epithelial types. Nevertheless, one of the commonest of all tumours, leiomyoma (fibroids) of the uterus, belongs in this category. Each neoplastic form will largely be determined by the cell type and any non-cellular material produced by those cells. Neoplastic connective tissue cells, especially if benign and well-differentiated, may continue to produce materials such as collagen fibres (fibroma cells) or the calcified matrix of bone (osteoma). Malignant tumours of connective tissue (sarcomas) are usually more diffuse and undifferentiated, and generally retain less of the features of the tissue of origin. They consist of masses or sheets of rapidly developing and invasive or metastatic cells. Malignant cells less frequently produce fibres or matrix than benign cells and the malignant tumours are therefore soft. Their growth may be so rapid that the stromal development of blood vessels is unable to keep pace and the blood supply becomes inadequate, resulting in patches of necrosis into which haemorrhages occur. Indeed, haemorrhage in a tumour is so characteristic of sarcomas as to be diagnostic. Ulcers or abscesses due to necrosis may also be features of larger or older tumours.

Malignancy: Invasion and Metastasis

A malignant neoplasm, not being effectively confined, tends to permeate adjacent tissues with strands of cells, particularly along lines of least resistance. The extent may thus be well beyond the macroscopically detectable. Tumours progress effectively in soft tissues with few physical barriers (e.g. parenchymatous organs, brain tissue, or bone marrow). Dense fibrous sheets (e.g. the fascia separating tissues, cartilage, and other compact masses) offer much more resistance, although penetration may still occur between or around such materials (e.g. between meningeal membrane layers or beneath the periosteum sheet covering bone).

More extensive spread occurs via natural channels. Lymphatic vessels in particular offer such routes and are frequently invaded, especially by carcinomatous cells. Some limitation to such spread may be offered by lymph nodes, but extensive lymphatic involvement, even into the main trunks, is quite possible. Blood vessels also provide the means for spread. Veins and capillaries are frequently occupied whereas arteries, with thicker walls, are less easily penetrated. Tumour cells in the vessels grow progressively in the form of solid cords extending along the channels. Tumour fragments are transported by lymphatic fluid or blood to produce metastases. Metastases arise from the deposition of these cellular emboli, usually where a constriction of flow occurs. Within lymphatics, spread between lymph nodes is usually by such emboli, with no intervening direct growth. Large secondary tumours in lymph nodes may form much more effective sources of both invasive and metastatic dissemination than an often small and constrained primary tumour.

Invasive or secondary growth within vessels may block the flow of blood or lymph. Thus, accumulating lymph may cause local oedema or ascites. Blocked blood supply may cause vascular congestion and areas of necrosis (infarct). An embolus reaching a main vessel may be large enough (or may secondarily grow to such an extent) to cause severe or even fatal ischaemia by blocking a vital artery or vein (e.g. coronary, pulmonary, or cerebral). Depending on the tumour type and its preferred means of spread, the subsequent dissemination from a particular site can to some extent be predicted. In blood vessels, embolic or tumour-carrying thrombi are arrested by the narrowing of vessels as the flow enters arterioles or capillaries. Most cells entering the venous system will find their next site of growth in the lungs; emboli in the portal vein will commonly be deposited in the liver. In contrast, arterial transport from a main vessel may give a very wide distribution to cerebral, visceral, or limb sites. Common patterns of dissemination are shown in Table 15.15.

Leukaemias and Lymphoreticular Tumours

These involve neoplastic change in the tissues responsible for generating blood cells, resulting in massively excessive production of one or possibly more types of cell. The cellular products may continue to pass into the

TABLE 15.15
Patterns of spread of malignant neoplasms originating in various parts of the body

Site of origin	Invasion of	Metastasis to
General distribution	local tissues	liver and lungs
Kidney	renal veins	regional lymph nodes, bones, liver, brain
Large intestine	local tissues	regional lymph nodes, liver
Lung	thoracic tissues	cervical lymph nodes, liver, adrenal glands, bones, brain
Mammary gland	overlying skin, underlying muscle	axillary lymph nodes, lungs, liver, bone
Oropharynx	head and neck	cervical lymph nodes
Prostate	local lymph nodes	bones
Skin	underlying structures (basal cell)	regional lymph nodes (squamous)
Stomach	duodenum, oesophagus, peritoneum	regional lymph nodes, liver, lungs
Thyroid	local lymph nodes	cervical lymph nodes, bones, lungs
Uterus	local tissues, vagina, bladder, rectum	pelvic lymph nodes, thoracic duct

circulation, particularly when the abnormality is seated in the haemopoietic bone marrow. When this happens, the neoplastic cell population usually becomes so dominant in the marrow and the blood that other cell lines are virtually obliterated. Thus, the blood may come to contain vastly too many of one cell type and marked deficiencies of others. When the proliferation produces erythrocytes, the condition is polycythaemia vera or, more commonly, neoplasia of a white-cell type causes a leukaemia.

The leukaemias arise in precursor cells of the bone marrow, which normally give rise to one of the different series of leucocytes: granulocytes (derived from myelocytes), monocytes, or lymphocytes (*see* Section 9.4). In many cases, the output allows some degree of cell development so that a proportion of the circulating cells have matured. However, cell production may be so rapid that immature precursor cells and even those actively dividing are forced into the circulation. Leukaemias are given the designations acute or chronic, depending upon the rate of progress of the disease and roughly indicating the prognosis. Acute leukaemias display larger proportions of the immature (blast) cells, corresponding to a much higher rate of increase in the population. Larger numbers of immature cells are detrimental to the numbers of normal functional leucocytes. Circulating leukaemic cells infiltrate body tissues generally. Cell replacement and further proliferation may proceed, causing tissue damage, hence the malignant character of the disease. In the acute forms, the radical blood alterations may alone be severe enough to cause death before any significant invasion of other organs.

Neoplastic disease of the lymphoreticular tissues (lymph nodes or lymphoid organs) may also involve excessive lymphocyte proliferation and may affect the important reticulum-cell population. Neoplasia in these structures results in the formation of more coherent tumours, although there may also be considerable spread of individual cell products. The simplest forms of lymphoreticular proliferative disorder (previously called reticulosis) are lymphocytic lymphomas or reticulum-cell sarcomas, one cell-type only being involved. A more complex form is Hodgkin's disease which involves reticulum cells and lymphocytic cells. Tumour masses in this disease are highly variable, containing large numbers of other cell types (e.g. neutrophils and eosinophils) and typically the double-nucleus giant-cell forms called Sternberg-Reed cells. Most forms of lymphoreticular proliferative disorder are malignant.

Mutagenesis and Causes of Neoplasia

Current views on the causes of neoplasia are mainly based upon the strong associations with the incidence of cellular mutations (i.e. the acquisition of genetic abnormalities in cellular chromosomal material). Mutagenic effects can be produced by diverse actions:

- chemical agents
- ionising radiation
- viral infections
- miscellaneous influences (e.g. persistent solid deposits of certain materials in tissues).

Depending upon the extent of the changes in the genetic material of a cell, functional defects may result which range from a minor decrease in activity to major disruptions severe enough to cause cell death. Qualitative changes may also take place (e.g. abnormal structural-protein or enzyme synthesis or inability of the cell to divide). Functional abnormalities may be attributed to the known forms of mutations:

- base-pair transformations (point mutations)
- base-pair addition or deletion (frame-shift mutation)
- chromosome deletions or rearrangements
- unequal partition/dysfunction (e.g. abnormalities in mitosis due to spindle-poison effects).

Essentially, these result in abnormal DNA which cannot be translated or, if it can, provides nonsensical information. Dividing cells are particularly vulnerable to such influences (cytotoxicity). Mutagenic influences can result in persistent abnormality, passed to subsequent generations of cells (cellular mutation) or to generations of offspring (reproductive mutation); either type might result in foetal abnormalities (teratogenic).

Among the many possible consequences, abnormal proliferation may be an exceptional event which can only result when the cell is not so badly damaged that it dies or cannot divide. When neoplasia does occur, it is thought that it results from relatively minor mutation which impairs the controlling mechanism inhibiting the cell's inherent tendency for division. Direct stimulation as an active influence is less likely, although it may be the way in which oncogenic viruses produce their effects. It has become increasingly apparent that some forms of neoplastic disease are caused by viral infections. Viruses replicating in host cells do so by insertion of their own nucleic acids into nuclear coding for production of viral DNA or RNA and protein (see also Section 14.3). Successful interpretation may be accompanied by an influence on cell division, resulting in production of further generations of virus-producing cells. Such a direct cause of cell proliferation, due to insertion of specific genes (oncogenes), may explain the excessive, persistent proliferation of neoplasia.

Carcinogenic effects of radiation or chemical agents are likely to be much more random events in which only a very small proportion of a cell population may be mutagenically damaged. The range of categories of chemical agents with carcinogenic properties is shown in Table 15.16. The most important common feature of

TABLE 15.16
Modes of action of carcinogenic agents

Class	Mode of action	Example
Genotoxic mutagen		
Primary carcinogen	reactive chemical, electrophilic, direct action on DNA	epoxides, ethyleneimines, chromates
Procarcinogen (inactive precursor)	activation by metabolic transformation to primary or ultimate carcinogen	benzo(a)pyrene, vinyl chloride, dimethyl-nitrosamine, β-naphthylamine
Alkylating agents, polynuclear hydrocarbons, azo-compounds, and aromatic amines are important general groups of carcinogenic chemicals, providing examples of both classes of mutagen.		
Epigenetic influences		
Hormonal imbalance	altered control on cellular proliferation and differentiation	oestrogens
Oncogenes	viral or inherited genetic material influencing affected cells to persistent proliferation	retrovirus sarcoma oncogene, Epstein-Barr virus
Solid-state or surface carcinogens	physical interaction, persistent contact effect, usually only mesenchymal cells affected	asbestos, metal implants, plastics, prostheses
Accessory effects		
Co-carcinogen	enhance genotoxic or possibly solid-state agents, during preliminary (initiator) stage	irritants, phorbol esters, pyrene, catechol, surfactants
Immunosuppression	neoplastic due to other factors; particularly viral infection permitted by inhibition of immunosurveillance	cytotoxic agents, lymphotoxic antibiotics, anti-lymphocyte serum
Promoters	promote neoplastic growth of cells previously subjected to carcinogenic influence	phenols, bile acids, phorbol esters

many of the known carcinogens is chemical reactivity, particularly when it is apparent that interaction with chromosomal material is a possibility. As with many other forms of toxicity, a large proportion of the known agents must be metabolised within appropriate tissues to produce a sufficiently reactive product. In most cases it is thought that the neoplastic cells are those directly exposed or those in which metabolic activation occurs. Similarly, with oncogenic effects of radiation, it is thought that the application of physical energy causes mutagenic chemical change in chromosomal structures. However, possible causes are even more diverse and it is apparent that the influence of contact with abnormal surfaces or some other physical interactions may be carcinogenic (e.g. effects of asbestos fibres or long-term prosthetic implants).

15.8 GENETIC AND DEVELOPMENTAL DISORDERS

Introduction

Preceding sections in this chapter have been concerned largely with ways in which damage may be inflicted upon established cells or tissues, together with their responses to these effects. In contrast, structural defects or malfunctions may arise in the development of cells and tissues, the faults being or becoming instrinsic features. Here, too, account must be taken of the various agents or influences which may constitute an original cause of the abnormality.

As currently understood, the normal development of tissues depends upon co-ordinated programmes of cell division. Also, the proper construction and functioning of the constituent cells depend upon precise programmed control mechanisms which determine the nature of their internal processes. It would appear that a great deal of abnormality of tissue construction or cell functions may be explained in terms of defects in these programmes or controlling mechanisms.

Developmental Control

Fundamental control of cellular function is exerted by its nucleus, the mechanisms being determined by the precise sequences of purine and pyrimidine bases incorporated in the nuclear nucleic acid constituents. This constitutes the genome, the information borne by all of the cells of the body and replicated at each cell division by the process of mitosis. The information of the genome

held in the structure of DNA, which relates to the performance of the cell, is transcribed to complementary sequences of bases, constituting the messenger RNA (mRNA). This, in turn, provides the information whereby the cytoplasmic structures of the cell employed for synthesis (microsomes on the endoplasmic reticulum) elaborate peptide or protein molecules by assembling sequences of amino acids. The exact order of amino acids within diverse peptides is determined by the linear sequences of bases (codons) arranged in threes (triplets) on the mRNA molecules. Such codon triplets correspond to similar coding triplets of the DNA from which the RNA is transcribed. Thus, particular parts of nuclear DNA chains (gene assemblies) provide coded RNA, which in turn translates to specific proteins or peptides, appropriate to cell structures or functions (enzymes or secretions). All of these processes thus have genetically predetermined control programmes. Genome information also programmes and controls the activation or suppression of particular syntheses and hence determines the timings, rates, or frequencies of the performance of subordinate functions. It also influences the construction of individual cells, their assembly in tissues, and ultimately the entire anatomical structure. Each feature of a body is determined by a corresponding assembly of gene DNA.

The genetic blueprint as a whole is referred to as the genotype, and its actual manifestation in terms of structure and function is known as the phenotype. The genotype depends upon the assembly of a number of individual components composed of strands of DNA (chromosomes). The nucleus of every cell contains the complete genotype information (normally assembled in 23 pairs of chromosomes) in its genome. The genome is passed on to further cell generations by mitotic division. Normally, the cell only expresses that portion of the information which concerns its particular function. It is only from the genotype of the germ-cells of gonads that this information is passed on to other individuals, to be inherited as part of their genotype.

Each chromosome contains the genes for numerous features, groups of genes for related features generally being linked on one chromosome. Chromosomes are present as paired strands, thus contributing pairs of genes (alleles) in matching locations along the length of each chain. Most chromosomes bear genes concerned with general body cellular structures (autosomes). A distinct pair of chromosomes is specialised, carrying genes concerned with sexual characteristics and reproductive functions (sex chromosomes).

Genotypic composition is inherited, via the mating and fertilisation process, from parents and their progenitors and may be passed on to subsequent progeny by further mating. The inherited genotype determines embryonic development, further growth to maturity, sexual development and, as explained in Section 15.9, may programme the ageing changes and influence lifespan. It is in the inheritance of genetic characteristics that the pairing of genes comes into special significance. In the production of ova and spermatozoa, the process of meiosis involves a reduction division in which the pairs of chromosomes are separated. Thus the paired genes on the diploid chromosomes of each parent become divided between the resulting haploid gametes. Fertilisation leads to new combinations by uniting pairs of haploid genetic chromosomes. The new, combined, diploid zygote will be composed of two different sets of chromosome chains bearing different but complementary ranges of genes. The phenotype of the progeny will thus reveal a combination of characteristics from each member of the preceding generation determined by their resulting gene-pairs. However, the influence of each of the genes in a pair is not always equal. As they are inherited, some genes are dominant in their ability to enforce the expression of that feature in the phenotype, while others are recessive and relatively weaker in their influence. Each autosomal or sex-linked characteristic expressed in the phenotype will depend upon whether the gene combination is homozygous or heterozygous. By such inheritance, it is possible that errors or defects acquired in previous generations may give rise to aberrations of cellular structure, anatomy, or function (*see below*). A recessive pathological character may be carried without expression but can be retained for transmission to a further generation.

Genetic Abnormality

The system described above is so precise in its determination of cell function that a defect is equally faithfully reflected in malfunction. The range of control exerted is also so wide that the scope for aberration is correspondingly very diverse. The potential for damage is attenuated by the operation of chromosomal repair mechanisms, but defects do occur and persist. Such defects will often have arisen in a previous generation, to be acquired and passed on by inheritance. Alternatively, aberrations may be caused during the life of the individual, affecting somatic cells, and may be revealed as malfunction or malformation expressed following division of those cells. Aberrations of immediate consequence or subsequently inheritable may range from alterations in the sequences of nucleotide bases, affecting coding for a single feature, to radical abnormality of whole chromosomes or changes in the numbers of chromosomes which constitute the genome or genotype. In many cases, these aberrations will almost certainly have resulted from

damage exerted by a recognised pathological influence (e.g. ionising radiation, toxic action, or viral infection). It is also recognised that some effects may arise as errors in performance through apparently spontaneous faults or other, random, unexplained adverse circumstances. Such aberrations, from whatever cause, are most common during cell division. The consequences of these genetic errors will involve alteration, addition, or loss of amino acids in the sequences of structural or functional proteins or peptides, further contributing to structural alteration of malfunction.

Mutations and other Genetic Abnormalities

The main defects in genetic control which account for human disease are mutation, clastogenesis, and aneuploidisation. The term mutation is applied to coding errors which are localised abnormalities of DNA (point mutation) limited to particular genes. Mutations occur mainly through changes in the sequences of hydrogen-bonded pairs of purines and pyrimidines (base-pairs), in which guanine (G) is paired with cytosine (C), and adenine (A) is paired with thymine (T). Errors take the form of base-pair transformations (e.g. AT in the normal sequence replaced by GC or the pairs in reverse order, TA or CG). Additions or deletions of any number of base-pairs in a sequence similarly alter the coding radically and are called frame-shift mutations.

More radical or extensive damage can be observed in DNA chains or portions of chromosomal structures. Clastogenesis describes the consequences of breakage and reconstitution of chains of genes in which portions are lost or rearranged into abnormal sequences. When the processes of separating and rejoining chromosomes occur during mitosis or meiosis, mechanistic defects may cause the passage of incorrect portions of a chromosome. Unequal chromosomal chain-separations may also occur.

More serious errors may involve the gain or loss of one or more whole chromosomes (aneuploidisation). The result is monosomy (one lost) or trisomy (one gained) of the normal paired chromosomes, and these defects are discernible by microscopic counts of chromosome preparations from cell samples. Even worse damage may be revealed as bizarre marker chromosomes, appearing in giant or elongated forms, with fused portions or eccentric junctions. Numerical abnormalities can provide between 40 and 50 chromosomes (heteroploidy) rather than the normal 46. The numbers may also be double or further multiplied (polyploidy).

Minor mutations may not be strikingly apparent in expression. A base-pair change and its effect on a codon sequence would result in the incorporation of an incorrect amino acid. This would be of significance only if it materially altered the physical character of a membrane protein or changed the specificity of an enzyme (*see* Inheritance and Congenital Abnormalities below). Conversely, a highly disorganised codon could result in nonsensical molecules or could present a synthesis-termination sequence, suspending an essential function. Depending on the numbers of abnormal genes, the range of abnormal consequences could vary strikingly. Nonsense sequences in control-mechanism genes could be expressed as congenital deformities, de-repressed neoplastic cells (*see* Section 15.7), or ageing changes (*see* Section 15.9).

Mutation could therefore cause abnormality of a single cell, development of an aberrant clone population, or the deformity of an anatomical feature. However, more radical chromosomal abnormalities might actually be less overtly expressed because severe aberrations may not permit the survival of the affected cell. Clastogenesis, aneuploidy, or polyploidy may constitute lethal mutations. Single cell death may be of no consequence, but the multiple cell effect might cause stillbirth or abortion of deformed foetuses. Heteroploidy accounts for 15% of spontaneous abortions in human pregnancies, and up to 30% feature some other detectable chromosome-associated aberration. It is rare for marked autosomal abnormalities to be live-born in humans because the phenotypic abnormalities are so severe that the foetal tissue is rejected. Even if live-born, survival is often problematic. A major exception, with survival despite notable aberration (poor cerebral development, and skeletal and other tissue defects caused by trisomy), is Down's syndrome.

Developmental Abnormalities

In many cases, the consequences of mutation, clastogenesis, or heteroploidy will be restricted to the individual in which the defect arises (i.e. non-heritable abnormalities). Other mechanistic defects may have similar results, causing individual abnormal body development (e.g. teratogenic effects). Toxicity, radiation, or infective agents may affect similar processes and, in-

TABLE 15.17

Defects of the skeleton, organs, or tissues arising as faults in development due to congenital or teratogenic influences

Cardiovascular	cardiac displacement	
	cardiac septal defects	
	coarctation of aorta	stricture or occlusion
	mitral or other valve stenosis	
	transposition of arteries	
Eyes and ears	anophthalmos or anotia	absent eye or ear
	coloboma	deformed eyelid or iris
	microphthalmos or microtia	small eye or ear structure
Gastro-intestinal	atresia	closure or lack of lumen
	fistulas	perforations or abnormally connected passages
	hernias of various parts	
	pyloric stenosis	sphincter muscle defect
Genito-urinary	absence of ovaries or testes	
	double ureters	
	ectopic displaced kidneys	
	polycystic kidney	deformed inflated nephron spaces
	renal agenesis	absence of kidneys
	undescended testes	
	vaginal or uterine atresia	
Nervous System	amyelia	absence of spinal cord
	hydrocephalus	brain distortion by fluid
	meningocoele	hernia of meninges
	microcephaly	reduced brain size
Skeletal	anencephaly	malformed cranium and brain
	cleft lip or palate	
	ectromelia	absence of one or more extremity
	peromelia	defective, stunted, or misshapen limbs
	spina bifida, rachischisis	absence of vertebral arches, open spinal canal
	syndactyly	webbed or fused fingers

a)   *Parents*

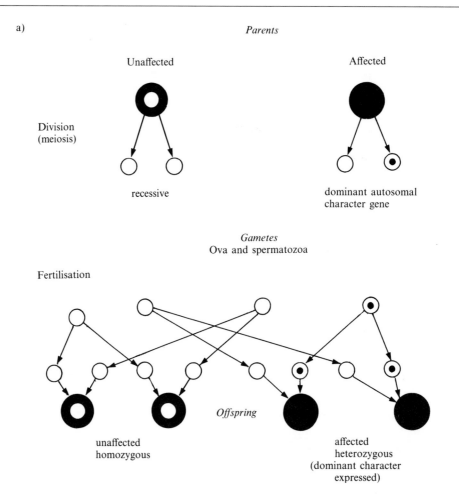

Fig. 15.14
Autosomal dominant trait inheritance from heterozygous parents: a) inheritance pattern when only one parent is affected and expressing the gene. Two of the possible combinations will lead to expression in the progeny. b) inheritance when both parents are affected. Three of the possible combinations may result in affected offspring.

deed, agents with recognised mutagenic actions can also act as teratogens. However, the outcome may eventually be of the same kind, whether teratogenic or congenital (due to cell-genome alteration); both cause a very wide range of abnormalities (Table 15.17).

Normally, the process of embryogenesis results in the precise development of every anatomical detail coded in the zygote genotype through an incredibly complex series of cellular activities. Series of divisions, cell migrations, selective cell death (apoptosis) on a large scale, and co-ordinated differentiation into tissues and organs are all programmed. However, many of the steps are vulnerable to interference. Eventually, this is revealed as partial (hypoplasia) or complete (agenesis) absence of particular tissue. These terms distinguish de-

velopmental failures from regressive changes later in life, which are called atrophy (partial) or aplasia (total). Otherwise, there may be failures of fusion, separation, or canalisation in forming organs. Structures may develop in abnormal sites (ectopia, heterotopia, or aberrance). Less frequently, there may occur simple overgrowth (hyperplasia) or formation of supernumary organs. Most of these originate in the embryo and are apparent at birth. Whatever abnormality occurs is less influenced by the nature of the teratogen, mutagen, or radiation than the timing and duration of the effect. Those particular mechanisms or stages of embryogenesis in operation at the time of exposure to the toxic influences are those most likely to suffer failure, as reflected in subsequent aberrant development.

b)

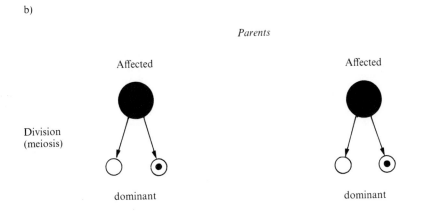

Parents

Affected   Affected

Division
(meiosis)

dominant   dominant

Gametes
Ova and spermatozoa

Fertilisation

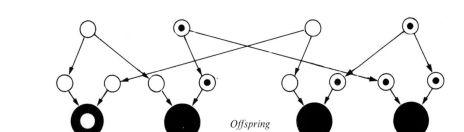

Offspring

unaffected   affected   affected
homozygous   heterozygous   homozygous
                       (dominant character
                       expressed)

Some aberrations do not appear until later life. Certain atrophies occur normally (e.g. closure of the ductus arteriosus or the ageing-involution of thymus tissue). Other delayed changes give rise to neoplastic features through persistent growth and cellular disorganisation (*see* Section 15.7). This may involve a single tissue (e.g. cartilage or blood vessels), producing a tumour-form (hamartoma). Accumulations of melanocyte cells also form hamartomas (the melanotic naevi) which are usually benign, but sometimes become invasive and metastatic (malignant melanoma). Other later developing tumorous malformations (teratoma) can be attributed to embryonic origins (e.g. nephroblastoma (renal nephron change), neuroblastoma (nerves), medulloblastoma (hindbrain) or retinoblastoma). Teratomas with multiple tissues can often display bizarre conglomerations of skin, muscle, bone, and even teeth. Ovaries or testes are also frequent sites of teratoma growth.

Inheritance and Congenital Abnormalities

The inheritance of gene-linked characteristics may be explained by Mendelian laws. These provide a basis for the assessment of chances of transmission and expression of characteristics, whether normal or abnormal. The determinant factors are the ways in which the genes from each parent are distributed at fertilisation and the relative powers of genes to exert their influence. For autosomal chromosomes, the pairing of identical (homozygous) genes ensures that the respective character gains expression. When the pairs differ (heterozygous), the relative potency is critical (Fig. 15.14). A dominant abnormal gene, causing such severe effects that it can lead to early death or impaired success of reproduction, would naturally become eliminated from the population. Many, less severe, genetic defects are persistent and widely distributed in the world's population. Of

TABLE 15.18
Disease, disorder, or malformation due to inheritance of genetic aberrations

Autosomal dominant gene inheritance

achondroplasia	intermittent porphyria
adult renal polycystic disease	neurofibromatosis
chronic familial neutropenia	osteogenesis imperfecta
familial periodic paralysis	polydactyly
haemorrhagic telangiectasia	polyposis coli
Huntington's chorea	tuberous sclerosis

Autosomal recessive inheritance

albinism	glycogen storage diseases
aminoacidurias	haemoglobinopathies
cystic fibrosis	lysosomal storage diseases
galactosaemia	types of dwarfism

Sex-linked gene inheritance (X-linked recessive)

agammaglobulinaemia	haemophilias A and B
alopecia	Hunter's syndrome
colour blindness	muscular dystrophy
glucose 6-phosphate dehydrogenase deficiency	nephrogenic diabetes insipidus

these, the dominant forms revealed in each individual (hetero- or homozygous) may to some extent be eliminated by choice of partner. The recessive genes will not necessarily be revealed in every generation and are thus less readily avoided and more insidiously widespread. Cultural, religious, or legal prohibitions on sexual intercourse between blood relations can be interpreted as attempts to avoid homozygous expression of recessive genetic defects. When a characteristic is dominant and rare or avoidable, it is probable that most individuals affected will be heterozygous.

Examples of disorders subject to various inheritance patterns are shown in Table 15.18. Some conditions are attributed to intermediate states of expression, and therefore dominance is not always absolute. Most characteristics are controlled by the autosomes and distributed irrespective of the sex of the offspring. However, certain aberrations carried selectively by the X- or Y-chromosomes will be sex-limited, although this limitation may be partial (e.g. gout, cleft palate, and megacolon are more common in males while spina bifida and congenital hip dislocation are more common in females). Sex-linked abnormalities are commonly carried on X-chromosomes but are mostly recessive; the defects are not expressed in heterozygous females, but are transmitted by them and expressed selectively in male offspring (Fig. 15.15). This arises because sons can receive X-chromosomes only from their mother; a recessive character on this chromosome, relative to normal X-chromosomes, may not have a corresponding dominant

gene on the much smaller Y-chromosome from the father. This explains the male expression of certain diseases (e.g. the haemophilias).

Some severe defects (aneuploidy, *see* Mutations and other Genetic Abnormalities above) may occur in sex chromosomes without impairing survival of the body as a whole. Such defects may, however, preclude further inheritance because of the consequent sexual malfunction. Klinefelter's syndrome arises through XXY aneuploidy. The Y-chromosome conveys male sexuality, but the development of male anatomy and function is poor because of the additional X-influence. The individual is infertile and poor production of male hormones results in failure of development of secondary sexual characteristics. Indeed, residual female influence may be apparent (e.g. gynaecomastia).

Otherwise, most common congenital disorders are autosomal. Often, these are instances of the relatively simple coding mutations in which the defect is expressed as abnormal protein production. Alterations in haemoglobin synthesis provide good examples. Sickle-cell anaemia derives from a point mutation of a single base, causing production of abnormal haemoglobin in which valine is substituted for glutamic acid in the peptide chains. Gene deletion may give a different version (thalassaemia) in which formation of α- or β-peptide chains of the globin component fails due to loss of the corresponding mRNA. Different examples are defective enzyme production (e.g. phenylketonuria) or inherited lack of functional protein (abetalipoproteinaemia), which are due to autosomal recessive genes. More varied consequences derive from another form of autosomal recessive gene (carried by 1 in 20 persons and expressed in 1 in 2000 live births) which produces excessive viscosity in secretions of exocrine glands (pancreas, intestinal crypts, salivary glands, and bronchial mucosa). The defect is caused by an increased concentration of glycoprotein. This condition develops into cystic fibrosis and is the most common autosomal recessive inheritance of disease in temperate climates.

15.9 AGEING AND GERIATRIC DISEASE

Introduction

Ageing is a complex process whereby the structures and functions of the body change, largely on a time-dependent basis. In the broadest sense, ageing could be considered to proceed from the time of birth or even from conception; from these points, quite clear chronological

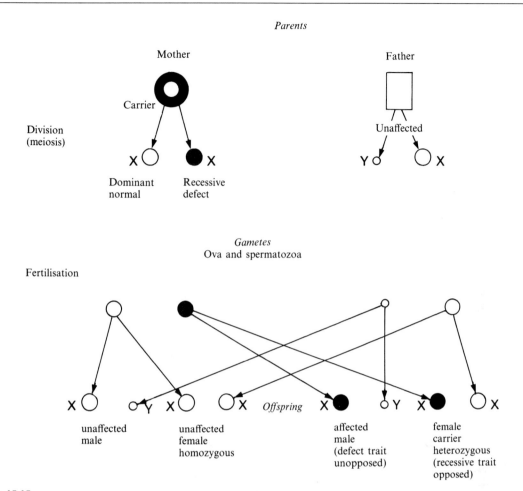

Fig. 15.15
Sex-linked inheritance of a recessive genetic abnormality, transmitted on the X-chromosome.

developments occur. However, both embryological and childhood growth obviously result in biological improvements in the system, firstly providing the differentation, organisation, and specialisation of tissues, followed by further growth in general functional capacity up to an optimal size. These advances in anatomy and physiological performance continue well into postnatal life. Apart from general growth, improvements of function occur with exercise, learning, and advancing co-ordination. Mental ability and the acquisition of knowledge and experience expand markedly during the early years of life. A later development long after birth is the commencement of reproductive activity, which is accompanied by further important modifications to the anatomy and physiology of the body. Thus, the optimal functional state of the body is attained with net improvements in most respects. The rates of these

developments differ markedly between different animals, although in general the period required for maturing is related to lifespan. In humans, the process requires approximately 20 years, approaching one third of the lifespan. Some would argue that biological improvements continue past this period, with continued mental experience or even physical training maintaining some further advance.

Improvements do not occur uniformly throughout this early period. Even in the embryological stage, substantial cell death occurs. This is necessary for the tissue-forming processes and is thus programmed and normal. After birth, further cellular loss occurs (e.g. atresia). Wear and tear of both external and internal tissues will also commence, introducing the possibility of net loss with time. In particular, no new production of neurones occurs from this time. Inevitably, some neuronal loss occurs from this time onwards and thus marks a potential deterioration with age. Age-related cell depletions or cessation of development early in life are of little adverse consequence and may even be of benefit. Most of the general deteriorations which commence when the optimal development is past still do not seriously impair the organism for a substantial time afterwards.

The time-dependent change or deterioration which represents ageing proceeds in a variety of ways. Not all of these aspects are obviously pathological. It is necessary to concentrate upon those which are clearly harmful or reduce functional efficiency. In general, the changes which occur progressively and predictably with age, becoming characteristics of later life, have to be considered as normal or inevitable (senescence). Some of these are harmless (e.g. white hair, wrinkled skin, and changed voice) and mark the typical appearance denoting advanced age. Most other aspects do, however, represent disadvantage, particularly when taken *en masse* and can therefore be regarded as being pathological. There are three main aspects to the pathology:

- deterioration of functions with or without overt tissue change
- increased susceptibility to death
- age-related diseases.

Functional Deterioration in Ageing

In advanced age there are clearly apparent alterations in the structures of the body, most of which are quantitative rather than qualitative. Most tissues decrease substantially in bulk with losses in the numbers of cells, although the changes are uneven (e.g. musculoskeletal shrinkage is greater than visceral decrease). Thus, body stature decreases with age once the optimal mature size has been achieved. Cellular numbers decrease (ageing atrophy) in most organs but this may not fully account for deterioration in functions. Generally, the vital organs have a very large excess functional capacity and geriatric cell-loss seldom comes near to exceeding the reserve until later on. Throughout life, cellular loss may be replenished by regeneration, except in muscular and central nervous tissues which lack such abilities. Hence, neuronal and muscular atrophy may be greater than in, for example, epithelial tissues. However, the rate of effective regeneration may decrease with age and thus disease or wear and tear may become more destructive.

At the cellular level, there are few marked changes in cell structure or general constituents. Cellular fluid, electrolytes, nitrogen, RNA or DNA, and cytoplasmic pH do not alter much. In old cells, deposits of ageing pigment commonly occur but are thought to have no special pathological significance. Some aberrations may develop in the production of intracellular enzymes, resulting in changes in specificity or loss of effectiveness. With time, these may lead to impairment of certain cellular functions and the effects of multiple aberrations may be additive. For whatever reason, functions generally do become defective, again in quantitative terms.

From maturity onwards, most functions undergo insidious adverse change. Detectable deviations from normality are observed in a number of functional parameters from 30 to 40 years of age (Table 15.19) and continue with an approximately linear decline. Even when resting level or average values for functional parameters are not markedly abnormal, they may become so when the system is required to change to meet rapid or severe demands. Thus, deviations in functional activity may be irregular, indicating aberrations of control mechanisms or alterations in capacity. In particular, the precision of control of homoeostatic mechanisms worsens with age, increasing variation and causing overshooting of required values when attempting to restore a function to normal or resting level (e.g. in blood pressure or blood-sugar levels).

Despite general and progressive deteriorations of this nature, major malfunctions are not usually apparent until advanced age (e.g. 70 years of age or more) unless caused by additional disease. Of particular note are the defects in musculoskeletal functions and in the nervous system. Muscular regressions are revealed relatively early as weakening, readier fatigue, and slower response to exercise or training. In later life, the debilities may progress to manual incompetence, locomotor disability, and changes in gait or stance. Similarly, most parameters of nervous function and mental capacity decline with age. Slower neuronal conduction and reflex-arc delays may account for inefficient control mechanisms. Neuromuscular control may become impaired, adding to the disabilities of weak muscles. Mental deterioration takes various forms, from minor loss of short-term memory and inabilities to concentrate or perform problem-solving tasks, to severe incompetence or gross senile dementia. Sensory impairment also becomes marked in advanced age (e.g. loss of tactile discrimination, hearing loss, limitation of adaptation for low-light vision, and intolerance of changes in temperature). Imperfect temperature control may be associated with more general senile decline, whereby lack of exercise and poor nutrition predispose to hypothermia or heat-prostration. Many problems of old age involve combinations of malfunction (e.g. faecal or urinary incontinence caused by loss of nervous control, reduced mental capacity, and manual incompetence). Alternatively, in many people

TABLE 15.19
Functional defects developing with age (see also Chapter 18)

Cardiovascular	decreased cardiac output
	delayed recovery of heart rate and blood pressure after exercise
	increased peripheral resistance
	slower heart rate
Endocrine	climacteric cessation of sexual functions
	decline in corticosteroid and testosterone production
	decreased iodine turnover in thyroid and thyroid atrophy
	greater variability of resting levels or irregular diurnal fluctuations
	increased vulnerability to stress
	pancreatic atrophy
	parathyroid hyperplasia
	pituitary enlargement
Musculoskeletal	delayed healing of fractures
	delayed recovery after effort
	loss of tensile strength and elasticity of bones and tendons
	muscle weakness and decreased endurance
	musculoskeletal atrophy
	postural changes
	slower benefit from muscular training
	unsure gait and instability
Nervous and mental performance	ability to see in low intensity light impaired
	concentration diminished
	decreased conduction velocity and reflex delays
	decreased temperature tolerance
	defective tactile perception
	fragmentation of cortical neurones and changes in morphology of Purkinje cells
	memory defects
	mental reaction times longer
	progressive neurone loss
	slower performance of thinking or calculating tasks
	visual and auditory acuities decreased
	worsening of motor co-ordination leading to impaired manual dexterity
Renal	lower glomerular filtration rate
	progressive nephron loss and compensatory hypertrophy
	reduced glucose tolerance
	renal blood flow decreased
Respiratory	delayed normalisation of respiration after exercise
	impaired ventilation and gas-exchange
	linear decline in basal metabolic rate
	reduced vital capacity

who retain most mental faculties, experience may enable an effective degree of adaptation to the problems of physical disability, and functional deterioration may be masked for long periods.

Connective tissues are subject to both qualitative and functional changes. In particular, loose (areolar) connective tissue (*see* Section 10.5) becomes degraded (e.g. loss of matrix components and molecular alterations in elastic and collagen fibres), causing altered physical properties. Loss of elasticity or shrinkage causes changes in tissues or organs. Skin is very obviously affected by underlying collagen-fibre degradation. In middle age, it tightens as the collagen shrinks and then relaxes to give the wrinkles of the aged. Failure of collagen fibres around capillaries leads to weakening and local haemorrhages, giving rise to the purple cutaneous blotches of senile purpura. Elsewhere, collagen degeneration weakens the tensile strength of tendons, while increasing collagen fibrosis impairs organ function. Bones become brittle due to changes in the elastic fibrous component and in their calcium deposits. In blood, there is an age-dependent decrease in numbers of lymphocytes and eosinophils, whereas neutrophils increase. Reduction in the supply of lymphocytes is reflected in a gradual reduction in the effectiveness of immune activity as well as less precise control over the direction of immune attack.

These defects may be related to the marked atrophy of the thymus as age progresses, thus losing the controlling influence of this tissue on some aspects of immunity.

Ageing and Death

Death is not due to age. As far as the event is understood, it involves the same circumstances at whatever age it occurs. It would appear that death must be due to fatal diseases, or to an imposed effect causing a lethal radical defect in one or more vital systems. Nevertheless, it appears to be an inevitable fact that death, in man and higher animals at least, is very strongly correlated with age. For each species the rates of ageing and the general lifespan are characteristic and relatively constant (i.e. short-lived animals age more quickly). As ageing is so clearly a determinant of general functional deterioration, it is likely that this contributes to decreased resistance to lethal circumstances. However, there must be many features of ageing pathology which are not directly involved in this. Clearly, white hair and wrinkles have little, if any, bearing on incidence of death, and even the radical loss of tissue masses or certain functions may not be directly lethal. Amputees, paraplegics, the blind, and persons who have lost one kidney, one lung, or 40% of the liver may survive for long periods, given appropriate assistance for the disability. What is necessary is that they escape a fatal disease or other lethal circumstances. Current experience demonstrates that life may be prolonged by counteracting a potentially lethal defect (e.g. heart failure), despite the concurrent progress of various and severe aspects of geriatric pathology.

The age-related factors most involved in death are probably those giving rise to functional errors, particularly in control mechanisms. One theory which goes a long way to explaining the death of cells and of the whole body is the error catastrophe. This accounts for the ultimate death of cell-lines after certain numbers of divisions, on the basis of accumulated errors in genetic control. The errors result in aberrations in enzyme production or disorganisation of vital functions, possibly with failure in gene repair processes. They lead to progressively worsening malfunctions, up to the stage at which the mechanisms cease to be mutually self-sustaining. The same concept may be applied to the whole body, where life depends upon nutrition and oxygenation distributed by the circulation in a controlled manner. Defects of individual vital components may be counteracted by the control and homoeostatic systems which optimise body functions in relation to environment. Systemic failure may, however, be caused by a lethal factor of sufficient severity, at any time and irrespective of any compensatory action that might be taken. This explains the ready possibility of deaths in healthy young people. If the protective or compensatory mechanisms are slow or inaccurate, the counteraction of lethal influence will be even less effective; hence the aged may succumb more readily. Failure or aberration of control mechanisms may contribute substantially to death if the errors are sufficient to cause a radically inappropriate response to an adverse provocation (e.g. circulatory collapse when normally blood pressure would be maintained). Yet another factor predisposing to death may be decreased resistance to infection. This may simply be the result of the aforementioned decrease in immune activity or it may be caused by other circumstances (e.g. the existence of chronic bronchitis, malnutrition, hypothermia, or cardiac defects).

A final point which is of great significance concerning the care of the elderly is that the longer people live the longer they take to die (i.e. terminal illness becomes more prolonged with age). This is now a well-recognised fact, albeit a generalisation. Thus, there are now larger numbers of people surviving to experience their expected lifespan and larger numbers living to experience senility. This produces a population of unwell people among whom, as a separate category, there are those who are dying.

Age-related Diseases

The incidence of a number of types of disease is clearly related to age, some having a particular correlation with childhood or early life, although most serious diseases occur more frequently with advancing age (Table 15.20). Certain of these may be severe enough to cause death, thus contributing to age-related mortality (e.g. myocardial or cerebrovascular necrosis, neoplastic disease, pernicious anaemia, or type II diabetes mellitus). Infections or neoplasias may be as fatal in the young as in the old

TABLE 15.20
Age-related diseases

Probably auto-immune aetiology	Varied or multiple aetiology
Addison's disease	atherosclerosis
megaloblastic anaemia	cataract
myasthenia gravis	chronic bronchitis
rheumatoid arthritis	and emphysema
systemic lupus erythematosus	hypertension
thyroiditis	neoplastic diseases
type II diabetes mellitus	osteoarthritis
ulcerative colitis	Parkinson's disease
	senile dementia and pre-senile dementia

but, generally, both incidence and vulnerability are greater with age. Pneumonia used to be notorious as the terminal illness of the aged ('the old-man's friend'). Other conditions (e.g. rheumatoid arthritis and parkinsonism) may be more disabling than fatal but have great importance as causes of disabilities, severely impairing the quality of life and rendering the sufferer much more dependent.

As with death, it is probably not these diseases themselves but susceptibility to other diseases which depends upon the general ageing process. Changes in the function of the immune system explain the aetiology of several auto-immune diseases (*see* Section 16.10). Defects in the immune defences against aberrant cell-lines probably also contribute to the behaviour of neoplastic cells or tissues; it may well be that malignant tumours are able

to behave in an aggressive manner because immune restraint is absent. This may partly explain why the incidence of malignancies increases with age. The other time of life when neoplasia may be highly malignant is during the first few months after birth, when immune function is undeveloped. However, it is likely that the basic cause of neoplasia is a mutational error in genetic control of cell growth. It is conceivable that such an error may even arise spontaneously, in the same manner as the changes which are thought to give rise to geriatric abnormalities generally. This is thus a stochastic process (*see* Section 15.2) which is cumulative and random.

Possible causes or mechanisms for age-related malfunctions, diseases, or mortality are listed in Table 15.21. Further aspects of the impact of the ageing population on pharmacy are discussed in Chapter 18.

TABLE 15.21
Mechanisms believed to contribute to geriatric malfunction, age-related diseases, and mortality

Programmed cell-death and determined lifespan control

- limitation of mitosis

   Most specialised (differentiated) cell-lines appear to have a limit to the possible number of mitotic divisions of approximately 50, after which proliferation ceases and the cells die. This is called the Hayflick Limit and may account for eventual atrophy of proliferating tissues. Neoplastic cells and germ-cells of some tissues do not have such limitation.

- programmed ageing

   Loss of cells (atrophy) occurs at characteristic rates and by a distinctive process (apoptosis), suggesting a genetically controlled, time-related mechanism.

Degradation of cell components at the molecular level

- somatic mutation

   Spontaneous defects arise in genetic control mechanisms (e.g. DNA and gene repair) due to random errors, radiation, virus DNA, oncogenes, or carcinogens (i.e. mutation provocation). As a result abnormal cell proteins are produced giving structural defects and ineffective enzymes resulting in cell malfunction or death. Abnormal cellular protein causes changed antigenicity and results in immunological incompatibility or neoplasia.

- auto-immune activity

   Altered cellular structures attract destructive attack (immunosurveillance) from the immune system eliminating mutated, aged, or neoplastic cells. Alternatively, defects in immune function may result in attack on normal cells due to lack of discrimination.

- macromolecular degradation

   Protein polymer molecules, particularly fibrillar structures, alter with age due to chemical denaturing, cross-linking, or free-radical substitution effects (e.g. in collagen, elastin, and contractile protein). Changes in tensile strength, elasticity, or tissue distortion and inactivities result. Chemical change may provoke auto-immune attack.

Control and adaptation defects

   Progressive inability to alter physiological functions in response to environmental change or operational demands. Inappropriate responses may lead to cumulative and worsening malfunctions, to the point of error catastrophe, giving cell or systemic death.

Chapter 16

PATHOPHYSIOLOGY

16.1 CARDIOVASCULAR DISEASE

16.1.1 CARDIAC PATHOLOGY

Introduction

Cardiac tissue is not subject to a wide range of disease forms as the heart is relatively well protected, especially from external influences. Infections and immune system attack are possible, but neoplasia is rare as a primary disease in the heart, generally occurring only as secondary growth from lesions elsewhere. The predominant pathology is of the degenerative-necrotic type, most often due to ischaemia (*see* Section 15.2). Usually, the nature of any lesion is less of a problem than the location or extent of damage in the heart. The heart is entirely muscular with minimal connective tissue components. Different parts of the structure (e.g. muscle-fibre bundles or tracts) differ only in their capacity to contract, conduct the excitation waves, or both. If muscle fibres are damaged, these capacities will be impaired. Excitation of muscular activity must be applied in a properly coordinated manner in order that consequent contraction spreads regularly through the atrial and ventricular muscle masses to give coherent pumping action. Lesions which alter the regularity of conduction may weaken the contractile performance more effectively than actual loss of muscle; contraction weakness of the muscle itself may require much more extensive damage. Damage to valves may be an even worse cause of deterioration of pumping performance.

Myocardial Degeneration and Necrosis

Necrotic lesions will most commonly result from ischaemia which is in turn usually due to coronary-artery disease (occlusion). Deprivation of blood results in anoxia and reduced nutrient supply. Clinically, the range of ischaemic heart disease extends from an asymptomatic reduction of flow, through the intermediate syndrome of angina pectoris, to extensive myocardial infarction. The latter causes death of a substantial number of cells; numerous others are less severely affected but degenerate sufficiently to become non-functional. If ischaemia is of minor severity, the oxygen supply will be deficient only when the muscle increases in activity beyond the limits of normality. If this is of short duration, no lasting harm may result as the relative ischaemia abates and the fibres recover rapidly after cessation of the increased effort. In the absence of oxygen,

anaerobic metabolism may only sustain the cell for a very short time. Longer anoxia results in damage so that degenerative changes (mainly hydropic, *see* Section 15.3) ensue. When deprivation is total, degeneration progresses rapidly to cell death (Fig. 16.1). Necrotic cells commonly occur deep in a severely ischaemic area. Surrounding, less severely deprived, cells display less damage but many may proceed to die over a longer period.

Circumstances which determine the progression to necrosis are total depletion of glycogen, build-up of lactic acid, and influx of calcium into the cell and its organelles. Cells vacuolate and swell, their energy resources are impoverished, and they lose contractile activity. Other metabolic changes result in additional fatty degeneration. Such changes may be reversible up to a point, if blood flow is re-established. Beyond this point, necrosis will be inevitable even if not immediate. A typical time-scale for the course of a severely ischaemic lesion is shown in Table 16.1.

The acid environment and release of lysosomal enzymes in the infarct promote autolysis of necrotic cells which is slow in cardiac muscle, although cell digestion may be greatly advanced by the action of neutrophils. Cell debris is removed by macrophage activity and is followed by growth of fibroblasts into the area to replace the disorganised structure with collagen fibrous scar tissue. This neither contracts nor conducts the excitation wave.

At the periphery of an infarct, some cells may remain viable although in a degenerate condition. In particular, those just within the endocardium have a greater survival

TABLE 16.1
Time course of pathological changes developing as myocardial infarction in severely ischaemic cardiac muscle

0 to 1 hours	Glycogen loss, lactic acid accumulation, calcium entry, myofibril weakness
1 to 3 hours	Cells swollen, organelles deformed, restoration of blood supply may be ineffective
1 to 6 hours	Necrosis established, infiltration of neutrophil cells at periphery
12 to 15 hours	Visible zone of infarction, pale and oedematous
24 hours	Cell-protein degradation
36 hours	Infarct borders haemorrhaged
3 to 4 days	Neutrophil numbers at peak, lysis of necrotic cells, macrophage infiltration; infarct soft and balloons under pressure
4 to 7 days	Infiltration of fibroblasts, collagen fibre deposition
3 to 6 weeks	Collagen scar formation, capillary regrowth
3 months	Fully formed and contracting scar

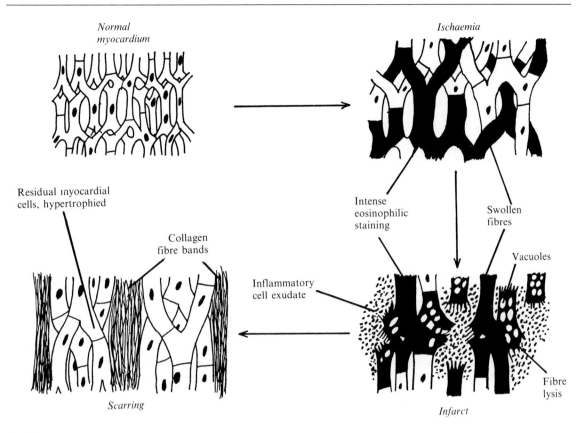

Normal myocardium

Ischaemia

Residual myocardial cells, hypertrophied

Collagen fibre bands

Intense eosinophilic staining

Swollen fibres

Vacuoles

Inflammatory cell exudate

Fibre lysis

Scarring

Infarct

Fig. 16.1
Myocardial infarct development.

rate than those deeper in the muscle. This may be due to oxygenation from blood within the chambers or via the internal channels called thebesian veins. Such surviving cells may eventually regain the ability to contract. They at least retain some tone and can help to maintain the muscle tension unlike flaccid necrotic tissue which tends to balloon under pressure. The viable but degenerate cells, although quiescent, may still transmit activation stimuli and help to preserve the regular passage of excitation waves. However, they can become the source of aberrant excitation activity and provide an ectopic focus of arrhythmic contractions.

Cardiomyopathy

A number of common diseases which affect the whole body exert their most serious effects on the heart. Unlike ischaemic damage, these effects depend upon a functional blood supply and inflammation is an additional component of damage. Almost any pathogen causing systemic infection may cause cardiac damage (infectious myocarditis) by direct growth or remotely by circulation of toxins. Diphtheria toxin provides a good example of a selective damaging effect resulting in necrosis, particularly of conducting fibres, and inflammation. Direct infection may be of bacterial origin (e.g. *Salmonella typhi*, meningococci, or gonococci), protozoal (e.g. trypanosomes or plasmodia), or parasitic (e.g. *Trichinella spiralis*). Viral infection of cardiac muscle is particularly important as a cause of widespread foci of necrosis and inflammation in the heart (e.g. caused by influenza, mumps, measles, and viral hepatitis). In poliomyelitis, the pre-paralytic viraemia often causes direct cardiac damage. It is now clearly recognised that common, low-grade, viral illness may leave a legacy of cardiac damage as revealed by paroxysmal tachycardia or other arrhythmias. Typical examples are ECHOvirus or Coxsackie B virus infections, generally associated with fever, malaise, and myalgia.

Other forms of infection result in the development of granulomatous lesions (*see* Section 15.5). One notable example is caused by syphilis, which was in decline but is now again prevalent. In its classical form, the later (tertiary) stages of this disease particularly caused nervous damage. However, the modern manifestations appear to affect the heart in preference to the nervous system. The typical granulomatous lesion of tertiary syphilis is the gumma (Fig. 16.2). Other focal inflammatory lesions in cardiac muscle are the Aschoff nodules associated with rheumatic fever. As a remote and delayed consequence of infection by β-haemolytic streptococci, mediated by antigen-antibody complexes (type III hypersensitivity) (*see* Section 15.6), the lesions are intially diffusely inflammatory but later become nodular. Granulomatous lesions ultimately become scar tissue.

Many of the most common cardiac lesions associated with infection occur in the valves. Both syphilis and rheumatic fever contribute to such damage, causing small diffuse patches of inflammation. Syphilis affects the aorta and its valves, causing valve cusp scarring with edge rolling or valve-ring deformities. The aortic wall may become scarred and weakened, to the extent that it becomes distended under pressure (aneurysm) or may even rupture. Rheumatic lesions may also damage valve cusps and rings, some occurring on the chordae tendineae anchoring the valves. Surface lesions acquire aggregates of platelets adhering to the inflamed surface. Other surface infection may be more widespread, extending from valves and chordae tendineae over the endocardial surface of the ventricles (infective endocarditis, Fig. 16.3). Arising from bacteraemias (e.g. *Streptococcus viridans*) or fungal infections, this condition is a dangerous feature of immunosuppression.

Cardiomyopathy may result from various toxic actions, either direct or due to hypersensitivity. Cardiac malfunction associated with fatty degeneration may be a result of chronic alcoholism. Other substances exerting toxic effects on the heart are phosphorus, lead, cobalt salts, and respiratory enzyme poisons (e.g. nitro compounds, cyanides, and heavy metals).

Heart Failure

Damaged muscle will suffer power failure because degenerate or necrotic cells are unable to contract and the affected chamber loses coherence of pumping function. Under the pressure exerted in systole, infarcted areas may stretch or balloon, decreasing blood expulsion. In diastole, such tissue does not readily return to its normal configuration after stretching. If there is substantial fibrotic scarring, the cardiac wall may be less compliant, again failing to conform to the tensions of surrounding beating muscle. In all of these cases the efficiency of pumping is decreased. Other efficiency impairing effects

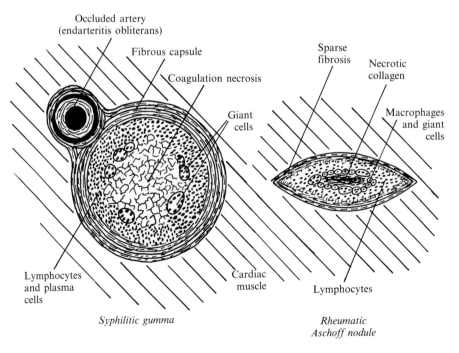

Fig. 16.2
Granulomatous nodular lesions.

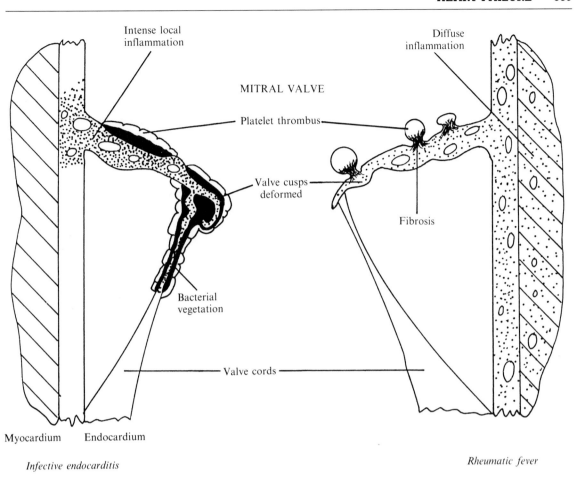

Fig. 16.3
Valvular lesions due to direct bacterial growth (infective endocarditis) or infection-associated immune inflammation (rheumatic fever).

accrue from the uneven passage of contraction-excitation waves through inflamed, infarcted, or scarred tissue. Arrhythmias may occur due to unco-ordinated firing of fibres or because some areas of muscle receive the stimulus from two or more waves at irregular intervals. Another possibility is that necrotic or scar tissue may rupture, allowing blood to escape which will then surge in and out of the pericardial space (cardiac tamponade) or may flow incorrectly from one chamber to another through a ruptured septum. Scarred papillary muscles may tear, giving mitral or tricuspid valve incompetence and backflow from the ventricles.

Like other vital organs, the normal heart is endowed with substantial reserve capacity. At rest, it performs more slowly and with much less force than it is capable of exerting to meet increased demand. A damaged heart may still retain the ability to function normally and even to respond to an increased load. Function may, therefore, be normal until the reserve capacity is exceeded and still be able to cope to a limited extent. This ability is illustrated by the Starling curves (Fig. 16.4). Ability to deal with the work load is particularly dependent upon the stretching of the muscle before contraction. Function may be markedly impaired by incorrect filling of the chambers, highlighting the importance of proper functioning of valves and co-ordination of atrial and ventricular beating. Even when the heart is not functioning properly and cardiac output is likely to fall, the circulation may be adequately maintained by other compensating mechanisms. However, severe or combined damage results in failure when any increase in performance is inadequate to satisfy increase in demand. Beyond a certain point, the performance actually worsens as the load increases.

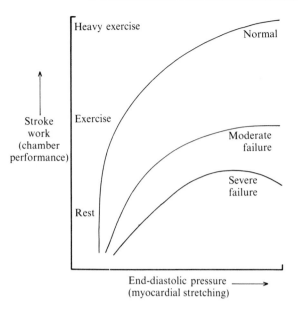

Fig. 16.4
Starling curves relating cardiac performance to circulatory load as indicated by the pressure of full ventricles.

Sudden and severe heart failure threatens the life of the whole body because the ability to maintain adequate perfusion of vital tissues is impaired. Decreased cardiac output, insufficient to maintain peripheral blood pressure, gives cardiogenic shock. Physiological priority is then given to the maintenance of flow to the brain and to the heart itself, calling on radical compensating mechanisms. The normally copious blood flow to the viscera, skin, and skeletal muscles will be shut down by extensive vasoconstriction, diverting flow to the brain and coronary circulation. The results of this include nausea and vomiting, and a cold, sweaty, blanched skin. Reduction of flow in the kidney reduces urine formation which will, if prolonged, give rise to kidney and liver damage. Total failure and cardiac arrest cause brain and body death if the circulation cannot be speedily restored.

Congestive Heart Failure

If failure affects the right side of the heart, the cardiac output falls because the left ventricle receives an insufficient supply. A similar effect will occur if the flow of blood through the lungs is obstructed. An unimpeded blood flow through the lungs is important because the entire blood volume must traverse them on each pass through the system. Should the failure be on the left side, pulmonary flow will be impeded and the right side of the heart will suffer congestion. Oxygenation of blood and

expiration of carbon dioxide will be affected, diminishing the quality of circulated blood. Respiratory distress may thus be an additional feature of heart failure.

When failure is gradual in onset or prolonged, longer-term consequences are added. The main feature will be a more radical redistribution of the blood and body fluid, accompanied by other compensating mechanisms. A useful compensation for incipient failure is cardiac hypertrophy, in which the surviving muscle fibres respond to a greater load by increasing in size and contractile ability. At the same time, the quantity of blood held by the ventricle increases (dilatation) which is helpful to a certain extent because the stretched fibres may contract more forcibly.

Further compensation may be required in the face of serious congestion of the circulation behind a failing ventricle. In all cases the systemic venous circulation will be affected (Fig. 16.5), causing congestion as a result of back-up of blood against the direction of normal flow. Increased pressure in the veins, extending back as far as the capillary networks, will act against the colloidal osmotic pressure of the plasma protein. Consequently, fluid cannot be held in the vessels and there is a net loss into the interstitial space (oedema, *see* Section 15.1), particularly of the lower extremities. This situation is worsened by the substantial increase in the body's sodium and water load resulting from kidney malfunction. As a result of low arterial blood pressure and compensatory vasoconstriction, kidney perfusion is maintained at a low rate. Glomerular filtration is thus decreased and the excretion of water and sodium reduced. This is an attempt to compensate for low blood volume but it also exacerbates the state of oedema. The overall situation is worsened by the activation of renin secretion, angiotensin production, and increased aldosterone secretion (*see* Section 6.6). The result is further sodium and water retention which adds to the increase in body water and the load on the failing heart.

16.1.2   VASCULAR PATHOLOGY

Introduction

In most instances, peripheral vascular disease results in decreased quantity or quality of blood flowing in a tissue. Consequent reduced oxygenation and nutrition will produce degenerative or necrotic effects (*see* Section 15.3), together with effects of inadequate waste removal and abnormalities in the fluid, electrolyte, or hormonal environment. Every organ and tissue is vulnerable and effects may be localised or widespread. Of the general consequences, the most important include atrophy, gan-

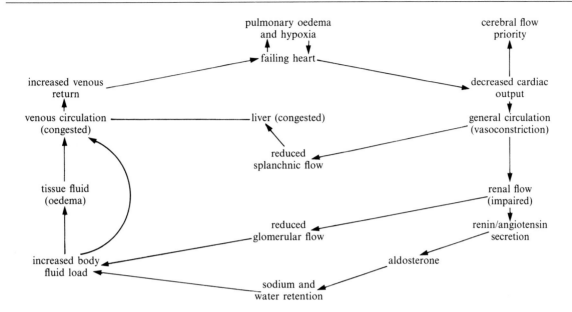

Fig. 16.5
Interrelated mechanisms operating in response to cardiac failure.

grene, swelling, oedema, intermittent claudication or other pain, paralysis, sensory loss, and autonomic disturbance. Any or all of these may occur (e.g. in an affected limb). The worst consequences, however, are those resulting from general vascular disease in which the function of the whole system may become disordered. In particular, increased resistance to flow may present an excessive load on cardiac function, leading to failure. Alternatively, serious malfunction may result from shock when circulatory pressure cannot be maintained. In this respect, it should be remembered that inflammation is essentially a vascular lesion, affecting both tone and permeability. Inflammation is involved in many disease processes and may occur on a widespread life-threatening scale, as well as being a localised effect. As this is considered in Section 15.4, the discussion here will be concerned with occlusion or wall-weakening damage.

Atherosclerosis

This condition may affect vessels throughout the system but is especially hazardous in the cerebral and coronary circulations. The complex development of atherosclerotic lesions starts with patches of thickening of the tunica intima (*see* Section 2.6) of affected arteries. This appears to be a proliferative process, resulting in excessive production of cells rich in lipid material, which are often visible as a thin, yellow, fatty streak. Further cell proliferation and more massive accumulation of lipid

produces the main form of the lesion, the atheroma (Fig. 16.6), a nodular structure with cell-breakdown at the centre. Within the coalescing lipid mass, crystals of cholesterol form. As the lesion enlarges, it encroaches upon the internal layer. Often, collagen fibres are deposited in a layer covering the luminal surface, originating in the inflammatory reaction which accompanies these changes.

An atherosclerotic plaque does not, by itself, cause arterial occlusion; in a properly pressurised vessel it protrudes outwards rather than into the lumen. However, other changes may lead to obstruction. One such effect results from erosion of the surface, the lesion rupturing so that the lipid mass escapes into the vessel. This material is viscous and capable of causing blockage (embolus) as it is forced into the narrower vessels. On the roughened fibrous surface of the atheroma, platelet attachment and fibrin clot formation frequently occur. The resulting thrombus protrudes into the lumen, obstructing flow at that point or detaching and causing blockage elsewhere, as another form of embolus. Finally, an old atheroma may become fibrosed and calcified; the plaque then becomes very hard and its extent may spread around the whole circumference of the vessel. Such calcification is generally a feature of ageing.

Thrombosis

During circulation, blood normally remains liquid as it is continually renewed and purified and is surrounded by

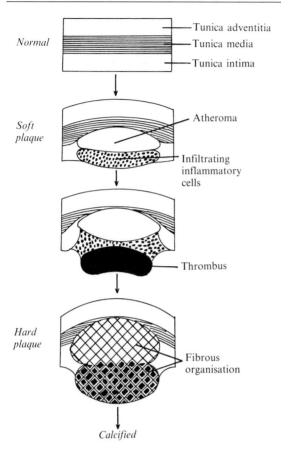

Normal — Tunica adventitia
— Tunica media
— Tunica intima

Soft plaque — Atheroma
— Infiltrating inflammatory cells

— Thrombus

Hard plaque — Fibrous organisation

Calcified

Fig. 16.6
Atherosclerosis developing in the inner layers of an artery.

healthy vascular tissue surfaces. When haemorrhage occurs or when the circulation fails after death, one or more of these requirements cease to apply and the blood commences to coagulate. Usually, the process occurs locally as a part of the process of haemostasis (*see also* Section 9.4). The blood flows through damaged tissues which interact with platelets and various plasma-borne factors to generate thromboplastins and start conversion of fibrinogen to fibrin. Such conditions also occur in inflammatory lesions, and in other circumstances in an apparently intact and active circulation. This is the process of thrombosis in which the sequence of reactions is the same as in coagulation but the nature of the thrombus differs from a haemorrhagic clot.

Coagulated blood consists of a mass of minute fibrin filaments enmeshing a residue of the original cellular and liquid components. Haemorrhagic clots of shed blood or in postmortem vessels are homogeneous, translucent, and gelatinous. A thrombus is not homogeneous; it develops in a flowing stream and consists of a number of layered components (Fig. 16.7). Firstly, a layer of platelets aggregates on the surface of the vascular endothelium. Clotting factors released from this mass cause the formation of fibrin. At the same time, further platelet aggregation may occur. The result is that a series of layers of fibrin and blood cells is superimposed on the basic platelet thrombus to give a complex (coralline) structure. As the growing thrombus ages, the trapped erythrocytes lose their haemoglobin and the thrombus turns a yellowish-grey. These layers protrude into the lumen, occluding the flow of blood with a growing barrier. Once the coralline thrombus impedes flow, further deposition of clotted material occurs (the occluding thrombus) which bears a closer resemblance to a homogeneous blood clot. When the vessel is completely blocked, stationary blood simply coagulates (the consecutive clot). Yet another stage may follow. When a consecutive clot extends as far as the junction with an actively flowing vessel it may attract platelet aggregation, forming the basis for another coralline thrombus. Thus, thrombosis and occlusion may extend along a series of vascular tributaries.

Portions of a protruding thrombus may break away to be carried onwards by the bloodstream and cause blockage, as an embolus, elsewhere. This may be particularly dangerous (e.g. in the case of large venous thrombi of the legs, when the whole mass detaches to cause an embolus in the pulmonary arterial bed). If not dislodged, a thrombus eventually becomes invaded by cells from the adjacent vascular wall. Endothelial cells grow over exposed surfaces and some thrombolytic activity may occur, resulting in the establishment of cell-lined cavities. Furthermore, endothelial growth may penetrate an occlusive thrombus, forming the route for growth of a new blood vessel. In time, such recanalisation may restore some blood perfusion. Alternatively, penetration of the thrombus by fibroblasts from the vessel wall leads to consolidation of the mass with collagen fibres. As in the case of atheroma, this may eventually become calcified. Fibrosis may also be beneficial in anchoring the thrombus more firmly.

Thrombosis is commonest in veins, probably because of lower pressures and rates of flow. When the condition is associated with reduced flow (e.g. in congestive heart failure, after pregnancy, after major surgery, or in bedridden patients), the thrombotic process is called phlebothrombosis. Lower-limb veins may be affected due to lack of muscular activity, external pressure, or incompetent valves. Phlebothrombosis is often clinically silent, particularly if it occurs in readily by-passed vessels. It may, however, block venous return sufficiently to cause tissue oedema or stasis ulcers.

Thrombosis in arteries is more commonly the result of

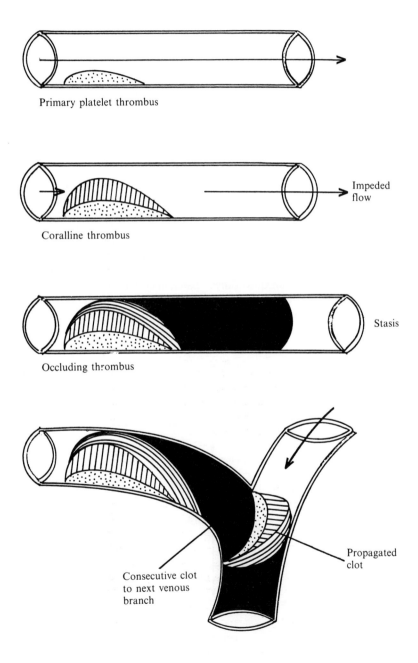

Primary platelet thrombus

Coralline thrombus

Impeded
flow

Occluding thrombus

Stasis

Consecutive clot
to next venous
branch

Propagated
clot

Fig. 16.7
Stages in the development of a thrombus.

inflammatory changes in the vascular endothelium (thrombophlebitis), and especially on atherosclerotic lesions. Other causes are infection, or vasculitis resulting from auto-immune or hypersensitive conditions. The process is essentially the same as in phlebothrombosis but the growth is usually less extensive as the blood flow is more rapid. Spasm of the affected vessel, ischaemia of supplied tissues, or severe pain may occur. The causative inflammation itself may be observable. Thrombosis is the ultimate cause of occlusion in most forms of vascular disease.

Systemic Hypertension

Abnormally increased resistance of peripheral arterioles due to vasoconstriction, but often superseded by other occlusive changes, gives rise to hypertension. This is pathological when maintained for prolonged periods and thus needs to be distinguished from temporary (pressor) effects caused by autonomic control mechanisms. As it is difficult to define precisely the limits of normal blood pressure, it is equally difficult to detect lower grades of hypertension. Furthermore, essential hypertension (the most prevalent form, accounting for 80% to 90% of all cases) is usually asymptomatic. The disease is diagnosed unequivocally only when it is progressive, severe, or causes obvious pathological effects. Initially, it is caused by persistent vasoconstriction which in theory is reversible, and

appropriate therapy is often successful. However, it appears that the normal blood pressure control is not operating effectively and later, more permanent constriction develops from structural changes in the vessel walls.

Essential hypertension may simply represent a functional error in pressure monitoring or reflex control mechanisms. Only in about 10% of cases is it possible to assign other, more definite, causes (secondary hypertension, Fig. 16.8). There is a particular association with occlusion of renal arteries, probably resulting in activation of the renin-angiotensin system (*see* Section 16.8); this produces the potent vasoconstricting polypeptide angiotensin and sodium- and water-retaining aldosterone (*see* Section 6.6). Other causes of vasoconstriction include adrenal gland malfunction, prostaglandin activation in vascular walls, and neurogenic overactivity.

In a minority of cases, hypertension progresses more severely with pressures becoming exceptionally high and with obvious adverse effects at an early stage. This is termed malignant hypertension, contrasting with the relatively benign aspects of the essential and secondary forms. All forms seem to have the initial vasoconstrictor effects but in malignant forms, this becomes severe. Later, in both benign and malignant conditions, distinct structural lesions develop in affected blood-vessel walls. In benign hypertension, deposits of abnormal material arise in the sub-endothelial layer of arterioles,

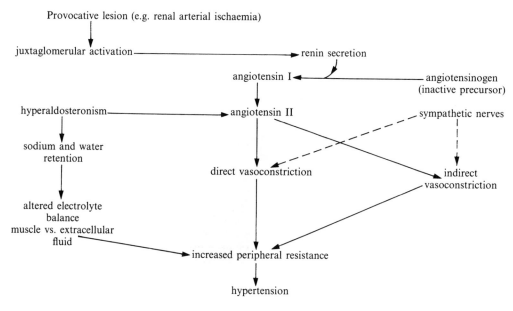

Fig. 16.8
Secondary mechanisms operating in hypertension.

spreading to replace the muscular and elastic components of the wall. As a result, the wall becomes much thicker and the lumen is constricted. These changes are arteriosclerosis, not to be confused with atherosclerosis. The deposits of arteriosclerosis are mainly of fibrin, leaked probably from plasma protein, with some lipid but no cholesterol (thus contrasting with the atheroma of atherosclerosis).

Structural damage ensues much earlier in vessels affected by malignant aetiology and may even be a part of the primary mechanism. Cells in the vessel walls undergo necrosis and the normal structure breaks down (arterionecrosis), to be replaced by fibrin-like deposits, again probably derived from exudation of plasma proteins. Once started, the process is progressive and the areas become further weakened. In between these areas, the lengths of arteriole are constricted producing an irregular 'bead on a string' appearance. Even in progressive lesions, some reparative activity takes place in the form of fibroblast-created fibrous scar tissue which may result in further occlusion. The tunica intima (*see* Section 2.6) becomes replaced by a series of concentric tubular layers of fibroblasts and collagen fibres to give 'onion-skin' thickening.

Essential and malignant hypertensive lesions are widely distributed along peripheral arterioles. Malignant necrosis extends even into capillaries. Blood vessels of the kidneys in particular, and also of the brain, pancreas, adrenal glands, and intestine, are markedly affected. Upstream, the occluded passage causes hypertension but downstream, the effects are ischaemic. Cerebral and renal necrosis are common long-term consequences. Heart failure in severe hypertension is attributed to the overwork against the excessive peripheral resistance. There is also an association between hypertension and atherosclerosis in coronary arteries, the consequent infarction exacerbating the risks of heart failure.

16.2 RESPIRATORY-TRACT DISEASES

Introduction

Although the passages, tubes, and cavities of the respiratory system penetrate deep within the head and body, the tissues are in direct contact with the atmosphere and, in effect, present an external surface. Thus there is an effective route of access for pathogens, toxic chemicals, and allergens. Medical statistics testify to the vulnerability of the tissues to their effects. What is more, the consequences of respiratory disease or the entry of disease via

the respiratory system may be catastrophic to the rest of the body, irrespective of whether they arise through blockage of the airways, neoplastic change, or the inhalation of toxic gases or vapours. Toxic effects are pronounced because materials are transported to cardiac muscle via the pulmonary and coronary circulations as well as being effectively distributed throughout the body. Furthermore, because the pulmonary circulation lies along the path between the right and left sides of the heart, it carries the entire blood volume during each pass through the circulatory system. Disease which impedes this flow may profoundly disturb cardiovascular functions; conversely, the lungs may be adversely affected by cardiac disorders. A further factor contributing to respiratory pathology is the connection between the respiratory and gastro-intestinal tracts. As a result, other harmful materials that the respiratory system may receive include food, drink, and regurgitated stomach contents.

Defence Mechanisms

Toxic, corrosive, irritant, or other harmful materials present in inspired air will be carried within the system. Some features serve to limit the access of these materials or to remove them from the system. Sensory nerves in the nostrils detect undesirable substances. Olfactory nerves detect many forms of impurity in the atmosphere, although an unpleasant odour does not necessarily correlate with damaging effect. More effective protection derives from sensory receptors of the trigeminal nerve, situated in the nasal passages. These detect irritants by producing stinging or painful sensations which reflexly momentarily suspend respiration. Sneezing and seromucous flow are also provoked to help expel offending agents. Irritants penetrating into lower airways also stimulate sensory reflexes, causing coughing to help the process of expectoration.

Toxic gases enter the same way as air and may pass into blood. Very soluble gases (e.g. sulphur dioxide) may dissolve in the liquid film on the surface of the respiratory tree so that effects are most prominent in the upper airways. Entry of airborne materials, dust, or liquid aerosols may be restricted by entrapment during flow through the nasal passages. Most smaller particles which may pass into the lower airways become deposited on the walls of the bronchi and bronchioles. As a result, deep lung tissues are protected from all but the smallest (mainly those less than one micron) particles. However, this may mean that upper airway surface exposure is correspondingly higher and may account for damage at particular locations (e.g. bronchitis and neoplastic change in bronchial mucosal tissues).

Most deposited material is removed by diffusion in solution or by adherence to the mucous layer secreted on airway surfaces. Tracheobronchial and nasopharyngeal mucus collects 99% of deposited particles, and 80% or more of lower-tract deposits are removed with the mucous sheet. Cilia on the surface cells of the airways act to propel the mucous sheet up and out of the tract (mucociliary escalator) to the pharynx from where it can be swallowed. Toxic or other adverse effects may impair movement of mucus so that it accumulates in the tract, although it may be removed by coughing and expectoration. Normal adult mucus production is about 100 mL per day but this may be markedly increased by irritant action. Clearance of material trapped in nasal passages is mainly by downward drainage of mucus.

Limited access and effective removal thus minimise chances of lung contamination. In the alveoli, populations of macrophage cells complete the process by phagocytosing particulate deposits. They digest or retain the material and much of it is transported in the cells to the mucociliary escalator or the lymphatic drainage channels. The clearance mechanisms are particularly important for the removal of infective material and normally the alveoli are maintained in a virtually sterile state. Impairment of defences or abnormally heavy contamination by pathogens or other noxious material may lead to serious disease.

Respiratory Infections

It is normal for the upper respiratory tract to be occupied by a varied population of micro-organisms in a commensal relationship with the host (*see* Section 15.5). A combination of physical barriers, immunosurveillance, and other defence mechanisms prevents invasion or spread. The terminal airways and alveoli, maintained free of micro-organisms, still possess similar defences. Nevertheless, if a virulent micro-organism is introduced into the non-pathogenic flora or the sterile spaces, infection may ensue. A reduction in defence mechanisms may allow infection from lower level contamination or from otherwise avirulent micro-organisms. In these circumstances the infection may even derive from the resident normal population.

The majority of upper respiratory-tract infections are of viral origin (Table 16.2). They arise from intracellular invasion and spread of virus on exposed surfaces or in the numerous cavities (e.g. the nasal sinuses). Inflammation and necrotic damage occur and the effects frequently predispose to secondary suppurative bacterial infections (e.g. sinusitis or otitis media). Bacterial growth is promoted by interference with drainage from the ear, sinuses, or other spaces as a result of virus-induced inflammation. In addition, viruses may decrease the normal oropharyngeal population of micro-organisms and activate epithelial-cell adherence sites to provide greater opportunity for colonisation by other bacteria. Further spread to bronchopulmonary structures may result from the aspiration of infected secretions draining from the nasopharynx.

Bacterial pharyngitis caused by Group A β-haemolytic streptococci is an infection worthy of particular note. These are virulent micro-organisms and further infection may develop in adjoining tissues (e.g. ear cavities or tonsils) or may spread via the bloodstream to distant tissues, which may lead to the inflammatory immunological lesions of rheumatic fever. Toxin-producing strains of Group A β-haemolytic streptococci may cause scarlet fever, which can be complicated by glomerulonephritis. Severe bacterial infections are relatively rare; viral infections predominate in the upper tract, as exemplified by the common cold. However, another normally commensal or self-limiting pharyngeal infection due to *Corynebacterium diphtheriae* may have virulent strains from which severe pharyngitis and diphtheria may develop. Colonisation and inflammation of the mucous membrane produces an adherent pseudomembrane of dead cells and coagulated secretions which threaten airway obstruction. Exotoxin-producing strains may cause distant organ damage (e.g. in heart or nerves).

Respiratory-tract infections (e.g. forms of pneumonia) have a life-threatening potential due to airway or al-

TABLE 16.2
Non-bacterial (usually primary) infections of the upper respiratory tract

Common cold	Oropharyngitis	Otitis media	Laryngitis
Rhinovirus	Rhinovirus	Respiratory syncytial virus	Respiratory syncytial virus
Coronavirus	Coronavirus	Adenovirus	Influenza virus
	Herpesvirus	Influenza virus	Parainfluenza virus
	Adenovirus	Parainfluenza virus	Adenovirus
	Coxsackie virus		
	Parainfluenza virus		
	Influenza virus		

veolar occlusion. Coccal, bacillary, and viral infections may cause inflammation of the alveolar parenchyma, resulting in the outpouring of fluid (plasma) and neutrophils from the blood vessels to fill the air spaces. As typifed by the primary pneumococcal form (lobar pneumonia), large volumes of the lung become consolidated by coagulated fibrin in the exudate, accompanied by blood-vessel engorgement. After several days, accumulated neutrophils commence the processes of liquefaction and ultimate reabsorption of the exudate, usually in conjunction with effective control of the infection. Cellular debris is phagocytosed, fluid drains away, and many alveoli become re-aerated whereby they recover their function. Thus, survivors from lung occlusion, septicaemia, and toxaemic effects may rapidly experience the resolution of the lesions.

An infection of major importance and located typically in the lungs is tuberculosis. Direct inhalation of *Mycobacteria* is the main cause, although entry may occur by other routes (e.g. gastro-intestinal) and infection may develop in many other tissues. The disease arises through competition between the generally resistant nature of the micro-organism and an often vigorous immune response. Following first exposure which usually occurs in childhood, micro-organisms may spread rapidly throughout the body unless resistance develops. Spread is usually restrained to the lymphatic system and this promotes immunity. In particular, cell-mediated immunity (*see* Section 15.6) develops through the action of T-cells against the bacilli. Subsequently, neutrophils and phagocytes (especially macrophages) are deployed in the infection sites. Macrophages accumulate in clusters or nodules (*see* Sections 15.4 *and* 15.5), and in tuberculosis are associated with an outer layer of lymphocytes to give the structure known as a tubercle. The infection becomes localised in these cells but because of the very resistant waxy coating on the micro-organisms, many may survive within the macrophages for long periods.

If the micro-organisms are eliminated from an actively immune host, the lesion may resolve without further damage. If they are not eliminated, the tubercle grows and acquires a central mass of coagulated necrotic cells (caseation). A layer of granulation tissue divides infected from normal tissue. However, in early disease, infected macrophages may escape or, at a later stage, a caseated tubercle may liquefy (cold abscess) and discharge infection via a sinus or ulcer to an exposed surface (*see* Section 15.5). Thus, lesions may become extensive and destructive and erode, compress, or obstruct vital structures. Ultimately severe scarring may result and scars may calcify.

Broncho-occlusive Disease

Acute infection or exposure to irritant or toxic agents may cause damage to the mucosa and submucosa of airways (laryngitis, tracheitis, bronchitis, or broncho-pneumonia). Epithelial cells degenerate or necrose and connective and vascular tissues become inflamed. An irritating raw sensation results which may provoke cough. Initially such a cough is unproductive but later, mucus is produced. Damage may occur as acute episodes, but long-standing inflammation, particularly bronchial, is common. In chronic bronchitis, permanent alteration to the epithelial surfaces may be accompanied by underlying tissue abnormality. The main change is striking hyperplasia (*see* Section 15.7) of mucous glands, covering up to two-thirds of the airway wall. This gives rise to copious, often very viscous, mucus which becomes purulent when infected. Bronchial wall damage may involve breakdown of cartilage and gives rise to dilatation and distortion. Irregular convolutions in the surface and saccular or cylindrical enlargements of the airway characterise bronchiectasis, and these cavities frequently become sites for more persistent infection.

It is thought that in many cases the airway obstruction in chronic bronchitis may be attributed to an allergic component, especially when infection is also present. Hypersensitivity may exacerbate the inflammation affecting the upper tract and may extend to the bronchioles. In these lower passages, an additional feature is the constriction of the lumen by contraction of the smooth muscle bands or sheets in the surrounding tissues. This bronchoconstriction is similar to that produced by inhaled allergens in persons suffering from type I hypersensitivity (*see* Section 15.6). Consequent reactions cause occlusion of the bronchioles, inflammatory swelling of the submucosa, and formation of tenacious mucous plugs which characterise extrinsic asthma (Table 16.3).

Emphysema is often associated with chronic bronchitis and is characterised by abnormal distension of alveoli, alveolar ducts, and terminal airways with breakdown of wall structures to produce cavities. These destructive changes can mainly be attributed to the abnormal pressures and hyperinflation resulting from occlusion of the proximal airways. Gas-exchange surfaces are reduced, ventilation across the alveoli is poor, and the pulmonary vascular network may be greatly reduced. This combination causes dyspnoea (the 'pink-puffer' condition) and has a worse effect on the patient's condition than the associated broncho-occlusive disease.

Pulmonary Fibrosis

Prolonged inhalation and deposition of the dust created by industrial activities can lead to the accumulation of

TABLE 16.3
Asthmatic or broncho-occlusive conditions affecting primarily bronchioles and caused by smooth-muscle bronchoconstriction and inflammation

Extrinsic (allergic or atopic) asthma

> Demonstrable allergy (type I hypersensitivity to inhaled allergenic/antigenic material), especially in atopic individuals, usually commencing in childhood.

Intrinsic (non-allergic or non-atopic) asthma

> No demonstrable allergy and unrelated to family histories of eczema or allergy. Attributed to changed tissue reactivity and in particular changes in autonomic nervous system control of muscle contractility, although it may have a psychosomatic component. Usually older adult onset.

Irritant asthma and exercise asthma

> Dyspnoeic effects of inhaled irritant material, often associated with an acquired hyperreactivity or irritant intolerance (e.g. to tobacco smoke or cold air). May have associations with intrinsic asthma.

Vasomotor rhinitis

> Inflammatory condition of upper respiratory tract characterised by episodic nasal congestion, copious secretion, and repetitive sneezing. Frequently associated with intrinsic asthma or irritant intolerance.

Cardiac asthma

> Bronchoconstriction (possible reflex) associated with left ventricular failure.

Status asthmaticus

> Severe, life-threatening, acute attack involving marked airway occlusion.

toxic materials in the lungs (pneumoconiosis). The action of particle-trapping and clearing mechanisms ensures that total quantities retained are small although local concentrations may be high. Certain dust deposits give rise to progressive fibrosis (collagen-fibre deposition) of the lung parenchyma, resulting in the loss of alveolar structure and adverse changes in its mechanical properties (e.g. decreased compliance). The main offending material is silica, a major component of many mineral dusts, which is especially damaging in the form of freshly-shattered crystalline particles. In silicosis, collagen fibres form concentric layers or nodular masses around the particle aggregates. In coal-dust pneumoconiosis, fibrosis occurs around particles deposited in terminal bronchioles provoked by the silica from the rock and not the coal itself. Asbestos fibres produce another characteristic form of fibrosis, and may also cause the neoplastic disease, mesothelioma.

Pulmonary fibrosis may also result from immune-system reactivity (type III hypersensitivity, *see* Section 15.6) activated in the alveolar interstitial tissue. Acute inflammatory damage (alveolitis or pneumonitis) and progressive and destructive collagen-fibre formation will result. Such effects are caused by numerous materials which usually take the form of very small organic particles gaining access into alveoli. Typical examples include mould spores (e.g. farmer's lung caused by

spores from mouldy hay), minute protein fragments, or industrial dusts (e.g. hard metal disease caused by allergy to the cobalt in inhaled dust from metal-grinding). The resultant fibrosis is a long-term change causing persistent respiratory difficulty which is often severely disabling.

Neoplastic Lesions

Primary tumours of the respiratory tract are among the most common examples of neoplastic disease, probably resulting mainly from contact with airborne carcinogenic pollutants. However the lungs also provide a common site for bloodborne metastatic tumours. This does not necessarily imply that the lungs filter the clumps of malignant cells arriving in venous blood but that they provide a suitable site for secondary development of tumours. Sarcomas are more prevalent than carcinomas as secondary growths in the lung.

Primary tumours of airways or lungs commonly occur in the epithelia and are thus carcinomas. Benign tumours are rare or, as in the case of bronchial adenoma, likely to progress to malignancy. Three types of carcinoma occur in the bronchi: the very variably differentiated epidermoid (squamous) carcinoma and two undifferentiated forms (small (oat) cell carcinoma and adenocarcinoma). Of the latter, the most important is the small (oat) cell carcinoma which develops as sheets or clumps of small cells and may secrete neuroendocrine hormones. Adenocarcinomas are more differentiated and develop deeper in the lungs. They usually retain glandular characteristics and accummulate masses of secreted mucus.

Lung carcinomas usually spread locally along airways or blood vessels and into alveolar spaces. Further direct spread along lymphatic vessels takes the neoplasm to lymph nodes of the lung-hilum, the pleura, and mediastinum. Metastases may form in cervical and axillar nodes. Direct invasion may extend the tumour in sheets beneath the pleural and pericardial membranes, leading to penetration of the heart and blood vessels. Bloodborne metastases occur in many cases, generating wide and complex spread to liver, brain, or bones. No organ is exempt and the ultimate consequences are severe.

16.3 GASTRO-ENTEROLOGY

Introduction

Through its direct connections with the external environment at two orifices, the gastro-intestinal tract constitutes a route of access to the rest of the body for disease-inducing agents (e.g. toxic materials and infectious pathogens). Disease of the tract itself may be the cause of considerable discomfort and harmful consequences (e.g. through ulceration or haemorrhage). Furthermore, impairment of function due to disease may severely affect general health, notably through malnutrition and affected excretion. Disorder may also result from abnormalities of surrounding tissues (e.g. compression of the oesophagus or rectum). Disease may also affect associated organs (e.g. the liver or pancreas).

Traumatic and Inflammatory Conditions

The tract in general, and in particular its upper regions, is vulnerable to physical injury caused by the entry of harmful materials or by direct damage. Swallowed foreign bodies (e.g. coins) may cause blockage; more seriously, other objects (e.g. fish bones or splinters) may cause penetration or tears in the walls. The escape of food, drink, saliva, or stomach contents into surrounding spaces may cause dangerous complications. Severe upper-tract injury may also result from ingestion of corrosive or toxic materials (e.g. strong acids or alkaline solutions). In addition to the immediate dangers, such injuries may produce fibrous scarring in or around the tubes, narrowing the lumen (stricture or stenosis), and obstructing the passage of food.

The oesophagus may be damaged by corrosive material in the reverse direction by reflux of gastric contents. The lower portion is usually affected, becoming inflamed through erosion of the mucosa (oesophagitis) followed by deeper ulceration and eventually scarring. The usual cause is hiatus hernia which is caused by enlargement of the space in the diaphragm through which the oesophagus passes. As a consequence, upward displacement of a portion of the stomach impairs efficiency of the gastro-oesophageal sphincter and results in the backflow of gastric contents. More than 50% of elderly people may suffer from hiatus herniation to some degree, although severe oesophagitis is rarer. Hiatus hernia and gastric reflux cause epigastric discomfort and pain (heartburn).

Irritants primarily affect the stomach although lower regions of the gastro-intestinal tract may not escape damage. The stomach may be severely affected by corrosive or toxic agents despite the protection afforded by copious mucous secretions. Less severe irritants may cause mucosal inflammation (gastritis), dyspepsia, or nausea and vomiting. Acute gastritis may be caused by food poisoning (e.g. staphylococcal gastro-enteritis), excessive alcohol intake, or drugs (e.g. salicylates and iron salts). The acute form seldom lasts more than 48 hours and features congestion of the mucosa and patches of haemorrhage but usually no deep glandular erosion. This contrasts with the more destructive, persistent chronic gastritis, which may present in two forms. In the less severe form, inflammation is prominent in association with mucosal atrophy; more severe pathology is characterised by loss of the mucosal peptic and parietal glandular cells and is less obviously due to inflammation. Chronic atrophy may be caused by an auto-immune mechanism associated with gastric auto-antibody. The resultant achlorhydria and lack of intrinsic factor can cause megaloblastic anaemia.

Ulcerative Lesions

The exposure of the intestinal mucosa to potentially destructive secretions and other damaging agents renders it liable to surface damage in most areas. Such damage may cause substantial loss of mucosal cells by atrophic processes, or take the form of erosion with penetration into underlying tissues (ulcers). Peptic ulceration is the most common and important form, with 1 in 10 of the population suffering at least one ulcer in a lifetime. The term peptic ulceration applies to the condition in any area of the tract exposed to gastric secretions. Thus, peptic ulceration may affect the stomach, duodenum, or even further down the tract, depending upon the reach of gastric secretions. Ulcers never occur in the absence of gastric acid and enzyme secretions and almost certainly depend upon this digestive combination. Ulcerative erosions initially affect mucosal tissues and progress deeper into submucosal connective tissue and muscle layers. In health, there is protection of the mucosa by the secretion of a mucous layer, regeneration of surface cells to replace those eroded, and a mechanism to prevent the diffusion of hydrogen ions back into the epithelium. Ulceration probably requires ineffectiveness of more than one of the above factors, plus alterations in the secretion of acid and digestive enzymes.

Inflammation generally precedes or accompanies ulceration but irritancy is not necessarily a primary cause. Drugs (e.g. corticosteroids, non-steroidal anti-inflammatory drugs, alpha-adrenoceptor blocking drugs, and cytotoxic drugs) have been linked to the development of peptic ulceration. Duodenal ulceration is now the more common form in the developed countries of Europe and North America, whereas gastric ulceration predominates in south-east Asia. Other aetiological factors are complex and imprecisely understood (e.g. mental stress appears to be contributory). Factors (e.g. drugs and stress) which exacerbate established peptic ulceration may cause deeper penetration which results in severe haemorrhage or perforation of the wall.

Ulceration in the lower regions of the gastro-intestinal tract may also have variable locations. Ulcerative colitis in fact usually arises in the rectum (strictly proctitis). However, most cases migrate to the colon and as many as 50% become 'universal' or 'total' colitis (i.e. involving the whole colon). Tissues of the mucosal and submucosal layers suffer vigorous inflammation and cellular infiltration (e.g. by immune-function cells including lymphocytes and plasma-cells). Accumulation of neutrophils (see Section 15.4) forms pus-filled cavities (crypt abscesses) leading to the breakdown and ulceration of the mucosa. Ulceration may progress from shallow lesions to deeper erosions which may ultimately perforate. Large areas may become ulcerated, although the disease may fluctuate and areas may be repaired by mucosal regeneration or fibrous scarring. Ulcerated and repaired surfaces may gradually become very ragged. The cause of ulcerative colitis is suspected to be auto-immunity and not infections. The condition is not painful although symptoms include bleeding diarrhoea, constipation, and abdominal cramps. Systemic illness is a feature especially of severe episodes; mental distress may also occur, although it is unclear whether this is cause or effect.

Crohn's disease is a similar condition to ulcerative colitis but is more variable in location. It can occur anywhere between the mouth and the anus, although the terminal ileum is involved in 80% of cases. The lesions are destructively inflammatory but involve accumulations of monocyte cells rather than polymorphonuclear neutrophils. Thus, granulomas are formed (see Section 15.5) rather than the pus of colitis. The character of the ulcers also differs. They cause deep fissuring of the mucosa and underlying structures. In contrast to perforations opening into the peritoneal cavity, the lesions of Crohn's disease produce penetrations connecting with other structures (e.g. fistulas) opening into the bladder or through the abdominal wall. The occurrence of immune cells in the lesions and the association with other severe inflammatory diseases (e.g. rheumatoid arthritis and ankylosing spondylitis) suggest auto-immune aetiology. No causative pathogens have been identified. In common with other immune reactions, general malaise, fever, rash, and growth retardation occur. Pain, diarrhoea, protein loss, anaemia, and vitamin B_{12} deficiency result from the intestinal damage.

Atrophy of the mucosa associated with immunopathology is the main characteristic of coeliac disease. This is less inflammatory in nature than the ulcerative conditions described above and is restricted to mucosal structural loss. Atrophic changes affect the jejunum and often the ileum, with total loss of the villi in advanced cases. These changes result from a dietary intolerance to gluten, the protein of wheat or rye flour. The presence of monocytes and plasma cells in affected mucosal tissues and antibodies to gluten in the plasma suggested a hypersensitive mechanism. However, immune activity appears to be impaired and it is suggested that the changes may be due to lack of a protective function of immunogobulin A. The result of mucosal deterioration is malabsorption of carbohydrates, fats, proteins, and vitamins, leading to malnutrition. The production of steatorrhoea is a typical sign.

Tropical sprue is not connected with gluten but results in similar mucosal atrophy, and is characterised by steatorrhoea or diarrhoea, and malabsorption. The major consequences are due to folic-acid deficiency. This disease is endemic in some sub-equatorial regions and probably results from infection or parasitic infestation.

Infections

The stomach, duodenum, jejunum, and ileum (see Section 1.10) are relatively free of micro-organisms. In contrast, micro-organisms can enter the gastro-intestinal tract through the orifices at both ends and they contaminate and constitute resident populations in the remaining portions of the tract. This is a 'normal' state and generally micro-organisms do not harm the host; in some cases there are mutually beneficial interactions.

Although entry is readily gained, many micro-organisms fail to colonise the buccal and pharyngeal cavities. These spaces are effectively flushed with saliva, well oxygenated and inhibitory to anaerobes, and subject to repeated changes in physical conditions (e.g. temperature and pH). Potential surfaces for microbial growth are scoured by tongue action, movements of lips and cheeks, and swallowing actions. There are also antibacterial substances in saliva. Microbial contamination of the mouth depends mainly on the presence and condition of teeth. Teeth provide surfaces to which microbes may attach and cavities for refuge. With tooth development in the child a permanent microflora becomes established.

Other microbes which enter the mouth and pass into the oesophagus find the protective epithelium normally unsuitable for colonisation. The stomach cavity is usually sterile due to the low pH, and gastric juice plus bile ensure the almost total sterility of the duodenum. Small populations of Gram-positive bacilli and cocci, lactobacilli, and diphtheroid micro-organisms are found in the jejunum. Bacterial species increase in the ileum but by far the major ileal micro-organism is *Candida albicans*. Massive populations of large numbers of different species occupy the colon and caecum and most of these micro-organisms are anaerobes. The rectum is contaminated but the micro-organisms are mostly transient. Even the main populations of the large bowel are normally commensal provided that their location is restricted to the lumen of the tract.

The presence of a permanent microbial growth (often streptococci initially) on teeth facilitates growth of more anaerobic micro-organisms. Colonies of these residents accumulate on tooth surfaces as the tenacious material, plaque. Acidic materials are produced by these growths and exert an insidious erosive action on enamel and dentine, which may penetrate into the pulp or deeper tissues (dental caries). Further extension of infection may cause abscesses, gingivitis, and other periodontal disease.

Alterations or replacement of the commensal populations of the tract give rise to the growth of pathogens. These may cause gastro-intestinal disease by growth in the tissues or by toxin secretion. The consequences of these are generally identified as gastro-enteritis. A variety of bacterial infections are associated with this condition but it is apparent that viral infections (e.g. parvovirus or rotavirus) explain many cases, especially in localised outbreaks. Infections usually produce mucosal inflammation (but rarely necrosis or ulceration), which results in diarrhoea and vomiting. Abdominal discomfort or pain is associated with general malaise and fever. Severe consequences are usually attributable to fluid loss which could result in dehydration, depletion of electrolytes, and metabolic acidosis. These may produce cardiovascular or neurological disorders which are especially dangerous in young children or in debilitated adults.

Effects similar to those described above may arise, not from microbial growth in the tract, but from the ingestion of an exotoxin formed by micro-organisms growing in foodstuff. Such food poisoning (e.g. by *Salmonella, Staphylococcus, Campylobacter*, or *Clostridium* spp.) takes the form of gastro-enteritis which rapidly follows the absorption of the preformed toxin but is of limited duration due to its ultimate dilution and elimination. Severity of the effects is in proportion to the toxin dose.

In more severe gastro-intestinal infections, diarrhoea becomes especially pronounced with the discharge of profuse watery stools. Toxins from strains of *Escherichia coli* or *Vibrio cholerae* are typical, the former accounting for 50% of the common acute diarrhoeas of hot countries and the latter for widespread outbreaks of cholera. The major effects are due to water loss rather than inflammatory or necrotic tissue damage. The enterotoxin reverses normal pathways of fluid and electrolyte flow in the intestinal vascular supply, resulting in fluid loss into the lumen.

Dysentery produces even more severe diarrhoea associated with inflammation and ulceration of the large bowel. Blood, pus, and mucus are added to the considerable fluid loss. In bacillary dysentery, *Shigella* spp. infect the large intestine, causing tissue destruction which may extend into the deeper layers of submucosa and muscle. Fibrotic scarring and stenosis may result. Intestinal damage also occurs in the more virulent salmonellal infections (particularly by *Salmonella typhi* or *S. paratyphi*) which cause enteric fever. Classical typhoid fever initially presents with systemic, not gastro-intestinal, symptoms following spread of infection from the tract to lymphatic tissues and blood. However, extension of the infection through intestinal lymphoid tissues and walls results in necrosis, ulceration, mucosal sloughing, haemorrhage, penetration, and peritonitis; thus virulent diarrhoea accompanies severe systemic illness.

Certain disease states derive from the microbial population which normally occupies the large bowel. Appendicitis results from the invasion of the mucosa of the appendix by micro-organisms changed in virulence or escaping due to defects in defence. The inflammatory lesions are accompanied by suppuration due to leucocyte accumulation and necrosis, resulting in perforation. Severe acute infection may develop into chronic appendicitis, resulting in fibrosis, structural defects (e.g. diverticulum formation), and persistent foci of infection.

Perforation of an infected appendix, puncture of the large intestine, or infection from any other abdominal site may spread through the peritoneal cavities and result in inflammation of membranes and suppuration (peritonitis). The cavity fills with pus and fibrin-containing inflammatory exudate. Long-term consequences are fibrous adhesions compacting intestinal folds and possibly stricture or obstruction. Abdominal abscesses may cause severe damage and be intractable.

Gastro-intestinal Neoplasia

Incidence of neoplasms in the small intestine and at the anus is low, but high in other areas of the gastro-intestinal tract. Colorectal cancer is very common in western countries; cancer of the stomach has a high incidence in the West and Japan. Some tumours are unusual (e.g. carcinoid or argentaffinoma of the appendix, ileum, and rectum, which secrete serotonin) or have special geographical distributions (e.g. oesophageal cancer in the Middle East).

Cancer of the stomach is probably largely attributable to the presence of carcinogenic substances in food or drink. There is also strong association with chronic gastric inflammation which frequently arises adjacent to ulcer scars. Benign growths (adenoma or papilloma) may arise but malignant change usually supervenes. Incidence of tumours is highest in the pylorus region, and cells from this area often retain their mucus-secreting ability (mucoid adenocarcinomas). Otherwise, gastric tumours display a variety of forms which, when accompanied by variations in cell differentiation, often give multiple features in the same tumour. Adenocarcinomas usually occur as solid tumours projecting into the stomach cavity, but other secretory forms (e.g. signet ring and spheroidal cell types) are more diffuse and invasive. Many others are poorly differentiated and associated with highly malignant characteristics. Such tumours show little or no glandular development, are soft, and frequently ulcerated or haemorrhagic. The malignant growths spread throughout the stomach and invade adjacent and remote organs. Extensive permeation of the lymphatic channels occurs from metastases which pass via the thoracic duct into the bloodstream. Spread to liver, lungs, and bones is common.

Neoplastic polyps grow in the colon and rectum as stalked lumps or finger-like projections. Initially, the growth may be confined to the mucosa and is regarded as benign, but the true state may be pre-malignant. Commonly the neoplasms break through into deeper wall structures and behave as carcinomas. They develop further as polyps or ulcers and frequently stenose or obstruct the lumen. Initial spread may be localised or limited to regional lymph nodes, and this indicates why 5-year survival rates are better than those for gastric carcinoma.

16.4   THE LIVER

Introduction

As with other organs or systems, the liver has special features which determine its relative susceptibility to pathological processes, including some very effective means for countering disease or damage. As it is remote from direct contact with the exterior, it has some degree of inaccessibility to infection or parasites unless they are bloodborne. At the same time, it is especially subject to toxic damage and this is probably the main cause of its pathology. About 80% of the hepatic blood derives from the portal supply which drains from the absorptive sections of the gastro-intestinal tract. Thus toxic substances ingested and absorbed into the blood will be carried directly to the liver in relatively high concentrations. Metabolic transformations in the liver may convert some of these compounds into even more toxic forms (first-pass effect), particularly through the action of the mixed-function oxidase system (see Section 15.2). Alternatively metabolism may result in detoxification. Toxic materials entering the general circulation and body fluids will reach other target tissues in much lower concentrations. At the same time, liver cells provide internal protective physiological buffer mechanisms against toxic effects (e.g. the glutathione/glutathione-transferase system and the availability of antioxidant substances), although such protection may be exceeded by high dosage of toxic material. Prolonged exposure may result in adaptive changes to give increased production of metabolising enzymes, protecting agents, or both.

The liver is adversely affected by other organ or system malfunctions, especially in cardiovascular and endocrine pathology. Because of its large functional demands for nutrient and oxygen supplies, the liver is susceptible to injury by impaired blood flow. The microstructural organisation of cells in the lobules of the liver (see Section 1.10) provides a special example of zonal vulnerability. Damage from toxic effects and defective blood supply or oxygenation affects the cells in the centre of lobules more than those at the periphery. The liver's special dual blood supply ensures that it receives well oxygenated arterial blood as well as the venous portal supply. It nevertheless suffers deprivation if either supply should be impaired (e.g. following heart failure, *see* Section 16.1, or if venous drainage is blocked). The liver is a richly vascular organ which transports a quarter of the normal cardiac output at one time. However, most of this reaches the liver at a low pressure and flow is easily impeded. Additionally, its flow characteristics and strategic location in the cardiovascular system render the liver liable to the secondary growth of malignant tissues (e.g. bloodborne metastases and spreading lymphoreticular malignancies).

The liver has functional versatility as exemplified by its metabolic, storage, secretory, and synthetic activities (Table 16.4). Any substantial impairment of liver functions may have severe consequences for the rest of the body. However, there are some important features of liver function which effectively reduce the incidence of severe disease or minimise the consequences. The versatility of the organ is both a weakness and a strength. Even following substantial tissue loss, the residual cellular mass can carry out almost all functions. Additionally, there is massive excess functional capacity of up to 8 times the quantity of tissue needed for normal function. If required, this cellular mass can be further increased by adaptive hyperplasia and hypertrophy (*see* Section 15.7). Importantly, the liver has greater capacity than most other tissues to replace damaged with normal

functional cells. The activities of individual cells may be enhanced in response to provocation.

Degenerative and Necrotic Damage

Within the liver, blood vessel tributaries deliver blood from the portal vein (1200 mL/min) and the hepatic artery (300 mL/min) to the peripheries of all of the functional lobules (*see* Section 1.10). Arterial and venous blood mingles as it percolates through the sinusoidal spaces between the plates of cells, draining inwards. The cells at the lobular peripheries (zone 1) thus receive the best oxygenated blood and richest nutrient. These supplies are depleted by absorption into the tissue as blood passes to the centre of the lobule (zone 3), but in health the central cells still receive adequate supplies. Should the flow become inadequate (e.g. in ischaemia) the innermost cells become deprived and sustain major damage. Thus, hypoxia gives rise to centrilobular zones of cells suffering from hydropic degeneration or necrosis (*see* Section 15.3). Damaged areas may be surrounded by intermediate zones of less severe damage often showing fatty change. This pattern is typical of damage from reduced blood flow for almost any reason (e.g. systemic shock, pulmonary embolism, prolonged surgery, sepsis,

TABLE 16.4
Functional consequences of severe hepatic damage with cirrhosis

Metabolic functions

    Decreased

- glycogen storage and glucose tolerance
- protein synthesis, including plasma albumin and coagulation enzymes
- metabolism and conjugation of waste products, drugs, and xenobiotic chemicals
- vitamin storage
- bilirubin excretion (causing jaundice)
- urea formation (causing accumulation of ammonia in blood)

    Increased

- serum enzyme levels (e.g. aminotransferases, lactate, and sorbitol dehydrogenases)
- gammaglobulin levels

    Systemic consequences

- anaemia, oedema, personality disorders, and coma

Endocrine malfunctions

- secondary hyperaldosteronism causes sodium and water retention, ascites, and oedema
- hyperoestrogenism (due to altered sex hormone metabolism) causes reversion of secondary sexual characteristics in males (e.g. testicular atrophy, gynaecomastia, fat redistribution, and hair redistribution or alopecia)

Cardiovascular malfunctions

- portal hypertension and mesenteric congestion cause oedema, ascites, oesophageal varices, and haemorrhages
- splenomegaly
- bone-marrow malfunction, anaemia, thrombocytopenia, and leucopenia
- impaired haemostasis

severe trauma, and myocardial infarction). It may also occur from general lack of oxygen in the blood or severe anaemia.

In congestive heart failure, pooling of blood in the veins causes back-pressure which especially impedes flow from the liver. Venous congestion extends as far as the centrilobular veins, and may cause tissue disruption and local haemorrhage in the lobules. Subsequent local necrosis extends away from central zones and may merge from one lobule to another (bridging necrosis). The whole of the liver may be affected and become swollen and tender. In contrast, localised obstruction may result from thrombosis of arterial branches which results in much more limited patches of ischaemic infarct.

A comparable pattern of degeneration and necrosis develops as result of many forms of toxic action. Again, zone 3 is mainly affected, giving centrilobular necrosis, lesser degeneration of the mid-zone, and little peripheral effect. The relatively poor oxygenation and nutrient supply to centrilobular cells may render them more vulnerable, particularly as these cells are mature and have higher functional energy demands. Toxic compounds affecting energy-producing mechanisms may particularly act in this way. The other determining mechanism is the requirement for preliminary metabolic activation to a more potent derivative (e.g. by the mixed-function oxidase system). Many materials (e.g. chlorinated hydrocarbon solvents) are converted into active radicals, epoxides, other oxidised or reduced products, superoxide, or hydroxyl free-radicals (see Section 15.2). These products may damage intracellular organelles or their associated vital mechanisms. The reason that such toxicity causes centrilobular lesions is that metabolic enzymes (e.g. mixed-function oxidases, cytochrome P450, and NADPH co-enzyme) are strategically located in the affected cells of zone 3.

Where damage is not centrilobular, it may depend upon other mechanisms (e.g. allyl formate and allyl alcohol cause necrosis in zone 1 cells, probably determined by location of alcohol dehydrogenase enzyme in these cells). Other toxic agents, and in particular those which cause fatty change rather than hydropic degeneration (e.g. ethionine or yellow phosphorus), may affect the whole lobule. Beryllium affects mid-zonal cells.

Ethanol is the cause of much hepatic damage but is not as such a substance foreign to the body. It may be formed in the liver itself from pyruvate or acetaldehyde, or in larger quantities in the intestine by microbial fermentation. Normally, it is rapidly and entirely converted to useful active-acetate, but excessive quantities cause toxic effects. The main toxic action is fatty degeneration (steatosis). This must be distinguished from the hydropic-necrotic effect of most other hepatotoxicants, although

lesions of both are centrilobular. Fatty degeneration is fully reversible but in more severe or chronic cases other forms of damage develop. Unlike steatosis, alcoholic hepatitis is less clearly dose-related, but is usually associated with a high intake (80 g daily) for at least five years. Steatosis, unlike hepatitis, does not appear to be dependent upon nutritional deficiency. Hepatitis involves mitochondrial and endoplasmic damage, swelling, formation of vacuoles and hyaline Mallory bodies, and polymorphonuclear infiltration. Distribution is initially centrilobular, but it may extend throughout lobules leading to centre-to-centre bridging into adjacent structures. Characteristically, pericellular fibrosis (collagen fibre deposition) occurs and spreads, which, in conjunction with bridging lesions, leads to cirrhosis.

Repair and Scarring in the Liver: Cirrhosis

When the period of cell destruction is short-lived and the extent of damage limited, substantial replacement by re-growth of normal functional cells can be achieved. The centrilobular location of lesions is important because proliferation of new cells usually occurs from the immature cells at lobular peripheries. Additionally, the framework of reticulin fibres necessary for the support of liver cells should be intact. Regenerating cells grow into the vacated spaces. Prolonged toxic influence can prevent cell production and recolonisation, and severe effects lead to tissue disruption, which prevents orderly regeneration. Instead, fibrous scarring becomes predominant as fibroblasts are much less susceptible to toxic or anoxic damage and replace damaged hepatocytes. Eventually numerous fibroblasts occupy damaged lobules, replacing the structures with strands of collagen fibres. Thus specialised liver tissue is progressively replaced and functional capacity is lost. Small groups of viable hepatocytes may remain isolated in the fibrous meshes and develop to form regeneration nodules, but this achieves only partial restoration of function. Over a period of several years, substantial permanent damage (cirrhosis) may be created. Chronic alcohol poisoning is a common cause.

Fibroblasts originate from connective tissue around the blood vessels of interlobular structures and the most extensive fibrous development occurs in these locations. In common with scar tissue elsewhere in the body, the fibres eventually contract and enclosed blood vessels become increasingly constricted. This initially impedes the low-pressure portal blood flow and, later, arterial supplies to liver tissue. Thus, perfusion of the portal vein blood through the surviving functional liver tissue progressively worsens. Metabolism, especially of ingested compounds, will be badly affected and therapeutic and toxic effects may be markedly and unpredictably altered (e.g. a normal dose of morphine may cause deep coma or death in a cirrhotic patient).

Another serious consequence is the loss of normal vascular supply through the lobules. With the destruction of the plates of hepatocytes, the narrow sinusoidal channels become wider and connect incoming and outgoing blood vessels. Blood will travel along the path of least resistance and therefore proceeds through the cavities, often at the expense of flow through relatively normal tissue. Thus, blood may pass through the liver without effective contact with hepatic cells. These cavities progressively become lined with fibrous tissue, creating permanent channels (shunts).

Infections in the Liver

Various patterns of damage may be caused by the growth or residence of pathogens in liver tissue. Most forms involve some degree of necrosis and the more severe or prolonged infections may cause typical lesions (e.g. abscesses or granulomas, see Section 15.5). Necrotic damage may give rise to cirrhotic changes.

Bacterial infections may cause liver damage through the action of toxins (e.g. the widespread necrotic focal lesions of typhoid fever or diphtheria). Infective microorganisms may initially be bloodborne or spread from elsewhere in the abdomen. When there is local tissue growth, the damage is mainly due to the activities of leucocytes which accumulate in response to immune influences and form pyogenic abscesses (see Section 15.4). In acute infections, little scarring results from these lesions which are rarely more than a few centimetres in diameter. More prolonged cases cause extensive fibrous scarring. Major problems are the spread of infection to the liver along biliary tracts or blockage of bile flow by pus. Granulomas are typical of chronic bacterial infections (see Section 15.5). Ineffectively controlled typhoid, syphilis, malaria, or tuberculosis cause these nodular lesions. Similar varieties of lesions can be caused by other pathogens (e.g. protozoal and fungal infections which are more common in tropical or underdeveloped countries). Amoebic abscesses affect the liver as a later development of common primary gastro-intestinal infections and the cavities produced may become large. Actinomycosis or candidiasis may spread from fungal infections (e.g. in the appendix), again causing liver abscesses. Other parasites colonise the liver as a special site for growth (e.g. schistosomes and liver flukes). The damage attributable to these infections accrues from biliary-tract blockage and from inflammatory (often fibrotic) reactions to resident parasites. Tapeworm infections,

especially the hydatid cysts of *Echinococcus granulosus*, may cause severe liver damage.

In the UK, viral infections (and in particular those responsible for hepatitis) are the most common cause of liver pathology. Hepatitis A virus is the most contagious variety, generally causing acute infection by faecal/oral spread. Hepatitis B virus produces infections of variable severity, often after long incubation periods. It frequently persists to cause a chronic-carrier condition, and is transmitted by blood. Non-A, non-B hepatitis virus is poorly characterised but is commonly spread in transfusions. The pathology of all three types is similar; the infections spread diffusely through tissues producing necrosis with considerable inflammatory cell activity. Damage may be extensive although regeneration is performed vigorously at the same time. However, widespread fibrosis may also occur which is persistent.

Other viral diseases commonly affecting the liver are yellow fever, infectious mononucleosis, cytomegalovirus infection, and herpes simplex (HSV type 2) virus infection. Again, variable degrees of liver cell damage occur due to growth of the viruses in the cells. Profuse lymphocyte and monocyte infiltration occurs and partly accounts for tissue damage.

Malfunctions due to Hepatic Damage

The overall consequences of liver disease may only become apparent when the extent of damage is severe (i.e. when adaptation and the reserve capacity can no longer compensate). Nevertheless, there are important manifestations of less severe liver damage which affect the patient adversely and provide diagnostic features. Probably the most readily apparent feature is jaundice, which is caused by elevated concentrations of bilirubin in the blood. Bilirubin is a normal constituent of blood, and hyperbilirubinaemia may be the result of other damage (e.g. haemolysis). However, bilirubin is considered a toxic waste product which is excreted by the liver. It is absorbed, conjugated into the readily excreted glucuronide, and eliminated into the bile by liver cells. If it is not excreted, bilirubin accumulates in the blood. The carrying capacity of the blood is largely dependent upon the ability of bilirubin to bind to plasma albumin. When this capacity is exceeded, bilirubin escapes into the tissues and produces the characteristic brownish-yellow discoloration. Adults normally tolerate the elevated bilirubin, although it probably contributes to the general feeling of malaise (see Section 15.1) and often causes severe pruritus. Bilirubin is toxic to brain and other nervous tissue but adults are protected by the blood-brain barrier. However, in neonates, bilirubin can pass into the brain and its toxicity may cause severe and usually irreversible damage.

Jaundice may result from almost any form of moderate to severe hepatic damage. It may be caused by blockage of bile flow (cholestatic jaundice) and by inability of damaged hepatocytes to process and excrete bilirubin (hepatocellular jaundice). Drugs or toxic agents may have a more specific action on certain components of the bile-producing mechanisms (e.g. novobiocin blocks bilirubin conjugation, and anabolic steroids cause occlusion of bile canaliculi).

Severe hepatic damage, characterised by the development of cirrhosis, is associated with much wider malfunctions (see Table 16.4). Overall the most severe results are anaemia, profound metabolic disturbances, and accumulation of toxic waste products (e.g. ammonia). Progressively, these may give rise to serious personality disorders (e.g. mania), coma, and death. In addition, malfunction of most of the major systems result in chronic general illness. Most notable are the effects on cardiovascular functions. Due to impaired blood flow through the cirrhotic liver, the drainage of the portal vein is prevented and causes congestion, which extends back into the mesenteric veins and results in portal hypertension. This in turn causes loss of fluid into the abdominal cavity (ascites). Furthermore, pressure on the vena cava impedes blood flow from lower extremities and leads to oedema of the ankles and legs. Ascites and oedema are aggravated by the impairment of plasma-protein synthesis which is normally carried out in the liver. Depleted plasma-protein concentration reduces the fluid-retaining ability of the vascular system. Compensatory elevated levels of aldosterone and vasopressin can be observed in cirrhotic patients. These in turn increase fluid retention which exacerbates the ascites and oedema.

Congestion of the portal vein impedes blood flow from the spleen and produces splenomegaly and impaired function. Some blood from the splenic and portal veins becomes diverted through normally unused, vestigial blood vessels remaining from the embryonic stage (i.e. the umbilical system). These vessels return blood to the vena cava via the oesophageal blood supply and in effect bypass the liver. Congestion of these vessels leads to oesophageal varices which often rupture, causing severe haemorrhage. Bleeding from varices may be persistent because prothrombin is lacking through liver damage. Loss of blood, impaired spleen function, and lack of stored vitamin B_{12} from the liver may give rise to anaemia.

The vital nature of hepatic functions ensures that effective protection and compensatory mechanisms guard against their loss. However, if these measures fail to prevent the consequences of more severe pathology, the subsequent mutually aggravating effects cause systemic failures so widespread and severe that they are matched only by the most catastrophic diseases of other organs. The liver is thus a vital organ ranking with the heart and brain in its functions.

16.5 NEUROPATHOLOGY

Introduction

For historical and other reasons, the study of pathology in the nervous system is regarded as a distinctive and highly specialised division of the discipline conveying an impression of separateness. In particular, the terminology employed in neuropathology is different. Certain important effects which may be analogous to those occurring elsewhere in the body are described by different names when they apply to nervous tissue. This may make it difficult for the uninitiated to comprehend descriptions of diseases in this system. However, there are special features of structure and function pertaining to nervous tissues which do justify special consideration. Therefore, while many of the general principles of pathology outlined in Chapter 15 can be seen to apply to nervous tissue, this system perhaps more than any other requires a separate discussion.

Like any other organ, the functions of nervous tissue depend upon specialised differentiated cells, in this case neurones. These are distributed throughout a coherent tissue mass in association with a limited variety of subsidiary cells, and this gives an appearance of some homogeneity. The nervous system is, however, much more highly organised and compartmentalised than any other organ and has widespread cellular interrelationships and multiple integrated functional activities. Because of the inherent complexities, it is not sufficient to possess only a general understanding of the pathological behaviour of nerve cells. The locations of affected cells within the system, their functional connections, and their varied and distinctive neurophysiological functions must also be considered. A complete knowledge of neuropathology requires detailed understanding of functional neuroanatomy to a degree well beyond the scope of this text. Therefore, by way of an introduction, this account will deal mainly with the changes affecting the individual neurones which are not only the principal functional units but also the cells most vulnerable to pathological influences. At this stage it need only be pointed out that the location of a nervous tissue lesion is of vital significance; a minute lesion strategically sited in an essential structure may have more serious consequences than an extensive patch of severe damage elsewhere.

Responses to Cell Damage and Cellular Change in Death

Neurones are very demanding and inflexible in their requirements for energy-producing nutrients and adequate oxygenation. Anatomically, the elongated extensions of nerve cells (axon processes) which require special provision separate from the cell body render satisfactory supply of nutrients problematic. The highly specialised structure and function of these cells impose severe limitations on their ability to adapt to adverse circumstances. Other subsidiary cells of nervous tissue are generally less vulnerable to unfavourable conditions, although all cells may be subject to pathological influences to varying degrees. Some cells (e.g. the phagocytic microglia) may become particularly active in circumstances which are lethal to neurones. Equally, non-neuronal cells (Table 16.5) may themselves be selectively damaged (e.g. by toxic or infective actions).

TABLE 16.5
Cellular components of central and peripheral nervous tissue

Cell	Role or function
Neurone	Various forms and sizes. Major functional components, specialised to respond to and transmit stimuli.
Neuroglia	Supporting and sustaining cells necessary to neurones. Out-number other cell types.
• oligodendrocytes	Surround and support neurones in central tissues. Provide myelin sheaths for central nerve fibres.
• astrocytes	Two main forms, involved in nutritional transport for neurones: protoplasmic or fibrous astrocytes. Have attachments to capillaries and fibril or leaf-like processes contacting neurones.
Schwann cells	Supporting and nourishing cells surrounding peripheral axons. Provide myelin sheaths.
Microglia (Hortega cells)	Macrophages from vascular supply. Phagocytic cells with protective and repair processes. Related to monocyte macrophages of other tissues.
Ependyma	Living cells in the cavities and passages in the CNS.
Meningeal cells	Occupy connective tissue sheets on CNS surfaces. Cells related to connective tissue (areolar and fascia) of the rest of the body.

As some of these cells support and nourish nerve cells, the dependent neurones may in turn be affected.

Neuronal damage may be apparent from changes in the cell body (perikaryon) or in the fibrous extensions, particularly the axon. The cell body responds to almost any adverse circumstance by undergoing degeneration, closely resembling the process of hydropic degeneration (*see* Section 15.3), as a result of impaired energy production or utilisation. Functional failure is associated with the inability of the cell to maintain its membrane in a polarised condition, hence it will be unable to transmit impulses. As in hydropic degeneration, swelling is caused by influx of water. Disruption of intracellular structures (e.g. the Nissl granules or the Golgi apparatus) is associated with loss of stain-attracting particles (chromatolysis); mitochondria also swell and disrupt. The combined effects cause radical biochemical and structural disorganisation and result in vacuole formation. In many cases, nuclear swelling may also occur.

Degenerative changes may be reversible if conditions speedily revert to normal so that, within a few days, cellular reorganisation and membrane depolarisation may restore excitability. More severe injury culminates in the death (necrosis) of the neurone. The immediate consequences are autolytic (i.e. destructive processes from within the cell). Disintegration of cytoplasmic contents involves particularly the lysis of neurofibrils. Characteristic nuclear changes may be seen (*see* Section 15.3). The nucleus becomes displaced to the cell periphery, distorts, and then disintegrates. When the neurone degenerates and dies, the associated dendrites and axons also shrink, distort, and fragment. Terminal structures (e.g. synaptic bulbs or sensory end-organs) swell and disintegrate.

In many cases, damage may be inflicted on the axon alone. The axon in central and peripheral structures is readily severed or crushed by various forms of traumatic injury. When axons in the brain or spinal cord are severed, the complete neuronal structure usually dies. Damage to the peripheral axons also affects the cell body but is usually not lethal. The cell body swells and there is chromatolysis and nuclear displacement (axonal reaction or retrograde degeneration), which affects the neurone from the break to the cell body. Wallerian degeneration (Fig. 16.9) describes the complete disintegration of the distal severed portion.

The larger axons usually have myelin sheaths which also disintegrate when the nerve fibres are damaged. On a peripheral nerve axon, the myelin is provided by processes from the Schwann cells. The myelin sheath is a multiple laminated layer of membranes wrapped around the axonal core (Fig. 16.10). Central nervous system axons are also myelinated (white matter) but

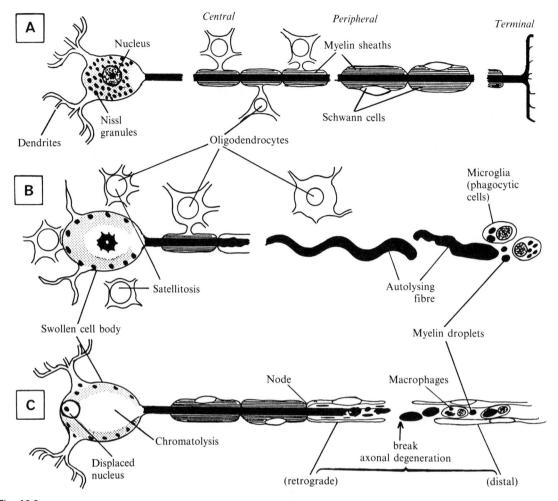

Fig. 16.9
Neuronal structures related to degeneration and neurosis in cell bodies and axon fibres.

from the accessory oligodendrocytes. Myelin degenerates over approximately 8 days into a residue of fatty droplets. Ultimately, degenerated myelin residues are usually ingested by microglia, but may remain for many months to mark the destroyed axonal tract.

Ischaemia, Hypoxidosis, and Toxic Damage

Without adequate oxygenation, neurones can survive only for a very short time before suffering radical damage (hypoxidosis), although the susceptibility to damage varies between nerve cell types. Cerebral cortical cells and the Purkinje cells of the cerebellum are very sensitive to hypoxia; the small pyramidal cells of the cerebral cortex may be damaged permanently within as little as 2 or 3 minutes. The cells of the basal ganglia are only slightly less vulnerable; thalamus and brainstem cells are somewhat less so. The anterior horn cells of the spinal cord and the Betz cells of the cerebral cortex are the least affected, but even these are able to withstand severe hypoxia for only about 15 minutes. Following hypoxia of 7 or 8 minutes, most cortical cells will have been affected and are unlikely to remain alive for more than a few hours even if apparently ideal conditions are restored.

The distribution of hypoxic lesions is dependent upon the circumstances, and functional consequences may therefore be diverse. Damage will be widespread if the whole of the nervous system is deprived of oxygen (e.g. following cardiac or pulmonary failure, general asphyxia, severe shock, or inhalation of nitrous oxide or

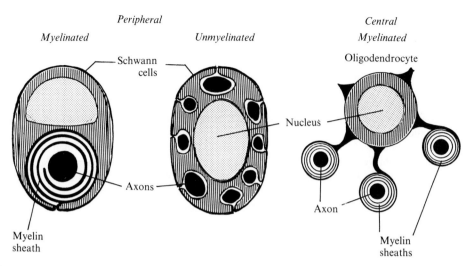

Peripheral

Myelinated   *Unmyelinated*

Central

Myelinated

Schwann cells

Oligodendrocyte

Nucleus

Axons

Axon

Myelin sheath

Myelin sheaths

Fig. 16.10
Myelin sheaths of central and peripheral nerve fibres (axons), provided by accessory cells: oligodendrocytes for central axons and Schwann cells for peripheral axons.

carbon monoxide). More localised lesions occur when restricted areas are deprived of blood (ischaemia) due to vascular blockage, severe constriction, or possibly haemorrhage. Wherever the site of damage, the extent of the lesion will spread; as the cells die, the disintegration proceeds into the fibrous extensions of the white matter of the brain or spinal cord.

Neuronal hypoxic degeneration and necrosis is most commonly due to a stroke which results from sudden deprivation of blood supply. It is uncertain whether the insidious chronic loss of neurones in approaching senility can be particularly attributed to vascular disease (e.g. arteriosclerosis). It is clear, however, that cerebro-vascular incidents do produce long-lasting effects. Actual pathological change will depend upon survival of the subject and whether there is continued cerebrovascular abnormality or circulatory recovery. Immediate effects of a stroke may not cause structural disorder, although there may be a considerable degree of malfunction. Although early malfunctions may include sensory and motor paralysis and coma or mental disorganisation, there may still be considerable functional recovery. Provided oxygen deprivation is not total, many neurones may remain alive although non-functional for considerable periods. Some degree of this degenerative change is reversible and restoration of adequate circulation could lead to cellular recovery.

The nervous system is wholly dependent upon the maintenance of supplies of glucose at a level above 60 mg/100 mL of blood. Hypoglycaemia causes neuronal damage akin to hypoxia (i.e. degeneration and necro-

sis) with similar relative cellular susceptibilities and likely distribution of lesions. The most common cause of hypoglycaemia, which may be severe enough to affect nervous function, is insulin overdosage. A number of toxic substances (e.g. cyanides and heavy metals) also affect the metabolism of neurones, preventing the proper utilisation of oxygen and glucose (*see* Section 15.2) and causing degeneration and necrosis. Neurones appear to depend upon astrocytes for nutritional support; toxic damage to astrocytes may, in turn, damage neurones.

Damage may affect peripheral fibres rather than the neurone as a whole. Localised ischaemia or toxicity may cause axonal damage which spreads back to the cell body. Peripheral damage may result from ethanol, hexane, organophosphorus compounds, or poisoning by arsenic and organic mercurials.

Demyelinating Disease

A special feature of a number of conditions is the destruction of the myelin sheath, often in conjunction with the cells which form it. In many cases this may be secondary to axon destruction, but in others it is the primary lesion.

The most important disease in this category is multiple sclerosis. Demyelination is associated wih numerous widely distributed inflammatory lesions in the white matter of the nervous system and is accompanied by loss of function. Lesions occur in the lateral and posterior columns of the spinal cord, giving sensory and motor paralysis. The optic nerves, brainstem, and temporal lobes are also often affected. Demyelination and the loss of function may be reversible, giving periods of significant remission, although the episodes gradually increase in frequency, severity, and extent. The disease is usually progressive to the stage of complete disability, coma, and death.

There is increasing evidence to suggest an auto-immune aetiology for demyelinating disease. Evidence also reveals associations with previous viral infection (e.g. demyelinating encephalopathy is an occasional sequel to measles, mumps, chickenpox, and vaccination). Demyelination is also caused by toxic agents (e.g. heavy metals, isoniazid, triethyltin, and hexachlorophene). Demyelination associated with retrograde axonal damage has been a feature of some major poisoning outbreaks (e.g. triorthocresylphosphate contaminating food or cooking oil).

Infection

Access to the central nervous system is not easily gained by infectious micro-organisms, unless facilitated by penetrating injury. Very occasionally, ear or nasal sinus infection may extend into the cranium. Otherwise, central nervous system infection is only likely to occur when there is septicaemia originating from a site of infection elsewhere. Even then, much of the development of the infection may occur only in the meningeal membranes. Rapidly growing bacteria (e.g. meningococci and staphylococci) may gain access from the blood vessels in the subarachnoid space (see Section 4.6) which contains cerebrospinal fluid (CSF), an excellent culture medium. Rapid growth of micro-organisms allows the infection to spread through the space causing meningitis. Further spread into cerebral ventricles and the spinal canal may lead to inflammation and accumulation of fluid and pus. Brain damage is usually attributable to pressure of accumulated pus, blocked blood flow, or more rarely, to invasion of the brain substance.

Some viruses have a predilection for growth in nervous tissues (neurotropic forms) and may readily gain access into neurones or accessory cells. Intracellular growth may cause damage and necrosis which may result in extensive damage to the system. Involvement of the brain is termed encephalitis, of the spinal cord, myelitis, and infection of both, encephalomyelitis. Poliomyelitis represents disease of this nature in which the nervous system is infected by bloodborne virions following growth elsewhere. The lesions may be restricted to meningeal inflammation, although in the most severe paralytic forms the viruses invade deeper tissue. The anterior horn cells of the spinal cord or the hindbrain (bulbar) nuclei, or both, are particular targets. As the nuclei of the hindbrain are concerned with respiration, paralysis of that function results. There are numerous other common viruses which may cause meningitis or encephalomyelitis (e.g. members of the Coxsackie and ECHOvirus groups, mumps viruses and herpesviruses). Insect, louse, or tick-borne viruses or rickettsiae (e.g. see Typhus Fevers) also affect the nervous system.

In common with other tissues, severe nervous damage may be the result of immune system activity secondary to the infection. Protection is provided against infection by the usual inflammatory mechanisms (see Section 15.4) by the action of cells from blood and adjacent connective tissues (meninges) and subsidiary cells of the tissue itself. Thus neutrophils, lymphocytes, plasma cells, and monocytes may be supplemented by local microglial cells in attacking the pathogenic micro-organisms. Granulomatous nodules (see Section 15.5) or collagen-fibre barriers may develop to isolate surface infections. In deeper tissue, astrocytes may be involved in the formation of an anti-infective barrier. Such mechanisms may effectively restrain the spread even of serious pathogens. However, severe inflammation may cause destruction of nervous tissue by direct erosion or as a result of extensive vascular damage. This is exemplified by the neuropathological manifestations of syphilis in which the standard pattern of septicaemia, meningitis, and neural damage by direct and inflammatory activites is characteristic of an uncontrolled secondary phase infection. Typically, meningeal inflammation may extend over the spinal cord, accounting for damage in the lumbar and sacral portions which provide innervation of the legs. Damage results in defects of posture and gait (e.g. locomotor ataxia). The later (tertiary) more widespread development of neurosyphilis is not attributable to direct reaction against infecting micro-organisms, because at that stage the presence of viable micro-organisms can no longer be detected. The very extensive neuronal destruction in the cerebral and cerebellar cortex or basal ganglia may be due to auto-immune reactivity or reaction against residues of dead micro-organisms.

Repair and Regeneration

The cells of connective tissue act with phagocytic blood cells to repair tissue damage within the cranium. However, this repair is limited to the meningeal membranes and tissues adjacent to blood vessels. In particular, fibroblasts may deposit collagenous scar tissue around foreign bodies or form adhesions between the brain and meningeal membranes after infection. Most of the brain substance is subject to different repair processes.

The general removal of necrotic neuronal material from a tissue is performed by the microglia. These mobile cells migrate into lesions, acting as macrophages and cause breakdown and phagocytosis of cell debris (neuronophagia). Laden with waste materials, they then move into CSF and drain into the bloodstream. The loss of neurones may be followed by proliferation of adjacent astrocytes which also participate in neuronophagia. Astrocyte extension processes elongate and pack the cavities of the lesions with masses of entwined fibrils or sheets (gliosis). Unlike collagen from fibroblasts, the glial material remains part of the cells, although the result is the same (i.e. closure of spaces by non-nervous scar material).

Full-functional healing could only be achieved by regeneration of neurones. There is in fact virtually no ability for neuronal proliferation after foetal development. With the notable exception of damaged neurohypophyseal fibres (*see* Section 16.6), regrowth of mature neurones is restricted to peripheral fibres. If a damaged neurone survives, regrowth by sprouting neurofibrils from the axonal stump to renew severed connections (Fig. 16.11) will be attempted. Success of regeneration is determined by the availability of a suitable supporting structure into which the fibrils can grow. In peripheral nerves a suitable structure is provided by

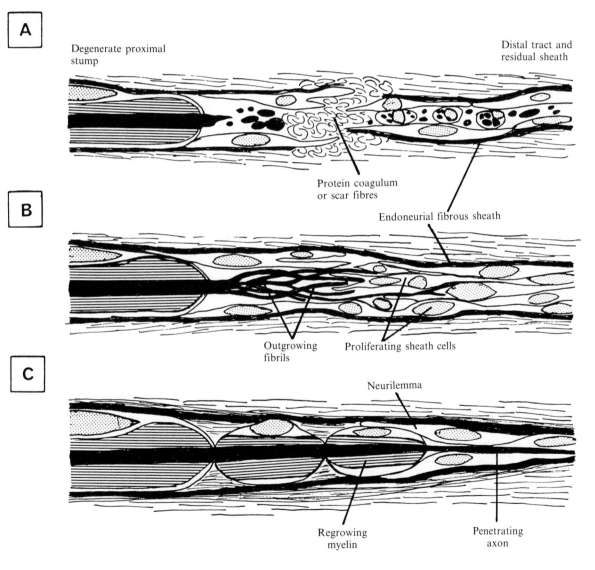

A

Degenerate proximal stump

Distal tract and residual sheath

Protein coagulum or scar fibres

Endoneurial fibrous sheath

B

Outgrowing fibrils

Proliferating sheath cells

C

Neurilemma

Regrowing myelin

Penetrating axon

Fig. 16.11
Regeneration of peripheral axon fibres.

the original connective tissue tubes (endoneurium) in which Schwann cells may survive. Schwann cells then provide a neurilemma to guide and allow further growth and survival of the neurofibrils. In these circumstances the fibrils will recolonise a severed nerve stump at the rate of 1 or 2 mm a day, ultimately enlarging to reform the typical axon cylinder. Where appropriate, the Schwann cells will grow around the axon to produce the layered myelin structure. Completion of the process will require the growth of nerve terminals to innervate the appropriate structure.

Nerves within the brain and spinal cord do not have the endoneurial fibrous support nor the Schwann cells to promote regrowth. The oligodendrocytes which form the myelin sheaths of central neurones usually perish with the disintegrating axon. There is no subsequent development of a suitable supporting structure and hence no effective regeneration. Restoration of function may not be perfect even in peripheral tracts. When regrowing fibrils at the end of a damaged nerve cannot find a receptive structure, a mass of tangled neurofibrils and sheath cells (neuroma) may be formed. A neuroma of sensory fibres (e.g. in an amputation stump) may become capable of generating impulses and give rise to the unwanted and often excruciatingly uncomfortable sensations of a 'phantom limb'.

Degenerative Diseases and Special Lesions

Confusion may arise from the use of the term degenerative; when used for systemic, and including nervous system, disease it implies cell loss from tissues rather than degenerative change in cells. Degenerative disease of the nervous system thus denotes progressive death of neurones as a primary lesion, with lysis of associated nerve fibre tracts as a secondary consequence. In many cases, the degenerative loss is selective, affecting widespread populations of particular neurones or limited target areas (e.g. selected nuclei). Two contrasting examples of neuronal populations which are selectively destroyed occur in Alzheimer's disease (affecting mental functions) (see Dementia) and motor neurone disease (causing loss of mobility). The causes are not properly known and may be unrelated, although infection with slow-viruses or auto-immune attack are possible offending mechanisms. Special pathological changes in the brains of patients with dementia are plaques of amyloid-like material and tangled neurofibrillary masses.

Not all severe nervous disorders are associated with overt structural defects. Some of the major psychiatric disorders (e.g. depressive disorders and schizophrenia) provide little or no evidence of organic disease. Other conditions may display major malfunctions but result from lesions of limited extent. Parkinson's disease provides a good example in which the functional defects (i.e. abnormalities of muscle tone or co-ordination of movement) may be widespread, although the major detectable pathology is restricted to lesions of neurones in the substantia nigra. There may also be loss of cells and myelinated fibres which pass from this area to other basal ganglia through the globus pallidus. Nerves of this tract liberate the neurotransmitter dopamine; parkinsonism results from markedly reduced levels of dopamine in the basal ganglia receiving these nerves (caudate nucleus and the putamen). Malfunction may be due to structural damage or to a less tangible pharmacological defect of neural transmission. Related conditions (e.g. Huntington's chorea) also involve damage in the caudate nucleus. Both the widespread neuronal degeneration and the targeted nuclear lesions may have multiple causes. Parkinsonism occurs in 'punch drunk' syndrome, after concussion and cerebral abscesses, and as a consequence of neurosyphilis. It may be caused by hypoxia, toxic damage (cyanide or carbon monoxide), or by manganese poisoning. Complex pharmacological interactions may also cause parkinsonism-like effects (e.g. with the use of reserpine, phenothiazines, and butyrophenones, and through methyldopa toxicity).

Manifestations of Neural Pathology

Nervous malfunction is dependent upon the particular area affected. If the affected tissue normally originates or transmits motor instructions or receives sensory information, damage is likely simply to paralyse these functions. In many cases, however, the result will not be that simple because of multiple interactions. A particular feature of nervous system organisation is the functional balance achieved by reciprocally inhibitory influences between opposing tracts of nerves. Loss of one system from nerve damage may therefore lead to exaggerated activity in its newly unopposed counterpart. Some pathology involves marginally adverse influences in which affected cells fluctuate between quiescence and activity, resulting in highly irregular discharged impulses. One overall result may be the uncontrolled overactivity of epilepsy.

16.6   DISORDERS IN ENDOCRINE DISEASE

Introduction

Pathological processes affecting any organ of the endocrine system are likely to increase or decrease the secretion of the hormone(s) normally produced by that tissue. Less commonly, the type of hormone secreted may change. However, changes in the amount of hormone secreted may cause significant malfunction in target tissues, or the structure of the hormone-dependent tissue may become altered. A notable feature of virtually all endocrine-dependent functions is the precision of the normal control mechanisms. The loss of this precision, through pathological influence, can result in inappropriate responses to physiological alterations and cause malfunction. In particular, complex hormone-mediated control of interdependent functions of several tissues or organs, operating as one system, may be vulnerable to altered production of any component hormone.

Hormone production is a specialist function of usually well differentiated mature cells, generally organised into a specific structure adapted for that purpose. Such tissue may be subject to failure or aberration during development, resulting in congenital defects. In some cases, especially the pituitary gland, special anatomical arrangements of nervous and vascular connections may be the basis for pathological vulnerability. In all cases, the biosynthetic mechanisms for hormone production may be subject to genetic, biochemical, or toxic alterations, while systemic factors may alter the transport of the hormones after production (e.g. change in plasma carrier-proteins). Tissues may also be affected by any of the general forms of pathology (e.g. traumatic, ischaemic, infective, or neoplastic).

Glands of the endocrine system are themselves controlled by the nervous system, the prevailing blood levels of particular substances and hormones, or by combinations of nervous and other influences. Thus, endocrine secretion may directly reflect integrated nervous functions (e.g. circadian rhythms or alterations in blood flow or homoeostatic control mechanisms for body fluid and electrolyte levels). Secretions of the pancreatic islets or the parathyroids are controlled respectively by glucose or ionic calcium in the blood, while general levels of thyroid activity are indirectly dependent upon the levels of thyroxine or liothyronine. Above all, the control of several major endocrine systems is achieved by reciprocal or feedback loop interactions between the anterior lobe of the pituitary (*see* Section 6.6) and the subsidiary gland. The release of trophic hormones from the anterior pituitary is in turn dependent upon neuro-endocrine control, in the form of releasing-factor neurohormones secreted by the hypothalamic neurones. The hypothalamic releasing-factors are carried to the pituitary by a special local blood supply. This integration of nervous and endocrine functions provides a good example of negative feedback control (Fig.

16.12). Elevated levels of the subordinate gland hormones (e.g. adrenal corticosteroids) decrease secretion of releasing factor and subsequently of trophic hormone (e.g. adrenocorticotrophin), thus reducing the stimulus to the target organ. Multi-hormonal interactions (e.g. those required for ovulation or parturition) are brought about by this versatile system. Faults in integration, secretory mechanisms, or any of the component structures can have far-reaching effects, impairing the whole system. However, such systems are very resilient and do have considerable ability to compensate for at least some of the malfunction which might arise from the component damage. Thus, overt clinical development of endocrine dysfunction may be lessened or delayed, although overcompensation following deficiency of one component may lead to excessive growth or overactivity of an associated tissue.

Secretory Malfunctions

Numerous endocrine disorders are recognised and named according to the abnormality of a particular hormonal secretion or its consequences to the body (Tables 16.6, 16.7, and 16.8). It should be noted that the disease classification does not refer precisely to the actual pathology of the gland or other defective mechanism. A variety of effects may produce the same result in terms of the level of hormones or target-organ malfunction.

Destructive lesions of endocrine tissues may be caused by ischaemia, compression, infection, auto-immune attack, or toxicity. The pituitary and adrenal glands are particularly vulnerable to ischaemia, which may arise as a result of mechanical ventilator hypoxia, postpartum haemorrhagic shock, or local interruption of blood supply (e.g. in pituitary stalk damage caused by head-whiplash injury).

Auto-immune damage may affect a number of organs and account for important and age-related endocrine diseases (e.g. Hashimoto's thyroiditis and some cases of Addison's disease). It is also becoming increasingly evident that auto-immune mechanisms play a causative role in Type I diabetes mellitus. Insulin antibodies and T-cell mediated attack may have wider effects, including the aetiology of the numerous systemic complications. Auto-immune antibody to cell-surface insulin receptors may also explain some cases of the more common Type II diabetes mellitus.

Infections also cause endocrine disease by direct damage; virus infections may result in auto-immune mechanisms. Tuberculosis was formerly a major cause of adrenal and other glandular damage; the adrenals may be particular sites of damage in other chronic granu-

TABLE 16.6
Pituitary gland malfunctions

Malfunction	Hormone	Consequence
Anterior pituitary		
• hyperactivity	growth hormone (somatotrophin)	gigantism, acromegaly
• hyperactivity	adrenocorticotrophin (ACTH)	Cushing's syndrome (hydrocortisone hypersecretion)
• Cushing's disease	ACTH secretion from basophil tumour	Cushing's syndrome (hydrocortisone hypersecretion)
• hyperactivity	thyrotrophin	hyperthyroid goitre
• hyperactivity	prolactin	galactorrhoea, amenorrhoea
• hyposecretion	growth hormone (+ thyrotrophin or gonadotrophins)	dwarfism
• hyposecretion	ACTH	adrenocortical insufficiency
• hyposecretion	thyrotrophin	hypothyroidism
• hyposecretion	gonadotrophins	male or female hypogonadism
• panhypopituitarism	total or general hormonal failure	general endocrine malfunction
Posterior pituitary		
• hyposecretion	vasopressin (antidiuretic hormone)	diabetes insipidus
• hypersecretion(?)	vasopressin (probably ectopic secretion)	water retention

TABLE 16.7
Hormonal abnormalities of peripheral endocrine tissues

Condition	Tissue	Result
Hyperactivities		
• Cushing's syndrome	adrenal cortex	hydrocortisone hypersecretion
• Conn's syndrome	adrenal cortex	primary aldosteronism (adrenal adenoma)
• secondary aldosteronism	adrenal cortex	aldosterone hypersecretion (compensatory)
• Graves' disease	thyroid	hyperthyroidism, goitre
• nodular goitre and toxic adenoma	thyroid	hyperthyroidism
• exophthalmic goitre	thyroid	hyperthyroidism, eye and orbital lesions
• thyroid storm	thyroid	life-threatening hyperthyroidism
• hyperparathyroidism	parathyroid glands	excessive hormonal secretion, hypercalcaemia
• insulinoma	pancreas beta-cell tumour	hyperinsulinism, hypoglycaemia
• glucagonoma	pancreas alpha-cell tumour	hypersecretion of glucagon, hyperglycaemia
• carcinoid syndrome	argentaffin cell tumour	hypersecretion of serotonin
Hypofunction		
• Addison's disease	adrenal cortex	hyposecretion of hydrocortisone and/or aldosterone
• congenital adrenal hyperplasia	adrenal cortex	hyposecretion of hydrocortisone and overproduction of androgen
• hypothyroidism (mainly Hashimoto's thyroiditis	thyroid	primary thyroid hormone deficiency and myxoedema
• hypoparathyroidism	parathyroids	hormone deficiency and hypocalcaemia
• type I diabetes mellitus	pancreas	primary insulin deficiency and hyperglycaemia
• type II diabetes mellitus	pancreas	end-organ resistance to insulin

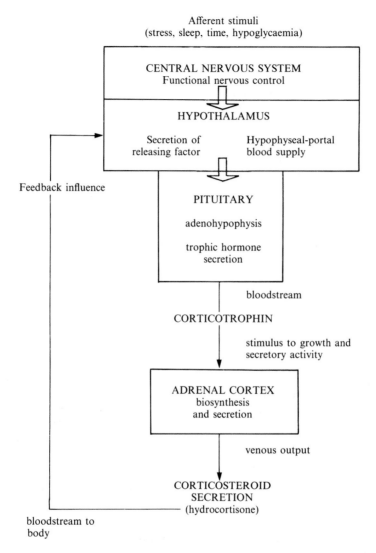

Afferent stimuli
(stress, sleep, time, hypoglycaemia)

CENTRAL NERVOUS SYSTEM
Functional nervous control

HYPOTHALAMUS

Secretion of   Hypophyseal-portal
releasing factor   blood supply

Feedback influence

PITUITARY

adenohypophysis

trophic hormone
secretion

bloodstream

CORTICOTROPHIN

stimulus to growth and
secretory activity

ADRENAL CORTEX
biosynthesis
and secretion

venous output

CORTICOSTEROID
SECRETION
(hydrocortisone)

bloodstream to
body

Fig. 16.12
Feedback control mechanisms exerted upon subsidiary endocrine organs by the hypothalamo-hypophyseal axis, involving secretion of pituitary trophic hormones, as exemplified by secretory activity of the adrenal cortex.

lomatous infections (e.g. syphilis, histoplasmosis, and coccidioidomycosis). However, endocrine damage due to uncontrolled infections is probably now much less common.

Genetic defects can result in developmental failure of endocrine tissues, giving total absence or glandular malformations (e.g. of thyroid, ovary, testis, or either lobe of the pituitary). Alternatively, genetic defects account for abnormal hormonal biosynthesis, causing reduced or qualitatively different secretions. End-organ deficiencies in which normal hormonal secretions are ineffective may be genetically determined, with target cells un-

reactive due to lack of hormonal receptors or related mechanisms.

Hypersecretion of hormones may be the cause of malfunction in target tissues and is equally as harmful as hyposecretion or total failure. Hypersecretion is closely linked to structural enlargement of the glands (hyperplasia) or neoplastic change (*see* Section 15.7). In some cases, hyperplasia and elevated hormone production occurs in glands subordinate to the pituitary through overstimulation by trophic hormones (e.g. Cushing's syndrome and adrenal hyperplasia). Hypersecretion of hormones may be due to abnormal stimuli (e.g. the

TABLE 16.8
Hormonally-mediated reproductive disorders

Disorder	Mechanism	Effect
Male and female		
• delayed puberty	failure of hypothalmic-pituitary function, gonadotrophin deficiency	absence of sex-hormone mediated body development
• precocious puberty	abnormal gonadotrophin or sex-hormone secretion	early development of sex organs and secondary sexual characteristics
• infertility	adult failure of hypothalmic, pituitary, or gonadal function	lack of secretion of gonadotrophins and/or corticosteroid hormones
• congenital adrenal hyperplasia	adrenocortical hyperplasia with failure of corticosteroid biosynthesis	corticosteroid deficiency with secretion of intermediate biosynthetic products (e.g. androgens)
Male		
• hypogonadism	hypothalamic or pituitary dysfunction	androgen deficiency and failure of testicular function
• hypogonadism	elevated gonadotrophin secretion ineffective because of diseased testes	androgen deficiency, testicular feminising syndrome
• cryptorchidism	undescended testes gonadotrophin failure	gonadal failure
• gynaecomastia	pituitary disturbance giving oestrogenic effects	mammary gland development, feminising syndrome
Female		
• hypogonadism	pituitary or ovarian damage and/or failure	primary amenorrhoea, oestrogen deficiency
• secondary amenorrhoea	pregnancy or abnormal gonadotrophin and/or sex hormone production (neoplasms)	impairment of normal cycles
• polycystic ovary syndrome	multiple follicle development	chronic anovulation and aberrant hormonal production (oestrogens and androgens)
• menopause	hypothalamo-pituitary-ovary axis, cessation of function	cessation of function, hypogonadism and infertility
• hirsutism, virilisation	androgen secretion	alteration of secondary sexual characteristics to male pattern

hypersensitivity caused by antibody effects on cytoplasmic membrane receptors, which produces hyperthyroidism). Cellular damage may also result in leakage of hormones, giving elevated blood levels.

Long-term overstimulation of endocrine tissue may cause hyperplasia to develop into nodular overgrowths and even neoplasia (e.g. adenomas of pituitary, adrenal cortex, or parathyroid tissues, which usually continue to overproduce hormones). Neoplastic changes produce a multiplicity of tumours in endocrine tissues and, again, hormonal hypersecretion often results (e.g. primary aldosteronism from tumours of the zona glomerulosa of the adrenal cortex). Hyperplastic or adenomatous tissues may continue full hormonal production in contrast to malignant tumours which may produce abnormal secretions. Abnormal structures or deficiencies of biosynthetic enzymes result in incomplete hormonal

synthesis. The aberrant secretion may represent overproduction of a precursor of the normal hormone which may be qualitatively different in action (e.g. the steroid precursors of adrenal glucocorticoids are oestrogens and mineralocorticoids). In phaeochromocytoma, adrenaline becomes predominantly replaced by the precursor, noradrenaline. Secretion of completely foreign hormones by endocrine tumours is less common, although it can occur from intrinsically non-endocrine tissue (e.g. adrenocorticotrophin secreted by small (oat) cell carcinoma of the bronchus).

General consequences of abnormal secretion depend upon the specific properties of the hormones involved. Quantitative hypersecretion produces hyperactivity in target tissues; hyposecretion produces underactivity. Changes in target-cell reactivity are also quantitative. Thus the diagnosis, interpretation, and treatment of endocrine disorders may generally rely on the principle that the abnormalities may be explained in terms of the normal secretions and their usual effects.

Pathophysiology of the Pituitary Gland

The most radical pathology results from the complete absence of the gland, although this is rare. Congenital absence usually involves only the anterior lobe. Substantial damage to either lobe may be a common result of severe head injury, with necrosis resulting from interrupted or severed blood supply. Equally, severed nerve connections from the hypothalamus can cause loss of function in either lobe. The pituitary tissue itself may become neoplastic; growth of chromophobe cell adenoma and secondary malignant growths (e.g. metastases from cancer of the stomach, lung cancer, or breast cancer) may obliterate other cells. Other important causes of abnormality include necrosis occurring in diabetes mellitus. Cellular damage in the anterior pituitary does not readily reverse as, unusually for epithelial cells, regeneration is poor (*see* Table 15.4). However, satisfactory function may be provided by small undamaged fragments, comprising as little as 10% to 20% of the lobe. There is also some ability of damaged posterior pituitary fibres to regenerate, which is unique amongst nerve fibres in the central nervous system.

The anterior pituitary has three cell types responsible for secretion of growth hormone, prolactin, adrenocorticotrophin, thyrotrophin, and the gonadotrophins (*see* Section 6.6). Loss or malfunction of one or more of the functional cell types causes disorders or combinations of disorders. Panhypopituitarism involves all types, giving partial or total failure of all subordinate endocrine organs and functions. Other hypopituitary combinations which have lack of growth hormone in common give rise to the various forms of dwarfism (*see* Growth Hormone Deficiency). Individual hormone deficiencies result in adrenocortical, thyroid, gonadal, and mammary gland changes respectively, involving tissue atrophy and functional failures.

Hypersecretion rarely involves more than one hormonal type and usually results from tumours of one particular cell type. One fifth of all anterior lobe tumours secrete growth hormone and cause acromegaly and gigantism. Tumours of neurosecretory cells do not occur and hypersecretion of posterior lobe hormones is therefore almost unknown. High vasopressin levels do however occur and cause water retention. These may be attributed to vasopressin secretion elsewhere (e.g. from bronchial carcinoma). Destructive loss of vasopressin-secreting neurones is much more common and gives rise to the opposite effect, diabetes insipidus.

Pathophysiology of the Thyroid

Thyroid neoplasms, and malignant forms in particular, are rare. They are a distinctive feature of the relatively small number of people who have been seriously contaminated with nuclear fallout, as the thyroid selectively takes up absorbed radioactive iodine. Hyperthyroidism is therefore most often due to excessive stimulation of the gland, which may sometimes be secondary to excessive secretion of thyrotrophin from the pituitary. The vast majority of cases, however, are classed as Graves' disease and are thought to be due to auto-immune influence. Circulating immunoglobulin auto-antibodies act as stimulating factors, causing hypersecretion of hormones and glandular enlargement (goitre). Secretion of thyroxine, liothyronine, or both, may be so high that severe symptoms (e.g. tachycardia, arrhythmias, and potentially fatal shock) may result.

Development of goitre is a feature of several forms of thyroid abnormality. The enlargement associated with hyperthyroidism may be diffuse (as in Graves' disease) or nodular (Plummer's disease). However, glandular enlargement may also occur with hypothyroidism. In Hashimoto's thyroiditis, the actual mass of glandular tissue may be reduced with small follicles, but the gland is swollen with active lymphoid tissue and fibrosis. Other goitres may be associated with relatively normal hormonal levels (euthyroid or non-toxic goitres). When glandular activity is low (e.g. due to iodine deficiency, as in endemic goitre) or inhibited (e.g. by antithyroid or goitrogenic drugs), a compensating elevated secretion of thyrotrophin occurs; thyroid glandular hyperplasia is provoked and hormonal production is restored. However, hypothyroidism may occur without goitre development and be due to failure of thyrotrophin secretion (secondary) or, more usually (90%), as the result of direct destruction of thyroid tissue by auto-immune attack, toxicity, or infection.

Diabetes Mellitus

This aspect of pancreatic pathology provides an excellent example of the way in which endocrine malfunction is increasingly recognised to be due to auto-immune mechanisms, with the damage not restricted to the primary organ and the overall adverse effects involving multiple-hormone interactions. The simplest circumstances occur in Type I (insulin-dependent, juvenile onset) diabetes which is the result of destructive attack on the beta-cells of the islets of Langerhans, causing severe insulin deficiency. The consequence of this is hyperglycaemia with complex metabolic abnormalities, which lead to ketoacidosis. Essentially, these disturbances result from the unbalanced effects of other hyper-glycaemic hormones (e.g. glucocorticoids, glucagon, or growth hormone). Type II (non-insulin-dependent, maturity-onset) diabetes results from reduced respon-siveness to the hormone in the tissues. The secretory tissue remains functional and insulin levels often high, although fibrotic and hyaline changes occur in the islets.

Longstanding and hence usually Type I diabetes often features widespread tissue damage based on underlying small blood vessel disease (microangiopathy). It seems very likely that the pancreatic islet damage is itself the result of microangiopathy. Resultant tissue damage typically affects the kidney, peripheral nerves, and the eye, particularly the retina. Ulcers or gangrene of the extremities and atrophic skin changes also occur. Metabolic disturbances probably also play a part in all of these. Viral infection, stress, and genetic and other factors probably determine the occurrence of the causa-tive lesions in this archetypal multifactorial endocrine disease.

16.7 DERMATOLOGY

Introduction

The integument (see Section 13.2) comprises the skin, with its glands and appendages, plus the subcutaneous connective tissue and the fat layer. It is especially subject to a variety of damage and disease because of its exterior exposure. Altogether, the integument represents the largest tissue mass of the body. Its functions of contain-ment, environmental control, and protection are of con-siderable importance. The component tissues are gen-erally affected by the whole range of pathological mechanisms outlined in Chapter 15, although there are special features.

The extent to which integumental functions are im-paired is largely dependent upon the extent and depth of penetration of the damage or disease. The most serious consequences to the whole body result from ineffective cutaneous participation in control of the internal environment and, in particular, fluid and electrolyte balance and temperature controls. If the skin's protec-tive functions become compromised, the consequences may also be serious; pathological effects (e.g. infection or toxicity) in other parts of the body may well depend upon an initial penetration of the barrier layers. Normally, within the limits of its physical properties, the integument does provide effective protection against physical erosion, adverse environmental change, infec-tion, chemical action, and some irradiation. However, at the same time as providing a barrier against entry of many harmful substances (e.g. water-soluble materials), it is permeable to a wide variety of lipid-soluble com-pounds and gases or vapours. As a second line of de-fence, cutaneous cells can metabolise many absorbed chemicals, often rendering them less toxic.

Additional protective roles against disease are varied. Cellular and humoral immune mechanisms (see Section 15.6) operate within the tissues. To counteract its vul-nerability to damage and disease, the skin is highly effec-tive at regeneration and repairing its defects. Thirdly, the outermost layers of the epidermal epithelium are dead and provide the impervious horny keratin layer.

The skin and its appendages have an important physio-logical role as a sense organ, as they carry the major proportion of the body's sensory nerve endings. Because these are affected by many of the pathological mechan-isms, the awareness of cutaneous pathology is particu-larly high. This is not restricted to the perception of pruritus and pain from lesions but encompasses more subtle mental and social considerations. The skin's appearance plays an important part in a person's self-regard, in interactions with other people, and especially in matters of sexual attraction. The visual effects of cutaneous lesions may transcend and magnify any sensory discomfort. Thus, the disfiguring effects of rela-tively minor cutaneous pathology, especially in cosmetically significant regions (e.g. the face), may cause mental and social distress to the sufferers and onlookers. Similar considerations may apply to abnormalities of the nails or hair, which are in no sense physically life-threatening but nevertheless of medical significance.

A large variety of skin disease is recognised and classified by dermatologists. Descriptive terminology is listed in a concise glossary (Table 16.9). The skin is an essentially simple structure and most manifestations of skin disease can be considered to be forms of inflamma-tion, with or without necrotic change, or involve abnor-mal cellular proliferation. In many cases and especially in inflammatory mechanisms, there will be a component determined by activity of the immune system. Thus, a limited range of mechanisms operate in the skin or in its associated connective tissues and blood vessels, to account for a wide range of diseases.

Allergic Diseases

Allergic or hypersensitivity reactions which are deter-mined by immune-system activity (see Section 15.6) are the most common group of cutaneous disorders. All four main classes of mechanism may be identified but types I, III, and IV are most usual. Urticaria is the typical form of type I reactions and is characterised by lesions dis-playing   the   classical   histamine-mediated   'triple

TABLE 16.9
Glossary of descriptive terms used in dermatology

Acanthosis	thickening of epidermis
Bulla	blister; a vesicle over 1 cm in diameter
Ecchymosis	a bluish-purple point-source haemorrhagic spot, larger than a petechia
Erythema	reddening due to vasodilatation
Eschar	necrotic tissue
Exanthem	rash; eruptive lesion
Excoriation	scratch or score; superficial damage removing epidermis
Furuncle	infection developing in or from a hair follicle; boil
Keratinisation	formation of the horny material by dehydration of epithelial cells
Lentigo	freckles
Lichenification	hardening and thickening of skin, with inflammation and scale formation, caused by chronic irritation or scratching
Macule	circumscribed discoloration (less than 1 cm), no change in thickness or texture
Nodule	well-defined solid lesion, dermal or subdermal
Papule	elevated lesion of surface, due to hyperplasia, infiltration, or material deposits (less than 1 cm)
Patch	lesion like a macule, over 1 cm
Pemphigus/pemphigoid	variety of conditions involving severe blistering
Petechiae	small, point-source haemorrhages
Plaque	lesion like a papule, over 1 cm
Pruritus	cutaneous itching
Purpura	purple or brownish-red discoloration due to sub-epidermal haemorrhage
Pustule	pus-filled vesicle
Scales or squames	flakes or sheets or horny, keratinised material
Scar or cicatrice	tissue replacement after damage to dermal tissue
Sclerosis	hardening of subcutaneous tissue (induration)
Striae	linear marks on skin
Telangiectasia	persistent visible vasodilatation
Vesicle	papule filled with exuded fluid
Vitiligo	depigmented patches
Wheal	oedematous white compressible elevation

response'. Lesions resemble 'nettle rash' and may be recognised by localised erythema, sharply defined wheal formation, heat, and intense pruritus. Such lesions usually resolve without permanent damage. They may be due to local exposure to allergenic material in subjects sensitised by the production of immunoglobulin E, and such reactivity occurs mostly in the predisposed atopic patient. Urticarial rashes do not play a large part in microbial pathology but may feature in some bacterial infections. Skin-sensitising antibodies have been found in sera of patients with systemic streptococcal infections, lobar pneumonia, tonsillitis, and after tetanus immunisation. Urticaria may also be caused by other natural antigens, including animal and plant protein or ingested foodstuffs (e.g. shellfish). It may also be due to the direct irritant effects of chemicals applied to the skin (non-allergic effects).

A number of localised or systemic infections feature rashes caused by damage in blood vessels beneath the skin (vasculitis). This is usually the result of immune complex formation following the development of type III hypersensitivity (*see* Section 15.6). The antibody complexes with antigenic material (e.g. infecting micro-organisms, toxins, or degradation products) in the circulation or in blood-vessel walls. Complement activation follows, attracting neutrophils and provoking the release of tissue-damaging enzymes and other inflammatory mediators. Vascular damage results, causing erythema or purpura, and may be followed by necrosis of surrounding tissues. In general, lesions of this type are more serious than urticarial reactions and tissue damage may be severe enough to cause scarring. Type III hypersensitivity to drugs (e.g. salicylates, thiazides, quinine, or tetracyclines) may cause such haemorrhagic damage and give the appearance of intense deep bruising (vascular purpura). Other causes are infections in which the immunity may be sufficient to restrain the spread of pathogens but not to eliminate them. Extensive vasculitis-based rashes are associated with systemic infections (e.g. meningococcal septicaemia, gonorrhoea, and streptococcal endocarditis) or with bacterial or fungal infections of the skin (e.g. *Staphylococcus aureus* or *Trichophyton mentagrophytes*). The more generalised rashes are often associated with systemic symptoms, including pyrexia, arthralgia, lymph node swelling, and glomerulonephritis.

Cell-mediated type IV hypersensitivity typically causes eczema, which is one of the commonest cutaneous lesions. The lesions represent severe inflammation of the skin and are characterised by red eruptions and small vesicles, developing towards the surface. Epidermal layers overlying the lesion become thickened and scaly (acanthosis) and the vesicles may coalesce to form bullae. Frequently the bullae erode and rupture to expose a tender weeping surface. Protein-rich fluid exuding from this surface tends to dry, leaving a crust. Both the drying surface and crust may crack and fissure. Exudate beneath the crust or in fissures provides a good medium for infection by bacteria or fungi. Pruritus, which is often severe, is a general feature of eczema; the provoked scratching erodes the surface, removes scales or crust, and further promotes infection. Continued scratching, even after the lesion has started to heal, may retard healing and cause chronic inflammation. This produces red, thickened, scaly areas (lichenification). Acute and chronic eczema is usually allergic in origin (*see* Section 15.6) but similar inflammatory changes may also be caused by irritant chemicals.

In a number of infections, lesions may arise in parts of the body remote from any focus of micro-organisms. It is usually impossible to detect infection in these lesions, and such id (pronounced 'ide') reactions are attributed to allergy. Id reactions are a common consequence of fungal infections (e.g. tinea infections) of skin, hair, or nails, with sterile vesicular lesions occurring on the palms, soles, or other skin (pompholyx). Other remote inflammatory id lesions are associated with streptococcal and meningococcal infections, tuberculosis, and syphilis. They may occur as secondary results of purely allergic disease (secondary sensitisation dermatitis). It is estimated that one third of patients with varicose ulcers and two thirds of those with nickel dermatitis suffer generalised reactions in other areas.

Infections

Infections (*see also* Section 15.5) generally cause direct tissue damage (degeneration and necrosis) accompanied by inflammation. Vesicles or pustules are also common in viral (herpes or pox viruses) or bacterial infections. Pustules may extend to become furuncles, carbuncles, or abscesses. These eruptions are due to exudation of fluid and the infiltration of neutrophils. This exemplifies infection by pyogenic bacteria (*see* Table 15.7) which infect hair follicles, sweat glands, or epidermal abrasions, releasing toxins and causing local necrosis and inflammation. The severity of the tissue response is determined in part by immune processes. Fungal growth in the epidermis is also associated with immunity-determined in-

flammatory eruptions and results in scaling, vesiculation, and sometimes suppuration with pustule formation. Such dermatophytes include *Microsporon*, *Epidermophyton*, or *Trichophyton* spp.

Some infections cause the development of granulomas (*see* Section 15.5) in or under the skin. Well demarcated subcutaneous nodules are features of bacterial (e.g. tuberculosis, leprosy, and syphilis), fungal (e.g. actinomycosis), or viral infections. Type IV hypersensitivity to very persistent intracellular parasites appears to be the determining cause.

Tuberculosis, more commonly considered a pulmonary infection, may also affect the skin as a primary infection and in secondary or reinfection cases (when some immune reactivity has developed). Secondary cutaneous lesions depend upon the degree of immune involvement. The condition in moderately hypersensitive individuals, lupus vulgaris, is characterised by aggregates of pin-head, deep, subcutaneous nodules, giving reddish-brown patches in the skin. Overlying skin may atrophy and the lesions ulcerate. More intense reactions cause epidermal hyperplasia over the lesion (warty lupus) with hyperkeratosis. Another form of tuberculosis with cutaneous involvement is scrofuloderma, a suppurating infection (usually in the neck) extending outwards to ulcers or fistulas in the skin.

Proliferative Lesions

One of the most important abilities of the integument is its ability to repair destructive damage. This depends upon the effective proliferation of certain component cells in the different layers. This is exemplified by simple wound healing, which involves granulation tissue formation in subepidermal structures and cellular regeneration in the epidermis. The repair of connective tissue layers is associated with inflammation, which activates plasma exudation and leucocyte infiltration. Plasma proteins coagulate in the wound, and phagocytic cells clear up debris and infection in and around the coagulum and scab. In the connective tissues adjacent to the wound, granulation processes commence with the proliferation of fibroblasts and their migration into the wound to form masses of collagen fibres. Advancing fronts of active fibroblasts gradually spread across the space and finally unite. These are followed by developing capillary networks. Thus, the deeper parts of a cutaneous wound are filled by new vascular connective tissue which replaces coagulated protein. Surface repair is by epidermal cell proliferation from adjacent sources (e.g. any remaining glands or hair follicles and epidermis at the wound edges). Increased cell division in the basal cell layer and migration of new cells from the prickle cell layer form a layer over exposed tissues. The cells move over one another until contact between opposing edges of new epidermal layers is established. Subsequently the epithelium becomes layered and the outermost cells become keratinised by dehydration. Further activity rearranges the subepidermal collagen and the surface layers become thinner, with components returning to a more normal state. Repair processes account for the ultimate healing of most kinds of cutaneous lesion. Excessive growth during wound healing may give rise to distortion and an unsightly scar (keloid).

Epidermal cell proliferation is normally a restricted process, in which mitosis occurs in the basal cell layer only to replace individual cells normally lost by keratinisation and wear and tear of the surface layer. Cell division is restrained by inhibitory substances (chalones), and mitotic activity at wound edges is thought to be due to their loss from damaged tissue. Other skin lesions which may lead to abnormal growth effects probably depend upon similar loss of control. In psoriasis the lesions are characterised by vigorous proliferative activity in the epidermis. This produces marked scale production (acanthosis), although the epidermis becomes thinner because the granulation layer is absent and the dermal papillae are elongated. These changes overlie inflammation in the dermis, and the condition produces inflamed macules or papules covered by silvery-looking scales of keratin. When the scales are scraped away, pinpoint bleeding occurs.

The skin is commonly affected by neoplastic change, especially in later life. This may be a consequence of the greater likelihood of exposure to carcinogenic influences or because of the continual cell proliferation. Effects range from benign forms to malignant tumours (Table 16.10), but some are considered to be only 'tumour-like'. The latter (polyp or papillary masses) are produced by excessive epithelial cell division and are particularly associated with viral infections. After a period of tumour-like growth they regress, apparently as a result of immune activity (e.g. common wart).

16.8 KIDNEYS AND URINARY TRACT

Introduction

The importance of the role of the kidneys in controlling the body's internal fluid compositions and the excretion

TABLE 16.10
Cutaneous neoplasms and other proliferative lesions

Benign	
• common wart, molluscum contagiosum, and condylomata acuminata	Epithelial neoplasms, papillary or polyp in form, probably caused by virus infection.
• keratoacanthoma	Self-limiting, squamous cell hyperplasia, associated with active inflammatory reaction.
• Senile warts (seborrhoeic keratosis)	Pigmented papilloma, common in elderly, only rarely become malignant.
Initially benign becoming malignant	
• chemical keratosis (arsenical keratosis, tar, or pitch warts)	Due to exposure to carcinogens.
• naevocellular naevus	Quiescent or localised collections of pigmented cells at or beneath the junction of the dermis and epidermis. May be migratory, but not invasive.
• solar keratosis	Associated with prolonged exposure to ultraviolet radiation.
Malignant	
• basal cell carcinoma	Raised plaque-like thickening in area between ear, eye, and base of nose; extends laterally and ulcerates in centre; inwardly invasive by cords of basal cells; ultimately erodes underlying tissues.
• malignant melanoma	Spreading, or aggressively invasive, pigmented cell patches or nodules, often arising in cutaneous naevi but behaviour is very variable. Some are associated with severe exposure to ultraviolet radiation, and some are caused by hereditary predisposition.
• squamous cell carcinoma	Invasive polyp or papillary neoplasms, with inward deep penetration by cords having core of squamous cells and keratin.

of waste products is reflected by the serious systemic consequences of malfunction. Conversely, systemic disease, and especially alterations of the cardiovascular system (*see* Section 16.1), may markedly impair renal function. The kidneys are major sites of pathological change; structures and mechanisms involved in renal function are complex and contribute to the varied pathology displayed.

The urinary tract is of major consequence only in relation to its fluid transporting role. Tract components (e.g. the ureters and bladder) are subject to general disease processes but little special pathology, and only obstruction or infection have particular bearing on renal pathology. The urinary tract may provide a route along which infection from the exterior may penetrate as far as the kidneys. Otherwise, the kidneys are readily accessible only to bloodborne agents or influences.

Because of relative inaccessibility, knowledge of kidney disease has been gained more from clinical functional studies than from structural studies. The identification of pathological change used to be dependent on postmortem or material extracted during surgery. Percutaneous renal biopsy now makes it possible to obtain samples from living kidneys for diagnosis and research. Nevertheless, it appears to be a feature of renal disease that each major clinical condition recognised may be due to several different causes, and each may damage the kidneys in various ways. Thus, the relationship of malfunctions to pathological lesion types are even less specific than those applying generally throughout the body.

A consideration of kidney structure (*see* Section 7.6) underlines the complexity of renal function and accounts for some aspects of the distribution of pathological damage. Differences in structure and function result in parts of the nephrons being special target sites for some pathology (Fig. 16.13).

Renal Malfunction

Numerous individual aspects of renal function may become defective, often without overt structural abnormality. These are predominantly biochemical disorders, resulting in renal tubular transport defects (Table 16.11) in the proximal or distal tubules or sometimes in the collecting tubes. These may often be congenital disorders with one or more types occurring together. Multiple metabolic pathway abnormality (Fanconi's syndrome) was originally associated with rickets and involved defects in the proximal tubular reabsorption of calcium, phosphate, and glucose. However, the term has been extended to include conditions of varied aetiology involving loss of protein, amino acids, peptides, bicarbonate, and potassium (e.g. drug or toxic effects and endocrine disorders). Abnormalities in urine content may result simply from fluid intake, nutritional, or metabolic circumstances (e.g. ethanol intake or solute overload due to excessive excretion of sodium or glucose). Excessive water loss (e.g. in diabetes insipidus) and changes in acid-base balance (due to respiratory or metabolic acidosis and alkalosis) are of particular note.

TABLE 16.11
Disorders in functions of renal tubules (with or without structural defects)

Function	Defect
Acid-base balance and pH control	alkalosis or acidosis, abnormal HCO_3^-, H^+ ion, or ammonia excretion
Amino-acid reabsorption	possible defects in active-transport mechanisms (four different groups) give aminoacidurias (e.g. cystinuria)
Calcium reabsorption	overload due to hypercalcaemia
General functions	Fanconi's syndrome (multiple failures giving amino acid, calcium, glucose, phosphate, bicarbonate, and potassium losses)
Magnesium reabsorption	usually secondary to drug or toxic action
Phosphate reabsorption	related to calcium excretion or conservation
Potassium excretion	both over- and underactivity possible
Sodium reabsorption (with chloride)	hyponatraemia and excessive sodium, chloride, and water excretion
Urate excretion	balance of reabsorption and active secretion upset. Gout may be associated with impaired excretion. Competition with lactic acid in pre-eclampsia of pregnancy and β-hydroxybutyric acid in diabetes mellitus
Urinary concentration	diabetes insipidus (excessive water excretion, polyuria)

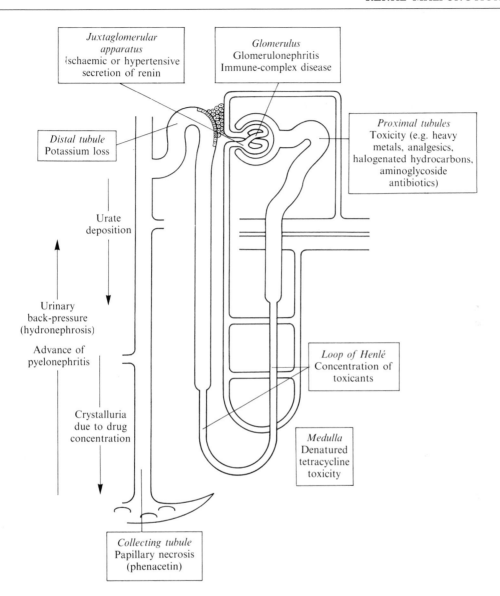

Fig. 16.13
Representation of nephron structure showing locations of particular forms of pathological lesions.

Electrolyte disturbances in body fluids and tissues may arise because of abnormalities in excretion of sodium (primary aldosteronism or corticosteroid deficiency), potassium (thiazide diuretics), or calcium (parathyroid disorders). Not all urinary changes are attributable to tubular malfunction; urea and creatinine levels reflect changes in glomerular function.

More serious or extensive malfunction, usually with distinct structural pathology, gives rise to renal failure in which urine production is decreased or excretion impaired. Urinary volumes may decrease to less than 400 mL per day (oliguria) but severe cases may produce less than 100 mL per day (anuria). Such failure may occur in the absence of renal damage from systemic causes which reduce blood flow and give very low urinary filtration. Thus, renal failure may be a feature of heart failure, shock, or conditions which reduce blood volume (e.g. haemorrhage, severe burns, dehydration, diarrhoea, or vomiting). Anuria or oliguria may also be due to obstruction. Acute renal failure occurs as a sudden change in urine production and a consequent rise in plasma-urea concentrations which may, in particular, be due to tubular necrosis. Most cases of acute failure, with or without tubular damage, are potentially reversible. In contrast, chronic renal failure is insidious in onset, more likely to be persistent, and radically alters body fluids. Generally, this results from progressive loss of nephrons due to a variety of causes which are mostly destructive but include obstruction.

Another important clinical disorder with a multiplicity of possible causes is nephrotic syndrome. In contrast to renal failure urine production continues, although failure may supervene. Protein is lost in the urine, which is due to glomerular membrane defects. As a result of loss of plasma protein, water cannot be retained in blood and passes out into the tissues, resulting in oedema. Associated renal tubular disorders, lipid accumulation, and sodium retention may or may not be directly due to the glomerular membrane defects.

Nephron Cellular Damage

Cells of the convoluted tubules are particularly vulnerable to a variety of pathological influences as a result of their active-transport functions. Active transport may cause the accumulation of high concentrations of toxic agents in these cells. Active-transport processes also impose high demands for energy, oxygen, and nutrient and these cells are further examples of tissues particularly susceptible to hypoxia and general cytoplasmic toxicity. Acute tubular necrosis leads to acute renal failure. Hydropic degeneration (with cellular swelling), necrosis (with cellular disintegration), and general protein loss with coagulation (producing protein casts in the lumen) are causes of tubular blockage. Tubular swelling and renal interstitial oedema also cause diminished blood flow which reduces glomerular filtration, resulting in anuria. Excessive fluid reabsorption is also a cause of anuria. Complete functional breakdown results when necrosis leads to tubular rupture in any part of the nephron (tubulorrhexis).

Locations of hypoxic or toxic damage in the renal tubules are quite specific and often both effects operate together. Nephrotoxicity causes lesions predominantly in the proximal convoluted tubules, with different agents affecting specific portions (e.g. chromates damage the initial third, chlorates the middle portion, and mercury salts or ethylene glycol the terminal third). Carbon tetrachloride and excessive alcohol concentrations affect convoluted tubules less specifically. Ischaemic necrotic effects may be even more extensive, with damage also occurring in distal and collecting tubules. Kidney tubular ischaemia is a common sequel to limb damage (crush injuries), surgical operations, burns, obstetric haemorrhage, and other conditions causing shock or hypotension.

Another location of toxic lesions is the mass of collecting tubules running through the medullary and pyramidal portions of the kidney. Urine passing through these tubules is progressively concentrated as water is lost, and toxic effects may become more severe or damage may occur from deposition of masses of crystals (e.g. from sulphonamides or following metabolism of glycol to oxalate). The consequent renal papillary necrosis is a notable effect associated in previous years with analgesic abuse, particularly by phenacetin consumption in high doses or for long periods.

Not all toxicity causes direct nephron damage. Interstitial nephritis, with numerous and varied causative agents (e.g. penicillins, cephalosporins, phenindione, allopurinol, or diphenylhydantoin), appears to be an immune-complex disease. Inflammation of the cortex and medulla, oedema, and cell infiltration lead to scarring fibrosis of the kidney parenchyma. Damage and atrophy of glomerular and tubular structures are secondary.

Renal Infection

Infections cause nephron damage with inflammation in the kidney and may produce blockage throughout the urinary tract. Kidney tissue infection may be generalised (pyelonephritis) or confined to the pelvic space (pyelitis). Further down the urinary tract, infection occurs as cystitis (bladder) or urethritis (urethra), and bacteriuria may occur. Normally the urinary tract remains sterile but pathogens may penetrate via the blood (bacteraemia or septicaemia) or by migration from the distal third of the urethra, which may readily harbour them. Reflux of urine from the bladder into the ureters is prevented by valves and downward peristalsis, but upward travel may be achieved by motile micro-organisms or when urine flow is obstructed (e.g. by stones, stricture, or prostate enlargement). Infection often originates from the perineum, where *Escherichia coli* predominates; *Proteus* spp., *Pseudomonas pyocyanea*, and *Streptococcus faecalis* may also cause such infection. Urinary-tract infections are commoner in females due to the very short urethra.

Pyelonephritis is likely when the medulla is damaged, this part being most susceptible as it has a lesser blood supply. Such infection may become chronic, causing scarring and renal papillary necrosis. Dead papillary tissue may slough away, contributing to obstruction downstream, while secondary shrinkage may occlude glomeruli or cause hypertension. Chronicity of pyelonephritis may be explained by the scarring and the transformation of micro-organisms into immunity- and antibiotic-resistant protoplasts.

Glomerulonephritis

The glomerulus differs from the rest of the nephron in possessing specialised blood vessels in the capillary tuft. Glomeruli are less affected by the general cellular pathology afflicting tubules, but are subject to special attack by immunological processes and vascular disease. Resultant glomerulonephritis is characterised as a group of conditions involving defective glomerular filtration function. In most cases, this is associated with distinctive and varied structural lesions; any associated renal tubular damage is usually secondary. Despite the limitation in the ways whereby a tissue can reflect damage (*see* Section 15.3), the lesions of glomerulonephritis display considerable variety, leading to complex classification. This is a reflection of the complexity of the structure. Unfortunately, discernible categories of glomerular lesion do not correlate precisely with the diverse range of causes or the resultant clinical manifestations. World Health Organization classifications recognise four classes of glomerulonephritis based on direct or indirect cause (Table 16.12), and five classes of clinical malfunction, including combinations of renal failure, nephrotic syndrome, and haemorrhage. The classification of glomerular features may range from minimal change glomerulonephritis, in which there is little or no structural abnormality, to nephrotic syndrome, with crescentic proliferative or sclerosing lesions, involving massive cellular or fibrous obliteration of the structures. It would appear that the various glomerulonephritis changes may occur in the kidneys on their own or in association with major systemic diseases, particularly of the blood vessels.

Mechanisms producing glomerulonephritis appear to be mainly based upon immune-complex disease (a type III hypersensitive reaction, *see* Section 15.6) in which circulating immunoglobulins complex with antigenic material and activate complement. This takes place in the walls of glomerular blood vessels or on and in the basement membrane, with components of these possibly comprising the antigen. Due to complement activation, neutrophils infiltrate the glomeruli and cause damage. Plasma-protein exudation and coagulation also occur, resulting in fibrin deposition. There is thus an inflammatory and fibrinoid necrosis combination which is often accompanied by proliferation of supporting (mesangial) cells. As a result, capillaries are occluded and glomerular flow blocked. In the filtrate space, deposited fibrin is phagocytosed by macrophages which gather in masses, giving further space-occupying (crescent) structures.

Other hypersensitivity mechanisms (types II or IV) may also operate and overall there is a strong association of glomerulonephritis with a wide range of immunological diseases (e.g. auto-immune, rheumatoid, and some chronic systemic infections).

TABLE 16.12
Classification of renal glomerular lesions or malfunctions

Structural lesions

- minimal change glomerulonephritis
  little or no observable structural pathology

- focal and segmental lesions
  different distributions in glomeruli

- diffuse glomerulonephritis
  divided into membranous or proliferative types; proliferation involves capillaries, and mesangial or monocyte cells; monocytes form crescents

Aetiological relationships

- primary glomerulonephritis
  direct immune attack

- secondary to systemic diseases
  infective endocarditis, syphilis, malaria, or auto-immune diseases

- secondary to vascular diseases
  also numerous auto-immune cases

- secondary to metabolic disease
  diabetes mellitus, amyloidosis, sickle-cell anaemia

Clinical manifestations

- acute nephritis

- chronic nephritis

- recurrent haematuria
  blood and protein in urine

- nephrotic syndrome

- rapidly progressive glomerulonephritis
  combination of nephrotic syndrome, renal failure, and haemorrhage

Renal Involvement in Systemic Disease

A wide range of renal diseases, particularly those caused by ischaemia or other vascular impairment, have a two-way causal relationship with hypertension. The association of chronic renal failure with progressively irreversible hypertension was recognised by Bright in 1827. Renal arterial occlusion (e.g. as a result of atheroma or thrombosis) or other blood deprivation may cause tubular atrophy, renal failure, and hypertension.

Reversible (essential) hypertension is partly explained by activation of the juxtaglomerular tissue in the kidney when the blood supply is reduced, so that the cells secrete renin and activate the hormone, angiotensin.

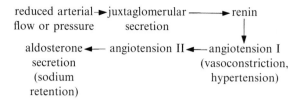

A reverse influence appears to operate as progressive arteriosclerosis develops in association with persistent (malignant) hypertension. This causes haemorrhage and fibrinoid necrosis in glomeruli, plus hyaline degeneration and necrosis in tubules. Thus, renal damage is caused and may be superimposed on existing lesions and renal failure.

The kidney may be affected by serious pathology in diabetes mellitus, in addition to functional renal disorders such as glycosuria, osmotic diuresis, and keto-acidosis. Renal failure is a common feature of Type I diabetes mellitus. Diabetic nephropathy affects the glomerulus, particularly with developing proteinuria. The lesions have some characteristics in common with glomerulonephritis although the damage mainly affects the capillaries. Larger blood vessels (e.g. renal arterioles) are affected by fibrinoid necrosis.

Chronic infection elsewhere in the body (e.g. tuberculosis or osteomyelitis) or chronic inflammatory disease (e.g. rheumatoid arthritis) may result in amyloid deposition in the kidneys and insidious development of substantial blood vessel and nephron damage. Amyloidosis may also occur in the kidneys as a primary disease.

Cystic Disease

Embryological development of the nephrons requires the growth and ultimate linkage of two sets of tubular structures derived from the ureteral bud and the metanephric blastema. The ureteral bud forms the ureter, renal pelvis, and collecting tubules of the kidney itself. The metanephric blastema forms the convoluted tubules, loops of Henlé, and glomeruli, which comprise the rest of the nephron structures. Genetic or teratogenic defects in these developments may lead to complete or partial omission of structures (e.g. ureters or even whole kidneys). Other abnormalities occur due to faults in the union of the two embryonic nephron components, typically giving rise to malformations with cysts and cavities. A variety of forms of polycystic disease may occur in infancy or adulthood, with single or multiple cysts (e.g. polcystic kidney disease) of variable sizes; kidney function is commonly impaired or totally absent.

Other Aspects

The kidney, like any other tissue, is subject to neoplasia and it is worthy of note that Wilms' tumour is one of the most common types of malignant tumour in children, in whom neoplasia are relatively rare. Carcinogen-induced tumours may occur in the bladder associated with urinary concentration of the agent or the excretion of a carcinogenic metabolite (e.g. β-naphthylamine or acetylaminofluorene).

Due to excessive excretion or urinary concentration, deposits of urates or calcium salts may occur, forming urinary calculi. These may cause obstruction in the tract or direct kidney damage.

16.9   OPHTHALMIC PATHOLOGY

Introduction

In relation to its size, a diseased eye can be the source of seemingly disproportionate discomfort or distress. Serious malfunction may be handicapping and loss of function disabling. Of course, some of the more dire possibilities are countered by duplication of the organ and the robust nature of the eyes. Nevertheless, world-wide figures indicate between 10 and 15 million blind people and immense numbers are afflicted by serious eye infections (e.g. trachoma). In developed countries the incidence of blindness is lower than underdeveloped nations, but still stands at about 200 per 100 000 of the population, with glaucoma, diabetes mellitus, and cataract among the main causes.

The vulnerability of eyes to pathological influences may be likened to that of other surface structures (e.g. see Section 16.7). Thus, there are possibilities of traumatic and foreign-body damage, contact with corrosive or irritant materials, access by infectious agents or allergens, and physical effects (e.g. damage by exposure to intense visible light). Ranged against these are special protective measures. These include shielding by the eyelids and the iris, very effective irrigation to wash away harmful materials (lachrymal secretion and drainage), provision of anti-infective influences (tear components including lysozyme), and avoidance or closure mechanisms carried out by sensory nerves and reflexes (e.g. iris closure, blinking, and tear secretion). The eyes are subject to disease resulting from the pathology of other systems (e.g. diabetes mellitus or hypertension) and are closely involved in any effects on surrounding or accessory structures (orbital, muscular, and secretory tissues). Sight itself depends upon a healthy optic nerve and the appropriate brain functions. Tumours, haemorrhages, infection, or ischaemia affecting these structures may all give rise to blindness.

Inflammatory Conditions

The most exposed surfaces of the eye (i.e. the cornea and conjunctiva) will be most frequently affected by influences which cause inflammation. Surrounding external structures (e.g. the eyelids) may also be affected and inflammation may occur in internal structures (e.g. the uveal tract). Inflammation affects vascular connective tissues (*see* Section 15.4) and will therefore occur only in those parts of the ophthalmic structures receiving blood. Mechanisms, signs, and symptoms will be much the same as those of inflammation anywhere and are apparent as a painful red eye. The eye is contained within relatively inextensible layers of tissue and its structures are maintained under tension by pressure generated internally. As a result, there is less scope for swelling than appears in looser tissues elsewhere. Local alterations of pressure due to inflammatory oedema may cause damage, malfunction, and discomfort.

Acute conjunctivitis is usually attributable to infection, particularly by bacteria (*Haemophilus aegyptius, H. influenzae*, and *Diplococcus pneumoniae*, which may account for epidemic episodes, or *Staphylococcus aureus*). Such micro-organisms may be derived from infections established in the eyelids (e.g. stye) or by finger or cough transmission associated with respiratory-tract infection. In some cases, skin commensals may gain access and thrive. Infection is aided by trauma or surface erosion (e.g. by foreign bodies). There is a groove in the under surface of each eyelid, running 2 mm from the margin, where grit or other particles become lodged and cause discomfort and damage. Infections invade the spaces beneath the conjunctival membrane which covers the sclera of the eye and lines the eyelids (*see* Section 11.2). The cornea is less readily affected because the conjunctiva is closely adherent. Elsewhere, the richly vascularised conjunctiva may become very red. Bacterial infections may cause pus-like exudation (e.g. the 'sticky eye' (ophthalmia neonatorum) of newborn babies). Eyedrops contaminated with *Pseudomonas pyocyanea* have been known to cause severe conjunctivitis. Other severe infections may result from gonorrhoeal and diphtheral infections, the former still being an important cause of blindness in children in some parts of the world.

Viral infections are also commonly associated with acute conjunctival infections (e.g. adenoviruses, measles virus, and rubella virus). Types 7 and 8 adenoviruses have been the cause of serious epidemic outbreaks of keratoconjunctivitis. These infections display the typical pattern of the inflamed red eye, causing a particularly 'gritty' discomfort. When there is corneal involvement (keratitis) the discomfort may be severe, with pain, photophobia, lachrymation, and blepharospasm. Haemorrhages are also prevalent in the cornea. Viral infections are generally spread by finger contact and eye rubbing following contagion contact. Local epidemics are especially associated with dirty occupations, with risks of eye damage due to foreign bodies (e.g. metalswarf particles). Family contacts and even medical treatment (e.g. eye-wash contamination or the use of an ophthalmic tonometer) can spread infection.

Other forms of conjunctival inflammation also result from access of harmful materials. Direct access of irritants and corrosive agents (e.g. gases, vapours, and aerosols of acids in the air) affect the eye surface at the same time as attacking the respiratory system. The other major cause of acute conjunctivitis is allergy, with probably any material provoking allergy in general also capable of affecting the eye. Drugs (e.g. physostigmine, atropine, and sulphacetamide) and cosmetic applications have been recognised as common sensitisers of this kind. The production of red watery eyes may be associated with eczema of surrounding skin. Bacterial allergy developing from tuberculosis or local staphylococcal infections of the eyelids (blepharitis) may cause a more persistent damaging (ulcerative) condition, phlyctenular conjunctivitis. Another very common form of allergy which usually occurs as part of allergic rhinitis is vernal keratoconjunctivitis. Seasonal and recurrent attacks associated with allergy to pollens in the air cause conjunctival inflammation, epithelial thickening, and some fibrosis if the attacks are prolonged. Surface ulceration may also occur. Inflammatory cell infiltrations cause a discharge from the eye and swelling of lymph nodules around the eye.

Most forms of inflammation develop chronic characteristics (*see* Section 15.4) if the causes are persistent, although in some cases causes are not readily apparent. One important infection, featuring scarring inflammation, is trachoma, which is caused by members of the *Chlamydia* genus. Initial symptoms of red eye and follicle formation develop into the growth of vascular fibrous pannus over corneal and eyelid surfaces, leading further to ulceration and causing blindness. Other forms of chronic inflammation may take the form of granuloma formation, usually as nodules. Persistence of foreign bodies or surgical sutures probably accounts for most of these lesions, whilst tuberculosis is another occasional cause. These effects may not be restricted to the conjunctiva.

Inflammation of structures deeper in the eye occurs particularly in the uvea (*see* Section 11.2) and comprises iridocyclitis or uveitis, although local variations do occur. This inflammation produces another version of red eye in which the associated pain is deep-seated and often severe. The main problems accruing from this inflammation are adhesion of the iris to the lens and internal pressure changes, due to vascular congestion and swelling or exudation in the ciliary body. Cataract and secondary glaucoma might be later developments. The sclerotic coat of the eye may also be affected by inflammation; episcleritis describes involvement of the layer beneath the conjunctiva and scleritis affects deeper layers. Infections are less common causes of inflammation of the deeper eye structures unless caused by penetrating injuries. Allergy or auto-immune mechanisms are thought to be the usual causes of uveitis and there is a recognised association of incidence of this eye condition with genital infections and arthritis (Reiter's syndrome). Uveitis and ankylosing spondylitis is another combination suggesting auto-immune aetiology.

Corneal Injury

The normal absence of vascular supply in the corneal area requires that responses to damage have to be considered separately from general inflammatory conditions. However, the cornea is continuous with surrounding structures and is frequently involved with other conjunctival pathology. Corneal ulceration is the main consequence of injury or infection and one frequently leads to the other. Ulcer development represents necrosis of the conjunctival epithelium, oedema, and inflammatory cell infiltration. The cellular infiltration, comprising mainly neutrophils, may lead to the accumulation of a cellular sediment (hypopyon) in the aqueous humour of the anterior chamber. Ulceration is accompanied by pain, blepharospasm, and lachrymation. Cavitation of the membrane may occasionally progress to a perforation, with more extensive internal damage to the lens and uveal structures. Otherwise, ulcers tend to heal by filling with fibroblasts and development of granulation tissue with blood vessels. These scarring changes in early life may regress without impeding vision, but more opaque plaques of scar tissue may be left from ulcers in later life.

Infections with herpesviruses in the eye cause herpetic or dendritic ulcers. Early herpetic infections may be readily confused with other conjunctival inflammation and corticosteroids applied as treatment. This exacerbates herpes infections and should be avoided. Herpesvirus infections are often not restricted to the cornea, and may be described as keratoconjunctivitis. The resulting ulcers are star-shaped or branching and, although the lesions are not purulent, secondary bacterial infections may change their character to include pus discharge and hypopyon. Infections may penetrate and affect the uvea, at which time the condition becomes especially painful. Secondary cataract or glaucoma may result.

Glaucoma

The flow of aqueous humour (*see* Section 11.2) is commonly impeded in two ways, either of which causes its accumulation and results in raised intra-ocular pressure. Open-angle glaucoma is due to impaired drainage of the aqueous humour, which causes distension of anterior and posterior chambers. Pressure elevations are usually not severe (from the normal 10 to 20 mmHg up to 25 to 35 mmHg). Closed-angle glaucoma results from confinement of fluid in the posterior chamber, usually also associated with drainage occlusion. Pressure may increase more severely and acutely than most open-angle cases, attaining levels of 40 to 100 mmHg or more. In either form, visual defects (e.g. blurring and coloured haloes) occur due to distortion and physical changes in the cornea or lens. Discomfort may be minimal in insidious or early cases but in acute closed-angle attacks, severe pain accompanies the marked and rapid ocular congestion. This produces an emergency situation requiring early control to prevent permanent damage or blindness. Prolonged or severe pressure may cause damage deep within the eye (e.g. death of optic nerve and retinal cells, and optic disc deterioration). Scotomas develop in visual fields. Corneal epithelial transparency may be affected by oedema, and stretching damage eventually leads to granulation or pannus-scarring and opacity.

Each form of glaucoma may occur as primary or secondary disease and there is also a congenital variety. Primary open-angle cases involve defects in the trabecular meshwork of the ciliary body and breakdown in the fibrous structure which channels filtration fluid into the canal of Schlemm. In secondary cases (e.g. iridocyclitis), these drainage channels may be blocked by foreign material, tissue debris, iron deposits, material from lens disintegration, or other forms of occlusion. Primary closed-angle glaucoma results from the development of an eye in which the anterior chamber is shallow, the lens is sited too close to the iris, or the iris is pushed forwards to close the filtration angle. Mydriatic drugs which dilate the pupil cause the peripheral iris to bulge forward and block the path to the drainage trabeculae. They are therefore contra-indicated in patients with closed-angle glaucoma. Secondary closed-angle disease may result from inflammatory, neoplastic, oedematous, or traumatic damage to ciliary body, iris, or lens structures.

Cataract

Degenerative changes in the lens which lead to loss of transparency are of a similar form, irrespective of the aetiology (i.e. developmental cataract or degenerative cataract). Changes occur through the action of proteolytic enzymes on the proteins of the lens. These protease actions are favoured in the moderately acidic environment (pH 5) which develops with age. The accumulation of smaller molecules (peptides and amino acids) increases osmotic pressure and water is drawn in, which results in swelling of the lens. One exception to the action of the proteolytic enzymes is the protein component, α-crystallin, which does not lyse but coagulates; water is also drawn in from this action. Water accumulates in vacuoles and fissures which separate the lens fibres. The fibres swell, disintegrate, and clump, ultimately forming rounded masses of degenerate material (Morgagni globules) and other more jagged fragments which float in the fluid. Thus, the lens undergoes partial liquefaction. It may initially remain transparent but the accumulated debris renders it milky. Loss of transparency is also due to proliferation of epithelial cells in an irregular layer, which surround the lens and gradually thicken (sclerosis). If this capsule becomes impermeable, the fluid is retained and the residue (nucleus) of the lens becomes displaced or completely dissolved. Alternatively, the fluid gradually passes out through the capsule wall, leaving the residual material, often calcified, within a shrunken wrinkled shell.

Inflammation may develop in or around a damaged lens with cataracts. Cells (e.g. neutrophils and macrophages) contribute to the enzymatic destruction of the lens fibres. Escape of material from the lens may give rise to further inflammation (lens-induced ophthalmitis or phacoanaphylactic ophthalmitis). There is evidence that this results from an allergic response (*see* Section 15.6) to antigenic lens material. A suppurative or granulomatous inflammation develops in the anterior chamber, affecting the lens and uveal structures. Unless the offending material is removed, damage may be severe with scarring. Blockage of the fluid drainage by lens or cellular debris may cause phacolytic glaucoma.

In lens-induced ophthalmitis only one eye is affected, unless the other subsequently acquires a damaged cataract. This is in direct contrast to sympathetic ophthalmitis, in which uveitis commences in one eye and is subsequently matched by similar activity in the other eye after 2 to 8 weeks. This combination is almost invariably associated with a penetrating injury of the eyeball involving the uvea. Severe inflammation affects the ciliary bodies, iris, and choroid layers of both eyes, producing scarring granulomatous damage usually with secondary glaucoma. Cell-mediated auto-immunity to uveal protein may be the cause; material released in one eye causes allergy which results in an attack on both.

Retinopathies

The light-detecting innermost layer of the main chamber, the optic or neural retina, is essentially an extension of the central nervous system and its pathology has similar features (*see* Section 16.5). The retina consists of layers of neuronal cells and processes (*see* Section 11.2) which are unmyelinated and thus resemble grey matter of the brain. Like cerebrocortical cells, they are particularly susceptible to deprivation of nutrients and oxygen. Hence, the retina is highly dependent upon its blood supply. Blood reaches the retina through the underlying ciliary blood vessels of the choroid coat and the surface vessels from the central retinal artery. Neither of these supplies are alone sufficient to maintain adequate oxygenation of the retinal neurones. Partial ischaemia and consequent hypoxia produce distinctive degeneration of the unmyelinated axons, which may be observed on the retinal surface as 'cotton wool spots'. These are due to local hydropic swelling (*see* Section 15.3) and occur when there is blood vessel blockage (e.g. by microthrombi, fat-globule embolism, or bacterial clumps). In the short-term this damage may be reversible, but neuronal necrosis results readily from more complete ischaemia. Occlusion of the retinal artery (e.g. by atheroma or thrombosis) causes extensive infarction because it is an 'end-artery' (i.e. it has no collateral branches or alternative blood pathways). Necrosis also results when the retina is torn from the choroid. Retinal neurones do not regenerate and the dead tissue collapses or is replaced by glial scar tissue (*see* Section 16.5). Blockage of the retinal vein also causes infarction and haemorrhages due to the continued arterial pressure. Eventually, new growths of blood vessels on the retina and outgrowths into blood clots attempt to establish new paths for blood flow.

Ageing changes in the arterial branches give rise to arteriosclerosis (*see* Section 16.1), which is characterised by distinctive ophthalmoscopic appearance and some retinopathy. Thickened vessels may be accompanied by 'cotton wool spot' swellings, haemorrhages, and retinal exudates (fatty deposits). If arteriosclerosis is systemically widespread, blood pressure will correspondingly be raised. Hypertensive retinopathy may be the result of benign or malignant hypertension or preeclampsia. Patches of vessel constriction, exudation, haemorrhage, oedema, and even retinal detachment may occur variably, depending on the severity of the hypertension.

Different pathology results from diabetic retinopathy, although this may often be complicated by simultaneous arteriosclerotic and hypertensive effects. Diabetic changes initially affect mainly the retinal capillaries, which develop microaneurysms. These globular swellings probably represent local weakness in wall structures, giving rise to expansion and subsequent nodular deposits of lipopolysaccharide. Other exudation of blood, lipid, or plasma protein also occurs. A distinctive later change involves arteriolar closures and new capillary formations, giving tufts or fronds of overgrown vessel loops. In all of these changes, loss of neurones from the retina accompanies the varying degrees of ischaemia and anoxia.

16.10   ARTHRITIC LESIONS, CONNECTIVE TISSUE DISORDERS, AND AUTO-IMMUNE DISEASE

Introduction

These conditions are generally characterised by aggressive inflammation causing damage to tissues. Several categories need to be considered, determined either by the typical distribution of the lesions or by what is understood of the mechanism of the disease. In arthritic lesions (rheumatoid disease) the damage especially involves the joints. The main examples are rheumatoid arthritis, osteoarthritis (osteoarthrosis), ankylosing spondylitis, rheumatic fever, and gout, although in some of these, the lesions are not restricted to the skeleton but also occur in various soft tissues. Another group of less well-known diseases presents inflammatory damage of various non-skeletal tissues, with mechanisms connected with rheumatoid pathology and are called pararheumatoid. Examples are systemic lupus erythematosus, systemic sclerosis, polyarteritis nodosa, and dermatomyositis. These conditions were formerly known as collagen diseases as deterioration in collagen (collagen necrosis) is a feature. Currently, a more generally applicable term, connective tissue disorders, is used.

Causes and mechanisms are still not fully elucidated, but for most of the examples there are increasingly strong indications that activity of the immune system is involved. In some examples there are also strong associations with various infections, which usually precede the rheumatoid or pararheumatoid development. The pathology primarily involves auto-immunity or immune reactivity determined in some way by the infection. This

indicates a strong link between rheumatoid and pararheumatoid diseases and other conditions which are most distinctly recognised as being of auto-immune aetiology (Table 16.13). Diseases of auto-immune aetiology display apparently specific, immune-based, tissue-damaging effects on particular target organs or tissues. In contrast, rheumatoid and pararheumatoid diseases produce more diverse effects. All three groups are probably distinct from conditions of allergy and hypersensitivity (see Section 15.6), although the likely immunopathological mechanisms are related.

Arthritic Lesions

Rheumatoid arthritis is typified by inflammatory lesions affecting the synovial linings of peripheral joints. The distribution of lesions is usually symmetrical and parts affected differ from those in comparable diseases (Fig. 16.14). Arthritic lesions start as acute inflammation marked by dilatation of blood vessels, congestion, oedema, and subsequent cellular infiltration. The inflamed membrane becomes swollen, folded, and hyperplastic and the whole joint swells. The synovial fluid becomes more viscous due to increased protein content, and coagulated fibrin forms a layer on the synovial surface, both of which impede the free movement of the joint surfaces, contributing to further damage.

TABLE 16.13
Auto-immune diseases

Specific organ or tissue malfunctions associated with aggressive immune cell or antibody-mediated damage, destroying apparently normal target tissues or related materials	
Organ or tissue	Disease
Adrenal cortex	Addison's disease (non-tubercular)
Brain (myelin)	multiple sclerosis
Cutaneous epidermal cells	pemphigus
Erythrocytes	haemolytic anaemia
Gastric parietal cells (or intrinsic factor)	pernicious anaemia
Islets of Langerhans (or insulin molecules)	diabetes mellitus
Lens	ophthalmia
Platelets	thrombotic thrombocytopenic purpura
Skeletal muscle	myasthenia gravis
Thyroid gland (or thyroglobulin or thyrotrophin molecules)	thyroiditis, Graves' disease, Hashimoto's thyroiditis, or hypothyroidism

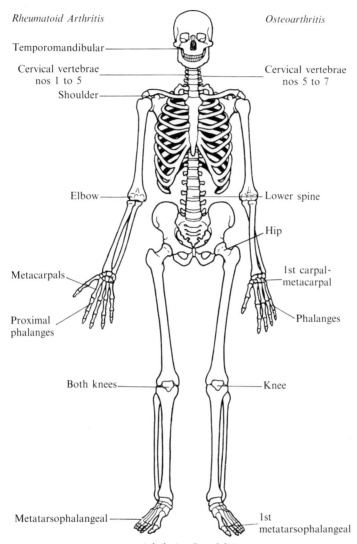

Rheumatoid Arthritis

Temporomandibular

Cervical vertebrae
nos 1 to 5

Shoulder

Elbow

Metacarpals

Proximal
phalanges

Both knees

Metatarsophalangeal

Osteoarthritis

Cervical vertebrae
nos 5 to 7

Lower spine

Hip

1st carpal-
metacarpal

Phalanges

Knee

1st
metatarsophalangeal

Ankylosing Spondylitis
(cervical, thoracic, and lumbar spine,
costosternal, sacro-iliac, hip, and knee)

Fig. 16.14
Diagram of skeleton showing the locations of joints particularly affected by rheumatoid arthritis, osteoarthritis, and ankylosing spondylitis.

Chronic or repeated development of the disease leads to scarring of the joints. Fibroblast infiltration of damaged membrane leads to pannus formation, a form of granulation tissue (*see* Section 15.4). Ingrowth of this fibrous tissue replaces the normal articular surface membrane, further limiting the movement and even forming connections between apposing surfaces. These fibrous adhesions account for the stiffness of rheumatoid joints, particularly in the morning or after a period of inactivity. Pannus formation can lead to distortion of the joint, and adhesion of surfaces can result in eventual consolidation and immobility (ankylosis). At the same time, articular cartilage beneath the pannus becomes eroded by inflammatory cells extending into the underlying bone. Such changes cause weakening, distortion, and immobilisation of the joint which may ultimately become permanently calcified.

Another feature of rheumatoid arthritis is the development of granuloma-type nodules in tissues other than the joints (i.e. in soft tissues). These rheumatoid nodules occur especially in tissues overlying prominent bony joints (e.g. knuckles, elbows, heels, knees, and buttocks). Unlike synovial lesions, soft-tissue lesions form around foci of necrotic connective tissue (fibrinoid necrosis). This is surrounded by a macrophage granuloma (*see* Section 15.4), usually also with lymphocytes and plasma cells and an outermost layer of fibrous granulation tissue. Nodules or more diffuse inflammatory lesions may also be found in internal viscera and account for serious complications. The heart may be affected by pericarditis, lesions in the coronary vessels, or nodules in the aorta. Similar damage may occur in lungs, eyes, and other tissues. Nodules in the brain are unknown, although nerve damage may occur when blood supplies are impeded by lesions.

Diverse vasculitis in both arterioles and venules may be common, with or without associated nodular lesions. There is a central focus of fibrinoid necrosis in the vessel walls, around which infiltrated monocytes and other inflammatory cells accumulate. Fibrosis may surround the lesion. These changes may cause occlusion of the vessel, with or without thrombus formation. Areas supplied by vessels with vasculitis are likely to suffer ischaemia and further necrosis. Infarcts of brain, heart, lung, kidney, and intestines may therefore be important complications of rheumatoid arthritis.

Ankylosing spondylitis is a similar condition although the lesions affect different articular structures (*see* Fig. 16.14). The lesions are characterised by destructive inflammation affecting the cartilaginous joints, particularly the intervertebral discs of the spine. The synovial membranes become acutely inflamed, followed by infiltration of inflammatory cells which spread and erode the cartilage. Other foci of inflammation occur in adjacent bone. Structural erosion is accompanied by formation of fibrous granulation tissue, which continues until the joint is completely fibrosed. Such joints ultimately become calcified and ankylosed, fusing the bones together. In this manner, the spine becomes united to give the completely inflexible and often deformed 'bamboo spine'. Joints connecting the ribs and spine are also affected. In addition, there are inflammatory lesions of soft tissue but not the distinctly nodular structures of rheumatoid arthritis.

Osteoarthritis is another form of degenerative joint disease which, like rheumatoid arthritis, affects the diarthrodial joints but with a different distribution (*see* Fig. 16.14) and no soft tissue lesions. The aetiology probably also differs. The lesions occur in the cartilage rather than in the synovial membranes, causing degeneration of the cartilage matrix. Joint movement results in shearing effects, causing fissuring and erosion of the cartilage until the underlying bone is exposed. Con-

tinued joint movement wears and polishes the bone until it is hard and ivory-like. In the bone itself, destructive mechanisms also operate. The bone structure is remodelled by osteoblast and fibroblast activity, forming dense fibrous and highly calcified bone with vascular channels. Cysts form in places and the surface layers may collapse and destroy the joint. Osteophytes or Heberden's nodes are excrescences of bone developing at the edge of osteoarthritic joints as a result of remodelling. Thus, osteoarthritis progresses to joint destruction, whereas the other rheumatoid conditions lead to joint fusion. An important distinction is that use of osteoarthritic joints aggravates the condition, whereas rheumatoid diseases benefit from exercise.

Gout also causes inflammatory lesions of joints and the damage extends into overlying tissues, thus superficially resembling rheumatoid arthritis. However, this is essentially a metabolic disorder, with excessive concentrations of uric acid in the blood resulting in precipitation of crystalline deposits in or around certain joints. These urate deposits provoke inflammation, joint destruction, and deformity and cause nodular distortions (tophi) around joints.

Not the least important example of a rheumatoid disease is rheumatic fever. This has a great deal in common with rheumatoid arthritis, showing similar inflammatory lesions in joints and soft tissues. However, the condition is essentially acute, although long-term consequences may remain from the scars of lesions. Moreover, it is mainly a disease of childhood and, more than any of the other rheumatoid diseases, is directly associated with infection. The first manifestation of the disease is usually a sore throat caused by Group A β-haemolytic streptococci. Sustained fever and migratory polyarthritis develop at least three weeks later. The joint lesions resemble the initial phases of rheumatoid arthritis, and are characterised by swelling, redness, pain, and warmth. In addition, there is vascular congestion, synovial membrane hypertrophy, and infiltration of inflammatory cells within the joint. Inflammatory lesions also affect other tissues, especially the heart. Nodular lesions occur elsewhere in the body, notably beneath the skin; in some individuals, there may also be a rash (erythema marginatum). The joint lesions, soft tissue damage, and rashes are transient and generally resolve without permanent scarring, in contrast to the chronic progressive effects of other rheumatoid conditions.

The one exception to the transient nature of extra-articular lesions is rheumatic damage in the heart. Focal inflammatory and necrotic lesions (Aschoff nodules) in the muscle give rise to various cardiac malfunctions, arrhythmias, and even to failure. The main long-term effects, however, come from lesions in endocardial structures, especially the mitral and aortic valves. Scarring of these structures may lead to distortion and permanent incompetence.

Connective Tissue Disorders

These conditions have features apparently related to the soft tissue lesions of rheumatoid arthritis but do not have a comparable degree of joint involvement. The typically inflammatory lesions are either diffuse or nodular and are usually widespread. Associated fibrinoid necrosis is a common feature.

Systemic lupus erythematosus (SLE) is a serious diffuse connective tissue disease, with diverse patterns of necrosis and inflammation affecting the skin, kidney, heart, pericardium, lungs, pleura, spleen, brain, and synovial membranes. Connective tissue and blood vessel damage (vasculitis) occurs.

Polyarteritis nodosa is as varied in its manifestations as SLE but with vasculitis as the main cause of tissue damage. Lesions of arteries, arterioles, and capillaries, with consequent ischaemic damage to dependent tissues, give complex, extensive, and bizarre varieties of organ damage (e.g. in kidney, heart, brain, skin, eyes, and abdominal viscera).

Systemic sclerosis is caused by the replacement of loose elastic connective tissue, muscle, and some epithelial cells by collagen fibres (fibrosis). Skin, kidneys, heart, and main blood vessels may be seriously damaged. Subsequent shrinkage of collagen may cause further abnormality.

Dermatomyositis is characterised by inflammatory lesions, fibrotic change, and various vascular defects, which cause muscular degeneration and dermal abnormalities. Polymyositis is a related condition restricted to muscles.

Immunopathology and Auto-immune Disease

Despite the often strong associations between many of the foregoing conditions and a previous serious infection, it is probable that the active disease mechanisms are not the direct result of infection. Even in rheumatic fever, which is caused by an initial streptococcal infection, the delayed and persistent effects cannot be explained by the growth of micro-organisms or the direct effect of toxins. It is much more likely that an immune mechanism is activated during the infection, probably by the antigenic effects of streptococcal toxins. Such toxins may form soluble complexes with the antibody, which deposit in walls of blood vessels and activate complement as in type III hypersensitivity (*see* Section 15.6).

Although many of the other conditions follow infection, the intervening periods are usually much more prolonged, thus reducing the likelihood of direct causation. In rheumatoid arthritis, the evidence for an immune mediation consists of:

- Presence of lymphocytes and plasma cells in joint and nodular lesions.
- High levels of antistreptococcal antibody in the plasma of some rheumatoid patients.
- Splenic enlargement and leucocytosis.
- A large molecular weight immunoglobulin (IgM) (rheumatoid factor) in the plasma of the majority of patients, which is directed against other antibody molecules (IgG) and able to form inflammation-provoking immune complexes.
- Demonstration of immune complex deposition and bound complement in blood vessel walls of affected synovial membranes, and in other lesions.
- Lymphocytes in lesions, indicating cytotoxic effector T-cell activity and helper T-cell interactions with antibody-producing B-cells (*see* Section 15.6).

Thus, humoral and cell-mediated immune mechanisms are implicated and there are strong indications that much of the activity is of an auto-immune nature. Similar features in the various connective tissue disorders and in specific organ targets (*see* Table 16.13) also indicate auto-immune mechanisms.

PART B
PATIENT ADVICE

INTRODUCTION

The ability of pharmacists to be able to relate to patients and to perceive their needs is one of the major requirements of successful pharmacy practice (and indeed of all health care). No amount of knowledge about diseases and drugs is sufficient in itself unless pharmacists can communicate with patients and medical personnel, and can recognise the special problems which individuals face.

With these factors in mind, two main components of **Part B** of the *Handbook of Pharmacy Health-care* have been devised. Firstly, it provides information on those groups of the population whose circumstances may require special skills, and outlines the most appropriate means by which information and advice may be imparted. Secondly, it emphasises the increasingly important concept of personal responsibility for health by identifying the benefits and problems of self-medication, and highlighting how pharmacists can contribute to self determination in minor illness. The importance of self-help groups must also be recognised and detailed information on a wide range of organisations is listed.

The speciality of child health has always been one in which pharmacists, particularly those within the community, have been intimately involved. Many of the regular visitors to pharmacies are mothers accompanied by infants and young children. The bewildering array of milk products, first foods, and feeding equipment can frequently confuse parents. It is therefore vital that pharmacists possess adequate knowledge of the types of products available and the rationale for their use. Awareness of the current recommendations concerning breast and bottle feeding, the advantages and disadvantages of each, and the most appropriate means by which bottle feeding can be carried out, may seem relatively straightforward to the pharmacist who has reared her own children, but can appear an intimidating minefield to newly qualified pharmacists of both sexes. **Chapter 17** provides information which is intended to be of use to both experienced and inexperienced pharmacists, enabling them to advise parents informatively and confidently.

The occurrence of minor illness in infants and young children, and in particular illnesses associated with feeding difficulties, can pose special management problems. The ability to distinguish minor causes of feeding problems from those of a serious nature is essential, and guidance is provided to assist pharmacists in this task.

An awareness of the importance of contributing towards the healthy development of children is often enhanced within the pharmacy by the prominent display of weighing scales and height charts. By themselves, they are of little value; but in conjunction with explanation of their purpose, and suggestion as to when it may be necessary to seek further advice, pharmacists can contribute to the early identification of developmental abnormalities. Advice is also given in Chapter 17 on the vexed questions of fluoride supplementation, use of sugar-free medicines, and immunisation. The emphasis within each of these Sections is on providing detailed information for pharmacists so that they may make constructive suggestions to parents on each of these matters.

At the opposite end of the spectrum of life, recognition of the needs of the elderly have become increasingly important for all personnel in the health-care professions, and many of these special needs are discussed in **Chapter 18**. The multidisciplinary (e.g. involving health visitors, district nurses, and home helps) and multifaceted (e.g. involving family practitioner services, hospital services, and social services) approaches to the care of this ever increasing group is highly complex, but pharmacists can play an important role in promoting health in this high drug-use group. In the UK, government recognition of the importance of input from pharmacists has been attained by the introduction of payments to pharmacists providing services to residential homes.

It is vital to recognise that the numbers of elderly people, and by assumption the incidence of problems that pharmacists will encounter, is bound to increase. Population forecasts in the UK up to 2011 predict that, during this time, the number of people over 85 years of age will double and the rate of increase of those aged 65 years of age or over is approximately twice that of the rest of the population. Identifying regular visitors to the pharmacy and assisting the elderly in their use of medicines can provide an invaluable and rewarding service.

The possession of a specialist knowledge in any area of expertise is useless unless that information can be imparted to others. In the health-care professions, the ability to be able to communicate effectively with patients and other health workers is essential. Various aspects of the social and behavioural skills required for the effective practice of pharmacy (including a knowledge of the means of achieving effective communication, and applying that knowledge in counselling) are explained in **Chapter 19**. Patients' perceptions of pharmacy and pharmacists are significantly influenced by the way in which they, the patients, are dealt with. Do pharmacists make themselves available for members of the public to make direct contact? Is the environment in which the 'consultation' takes place conducive to personal exchange of information? Do pharmacists make a pro-active attempt to talk with patients, or is communication nearly always initiated by patients? Are opportunities taken to offer general health advice at the same time as responding to patients' specific enquiries?

One of the most important ways in which pharmacists can contribute towards health-care is by emphasising the correct use of drugs and medicines, and helping to ensure that patients comply with their dosage regimens. Factors which can reduce compliance are extremely diverse, but recognising that there is a problem in the appropriate use of medicines is an important step along the path to achieving optimum compliance.

Many patients are reluctant to consult their doctors about symptoms which they themselves consider trivial. In fact, it has been estimated that only about 1 in 3 symptoms experienced by patients are referred to doctors. Many of the submerged 'iceberg' of symptoms which are not referred to doctors are often brought to the attention of pharmacists; this ability to screen out minor illnesses by pharmacists is an important element in maintaining the viability of the health services, and is discussed in **Chapter 20**. Many of the symptoms reported to pharmacists require no medical treatment, often only requiring advice on lifestyle matters (e.g. diet, exercise, or reassurance). Guidance on self-medication can be usefully given for those minor symptoms which might benefit from use of non-prescription medicines. At all times, however, pharmacists should be alert to the possibility of reported symptoms being one manifestation of more serious disease, and in such cases, the importance of seeking immediate medical advice should be stressed to patients.

Every individual ultimately has the right to self-determination in matters of health, and, whenever possible, pharmacists should be encouraging patients to take full responsibility for their own health. Equally, it is important that patients participate in decisions taken about their health so that they can develop this self-determination and autonomy. It should be recognised that compliance with a particular course of action (e.g. taking medicines, or adopting a healthier lifestyle) is considerably easier to achieve if patients have been intimately involved in the decision-making process. One potent manifestation of the desire by patients to participate in maintaining their own health is the proliferation of self-help organisations (**Chapter 21**), which operate in parallel to the 'official' health services. Pharmacists are frequently approached by members of the public for information on specific groups, or for advice about whether other patients in a similar predicament can be contacted. Pharmacists should recognise the importance of such groups; referring patients to them can be just as important in the overall care of patients as handing out prescription and non-prescription medicines.

All cross-references specified within Part B are to BNF No. 19 (March 1990).

Chapter 17

CHILD HEALTH AND IMMUNISATION

17.1 INTRODUCTION

As emphasised in Chapter 19, the pharmacist is a readily accessible health-care professional, a fact confirmed by the approximately six million visitors to pharmacies each day. A large number of these visitors are mothers accompanied by infants and young children. Pharmacists can be a valuable source of information for parents who may be concerned about the health of their children, by providing advice on a wide range of paediatric issues (e.g. feeding), and recommending an appropriate course of action.

It is vital that pharmacists can distinguish between minor ailments and potentially serious childhood conditions. In determining the potential severity of the symptoms, it is essential that pharmacists listen to what parents tell them, and in particular what form of treatment (if any) has already been tried. In this respect, there is little difference between the range of questions which should be asked for an adult illness (*see* Section 20.3) and one occurring in a child. What may be more important is the fact that the child may be causing the parent emotional stress and distress. Pharmacists should therefore be capable of reassuring the parent with a calm confident manner that recognises the parent's concern but confirms the best course of action.

Many community pharmacies also stock a wide range of babycare products, and pharmacists should be prepared to assist the parent in the selection of foods, feeding utensils, and sterilisation equipment, especially for the mother of a first-born child.

This chapter will detail some of the problems most commonly presented to the pharmacist and outline the action to be taken in each case. The terms infant and baby are used here to define a child under one year of age, and a young child is classed as between 1 and 3 years of age.

17.2 INFANT FEEDING

Breast vs. Bottle Feeding

The vital importance of adequate nutrition during the first 12 months of life is highlighted by the facts that a baby trebles its weight and that 50% of postnatal brain growth takes place during this time. In underdeveloped nations of the world, the lack of resources and an unpredictable supply of alternative forms of milk have maintained an almost total reliance on breast milk for newborn babies. In the developed nations, however, this dependence on breast milk has diminished through increased wealth, changes in maternal lifestyle (e.g. returning to work immediately after a baby has been born), and a reluctance to feel tied to the baby for long periods. Many more women have elected to bottle-feed the baby at the earliest opportunity, although active education campaigns have marginally increased the proportion of breast-feeding women in developed countries at different stages after the birth. There is now a strong correlation between the incidence of breast feeding and continued education after 18 years of age, a high social class grading (i.e. professional and managerial as opposed to unskilled women), and living in more affluent parts of a country. Conversely, unhappy experiences or difficulties with breast feeding a first-born child reduce the likelihood of subsequent children being put to breast.

TABLE 17.1
Mean composition of mature mother's milk per 100mL

Energy (kcal)	70
(kJ)	293
Protein (g)	1.3
Lactose (g)	7
Fat (g)	4.2
Vitamins	
A (μg)	60
D (μg)	0.01
E (mg)	0.35
K (μg)	0.21
Thiamine (μg)	16
Riboflavine (μg)	30
Nicotinic acid (μg)	230
Pyridoxine (μg)	6
Cyanocobalamin (μg)	0.01
Total folate (μg)	5.2
Pantothenic acid (μg)	260
Biotin (μg)	0.76
Ascorbic acid (mg)	3.8
Minerals	
Sodium (mg)	15
Potassium (mg)	60
Chloride (mg)	43
Calcium (mg)	35
Phosphorus (mg)	15
Magnesium (mg)	2.8
Iron (μg)	76
Copper (μg)	39
Zinc (μg)	295
Manganese (μg)	1.2
Chromium (μg)	0.6
Selenium (μg)	1.4
Iodine (μg)	7
Fluorine (μg)	7.7

The characteristics of human milk   The structure of the breast and a description of the secretion of milk is given in Section 7.6. Immediately after birth, the initial secretion from the mammary gland is a thin yellow fluid, colostrum, which is high in protein, vitamin A and cyanocobalamin, lymphocytes, and macrophages but low in fat content. Colostrum also contains a polypeptide (the mucosal growth factor) specific for intestinal mucosa, and this stimulates DNA synthesis and activates cell division. The presence of the polypeptide leads to the rapid growth of the jejunum and ileum necessary for the adaptation of the infant's intestine to milk feeding. Colostrum also contains a high concentration of immunoglobulins, and in particular immunoglobulin A (IgA), which retard the multiplication of bacteria and viruses within the gastro-intestinal tract. Early suckling by the baby increases the secretion of colostrum, but within 72 to 96 hours the thin fluid is gradually replaced by milk. The term mature milk is used for the milk produced by about the tenth postnatal day.

Breast milk contains all the ingredients necessary to sustain the baby during the early months of its life (Table 17.1). Carbohydrate is present predominantly in the form of the disaccharide, lactose, which is broken down in the intestine into galactose and glucose by the enzyme lactase (*see* Lactose Intolerance). About half of the baby's energy requirements are provided by fat (predominantly triglycerides surrounded by lipoprotein) and approximately one quarter from saturated fatty acids. The fatty acid content of breast milk largely reflects the content in the maternal diet. By comparison, the protein content of breast milk is low and about 60% of this is comprised of easily digestible whey rather than relatively indigestible curds (casein). The benefits of whey are that it also supplies albumin, lactoferrin (a protein which binds iron and makes it unavailable for bacterial multiplication), lysozyme, and IgA. Other constituents include minerals, enzymes (e.g. lipase), and cellular components (e.g. macrophages) which help to resist the development of infection in the milk ducts and in the infant's intestine. The vitamin content of a healthy and well-nourished mother's milk should be adequate to supply all of the infant's requirements. However, if the vitamin D and vitamin K status of the mother is low, there is a risk of the development of rickets and late haemorrhagic disease.

Other forms of milk   It is also useful at this stage to briefly consider the different types of milks which are available for purchase. Pasteurised (household or doorstep) milk is whole cow's milk which has been heat treated to remove potentially pathogenic microorganisms (e.g. *Brucella melitensis* and *B. abortus*, *see*

Brucellosis). Cow's milk is unsuitable for children under 6 months of age, and is not recommended for children under one year of age. If the milk is not pasteurised or there is no refrigerator in the home, the milk should be given to children under 12 months of age only after it has been boiled. The main disadvantage of heat treatment of cow's milk is that destruction of its useful components (e.g. lactoferrin and IgA) also takes place. Almost all infant feeding with cow's milk has now been replaced with modified formula dried milk powders or evaporated milk. Whole cow's milk should be a staple component of the diet in all children over one year of age, but under school age.

Homogenised milk is a form of pasteurised milk which has been further treated to evenly distribute the fat throughout the milk. Sterilised milk is homogenised milk that has been further treated, and has a thickened texture. The partial removal of water from pasteurised milk by evaporation forms evaporated milk, and the addition of sugar to evaporated milk produces condensed milk. The content of all of these milks is essentially the same as cow's milk, and the same limitations on its use in children under one year of age apply.

Other milks are available in which the nutritional content can vary significantly from its original value. Skimmed and semi-skimmed milk are by-products of the butter- and cream-producing industries which utilise the fat in milk. Almost all of the fat has been removed from skimmed milk, while about half is removed to produce the semi-skimmed form. Although these milks contain a high proportion of proteins and calcium, the lack of fat and fat-soluble vitamins leads to energy and vitamin deficiencies. Skimmed and semi-skimmed milk should not be given to children under 12 months of age and are not recommended for those under five years of age. Semi-skimmed milk may be introduced from five years of age provided the overall nutritional status is adequate.

Dried milks may provide a convenient form of milk in situations where refrigeration is lacking or ineffective. Low-fat milks and many of the infant formulae are available in this form. They are reconstituted by the addition of water, although the manufacturer's instructions must be closely followed.

Ultra heat treated (UHT) milk has been subjected to higher temperatures than pasteurised milk and, when it is aseptically packed, it may remain drinkable without refrigeration for up to three months.

Goat's milk is of a similar composition to cow's milk and has been used in an attempt to overcome allergy to cow's milk. However, like cow's milk, its use is not recommended for babies under 6 months of age as it is deficient in many vitamins and pasteurisation cannot be guaranteed.

Advantages of breast feeding   It is recognised that breast milk is the best source of nourishment for the newborn baby and for the first six months of life. Most mothers can provide adequate nutrition from the breast to nourish their infant for the initial 4 to 6 months of life. It also encourages the development of a close maternal-child bond and allows the mother the opportunity to rest and relax. Mother's milk provides an excellent source of nutrition, it is sterile, and is normally readily available at the correct temperature. The presence of breast milk in the infant's intestine encourages the growth of *Lactobacillus bifidus* which promotes the absorption of nutrients (the bifidus factor). The resultant intestinal acidification limits the growth of *Escherichia coli* and reduces the incidence of gastro-enteritis.

Equally important is the protective role afforded by the transfer of immunoglobulins in the milk which are recognised by the infant as 'self', and this may reduce the risk of eczema in infancy and asthma in later life. There is also a decreased tendency to obesity in breast-fed infants and this is important as obese babies are liable to grow into obese adults. One consequence of breast feeding is reduced fertility, which results in ovulation in only about 10% of women, although breast-feeding mothers should be warned that this is not an efficient means of contraception. The choice of contraception after the birth of the child may be determined by the reduced inhibitory effect that progestogen-only contraceptives have on milk flow in comparison to combined oral preparations.

The reasons for not breast feeding   Social and domestic reasons are commonly cited for the reluctance to start or continue breast feeding. Bottle feeding allows the mother to return to work and may also be carried out in public places (e.g. at work or in shopping centres) where breast feeding can be unwelcome and inconvenient. The mother may also be uncertain whether the infant is getting sufficient nourishment and have greater confidence once a bottle of milk has been seen to be taken.

Insufficient milk is often stated as a cause of stopping breast feeding at an early stage after the birth. Mothers should be advised that the hormonal stimulation of milk flow will only occur if attempts to breast feed are continued, perhaps with decreasing intervals between attempts. If bottle feeding is introduced at the first sign of limited flow, the lack of demand for breast milk will aggravate the situation.

Medical reasons which preclude breast feeding are rare. They include the presence of galactosaemia and phenylketonuria in the infant, serious maternal diseases (e.g. heart disease, depressive disorders, and glomerulonephritis) which inhibit lactation, and the presence of the human immunodeficiency virus (HIV) in the mother. However, maternal infection with hepatitis B virus is not a contra-indication, with appropriate immunisation of the infant. Difficulties in breast feeding are compounded with twins and multiple births, as the demand for milk cannot be met. Some women may develop painful engorged breasts, particularly in the first days after birth, because the supply is greater than demand. The pressure and pain generated further reduces the flow of milk and the swollen nipple limits the infant's ability to suckle. The milk may be expressed using a breast pump (*see below*) following warm bathing of the breast, or gentle palpation to reduce the build-up and relieve symptoms. Sore or cracked nipples may arise through incorrect positioning of the infant at the nipple. Application of a skin disinfectant or cleansing agent (BNF 13.11) may be beneficial, in conjunction with avoidance of the affected breast.

Accessories for Breast Feeding

Breast pumps   One method of overcoming some of the social problems cited as reasons for stopping breast feeding, and which may be particularly useful for the mother who wishes to return to work, is to express the milk so that it may be given at a later time, possibly by someone other than the mother. Milk may be expressed manually or with a breast pump. The manual method will be demonstrated to the mother by the midwife or a nurse. Breast pumps can be purchased from a pharmacy and it is important that pharmacists should be aware of their mode of action in the event of queries from the mother.

Milk should ideally be expressed in the early morning or, if night-time feeds have ceased, in the evening. The two most common types of breast pump are the bulb pump and the syringe pump. The bulb pump consists of a plastic or rubber bulb which is gently squeezed to draw milk from the breast into a reservoir. In the syringe pump, the suction necessary to draw milk from the breast is provided by the downward movement of a piston, and milk is drained into the body of the syringe. Cleanliness in the use of both types of pump is essential. Hands should be washed, and the pump and receiving containers washed and sterilised. Once the milk has been collected, it can be stored for up to 48 hours in a refrigerator. The milk can also be frozen and kept for up to 6 months.

Nipple shields   The presence of a prominent nipple is obviously essential for successful breast feeding. If the nipple sits within a pit, or retracts into a depression when the areola is gently squeezed, the nipple is described as inverted or pseudo-inverted respectively. This may be corrected by the use of a nipple shield, which consists of a saucer with a central orifice through which the nipple is inserted. A plastic cup fits over the saucer and the complete assembly is worn inside the bra to exert continuous pressure on the areola and encourage the nipple to stand proud within the shield. Women should be advised to wear the shields for short periods initially from about half way through the pregnancy, and gradually increase the wearing period until they can be tolerated throughout the day. They should not be worn at night.

Nipple shields may also be worn if the nipple is cracked or sore. In this case, the shield may be positioned over the nipple and held in place whilst the infant feeds through it.

Bottle Feeding and Infant Formula Milks

Infant formula products are manufactured so as to approximate the composition of mother's milk. Most products are based on cow's milk, even though cow's milk has a different composition to human milk. Some formulas are based on other proteins (e.g. soya protein) for infants with special nutritional requirements (*see below*). Energy values, the ratio of saturated to unsaturated fatty acids, and the levels of carbohydrates, essential fatty acids, and most major minerals and trace elements are similar in breast milk and infant formula products. The main differences in composition of manufactured milks occur in the increased energy content derived from protein; the absence of immunoglobulins, lymphocytes, and macrophages; the lack of non-protein nitrogen (e.g. urea, creatinine, uric acid, and free amino acids); and increased concentrations of vitamins and iron.

Modifications to cow's milk (*see* Table 17.2)   The modifications to cow's milk involve changes to carbohydrate, fat, or protein content.

- added carbohydrate, substituted fat, or both

  Cow's milk contains considerably less carbohydrate, more protein, and slightly less fat and provides roughly the same energy value as human milk. The addition of carbohydrate is the simplest modification made to cow's milk in the preparation of infant formula milks. Dilution with carbohydrate reduces the overall concentration of protein and minerals, and reduces the risk of renal overload produced by excess protein (*see also below*). Lactose is not used as the sole diluent, as overloading the infant's intestine with this carbohydrate may lead to frothy diarrhoea and reduced absorption. Instead, maltodextrins, singly or in combination with sucrose, are used to supplement the additional lactose.

Another alternative is to substitute cow's milk fat by vegetable and animal fats that are more easily digested. This modification is in addition to the extra lactose. Examples of substituted fat and added carbohydrate products (also described as less highly modified formulas) available in the UK are SMA White, Ostermilk Complete, Milumil, and Cow and Gate Plus.

- demineralised whey formulas

Cow's milk contains more protein than human milk, and a much higher percentage of the protein is curds. Milk in which the fat and the curd protein has been removed is referred to as whey. It consists of water-soluble whey proteins, lactose (which constitutes all the carbohydrate content), and minerals. Demineralised whey is formed when the mineral content of whey is reduced by ion exchange, electrodialysis (the passage of an electrical current through whey), or ultrafiltration (the total mineral content is not eliminated completely).

Demineralised whey formulas are prepared by the addition of skimmed or semi-skimmed milk (which re-introduces curd protein but in a smaller concentration, lactose, and minerals), a blend of butterfat (or modified beef fat) and vegetable oils to provide a fat content similar to breast milk, and vitamins. Examples, which are also referred to as highly modified formulas, available in the UK are SMA Gold, Cow and Gate Premium, Aptamil, and Osterfeed.

Infant formula milks are manufactured as ready-to-use preparations or as liquids or powders to which water must be added. It is essential that the manufacturer's guidelines for preparing feeds are rigidly followed. Some preparations are reconstituted by the addition of a stated volume of water, while others must be made up to the required volume by adding a sufficient quantity of water. Incorrect preparation (e.g. adding too much powder by compressing or not levelling off the powder in the scoop) is potentially harmful and carries the risks of hypernatraemia and obesity. Hypernatraemia can arise because the sodium content of cow's milk is about three times that of mother's milk. Obesity may be more common in bottle-fed babies because the mother may not respond to the baby's satiety when given a bottle, whereas on the breast the baby will determine its own degree of satiety. Parents should also be reminded that scoops are invariably **not** interchangeable between different product manufacturers, and the use of an inappropriate scoop may also lead to errors in quantities given.

The water used to reconstitute feeds should be boiled and allowed to cool to about 60°C. Water should be used direct from the mains and not from a water-softened supply, as the sodium content may be significantly increased in the latter. Water from a kettle which has been repeatedly boiled should not be used as repeated evaporation can lead to concentration of minerals.

The different characteristics of whey proteins and curd proteins have already been mentioned. In addition to the classifications mentioned above, infant formula milks may also be termed whey-based milks and curd-based milks (in which the dominant protein is casein), the latter containing higher concentrations of protein and minerals. The curd-based milks correspond to the added carbohydrate and substituted fat (less highly modified) milks, and the whey-based milks to the demineralised (highly modified) products. It is common for mothers to change from one milk formula to another, sometimes more than once, usually on the basis that the infant does not appear to be satisfied on the current product. The proportion of babies receiving curd-based milks increases with age, presumably because the relatively indigestible curds provide an increased sense of satisfaction within the intestine, although there appears to be little nutritional difference between the two types.

TABLE 17.2

Comparison of the two main types of infant milk formulas used in the UK, derived from cow's milk

	Added carbohydrate and substituted fat ('less highly modified formulas')	Demineralised whey ('highly modified formulas')
Protein (whey:casein ratio)	20:80	60/70:40/30
Carbohydrate	Lactose, often with maltodextrins and sucrose	100% lactose
Fat	Blend of vegetable oils, cow's milk fat, and occasionally animal fat (e.g. butterfat)	
Examples in the UK	Cow and Gate Plus SMA White Ostermilk Complete Milumil	Cow and Gate Premium SMA Gold Osterfeed Aptamil

Follow-on milks   A follow-on milk is one which can be used to satisfy the nutritional requirements of an older infant (over four months of age) and the young child. These milks differ from the infant formula milks described above in that they contain a higher concentration of electrolytes and and protein, although the content is still less than that of cow's milk. Iron and vitamin D levels are greater than in infant formulas and cow's milk and this may be of especial benefit to Asian children who are often found to have these specific deficiencies.

It is doubtful whether there is significant benefit of changing an infant to a follow-on milk if the child is satisfied with its current feed. Breast milk or infant formula milk, supplemented as required by intermittent solids, should provide all the nutritional requirements. If the mother insists on a change, follow-on milk is preferable to cow's milk.

A reference guide to the suitability of different milks in infants and young children is given in Table 17.3.

Cow's milk substitutes   Some infants may develop sensitivity to the protein of cow's milk present in infant formula products. True allergy is rare (with an incidence of less than 1%) and efforts should be made to dissuade mothers from choosing cow's milk substitute products in the absence of medical diagnosis. Other conditions may also benefit from the temporary or more prolonged withdrawal of cow's milk protein, although all indications must be medically supervised by the child's doctor or dietitian, or both. The most common indications for the use of cow's milk substitutes are:

- atopic disease with suspected food allergy
- cow's milk-protein intolerance
- following gastro-intestinal surgery
- galactosaemia
- intractable diarrhoea in infancy
- lactose intolerance.

Gastro-intestinal symptoms of cow's milk-protein intolerance include diarrhoea (which may be bloody and accompanied by mucus), vomiting, and colic. The presence of atopy may be characterised by eczema, urticaria, erythema, and rhinitis.

Cow's milk substitute preparations contain casein hydrolysate or soya protein. They contain no lactose, and reduced absorption of minerals from these formulas has been reported. Methionine, vitamin K, and iodine are additions made during manufacture. Casein hydrolysate preparations are hypoallergenic and are preferable to soya products for the treatment of gastroenteritis, as the intestinal mucosa may also be sensitised to soya protein. Cow's milk substitutes should not be used in an attempt to prevent the development of atopic disease in a child who may be at increased risk of hypersensitivity (e.g. an infant with one or both parents known to have a history of atopic disease). Additionally, it is essential to ensure that the product is suitable as a sole source of nutrition for an infant (e.g. comminuted chicken meat must be supplemented with carbohydrate, fat, vitamins, and minerals, whereas other sources are nutritionally complete). The consumer should also be aware of the wide variety of other soya liquids and powders available. These must under no circumstances be used instead of nutritionally complete soya preparations for infants. Soya milk drinks are also inadequate substitutes for cow's milk for infants under 5 years of age and should not be recommended.

Parents of infants with cow's milk-protein intolerance may require special guidance on the purchase of other nutritional products for their child, especially once weaning starts. Beef (which possesses a range of antigens similar to milk), milk, and milk products must be avoided, and it is essential that the labels of all products are carefully scrutinised. Some manufacturers have increased the range of information on labels to assist in the correct choice.

TABLE 17.3
Quick reference guide to the use of milks in infants and young children

	Under 6 months	6 to 12 months	Over one year
Breast milk	Ideal, for at least four months	May suffice in conjunction with other foods	Not suitable as a sole source of nutrition
Whole cow's milk	Unsuitable	Pasteurised milk may be given; non-pasteurised only if boiled and cooled	Essential component of diet
Skimmed milk	Unsuitable	Unsuitable	Not recommended for under-fives
Semi-skimmed milk	Unsuitable	Unsuitable	Not recommended for under-twos
Infant formula milks	Some formulas are suitable but not recommended	Suitable on their own or to supplement breast milk	A useful adjunct to solids

Feeding equipment   The basic feeding equipment necessary for non-breast milk feeding is a bottle and a teat. However, there is a bewildering array of shapes and sizes of these items and many mothers may be confused about the differing claims made by manufacturers. Pharmacists should be familiar with the range of equipment (a complete list is given in Table 17.4) and act on their own experiences as parents or, equally importantly, listen to others with experience so they can form an opinion about its suitability.

Bottles should be wide-necked to allow easy cleaning and made of unbreakable plastic. Graduation marks are often included on the outer surface but their accuracy cannot always be guaranteed, especially on bottles without straight sides. The bottle should have a cap to allow the teat to be inverted and covered during travelling.

The selection of the correct size of teat and teat hole is more critical. If the teat hole is too small, the infant will swallow air and develop gastric distension which can cause underfeeding. The child will also become frustrated because of the effort necessary to take milk, and feeds can take as long as 60 minutes. Ideally, the milk should drip out of the teat in a fine, steady stream at the rate of about one drop per second, and feeds should take no longer than 30 minutes. Teat holes which are too small may be enlarged by using a red-hot needle. One end of the needle should be placed in a cork which is held while inserting the other end of the needle into the blue part of a flame. When the tip of the needle glows it should be pushed through the rubber teat.

Repeated washing and sterilising of teats will cause their gradual deterioration and softening. Conversely, a new teat can be firm and relatively inflexible and may benefit from gentle squeezing in warm water to soften it.

Sterilising feeding equipment   It is essential to ensure impeccable standards of hygiene during the preparation of bottle feeds for infants and young children. The ability of the child to counteract the accidental introduction of micro-organisms is poorly developed, and gastroenteritis can easily result from poor hygiene. Before feeding utensils are sterilised, it is important to remove any remnants of dried milk as these can inactivate sterilising solutions. Bottles and teats should ideally be rinsed in cold water immediately after a feed to prevent the deposition of a thin dried film of milk on their inner surfaces. At a later convenient time, the bottle should be cleaned with washing-up liquid and warm water using a brush kept exclusively for this purpose. Thorough cleaning of the teat can be ensured by everting it, sprinkling the inner and outer surfaces with salt, and rubbing between the fingers. Teats and bottles should be rinsed after cleaning.

Equipment used to give the feed must be sterilised by chemicals (e.g. dichloroisocyanurate and sodium hypochlorite) which release chlorine, or by boiling. Sterilising agents may be purchased as a solution, crystals, or tablets and made up according to the manufacturers' instructions. Fresh solutions must be made up every 24 hours. A large plastic container (of capacity sufficient to hold at least two feeding bottles) is filled with water and the sterilising agent added according to the manufacturers' instructions. Bottles and teats must be completely submerged within the sterilising solution. Pinching teats to release trapped air bubbles assists in preventing them from floating to the top of the solution. The time taken to achieve sterilisation with chemical agents varies, and the utensils should be left in the solution until they are required. The manufacturers' instructions about rinsing before use with boiled and freshly cooled water must be followed.

An alternative form of sterilisation is to boil the feeding equipment. The bottles should be immersed completely in water in a large saucepan used exclusively for this purpose. The water should be heated to boiling point, the saucepan covered, and teats added once the water has started boiling. Teats and bottles should remain in the boiling water for at least five minutes, after which time the teats should be transferred to a sterile lidded jar. The bottles may be left in the covered saucepan until required.

Microwave ovens should not be used to sterilise feeding equipment immersed in water or in sterilising solutions.

Introducing Solids

The gradual introduction of semi-solids to a milk diet is termed weaning. This should not be attempted until the infant is at least four months of age, and ideally not later than six months of age. Before four months of age, the intestine of the infant is immature and has an increased permeability, especially to protein. Excessive absorption of protein may trigger allergic reactions in suscep-

TABLE 17.4
The range of equipment necessary for bottle feeding

Bottles (6 to 8)
Teats (the same number as bottles +1)
Bottle-cleaning brush
Sterilising solution/tablets/crystals
Sterilising vessel
Flat-edged knife (for levelling off powder scoop)
Salt
Graduated measuring jug (if feeds are not prepared in the bottle)

tible individuals, and the lack of maternal IgA in infants who have been bottle-fed almost from birth may render them more vulnerable to this effect. Solids also contain a higher electrolyte (e.g. sodium) concentration than breast milk. The concentrating ability of the infant's kidneys is not fully developed in the early months of life and therefore high levels of fluid intake are essential to allow the complete excretion of excess dietary electrolytes. Although the kidneys of most infants may adapt satisfactorily in health, any degree of dehydration (e.g. caused by infection, diarrhoea, or vomiting) will considerably overstress their function and lead to hypernatraemia. A third reason to delay the introduction of solids for as long as is practical is that the presence of baby foods may have a deleterious effect on the absorption of iron from breast milk.

Infant boys are commonly weaned at an earlier date than girls because of more rapid growth and hence greater nutritional demands. Mixed feeding is the provision of food other than human or infant formula milks.

The earliest foods given during weaning include rusks and cereals or commercial weaning foods. Cereals are popular as they provide a soft texture and familiar flavour when mixed with milk. Alternatively, cooked and puréed vegetables and fruits may be equally appropriate. The introduction of puréed home-prepared meals may be a useful means of familiarising the baby with the family's diet. Small amounts only (e.g. 1 to 2 teaspoonfuls) should be given initially and limited to one meal a day. The quantity may be gradually increased to about 3 to 5 teaspoonfuls within two weeks (although individual requirements may vary significantly), and subsequently to 2 to 3 meals a day by 6 to 8 months.

Most pharmacies offer a wide range of strained or homogenised foods specially manufactured as 'first foods', and these offer a wide variety of choice (e.g. from beef broth with vegetables to fish in cheese sauce) and flavours (e.g. bland and savoury). Manufactured products are also available as gluten-free, milk-free, egg-free, vegetarian, and sugar-free (e.g. all savoury foods). Many are also advertised as free of preservatives, colourings, and artificial flavourings. Their use can be ideal for busy mothers, in situations where adequate hygiene may be lacking, or as temporary measures (e.g. on holiday), but it is preferable to recommend that mothers introduce a puréed form of the rest of the family's food at the earliest opportunity. Although high standards of cleanliness and hygiene must be maintained, sterilisation of feeding equipment is not necessary once weaning has started.

17.3 FEEDING AND GASTRO-INTESTINAL PROBLEMS

An infant who appears to be healthy may suffer from a variety of gastro-intestinal problems. These problems may be related to the intake of food or they may be a consequence of underlying illness. It is important that pharmacists can recognise the possible cause and suggest appropriate action.

Colic

Incessant crying by an infant, especially in the early evening, can often be attributed to colic. The infant may cry and even scream at the same time as drawing the knees up to the chin and going red in the face. The phenomenon occurs commonly in infants of between 1 and 4 months of age without any outward signs of accompanying illness or distress. Cuddling and picking up the child may produce little improvement and many parents become considerably upset at its daily recurrence.

A wide range of factors have been linked to the development of colic (e.g. under- and overfeeding, tension, allergy, and under- and over-cossetting), but the pathophysiology is unknown. Gripe waters containing carminatives (e.g. dill) are traditional remedies, but reassurance and checking the suitability of feeding teats may be more constructive advice.

Regurgitation and Acute Vomiting

After a feed, many babies will regurgitate small quantities of food, especially if winding is encouraged. This is described as posseting and may be due to aerophagia caused by inappropriately sized teats (*see* Section 17.2). If the regurgitation is more voluminous, it may be caused by over-zealous feeding and should be discouraged to minimise the likelihood of obesity. Positive action which may be taken to encourage the retention of feeds is to thicken the milk (e.g. with carob flour) and to feed the child lying down but tilted up at an angle of 10 to 20 degrees. Frequent small volume drinks can also help to prevent the risk of dehydration caused by regurgitation.

Vomiting which is more persistent and forceful and stained with blood or bile, but not always directly related to the intake of food, may indicate a more serious problem which should be referred. Common causes include a mild infection (e.g. upper-respiratory tract infection or gastro-enteritis) or, more rarely, a serious infection (e.g. meningitis), gastro-intestinal obstruction (e.g. pyloric stenosis), and metabolic disease (e.g. galactosaemia). Other conditions which may produce vomiting include intolerance to the feed and concomitant drug administration. Infants suffering from any of these conditions will be clearly less well than those who are posseting.

Diarrhoea and Constipation

As in adults, definitions of diarrhoea and constipation are only valid when an individual's normal bowel movements are considered (see Section 20.3). Like adults, there is a wide range of frequency of bowel movements, although, in general, there is a gradual decrease as the neonate progresses through the first few weeks of life. When the infant is fed solely on breast milk, the stools are light yellow and pasty, and may be passed as frequently as after every feed or as infrequently as once every three days. Bottle-fed infants tend to have more frequent and malodorous stools which are firmer and more brown than those of breast-fed infants. If the stools appear too compacted, extra water may be advisable between feeds.

On the rare occasions when mothers seek advice from pharmacists about diarrhoea in infants under three months of age, the child should be immediately referred to the doctor or to the local casualty department. The loss of fluid and electrolytes at this age can be potentially fatal. Similar action should be taken with older infants with diarrhoea who appear listless, or who are excessively irritable and display a cold grey skin that is dry or clammy. These are the cardinal signs of dehydration.

Acute diarrhoea may be treated by the administration of an oral rehydration solution (BNF 9.2.1.2). Instructions issued with proprietary preparations should be followed, but pharmacists may usefully give additional advice. About 50 to 100 mL of oral rehydration solution should be given for each loose stool for initial rehydration. Breast-fed infants will derive an adequate volume of fluid from the mother's milk, but it is important to supplement the fluid intake of non-breast fed infants with water, giving a volume equal to about half the volume of rehydration solution administered. This supplement should be given about 2 to 3 hours after administration of the rehydration solution. Older children may prefer weak tea or dilute fruit juice and they should be encouraged to drink as much as they want.

Breast feeding can be continued during the period of diarrhoea but bottle feeding should be temporarily stopped or reduced to half-strength (to maintain an adequate intake of protein but decrease the risk of lactose overload). Young children who have been weaned onto solids should be starved for only as long as they refuse food, after which time mild bland foods may be gradually reintroduced. Extra foods should be given in the convalescent period following diarrhoea to allow growth catch-up. Preparations containing kaolin should be avoided in infants in deference to the prime objective of rehydration. If diarrhoea is persistent but relatively mild, the child should be referred to investigate possible causes (e.g. coeliac disease, cystic fibrosis, lactose intolerance, and milk-protein intolerance).

Constipation in infants and young children is rare and is commonly caused by inappropriate fluid or dietary intake or by changing from breast to bottle milk, and less commonly to disease (e.g. megacolon and Hirschprung's disease). Treatment should be directed to the underlying pathology, or at modifying fluid or dietary intake. In the young child who has been weaned, constipation may be rectified by an increase in the intake of fibre, fresh fruit, and vegetables. If no significant improvement is seen following these measures, the child should be referred.

17.4 GROWTH, DEVELOPMENT, AND FAILURE TO THRIVE

Height and Weight

Some pharmacies offer public use of weighing scales and devices for measuring height. However, all pharmacists must be prepared to respond to queries from mothers about the 'normal' and 'abnormal' weight and height for an infant of a particular age.

Growth is measured in terms of height and weight. In a child under two years of age height is measured with the child lying down, although at this age weight is a more useful (and more accurately taken) measure of growth. Growth is most rapid during the first six months of life and gradually slows towards 12 months of age.

Many mothers plot the infant growth on height and weight (anthropometric) charts and compare progress with average charts. Average charts display the height and weight of the average (50th percentile), and the normal range of weight and height (which extends from the 3rd to the 97th percentile, i.e. 3% of children fall above or below the normal range). If the mother queries the growth of her child when plotted on such a graph, it is important to remember that individual measurements are of little value and that all charts are constructed for the average normal child. A non-average child is not necessarily abnormal. The greater importance of **trends** in growth rather than individual measurements should be stressed, but if the mother requires further reassurance she should be referred to her health visitor or doctor.

Developmental Milestones

Although timing may be subject to wide variations, an infant will reach different milestones in development in a well-defined sequence. It is important to remember that development always proceeds from head to toe. The earliest milestones reflect the control gained in posture and movement of the head, followed by increased grasping and manipulative control of the hands, and culminating in the ability to crawl, stand, and eventually walk. The major milestones during the first 12 months of life are outlined below:

1 to 2 months responds to speech by smiling and, when placed on his stomach, can lift and maintain head in the same plane as the body for a brief period. Reflex grasping will be gradually replaced by more voluntary holding.

3 months will grasp hands for short periods and, when lifted upright from a horizontal position, can support his head. A rattle can be held when placed in the hand and there will be a directional response to noise.

4 months when placed on his stomach, the infant will be capable of lifting up his head and chest by propping himself up on his arms. He will also be capable of sitting when supported.

5 to 6 months capable of rolling from his back to his side and can successfully reach for an object. Will grasp items between both hands (e.g. often suck his own toes).

7 months can sit upright briefly when unsupported, although is dependent on his hands for support. Can feed himself by holding a biscuit.

8 months can sit upright without support, although cushions should be placed around the child as a precautionary measure. Larger items (e.g. play-bricks) can be picked up and grasped.

9 months crawling may be attempted when the child can support himself on his hands and knees. He can also pull himself to a standing position, hold his feeding bottle, and be capable of imitating words such as 'mama' and 'dada'.

12 months may be able to walk when supported (although walking can start anytime between 10 and 18 months of age), say several words, feed himself, accept and give objects, and speak 2 or 3 meaningful words.

Failure to Thrive

A child who is healthy looking, alert, and responsive is thriving and should give no cause for concern. However, one who is continually crying, lethargic, who consistently falls outside the third percentile on the growth chart, or who develops a sudden decline in a previously acceptable pattern of growth, is described by the term 'failure to thrive'. Other indications of illness in infants and young children are an inability to attract or maintain the child's attention, irritability, or restlessness.

Prenatal causes of failure to thrive may be a consequence of maternal intake of drugs and alcohol, smoking, or viral infection. After birth, it may be caused by inadequate food offered or taken (*see* Section 17.2), chronic infection (e.g. of the urinary tract), or malabsorption (e.g. caused by coeliac disease or cystic fibrosis). Rarer causes include milk-protein intolerance, congenital heart disease, cirrhosis, or renal insufficiency. Occasionally, rejection of the child by one or both parents, or marital discord, may contribute to the condition. In all cases of failure to thrive, the mother should be referred to the doctor.

Teething and Fluoride Supplementation

Teething   In child health, the eruption of the deciduous (milk or baby) teeth commonly starts at 6 months of age and is generally completed by two years of age, although there can be wide variations in timing. The earliest signs of the gradual movement of the teeth from their prenatal position beneath the gums are increased salivation and crying.

The first teeth to appear are commonly a pair of central lower (mandibular) incisors followed after about 6 to 8 weeks by the corresponding upper (maxillar) incisors. In all subsequent eruptions, the upper usually precede the lower teeth. A further pair of lateral incisors subsequently erupts, one on each side of the initial pair. The first pair of molars appear on the upper jaw at between 12 and 15 months, and the spaces between these and the incisors are filled by the canine (eye) teeth at 16 to 20 months of age. Finally, the 4 second molars penetrate the gums to the rear of the first molars at about two years of age, with one on each side and on each upper and lower surface. The 20 deciduous teeth are lost steadily between 6 and 12 years of age and replaced by 32 permanent, slightly larger teeth.

Teething can be a traumatic period for children and their parents. In addition to the symptoms described above, the cheeks and gums may become inflamed and reddened and there may be pyrexia, loss of appetite, and disturbed sleep patterns. Although dribbling may occur, particularly during eruption of the front teeth, other symptoms may be worse when the rear teeth push through. General measures which may help relieve discomfort include providing a firm object to chew (e.g. a teething ring, rusk, or raw carrot) and gentle rubbing of the surface of the gums by the parent with a washed finger.

Fluoride supplementation   Pharmacists are often asked about the fluoride content of the drinking water in their locality, and to advise on the necessity of dietary supplementation in infants. If doubt exists as to whether the local water supply is supplemented with fluoride, the local water authority should be contacted. Fluoride has been shown to significantly reduce the incidence of dental caries by reducing the solubility of enamel, remineralising any early lesions of dental caries, and directly inhibiting plaque bacteria. Daily administration of tablets or drops may be beneficial where the fluoride content of drinking water is less than 0.7 parts per million (700 μg/L)(Table 17.5). The importance of the local action of fluoride at the site of application is emphasised by the greater benefits which are conferred by dropping the fluoride onto the tongue or sucking the tablets, rather than swallowing. Pharmacists should advise that fluoride supplementation should **not** be given to infants less than 6 months of age (BNF 9.5.3). No benefit in the prevention of dental caries in children has been demonstrated from the mother taking fluoride supplements during pregnancy.

If the water supply is fluoridated, parents must be warned that additional fluoride administration is unnecessary. Excess fluoride can lead to dental fluorosis, in which the enamel becomes demineralised, pitted, and has a white mottled appearance on the surface of permanent teeth (which start to develop within the gums from birth).

Pharmacists should be prepared to advise parents on the supply of fluoridated toothpastes which comprise almost all sales of dentrifices. Most young children start to use toothpaste by 18 months of age, although appreciable quantities may be swallowed by children up to three years of age. To prevent ingestion of excessive quantities of fluoride and the resultant dental fluorosis, the amount of toothpaste used by a child living in an area where the water is fluoridated should be limited to the size of a small pea. Once a child has reached 6 years of age, effective spitting out after teeth-cleaning is possible and the amounts ingested are minimal. Fluoride is present in toothpaste at a concentration of 1000 parts per million as sodium monofluorophosphate (0.8%), stannous fluoride (0.4%), or sodium fluoride (0.25%). Mouthwashes and topical applications (e.g. gels, varnishes, or solutions) may also be applied by dentists. However, because they are packaged in large volumes (e.g. 250 mL) and contain a lethal quantity of fluoride, they are not recommended for home use.

Sugar-free Medicines for Children

A greater public awareness of the potential cariogenic effects of regular intake of glucose, sucrose, and fructose

TABLE 17.5
Dosage recommendations for administration of fluoride supplements to infants (BNF 9.5.3)

Fluorine content of water (micrograms per litre or parts per million)	Age of infant	Dose of fluoride ion daily (micrograms)
less than 300	under 6 months	none
	6 months to 2 years	250
	2 to 4 years	500
	over 4 years	1000
300 to 700	under 2 years	none
	2 to 4 years	250
	over 4 years	500
more than 700	all ages	not recommended

has led to the increased introduction of sugar-free for-mulations of medicines for children. While any attempts to reduce the dietary intake of sugars is to be welcomed, it must also be borne in mind that many of the prepara-tions for children are given for short-term treatment only. The presence of potentially cariogenic carbo-hydrates will have little effect on the overall develop-ment of dental decay. Reformulated preparations must retain the properties conveyed by the sugar-containing ingredient (e.g. syrup), which may include preservation, viscosity, and sweetening.

The greatest benefit of the use of sugar-free formula-tions is for the chronic administration of medicines to children (e.g. in the treatment of epilepsy, cystic fibrosis, and asthma) or in giving those which are to remain in contact with the teeth (e.g. teething gels). The replace-ment of syrup BP by an alternative vehicle for prepara-tions in chronic use has been encouraged by the BP Commission, although sugar-based extemporaneous preparations have not been subject to amendment. It is obviously essential that pharmacists are aware of the correct diluent for reformulated products.

The BNF includes information on those preparations which are sugar-free.

17.5 IMMUNISATION OF INFANTS AND YOUNG CHILDREN

Pharmacists can play a vital role in advising parents of the importance of immunising their children against in-fectious diseases. Parents may be concerned about the relative merits and potential drawbacks of immunisation (e.g. to protect against pertussis) and may ask phar-macists, as readily accessible health-care professionals, for advice. Pharmacists should be familiar with immunisation schedules and, in particular, be prepared to respond to items in the local and national press about the use of vaccines. They should also be aware of the contra-indications to immunisation and the possible re-actions which may be caused by the administration of a vaccine.

This section will not detail the causes and symptoms of the diseases for which childhood immunisation is recommended. These may be found in the relevant monographs in Chapter 5. Detailed information on the preparations available and their administration is given in BNF, Chapter 14.

The Importance of Immunisation

At birth, an infant is protected initially from pathogenic micro-organisms by the transfer of maternal IgG anti-bodies across the placenta. Consequently, the infant may be passively immunised against a range of infections (e.g. chickenpox, measles, and mumps), although significant by its absence from this category is pertussis. However, antibodies derived from the mother gradually decline during the first 6 months of life and are replaced by the infant's own antibodies produced in response to anti-genic challenge. This explains why infants of under 6 months of age rarely contract infectious illnesses but the incidence gradually increases with age. An infant below 6 months of age which the mother considers is showing the signs of an infectious disease must always be referred, particularly as severe complications may develop in very young babies.

Active immunity is promoted in the young child by the administration of inactivated or live attenuated micro-organisms or their products (e.g. toxoids) (Table 17.6). The administration of these products stimulates a pri-mary response, the production of predominantly IgM antibodies. Subsequent injections cause an accelerated response, resulting in high levels of IgG antibodies which can remain in the circulation for months or years. Even if the levels fall off, the mechanism for their pro-duction has been sensitised and a rapid increase in anti-body levels will follow reinforcement (booster) vaccination.

The concept of herd immunity is important in immunisation programmes. Herd immunity is the im-munological status of the community against a par-ticular infectious disease. It is desirable to ensure that the uptake of vaccination is as high as possible. This helps to ensure that protection is afforded not only to those who have been immunised, but that the overall reduced inci-dence of the disease in the population significantly lowers the risks of infection to those who cannot, or will not, be immunised. Additionally, most infectious dis-eases are rarely completely eradicated from the environ-ment or healthy carriers and, if the level of herd immun-ity falls, epidemic outbreaks quickly develop.

Rates of uptake of vaccines are extremely variable but the UK figures stated here are intended to illustrate the potential for improvement to which pharmacists may

TABLE 17.6
Types of vaccines

Live attenuated	Inactivated	Toxoid
Polio (oral form)	Pertussis	Tetanus
Measles	Polio (parenteral form)	Diphtheria
Rubella		
BCG (tuberculosis)		
Mumps		

usefully contribute. In 1987, the uptake for measles vaccine was just below 70% and about 65% for pertussis vaccine. About 85% of all children received the triple vaccine (diphtheria, pertussis, and tetanus) and the polio vaccine. The combined measles/mumps/rubella (MMR) vaccine may eliminate the risk of pregnant women being infected with rubella, especially by their own children, and increase the uptake of measles vaccination.

The Role of Pharmacists

Pharmacists can play an important role in advising parents on the importance of immunisation and help increase the uptake of vaccine use. However, in order to be capable of responding to enquiries from parents, pharmacists must be aware of current information on the relative risks and benefits associated with individual vaccines. In particular, they should bear in mind that sensationalised media reports (which commonly provoke enquiries by anxious parents) are invariably unbalanced and stress only the rare adverse reactions to a vaccine. The positive contribution to health of the immunisation programme has meant that many young parents are happily unaware of the dangers to their children of infectious diseases. They may not have witnessed the trauma undergone by a child with pertussis and are ignorant of the congenital malformations (e.g. deafness, cataracts, and heart problems) which may result from an attack of rubella in the mother during pregnancy (see below). Similarly, the perception of measles as a minor illness (despite the associated risks of permanent brain damage which may be fatal) may contribute to parents' belief that the risks of vaccination are greater than the condition itself. In immunisation, perhaps more than any other health topic, it is important that all health professionals give uniform advice to parents. Conflicting advice (e.g. from pharmacists, health visitors, and doctors) confuses parents and can undermine their confidence in the health-care team. The importance of uniform advice illustrates the benefits of maintaining good relations and communications between professionals at all times. Pharmacists could usefully be encouraged to contact other members of the team to clarify what advice they are giving.

A brief description of some of the facts concerning the use of specific vaccines is presented below.

The Use of Specific Vaccines

The contra-indications to vaccination are specified in the BNF and pharmacists should consult this source for current information. Parents may ask a range of questions about other aspects of childhood vaccination and some of the following points have been confirmed by the Joint Committee on Vaccination and Immunisation. All children with asthma, eczema, allergic rhinitis, and any history of allergy or minor upper respiratory-tract infections should follow the standard vaccination schedule. Treatment with antimicrobials, topical or inhaled steroids, and breast feeding are also not contra-indications. Adherence to the immunisation schedule is preferable, but a child over a particular age will still be immunised. No allowance is necessary for premature infants, who should be immunised at three months of age and not three months after the expected date of delivery. Mothers who report that the child has already had pertussis, measles, or rubella should be advised that immunisation for these diseases is still necessary. A child who has missed one dose in a course of vaccination should continue the course immediately with the previously missed dose and subsequent recommended dose intervals. No attempt should be made to 'catch up' on the original dosage schedule by increasing the dose or reducing the dosage interval.

Pertussis   Although concern had been previously expressed, the publication of and widespread publicity given to a paper in 1974 which linked pertussis vaccination and neurological damage had a dramatic effect on the uptake of the vaccine. Vaccination rates dropped from 80% in 1968 to 30% in 1976, but have since regained some ground. Parental fears, however, of the production of convulsions, cerebral palsy, and mental retardation can be countered by an incidence of less than 1 in 100 000 injections. In the UK, the Joint Committee on Vaccination and Immunisation has advised that absolute contra-indications to pertussis vaccine are any severe local or general reaction to a preceding dose. In cases of a history of cerebral irritation or damage in the neonatal period, a history of convulsions, or children with parents or siblings that have a history of idiopathic epilepsy, special care must be taken in the administration of the vaccine. In each of these cases there may be an increased risk from vaccination, but this must be balanced against the potentially greater risks from an attack of the disease. Vaccination may be postponed if the child has an acute febrile, and particularly respiratory, illness but these are not contra-indications.

Measles   Although measles has the reputation of a minor illness, it can produce a range of complications (e.g. otitis media, respiratory-tract conditions, and rarely encephalitis) which warrant strict attention to its prevention. An attack of measles has particularly high mortality in children with malignant disease (e.g. acute lymphoblastic leukaemia), even during remission. This can be an especial problem as these children cannot be given live vaccines.

A vaccine for measles has been available since 1968 and post-vaccination complications (e.g. encephalitis and convulsions) are extremely rare. Despite early doubts concerning the efficacy and side-effects of the early products, parents can be reassured that the current product is safe and effective, and produces only a mild measles-like syndrome. A trivalent vaccine for measles, mumps, and rubella is also available.

Rubella   Rubella in a young child is itself a relatively minor illness and would not be a case for urgent and effective immunisation programmes. However, rubella contracted during pregnancy can have devastating effects on the health of the unborn child, as characterised by the congenital rubella syndrome. Since its introduction in 1970 for schoolgirls between 11 (later reduced to 10) and 14 years of age, the uptake of vaccination has risen to almost 90% of this selective population. The programme of vaccination, however, is not intended to completely eradicate the disease. Rubella virus stills circulates within the community and may induce natural immunity in up to 80% of women by the time they reach child-bearing age. The vaccination programme can therefore be considered a safety net intended to protect that portion of the remaining population that has not previously come into contact with the disease.

It is uncertain how long immunity is provided by active immunisation. Immunity may diminish with time, and immunisation is delayed from early childhood to ensure that girls are covered during their fertile years. (In the USA immunisation is given between 12 and 15 months of age and is a prerequisite of school entry.) The benefit of rubella virus within the population is indicated by the boost it can provide to the level of immunity in women before pregnancy. Active immunisation is also offered to seronegative women after pregnancy, although strict contraceptive cover must be ensured for at least three months after vaccination.

Poliomyelitis   The risks of paralysis produced by poliomyelitis have been almost completely eradicated through effective immunisation programmes introduced at the end of the 1950s. Protection can be given by an oral live attenuated vaccine (the Sabin vaccine), or a slightly less vigorous response may be obtained by an inactivated vaccine (the Salk vaccine), given parenterally. In the UK, the injectable form is given only if the patient requiring protection is pregnant or immunocompromised. There is a very small risk of developing poliomyelitis following oral vaccination, and there is also a risk that the disease can be passed on from an individual who has

been recently immunised to an unprotected person. Theoretically, the virus can become strengthened on transmission and may lead to full-blown poliomyelitis, although this occurs in only about 1 in 5 million immunisations. To minimise this risk, parents who are uncertain of their immune status should also receive vaccination at the same time as their children. The household contacts (e.g. parents and siblings) of immunosuppressed children should, therefore, receive only the injectable form.

Mumps   A mumps vaccine has been available in the USA since 1967 and in the UK since 1971. The uptake of mumps vaccine should increase as a result of the introduction in October 1988 of a trivalent vaccine for mumps, rubella, and measles (MMR). A similar triple vaccine is given to infants in the USA at 15 months of age. It may be effective for up to 12 years.

Diphtheria   In the UK, diphtheria vaccination has resulted in the virtual elimination of the infection. Natural immunisation, therefore, cannot occur and the high acceptance-rate must be maintained to protect the population from a resurgence of the disease. This may occur especially following introduction from overseas.

Tetanus   Tetanus vaccination, since its introduction in the UK in 1961, has resulted in a sharp decline in the incidence of children developing tetanus. However, adults continue to be affected at a higher rate because of the lack of vaccination in their childhood. This emphasises the need to maintain a high acceptance-rate.

Tuberculosis   The incidence of tuberculosis has declined but fatalities still occur in the UK. In addition to the recommended schedule for vaccination against tuberculosis, BCG vaccination may be offered when an infant is known to be in contact with a case of active respiratory tuberculosis, to children in immigrant communities who exhibit a higher incidence of tuberculosis, and if an infant is to travel to a high-risk area or where crowded conditions prevail. Vaccination is also offered to children between 10 and 13 years of age.

17.6   OTHER INFECTIOUS ILLNESSES IN CHILDREN

The information in Table 17.7 summarises the characteristics of common infectious illnesses in children and is intended to act as an *aide-memoire* for pharmacists. More detailed information on the individual diseases can be found in the relevant monographs in Chapter 5.

TABLE 17.7
Characteristics of infectious illnesses in children

Infection	Incubation period (days)	Distinguishing features	Degree of infectivity	Isolation required?
A. Bacterial infections				
Diphtheria	2 to 5	Wide range of symptoms from mild pyrexia, headache, and fatigue to difficulty in swallowing caused by a greyish-white membrane over the tonsils. In severe cases the membrane may spread to the trachea and bronchi, and may cause death if breathing is obstructed.	Very	Yes
Erysipelas	2 to 5	Tender red swollen areas over the face, arms, and legs preceded by headache, fever, malaise, and vomiting.	Rendered non-infective if treated	Necessary until treated
Meningococcal meningitis	1 to 5	Upper respiratory-tract infection may occur 2 to 3 days before severe symptoms. Early signs include fever, lethargy, drowsiness, crying, irritability, neck stiffness, and dislike of bright lights. Confusion and coma can follow within 12 to 24 hours. A macular rash occurs in about 50% and can develop into petechiae.	As long as micro-organisms are in the throat and nose	During initial 24 hours
Pertussis	7 to 10	Catarrhal stage of 7 to 14 days characterised by symptoms of an upper respiratory-tract infection followed by a dry cough. In the paroxysmal stage, cough becomes more severe and spasmodic and is terminated by a whoop. It may be accompanied by vomiting and convulsions.	Mainly during catarrhal stage	Avoid contact with babies
Scarlet fever	2 to 3	Sudden onset with sore throat, fever, malaise, vomiting, and 'strawberry tongue'. Rash appears after 24 to 36 hours on chest, neck, and arms and spreads to rest of body. The rash is formed of red dots on pink skin. The tongue is white but peels to leave a red raw surface. The skin may peel after three days.	Non-infective after starting antibacterial treatment	Until treatment
Tetanus	1 to 14	Muscular rigidity of jaw and face, and stiffness of neck, back muscles, and abdomen. Spasms may occur on external stimuli.	None	No
B. Viral infections				
Chickenpox	14 to 16	Early signs are fever, malaise, and anorexia. Macular rash develops into fluid-filled blisters in crops over the trunk, face, and scalp. Limbs are rarely affected. Blisters encrust and the scabs formed gradually fall off.	Highly infectious before rash appears – less so later	No
Infectious mononucleosis	28 to 49	Early signs of headache, fatigue, and malaise are followed by sore throat, fever, and lymphadenitis usually in the neck. Faint rash may occur.	Low	No
Measles	8 to 14	Prodromal symptoms include fever, sneezing, cough, catarrh, and conjunctivitis. White spots surrounded by a red ring (Koplik's spots) occur on the buccal mucosa. Fever declines, spots disappear, and are replaced by a rash starting on the neck (behind the ears) and face and spreading to the rest of the body. Fever rises again with the rash.	Catarrhal stage is very infectious	No
Mumps	14 to 18	Pain and swelling of the salivary (and especially parotid) glands. Dry mouth, malaise, fever, and chills.	14 to 21 days	No
Roseola infantum	5 to 15	Abrupt onset fever with lethargy and occasionally convulsions. Fever abates on appearance of macular rose-pink rash on trunk. The rash fades on pressure and may last a few hours or several days.	Unknown	No
Rubella	14 to 21	Tender lymph nodes in the neck with malaise, headache, slight fever, sore throat, and conjunctivitis. A fine red rash starts on the face and trunk and fades as the areas of erythema merge over the rest of the body. The rash fades within three days.	Until the rash disappears	No

Chapter 18

CARE OF THE ELDERLY

18.1 CONCEPTS IN AGEING

Ageing is an inescapable fact of life. The inevitable sequel to ageing is death, which is necessary for the prolonged vigour and health of the species. Death prevents a population explosion and allows youth to develop its full potential.

The process of ageing may be described as either primary or secondary. Primary ageing represents a natural decline in efficiency characterised by loss of homoeostasis and weakening of structure. Both effects eventually lead to a breakdown in health, followed by death. Secondary ageing results from disease and trauma, causing irreversible degeneration. Although it is impossible to slow the rate of primary ageing, the incidence of disease, and by inference longevity, can be affected by life-style and medical care.

It has been suggested (*see* Section 15.9) that ageing arises from an accumulation of errors of metabolism throughout life. Essential biological materials (e.g. RNA and DNA) may be damaged by environmental and chemical factors (e.g. radiation and drugs). If the number of accumulated errors exceeds a predefined level, cells and tissues may lose their functional capacity and perish.

Why has the Elderly Population Increased?

The average life expectancy at birth in the UK has risen by more than 20 years since the beginning of the century. The infant mortality rate has dropped radically from 200 per 1000 live births last century to the present rate of approximately 15 per 1000. This upsurge in survival rate can largely be attributed to better environmental and health conditions. The net result of these changes is that there has been a shift in the population distribution, with considerably greater numbers of people over 65 years of age. Closely allied to this is an increase in the incidence of morbidity.

As a direct consequence of these changes, there has been a population explosion. While the world population more than doubled to 2500 million between 1850 and 1950, it is predicted that over 6200 million people will be alive by the end of this century.

Why does Care of the Elderly Create Special Problems?

Many problems of the elderly are socio-economic as well as medical. The background to such problems should be borne in mind by pharmacists in their day-to-day contact with the elderly.

Historically, elderly people in a community were often treated with great respect as a result of their accumulated knowledge and experience, which could be passed on to younger members. Such consideration was given despite the inability of older members to contribute directly to the survival of the community. However, since the development of modern technology, and the exponential increase in information stored in books and other media, this role for the elderly has steadily declined.

Lack of status and loneliness contribute to undermine the confidence of old people. Almost half the over-75s live alone. Nearly one-third of this group have never had children, and of those that have, nearly 40% have outlived their progeny. Many are therefore condemned to live out their lives without any direct family contact or support, relying on friends, neighbours, and other members of the local community for their social contacts. The support of health and welfare organisations, either directly or through families, friends, and neighbours, provides a tremendous asset in promoting happiness.

The problems caused through inadequate social contacts are increased when considerable age is attained. It has been estimated that 80% of the over-85s need assistance with everyday living. Other elderly, but perhaps slightly younger, groups who may be equally dependent include the recently bereaved, and those discharged from hospital who must re-adapt quickly to their home environment if they are to survive.

Despite these major problems, less than 5% of over-65s receive long-term institutional care. Such care that is given is divided between hospitals, residential homes, and nursing homes. Hospitalised patients are located either in geriatric wards, psychiatric hospitals, or in acute services.

A significant majority of the elderly therefore live in the community, either coping independently, living with relatives, or relying on the social, welfare, and health services. The pharmacist, in providing a vital link in the health-care team, can make a significant contribution to the health and quality of life of this ever-increasing group.

18.2   HOW DOES AGEING AFFECT BODY SYSTEMS?

Ageing comprises many physiological changes which are reflected by alterations to body composition from 40 years of age. These changes occur in the absence of any associated pathology. Table 18.1 lists the common diseases of the elderly by physiological system.

Gastro-intestinal Tract

Salivary secretion is reduced, causing dry mouth and difficulty in swallowing. Gastric acid secretion is also decreased, and may be associated with atrophy. Malabsorption may develop, affecting particularly iron and calcium absorption.

Intestinal motility can become disorganised, causing constipation, and this may be aggravated if the elderly person is immobile.

Cardiovascular System

Reduced lean body-mass decreases metabolic demands, which in turn reduces cardiac ouput. Consequently, regional blood-flow is altered, with a greater proportion of the available supply going to the heart and brain at the expense of the kidneys and muscle.

Fibrosis occurs everywhere, producing increased rigidity and decreased elasticity. The pressure within the system, and hence the work required by the heart to eject the stroke volume, is raised.

The heart is less able to respond to stress because the cardiac reserve capacity is reduced. The older person will notice this particularly during exercise.

Respiratory System

Atrophy of lung tissue produces an increase in the size of the alveoli, thinning of their walls, and loss of elasticity. Chest diameter may increase while residual volume and vital capacity are reduced. The risks of respiratory infection are increased due to unsatisfactory functioning of the cilia, reduced cough efficiency, and increased dead space.

Nervous System

The effects of ageing on the nervous system are amongst the most important in considering the care of the elderly.

Manifestations of degenerative CNS changes (e.g. forgetfulness and movement disorders) are due primarily to faulty neurotransmitter metabolism rather

TABLE 18.1
Common disorders of the elderly

Classification	Example
Gastro-intestinal tract disorders	Cholestatic jaundice Constipation Crohn's disease Diverticular disease Dysphagia Gallstones Malabsorption syndromes Peptic ulceration Pyloric stenosis Reflux oesophagitis Ulcerative colitis
Cardiovascular system disorders	Arrhythmias Arteriosclerosis Hypertension Ischaemic heart disease
Respiratory system disorders	Chronic bronchitis and emphysema
Nervous system disorders	Depressive disorders Insomnia Parkinsonism Stroke Transient ischaemic attacks
Infections:	
• bacterial	Infective endocarditis Pneumonia Pulmonary tuberculosis
• viral	Herpesvirus infections Influenza
Endocrine system disorders	Diabetes mellitus Hyperthyroidism Hypothyroidism
Genito-urinary system disorders	Renal failure Urinary incontinence Urinary-tract infection
Malignant diseases	Bladder cancer Breast cancer Gastro-intestinal tract tumours Gynaecological tumours Haematological malignant tumours Lung cancer Prostate cancer
Blood disorders	Anaemias Thrombocytopenia
Musculoskeletal and connective tissue disorders	Giant cell arteritis Gout Osteitis deformans Osteomalacia Osteoporosis Polymyalgia rheumatica Rheumatoid arthritis
Eye disorders	Cataract Glaucoma

TABLE 18.1 *(contd.)*

Classification	Example
Ear, nose, and oropharynx disorders	Impacted wax Otosclerosis Speech disorders
Skin disorders	Decubitus ulcer Eczema Pruritus Psoriasis

than loss of neurones. Increased confusion may be related to decreased cerebral blood-flow. Sleep disorders increase in frequency, particularly the incidence of awakening during the night.

Changes in autonomic function cause bradycardia and a significant incidence of thermoregulatory disorders. The failure of vasoconstriction during cold weather can produce hypothermia, while inefficient vasodilatation or sweating in hot conditions produces overheating.

Endocrine System

Plasma-thyroid hormone concentrations are marginally reduced in the elderly. The rate of secretion of insulin in response to glucose loading is also decreased. Normal fluid intake should be maintained to prevent dehydration because the ability of the kidney to respond to the secretion of vasopressin is reduced. Conversely, compensatory thirst mechanisms are impaired as a result of ageing.

In general, other endocrine functions are not significantly affected by ageing.

Renal Function

There is an age-related decline in kidney function even in the absence of disease. The kidneys lose approximately 20% of their weight and 30% of their functioning glomeruli between 40 and 80 years of age. Despite compensatory hypertrophy, renal function decreases by up to 50% by 80 years of age. Such changes are particularly important in the pharmacokinetic assessment of drug administration (*see* Section 18.3 below).

Reproductive System

In the female the decline of ovarian function at the menopause is one of the most dramatic indications of ageing. This change is accompanied by variable degrees of atrophy of the hormone-dependent organs (i.e. the vulva, vagina, cervix, corpus uteri, Fallopian tubes, and ovaries).

In the male, gonadal function may remain intact or decrease only slowly with age.

Blood

Blood elements are remarkably durable. Age-related degeneration does not occur unless it is a consequence of associated pathology (e.g. iron depletion).

Any increased tendency towards thrombus formation is usually due to the effects of arteriosclerosis rather than an increased platelet count. This tendency is further increased with lack of mobility.

Musculoskeletal System and Connective Tissue

A progressive reduction in muscle strength results from cell loss and disorganisation. Lost muscle is replaced by fat and connective tissue, maintaining or even increasing total body weight.

The effects of ageing on connective tissue are widespread. Cross-linkages are formed within the collagen macromolecule, causing loss of elasticity of blood vessels, muscle, and joints. Damaged cartilage has little capacity for repair, resulting in osteoarthritis.

Changes in the skeletal structure can be profound. Reabsorption of bone exceeds its formation, especially in postmenopausal women and, as a result, fractures develop (e.g. in the hip).

Skin

The appearance of the skin is one of the most obvious indicators of increasing age. It sags, thins, and becomes wrinkled. Loss of melanin may produce skin with a white translucent look, or of a yellow appearance with blotches. Subcutaneous fat and vascularisation are reduced, increasing the likelihood of the development of decubitus ulcer.

Eye

Symptomatic visual changes develop from middle age. Presbyopia, due to hardening of the lens, is one of the most common. It renders accommodation for reading small print and other forms of close work more difficult. The symptoms of this degenerative process, which is normally complete by 65 years of age, can benefit from the use of appropriate spectacles.

After this age, visual changes are more subtle and increasingly occur as a consequence of associated degenerative and pathological processes. Examples of such changes include increased opacity of the lens, and pupillary deterioration. The size of the pupil and its ability to react to alterations in light intensity are reduced. Changing glasses at this stage is not usually of significant benefit.

Ear

Presbyacusis is a natural consequence of ageing. It is characterised by high-tone deafness, and affects mainly those over 60 years of age, especially men.

Although wax volume is not increased, its consistency is changed. It thickens and impacts as it dries, resulting in hearing difficulties.

18.3   HOW DOES AGEING AFFECT DRUG HANDLING?

Even in the absence of disease, age-related changes occur in the absorption, distribution, metabolism, and excretion of drugs. The existence of multiple pathologies further complicates these pharmacokinetic parameters. Exaggerated drug action and side-effects are examples of resulting pharmacodynamic changes.

Absorption

The oral route is the most common route for drug administration. However, impaired drug absorption in the elderly is due to a reduction in the volume of secretions, blood-flow to intestinal tissue, and the number of absorbing cells. Delayed gastric emptying also occurs.

Drugs actively transported from the gut (e.g. calcium, thiamine, and iron) are more susceptible to these changes than those which enter the circulation by passive diffusion (e.g. aspirin and paracetamol).

In common with patients of any age, elderly people with renal disease may suffer from nausea, vomiting, and diarrhoea. Cardiac disease causes poor tissue perfusion. In both instances, drug absorption will be reduced.

Distribution

The distribution of drugs is influenced by plasma-protein binding, blood flow-rate, and tissue-fat content. Circulating drugs are bound largely to the plasma protein, albumin. Plasma-albumin concentrations decrease with age, particularly in patients with chronic liver and renal disease. As a result, the amount of free (and therefore active) drug is increased, resulting in enhanced therapeutic effects.

The blood flow-rate is an important determinant of drug uptake by tissues. The total systemic perfusion and cardiac output decrease with age. As a result, the proportion of blood entering the liver and kidneys is reduced, significantly affecting drug kinetics.

The amount of body fat increases with age, while body water, intracellular water, and lean body-mass decrease. This may be significant in drug kinetics, producing an increase in the half-life of highly lipid-soluble drugs (e.g. benzodiazepines). When great age is attained (>85 years of age), the increased amount of body fat reverts to normal.

Metabolism

In the aged, the capacity of the liver to metabolise drugs is reduced by up to two-thirds of the normal adult capacity. Consequently drugs for whom the liver is the major site of metabolism (e.g. non-steroidal anti-inflammatory drugs, antiepileptics, and analgesics) exhibit increased plasma concentrations and a longer half-life.

The rate at which drugs are delivered to the liver is an important factor in metabolic capacity. In the elderly, liver perfusion can fall by 40% to 45%, and this significantly affects the metabolism of hypnotics (e.g. chlormethiazole) and antipsychotic drugs (e.g. chlorpromazine).

The effects of microsomal enzyme induction are reduced by ageing, possibly causing toxic effects through increased plasma concentrations. Alternatively, enzyme inhibition may be reduced, thus increasing the rate of metabolism of a second drug, and rendering the dose ineffective. Such considerations emphasise the problems of polypharmacy in the elderly.

Excretion

As a result of the decline in renal function with age, the excretion of many drugs and metabolites is significantly impaired. However, the use of creatinine clearance values as an indicator of the glomerular filtration rate may be misleading in the elderly as creatinine production decreases with age. In conjunction with decreased kidney function, almost normal plasma-creatinine concentrations may be measured even in the presence of considerable kidney disease.

Pharmacodynamics

Many elderly patients exhibit altered responsiveness to drugs. The brain shows particularly increased sensitivity, and patients become confused and disorientated at doses normally well tolerated by younger patients. Drugs which cause particular problems are hypnotics, antimuscarinics, dopamine agonists, and warfarin. Conversely, decreased tissue sensitivity may occur on ageing (e.g. to isoprenaline or propranolol).

18.4 HOW DO THE PROBLEMS OF AGEING AFFECT PHARMACY?

A recent report of the Royal College of Physicians highlighted the important role that pharmacists can play in the care of the elderly both in the community and in hospital.

In the community, the total numbers of prescriptions dispensed in England and Wales in 1985 was approximately 343 million, averaging 6.9 prescriptions per head of total population. The average number of items dispensed for pensioners was double the average figure, suggesting that the elderly comprise a large proportion of patients visiting the pharmacy each day. The disproportionate use of services by this group is further emphasised by the fact that in 1985 the over-65s accounted for 43% of total NHS expenditure while comprising just 15% of the total population.

It has been estimated that advice on symptoms is sought from the pharmacist by between 15 and 25 people each day. While the proportion of these who are elderly is not clear, experience has shown that their requests are more common and frequently require more time than those from the general population.

Counselling the Elderly Patient

Various studies have shown that talking to patients for up to 15 minutes about their medicines significantly improves compliance. While this is clearly practical in only a minority of cases, it should be remembered that new information is assimilated less readily by the elderly, and advice may need re-iteration, particularly if the patient seems confused. (For a further discussion of counselling, *see* Section 19.3.)

Commonly Reported Symptoms

In the pharmacy, the conditions most commonly reported by the elderly are arthritis and related conditions, followed closely by difficulty in walking and unsteadiness, forgetfulness, and poor vision. Old folk will often also describe deafness, back pain, breathlessness on slight exertion, swollen feet, and indigestion. However, patients are frequently unable to describe their symptoms because of restricted knowledge and vocabulary. The elderly have been shown to be especially poor at describing detail and depth of symptoms, and pharmacists must therefore be patient and often penetrating in their questioning. (For further discussion on all aspects of responding to symptoms, *see* Section 20.3.)

Compliance

The problems of poor compliance in the elderly are now well recognised. Amongst the causes are polypharmacy, impaired mental ability, inability to open containers, and inadequate labelling.

A further complication which leads to confusion in tablet selection is the tendency to hoard medicines. Many pharmacists will have experience of vast quantities of medicines returned by relatives of recently deceased elderly patients, and this is also reflected in campaigns to encourage the return of unused and unwanted medicines.

Memory aids have been developed to improve compliance (*see* Fig. 19.6), together with supplementary written instructions. While these aids do not provide containers of BP standards, their use may be of benefit to some patients.

Self-medication

While polypharmacy in prescribed medicines has been recognised as a problem in the care of the elderly, concurrent self-administration of non-prescription medicines has only recently been acknowledged as a factor which can aggravate management. Pharmacists should be alert to requests for non-prescription medicines, especially if a prescription has just been dispensed.

Repeat Prescriptions

Guidelines on the issue of repeat prescriptions vary considerably between doctors' practices. Doctors may require patients to make an appointment after one or two repeat prescriptions have been issued. However, many chronic conditions of the elderly demand continuous therapy, and repeat prescriptions are a common occurrence.

Pharmacists should be wary of the elderly patient who 'doesn't need the water tablets this month'. This may indicate problems in compliance, or the presence of unwanted effects making the patient reluctant to continue treatment.

Hospital Pharmacy

Elderly in-patients have their medication administered at preset times by nursing staff. However, discharge medication must usually be self-administered, or given by the patient's family or friends.

Several studies have shown that counselling by the pharmacist immediately before discharge reduces medication errors at home. Elderly patients are also encouraged to supervise their own medication while still in-patients so that potential problems can be detected and remedied before discharge.

Residential Homes and Nursing Homes

Homes for the elderly may be classed as residential homes or nursing homes. In England and Wales, residential homes are not required to employ medical or nursing staff, and are registered and inspected by the Social Services Department of the Local Authority; nursing homes provide professional care by registered nurses, and are registered and inspected by the District Health Authority.

In nursing homes, medicines are administered under the control of the registered nurse in charge. The pharmaceutical input in nursing homes may be provided by community services pharmacists based at a nearby hospital. In residential homes, staff may supervise the administration of medicines, but many patients are encouraged to take charge of their own medicines and administration whenever possible. All prescription-only medicines should be supplied on a named-patient basis, with full directions on each container.

It is important that pharmacists visit residential homes to ensure that records are kept correctly, check and advise on the storage of medicines, and provide any further professional advice needed. Pharmacists should also take note of any non-prescription medicines stored in the residential home, confirming that their administration and storage is appropriate, and that there are no potential interactions between prescription and non-prescription medicines.

Chapter 19

COMMUNICATION, COUNSELLING, AND COMPLIANCE

19.1 INTRODUCTION

The role of the pharmacist, especially in the community, has always involved communication. Most pharmacists, through experience, have become adept at adjusting their verbal comments to the appropriate level necessary for effective understanding by the other party.

Hospital pharmacists have established an active role as communicators, not only to medical personnel and patients, but also to other health-care professionals working in, or from, the hospital environment. This extended communicator role has been further facilitated by the appointment in many health districts of community service pharmacists.

The importance of communication in pharmacists' roles has largely been taken very much for granted. In the past, little, if any, attempt was made to include instruction in undergraduate pharmacy courses, leaving it to the pre-registration training period. The Nuffield Report (1986) made several recommendations about communication skills and counselling services, which have encouraged and confirmed some of the changes already carried out in recent years in pharmaceutical education. The need for modern therapeutic agents to be used correctly and safely to minimise the risk of adverse effects is obvious. Greater demands than ever before are being placed on the prescriber and pharmacist to communicate with, and counsel where necessary, all patients to improve compliance. Those particularly at risk may have reading or language difficulties, or be mentally confused.

Although all human beings start to communicate from birth, some acquire greater expertise than others, reflecting the conscious effort required to achieve effective communication. The fundamental requirement in effective communication is that the information received is the same as that sent, and is understood in the way intended by the sender. From this statement it can be seen that communication consists of three components:

- a sender
- a message
- a receiver.

When applied to communication between pharmacist and patient, pharmacist and prescriber, or prescriber and patient, the sender and receiver are individuals while the message may be conveyed orally, or in writing as a prescription, a label, or a leaflet.

Remarkable changes have occurred over the past three decades in the way in which medicines are presented. No longer are patients supplied solely with mixtures to be taken a spoonful at a time or lotions to be applied to the skin. Instead, they are treated with the sophisticated products of pharmaceutical research and development, ranging from sustained-release tablets and capsules, through metered-dose inhalation aerosols, to percutaneously absorbed drugs impregnated in plaster patches. The continued development of communication skills by the pharmacist is necessary for counselling in the correct and effective use of medicines.

The dictionary definition of the word 'counsel' is consultation or advice, but the verb may also mean 'to warn', and the noun 'counselling', of American origin, means 'a service consisting of giving advice on miscellaneous problems to citizens and others'. In spite of the breadth of meaning of the term, it can more specifically be seen as part of the interaction which can usefully occur between pharmacist and patient. It also includes the potential for contributing to the most suitable choice of medication and resolving problems of administration or use of medication. Throughout this discussion, the term 'patient' will be used to include either a member of the public who presents a prescription, or one who requests advice about a non-prescription medicine.

Just as the acquisition of effective communication skills requires effort, so too does the development of the ability to be an effective counsellor. Probably the most important attribute is a willingness to listen as well as to talk.

The third term included in the title is compliance, which can be defined as 'agreement, consent, or yielding to the wishes of another'. Patient compliance is the extent to which patients take or use their medication in accordance with the advice given. People's behaviour and acceptance of associated dietary or life-style constraints may often be involved.

It is through effective communication and counselling by pharmacists that they can make an invaluable contribution to the correct and safe use of prescribed medicines, medicines purchased from the pharmacy, or those supplied by the pharmacist in response to symptoms described by the patient.

The association of the three terms communication, counselling, and compliance represents factors which may significantly contribute to enhancing patient care and to the greater fulfilment of the pharmacist's professional role.

19.2   COMMUNICATION

Communication is a complex process which, to be effective, depends greatly on the continuing transmission and feedback oscillating between sender and receiver. There are also important non-verbal reactions which must be in sympathy with the verbal messages if the latter are to be correctly understood prior to any response.

Barriers to Effective Communication

Some common barriers to effective communication can be readily identified and are listed in Table 19.1.

This short summary attempts to highlight the major problems which practising pharmacists may encounter and, by inference, how communication may be optimised for the patient's benefit and the more effective use of pharmacists' time.

It is the need to be able to adapt and respond to the individual patient's mood which makes the use of learning aids (e.g. a pre-recorded videocassette explaining how to use suppositories) a less than ideal substitute for personal communication.

Recognising and Overcoming Barriers

Communication invariably prompts questions from one or both participants. Pharmacists must be sure to ask the right questions while avoiding the threat of appearing to interrogate.

The message   Pharmacists must avoid giving the impression that they are sorry for the patient or, that by using lay terminology and speaking in short sentences, they appear to be talking down to the patient.

The environment   The environment must be conducive to the communication process. If the pharmacist is literally speaking down to a patient from a raised platform, this may appear threatening and create difficulties, particularly for the elderly, to either hear or to respond. Many pharmacies built with raised dispensaries to make them more conspicuous, and which help the pharmacist to literally oversee the pharmacy, are now being refitted at floor level.

Physical barriers (e.g. a pharmacy counter or prescrip-

TABLE 19.1
Common barriers to effective communication

The message
- the message is too faint or inaudible
- the language used is not understood
- the vocabulary is too sophisticated to be understood
- the accent is unfamiliar

The environment
- background noise or distraction
- lack of privacy

Attitude
- human characteristics such as impatience
- sender or receiver conveying the impression that 'they haven't time'

tion reception point) may militate against relaxed conversation. If the pharmacist moves around the end of the counter, the patient may feel more at ease and in less of an interview-type situation. For most people there is an optimum distance to be kept between communicators. Standing close to strangers may appear threatening and invasive, and is normally reserved for family and close friends. The optimum acceptable distance apart also varies with age group, culture, and sex.

Attitude   It is obviously essential that the pharmacist possesses a sound and adequate knowledge of the patient's medication and an awareness of the most useful information sources to which the pharmacist may refer. The patient will therefore be reassured by the pharmacist's confidence and manner.

Only a small part of the impact of any message communicated is attributable to the verbal content. Emotion, tone of voice, gestures, and body language are equally powerful influences.

The patient must perceive that the pharmacist has time; that he is genuine and wishes to establish an empathy with, and for, the patient; and that he is sympathetic and can encourage the patient to have trust and confidence.

The manner of expression may be dramatically influenced by anger, joy, despair, or weariness. The pharmacist must be sensitive to mood and be aware of the need to listen carefully to the patient before responding in a calm, resilient, non-aggressive, and supportive manner. The need to gain the patient's confidence is paramount. In body language, the way in which the participants use their eyes in face-to-face communication may be crucial (although there may be significant differences between races in the way in which eye contact is used). If either party fails to make eye contact, it can be extremely disconcerting to the other person and may easily convey disinterest. However, if one person stares hard and unwaveringly at the other, the effect may be equally disquieting and even threatening.

Eye contact conveys that the speaker has, even if only momentarily, the attention of the listener. In effective communication the skill is to regularly reaffirm attention by eye contact of varying duration, sensitive to avoiding either any threat, or any loss of attention by turning the head and eyes away to a distracting extent.

The timing of eye contact may also act as a means of emphasis and a vital feedback mechanism capable of registering the listener's reaction to what he has heard. Communication with patients who are blind or partially sighted may benefit from contact (e.g. touching the arm) as a substitute for eye contact.

The movement of head, arms, and legs may all con-

tribute to, or distract from, communication. The angle of the head may convey enquiry or, if tilted back, superiority or a haughty or aggressive attitude. A nod or a series of nods can confirm undivided attention and agreement on the part of the listener, although nods which appear too repetitive may be distracting.

Folded arms may convey, or at least exaggerate, a defensive reaction (i.e. a holding-at-arms-length type of response). However, facial expression in most people is very explicit, and in meaningful communication is a powerful indicator and feedback mechanism, showing emotions like happiness, anger, agreement, disagreement, interest, and disinterest. A fixed permanent smile may convey insincerity, whilst an encouraging smile confirms a willingness to start or advance a dialogue.

It is also most important to avoid any distracting tics (e.g. repetitively touching part of the head or face with a finger, the repetitive furrowing of the brow, or playing with spectacles).

Communication technique may be effectively studied and improved by role-play exercises, preferably aided by video filming and playback.

Communication with Prescribers

The principles of communication are no different when the pharmacist telephones a prescriber with a prescription query than when explaining the dosage directions for a dispensed medicine to a patient. In both, it is necessary to avoid language which appears to threaten. No pharmacist would, when querying an unusually high dose, normally state that an overdose had been prescribed. Instead, having first identified himself and supplied the patient's name and address, the pharmacist should seek clarification whether or not the prescriber intended a dose in excess of that recommended in the BNF or by the manufacturer. These independent, authoritative sources, quoted objectively from one professional to another, are much more likely to elicit a constructive response. This is no subservient strategy. In the highly unlikely event of the prescriber being unable or unwilling to adjust the dose appropriately, or providing an adequate explanation for an unusually high dose (which should preferably be initialled and endorsed by the prescriber), the pharmacist should professionally consider whether the patient would be put at risk. In such circumstances, it may be wise to seek a second opinion (e.g. from the Royal Pharmaceutical Society, the National Pharmaceutical Association, or another pharmacist) before proceeding. Sensitivity to adjust the particular communication strategy to fit the situation is what is required.

It is worth noting that interprofessional communication and understanding is immeasurably enhanced when the pharmacist personally knows the prescriber. Attendance at local professional meetings may provide an excellent opportunity for social interaction.

A summary of influences on effective communication and the characteristics of successful communication is given in Tables 19.2 and 19.3.

Enhancing Communication Skills

The use of communication skills in counselling by the pharmacist has wide ranging application, from the supply of dispensed medicines to health-care advice and health promotion. However, it is most important to recognise that the label, verbal instruction, or counselling and a leaflet are not alternatives but are all complementary to each other and essential for optimising the patient's understanding and compliance.

Labelling   The labelling of medicines is concerned with the communication of information. The pharmacist should preferably check with the patient to ensure that the directions for use are properly understood, and reinforced where necessary by the opportunity for verbal interactive response. Where essential additional information cannot be included on a label, it may be supplied in the form of a leaflet.

In the UK, cautionary advice has been incorporated into a range of 'Cautionary and Advisory Labels for Dispensed Medicines', included as an appendix in the BNF. The recommendation for their use reflects the growing recognition that patients should be given better information about their medicines. It also stresses the importance of counselling by pharmacists, reinforcing the care that should be taken during treatment (e.g. about the avoidance of alcohol, the risks of drowsiness, or the need to take the medicine with water, not milk).

The wording of additional labels has been carefully chosen, attempting to provide the information concisely but intelligbly. However, even with their use, it is vital that the pharmacist counsels the patient to confirm the information given on the label.

Occasionally, it may be preferable to counsel the patient rather than provide a cautionary label (e.g. about the risk of the medicine staining either clothes or the skin). The BNF includes additional recommended counselling advice for some products.

Much work has been done, and ingenuity used, to support verbal communication and medicine labels (e.g. Braille labels for blind patients reproducing simple directions like 'one to be taken three times a day' on semi-rigid plastic strips).

TABLE 19.2
Summary of influence on effective communication

- Create a suitable atmosphere for the patient or customer to be receptive including the absence of distracting noise, a sense of privacy, and the minimum of physical barriers.
- Be prepared to listen carefully and patiently.
- Ask logical questions where necessary in a systematic manner.
- Ensure that the information conveyed is correct, relevant, and reliably up-to-date.
- Facilitate communication by recognising the influence of non-verbal communication factors (e.g. body language, facial expression, gestures, head movement, and posture).
- Avoid distracting tics.
- Be sensitive to and keep to an acceptable distance apart.
- Ensure that the language and vocabulary, including any technical terms used, are right for the receiver.
- The quality of the communication depends more on interaction than on duration. Be ready to respond to non-verbal clues.
- Maintain empathy.

TABLE 19.3
The characteristics of successful communication

- The purpose of communication is not just to deliver a message but to effect a change in the recipient, in respect of his knowledge, attitude, and eventually behaviour.
- The value of communication is to be judged not on its purpose or content, but on its effect on the recipient.
- Good communication is difficult.
- Communication must be matched to the knowledge, social background, interest, purposes, and needs of the recipient.
- Communication is effected not only by words, which must have the same meaning for giver and receiver, but also by attitudes, expressions, and gestures.
- If communication is to change behaviour, the required change in the recipient must be seen by him to have more advantages than drawbacks.
- To make sure that communication has succeeded, information about its effect (feedback), both immediate and subsequent, is needed.
- Communication demands effort, thought, time, and often money.

Leaflets   Leaflets play an important part in the communication of information which is too detailed to include on the medicine label. The physical dimensions of many medicine containers are insufficient to allow the necessary information to be affixed to the surface in a print size which can be easily read. The advantage of leaflets derives from fewer constraints on space compared with labels, increasing the ease of readability and illustration potential. They are also more permanent than the spoken word and can be referred to at a later date by the patient. Product-specific leaflets and those which help patients in the use of particular preparations (e.g. eye ointments or nasal drops) have been devised. Many leaflets include illustrations (pictograms), which may be especially helpful and easier to comprehend by the poorly sighted and those with literacy or language difficulties. The main disadvantages of leaflets, however, are that they may become detached from the product to which they apply and, unlike verbal advice, they are not interactive.

A wide variety of leaflets has been produced, primarily by manufacturers of proprietary products as package inserts for the information of users. In prescription-only medicines, leaflets are often written for the prescriber or pharmacist and include data sheet style information as well as some information relevant to patient use. Pads of leaflets have been produced for bulk dispensing packs, written specifically for patient guidance and information. Unfortunately, there is no co-ordination in the production of information leaflets of this type between manufacturers of similar products, but with the introduction of original pack dispensing many more leaflets will become available.

Leaflets containing more specific information on product use are supplied with unit pack items (e.g. pressure inhalers). They are usually very well produced, often with colour printing, and frequently include step-by-step illustrations to aid comprehension. However, some leaflets may be too detailed to be meaningful without careful explanation by pharmacists, especially when issued to the elderly and when a medicine is first supplied. It is very important for pharmacists to have studied such leaflets before giving them out, enabling them to go through the salient points confidently. In

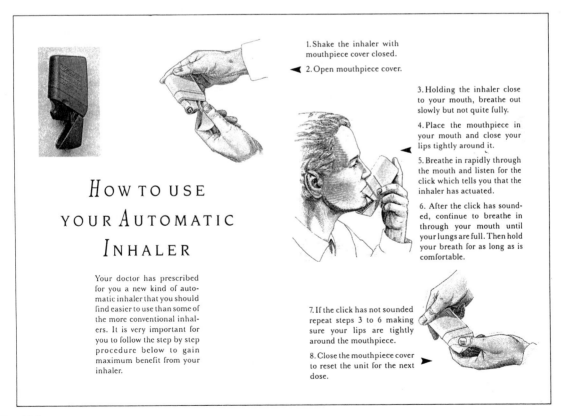

1. Shake the inhaler with mouthpiece cover closed.

◄ 2. Open mouthpiece cover.

3. Holding the inhaler close to your mouth, breathe out slowly but not quite fully.

4. Place the mouthpiece in your mouth and close your lips tightly around it.

5. Breathe in rapidly through the mouth and listen for the click which tells you that the inhaler has actuated.

6. After the click has sounded, continue to breathe in through your mouth until your lungs are full. Then hold your breath for as long as is comfortable.

How to use your Automatic Inhaler

Your doctor has prescribed for you a new kind of automatic inhaler that you should find easier to use than some of the more conventional inhalers. It is very important for you to follow the step by step procedure below to gain maximum benefit from your inhaler.

7. If the click has not sounded repeat steps 3 to 6 making sure your lips are tightly around the mouthpiece.

8. Close the mouthpiece cover to reset the unit for the next dose. ►

Fig. 19.1
Use of an Aerolin pressure inhaler.

practice it has been found that a maximum of 5 or 6 main points may be retained by the patient (e.g. for pressure inhalers, Fig. 19.1).

A number of investigations have studied the requirements for format, wording, and range of leaflets.

The Department of Health's treatment card for patients on monoamine-oxidase inhibitor drugs, and the Royal Pharmaceutical Society's treatment card for patients on oral anticoagulant therapy, have each fulfilled an important need. As long ago as 1977, the Medicines Commission recognised the importance of written information for patients as a supplement to oral advice from the prescriber and pharmacist, and to remind patients how to take the medicine and on actions to avoid. Treatment cards and leaflets issued by pharmacists are an appropriate means of communication and will continue to be so even when original pack dispensing becomes the rule rather than the exception.

Attention must be given when designing leaflets to ensure that sentences are short and technical terms are avoided. Phrases like 'one drop to be instilled into the conjunctival sac' are better replaced by 'put one drop in each eye'. Some words and phrases are more easily substituted than others. 'Thinly' may be considered to be more widely understood than 'sparingly', where the latter word is used in relation to the application of topical corticosteroids. It is not, however, easy to find an entirely satisfactory word for 'discard' when giving advice about the disposal of a medicine that has expired. 'Do not use after ...' is negative and does little to discourage hoarding while 'Throw away ...' may be seen as an unfortunate choice of words.

Other important design factors are page and type size, line spacing, margins, contrast and colour, illustrations or graphics, and, inevitably, cost. Type size variation and contrast can aid readability.

It was originally hoped that the introduction of type-written and machine-produced labels, required on all dispensed medicines since 1 January 1984, would have eliminated unreadable directions on labels. On the contrary, there are still many labels produced with type-face lettering which is too small, too faint, or both, and which is either difficult to read or actually unreadable by many elderly patients. Leaflets should be designed to avoid these problems.

Examples of leaflets include the Department of Health's monoamine-oxidase inhibitor card (Fig. 19.2), and the more elaborate lithium treatment card (Fig. 19.3) published by the Royal Pharmaceutical Society.

For those who may not speak, write, or read English there are additional difficulties. In many cases, patients may be accompanied to their surgery, and later to the pharmacy, by a family member who does understand

TREATMENT CARD

Carry this card with you at all times. Show it to any doctor who may treat you other than the doctor who prescribed this medicine, and to your dentist if you require dental treatment.

INSTRUCTIONS TO PATIENTS
Please read carefully
While taking this medicine and for 14 days after your treatment finishes you must observe the following simple instructions:-

1   Do not eat CHEESE, PICKLED HERRING OR BROAD BEAN PODS.
2   Do not eat or drink BOVRIL, OXO, MARMITE or ANY SIMILAR MEAT OR YEAST EXTRACT.
3   Eat only FRESH foods and avoid food that you suspect could be stale or 'going off'. This is especially important with meat, fish, poultry or offal. Avoid game.
4   Do not take any other MEDICINES (including tablets, capsules, nose drops, inhalations or suppositories) whether purchased by you or previously prescribed by your doctor, without first consulting your doctor or your pharmacist.
    NB *Treatment for coughs and colds, pain relievers, tonics and laxatives are medicines.*
5   Avoid alcoholic drinks and de-alcoholised (low alcohol) drinks.

Keep a careful note of any food or drink that disagrees with you, avoid it and tell your doctor.
Report any unusual or severe symptoms to your doctor and follow any other advice given by him.

| M.A.O.I. | Prepared by The Pharmaceutical Society and the British Medical Association on behalf of the Health Departments of the United Kingdom. |

Printed in the UK for HMSO 8217411/150M/9.89/45292
Revised Sep. 1989

Fig. 19.2
Monoamine-oxidase inhibitor card.

English. Sometimes, however, it is a very young member of the family who has to act as interpreter and the quality of translation due to a child's inexperience may be less than satisfactory. Some studies have shown that, unfortunately, many elderly immigrants unable to speak any English are frequently also illiterate in their own language. In such cases the otherwise excellent multi-lingual leaflets produced by some pharmaceutical companies (Fig. 19.4) and health authorities may be of limited value. The pharmacist must take responsibility to check that such directions are understood and be alert to some alternative means, however basic they may appear (e.g. the use of hastily designed pictograms) to ensure that the patient is not left in ignorance about his medicine and its regimen.

It must, however, be re-emphasised that, only if the

THINKING ABOUT STARTING A FAMILY?

Because Lithium can effect the unborn baby do NOT become pregnant without first talking to your doctor. If you are pregnant tell your doctor now.

Published by the Royal Pharmaceutical Society of Great Britain, 1 Lambeth High Street, London, SE1 7JN.
Printed April 1989.

The Society gratefully acknowledges the co-operation and sponsorship of Delandale Laboratories Ltd., Norgine Ltd., Smith Kline and French Laboratories Ltd., and Lagap Pharmaceuticals Ltd.

KEEP YOUR TABLETS IN A SAFE PLACE WELL OUT OF THE REACH OF CHILDREN.

PLEASE RECORD YOUR BLOOD LEVEL OF LITHIUM

DATE TAKEN	BLOOD LEVEL	DAILY DOSE

LITHIUM TREATMENT CARD

CARRY THIS CARD WITH YOU AT ALL TIMES. SHOW IT TO ANY DOCTOR OR NURSE WHO TREATS YOU AND ANY PHARMACIST YOU BUY MEDICINES FROM.

NAME ....

PREPARATION OF LITHIUM ....

Should a different proprietary product be prescribed, the card must be suitably endorsed.

HOW SHOULD I TAKE THE TABLETS?

Swallow each tablet whole or broken in half, with water. Do NOT chew or crush it. Try to take the dose at the same time each day.

WHAT SHOULD I DO IF I MISS A DOSE?

Do NOT double your next dose. If you find you have missed a few doses, start taking your usual dose on the day you remember and tell your doctor.

WHY MUST I HAVE A BLOOD TEST?

This is to check the amount of lithium in your blood. It is very important to have the correct amount because too much can be dangerous. Take the blood test ABOUT 12 HOURS AFTER the last dose of lithium.

CAN I DRINK ALCOHOL?

It is safe to drink SMALL quantities.

CAN I TAKE OTHER MEDICINES WITH LITHIUM?

Some medicines can change the amount of lithium in the blood. These include diuretic (water) tablets and capsules, some pain killers and some indigestion mixtures and laxatives. So check with your doctor or pharmacist before taking other medicines.

Please note: It is safe to take aspirin and paracetamol but not ibuprofen.

WHAT ELSE ALTERS THE LITHIUM LEVEL?

The level can be altered by the amount of fluids you drink, changes in the amount of salt in your food, sweating more than usual (in hot weather, fever or infection), severe vomiting, severe diarrhoea and a low salt diet. Check with your doctor if any of these things happen.

SIGNS OF A HIGH LITHIUM LEVEL

Vomiting, severe diarrhoea, unusual drowsiness, muscle weakness and feeling very giddy may mean that your level of lithium is too high. Stop taking the tablets and talk to your doctor IMMEDIATELY.

DOES LITHIUM HAVE SIDE EFFECTS?

Some slight effects (such as sickness, shaking) may occur at first but they usually wear off if blood tests are normal. Discuss this with your doctor. Some patients may gain weight but this can be prevented with a sensible diet.

HOW LONG WILL I HAVE TO TAKE LITHIUM?

Lithium is a way of preventing illness so you may have to take it for many years. Never stop taking the tablets without asking your doctor.

Fig. 19.3
Lithium treatment card.

content of a leaflet or warning card is drawn to the attention of the patient by the pharmacist, is the information likely to be of effect.

19.3   COUNSELLING

This term has been increasingly used to describe the sympathetic interaction between pharmacists and patients, which may go beyond conveyance of straightforward information about the medicine and how and when to use it.

Much greater attention is being paid to counselling and training for counselling by all health-care professions. This is especially so since the greater awareness of, and attention given to, holistic health, which is concerned with the integrated health and well-being of the person as a whole. While there are many forms of counselling it is generally a way of relating to a person in need of guidance, using understanding, sympathy, and sincerity. Most counsellors are eclectic, drawing from different types of counselling such as 'behavioural', which is concerned with modifying behaviour from the unacceptable to the acceptable, and 'humanistic', which is more concerned with personal growth and human potential.

START DAY

Mon
Tue
Wed
Thu
Fri
Sat
Sun

How to take Minulet®

1. Begin taking Minulet on the first day of menstrual bleeding. For example, if your first day of menstrual bleeding is Tuesday, start by taking any pill marked "Tue."

2. Under "Start Day," scratch off the silver indicator (▶) next to the day on which you take your first pill. This will also be your start day for every new pack of Minulet.

3. Take **one** pill each day. Follow the arrows in the direction shown. For your convenience, establish a routine of taking the pill at the same time each day; for example, at bedtime.

4. After you finish the pack, wait seven days before beginning the next pack.

Complete information about Minulet is available to you from your physician.

(શરૂઆતના દિવસો

સોમ
મંગળ
બુધ
ગુરૂ
શુક્ર
શનિ
રવિ

(મીનુલેટ કેવી રીતે લેવી?)

(૧) માસિક શરૂ થાય તે દિવસથી જ મીનુલેટ લેવાની શરૂ કરવી. દા.ત. જો તમારો માસિક શરૂ થવાનો દિવસ મંગળવાર હોય તો "મંગળવાર"ના નિશાનવાળી ગોળી લેવી.
(૨) "શરૂઆતના દિવસ"ની નીચે તમે જે દિવસે ગોળી લીધી હોય તે દિવસની આગળ જે તીરની નિશાની (▶) હોય તે ભૂંસી નાખો. આજ દિવસ તમારો મીનુલેટનું નવું પેકેટ શરૂ કરવાનો દિવસ હશે.
(૩) દરરોજ એક ગોળી લો. જે પ્રમાણે ગોળીની સંખ્યા અને તીરની નિશાની દેખાડી છે તે પ્રમાણે તીરનું અનુકરણ કરો તમારી સગવડતા માટે દરરોજ એક સરખા જ સમયે ગોળી લેવાની ટેવ પાડો. દાત. સાંજે સુતી વખતે.
(૪) ગોળીઓનું એક પેકેટ તમે પુરૂં કરો એટલે બીજું નવું ગોળીઓનું પેકેટ શરૂ કરતાં પહેલાં સાત દિવસ ગોળી લેવાનું બંધ રાખો.
તમને મીનુલેટની પૂરેપૂરી માહિતી તમારા દાકતર પાસેથી મળી શકશે.

Gujarati

ਆਰੰਭ ਦਾ ਦਿਨ

(ਸੋਮ)
(ਮੰਗਲ)
(ਬੁੱਧ)
(ਵੀਰ)
(ਸ਼ੁਕਰ)
(ਸ਼ਨੀ)
(ਐਤ)

ਮਿਨੂਲੈਟ ਕਿਵੇਂ ਲਈ ਜਾਵੇ

1. ਮਾਹਵਾਰੀ ਆਉਣ ਦੇ ਪਹਿਲੇ ਦਿਨ ਤੋਂ ਮਿਨੂਲੈਟ ਲੈਣੀ ਸ਼ੁਰੂ ਕਰੋ। ਮਿਸਾਲ ਵਜੋਂ, ਜੇਕਰ ਤੁਹਾਡੇ ਮਾਹਵਾਰੀ ਆਉਣ ਦਾ ਪਹਿਲਾ ਦਿਨ ਮੰਗਲਵਾਰ ਹੈ ਤਾਂ Tue ਦੇ ਨਿਸ਼ਾਨ ਵਾਲੀ ਗੋਲੀ ਲੈ ਕੇ ਅਰੰਭ ਕਰੋ।

2. ਜਿਸ ਦਿਨ ਤੁਸੀਂ ਪਹਿਲੀ ਗੋਲੀ ਲਈ ਹੈ, ਉਸੇ ਦਿਨ "Start day" ਦੇ ਨਾਲ ਲੱਗਾ ਚਾਂਦੀ ਰੰਗਾ ਨਿਸ਼ਾਨ (▶) ਕੁਰੇਦ ਦਿਓ। ਮਿਨੂਲੈਟ ਦੇ ਹਰ ਨਵੇਂ ਪੈਕ ਲਈ ਇਹੋ ਤੁਹਾਡਾ ਅਰੰਭਕ ਦਿਨ ਹੋਵੇਗਾ।

3. ਹਰ ਰੋਜ਼ ਇਕ ਗੋਲੀ ਲਓ। ਤੀਰ ਦੇ ਲਗੇ ਨਿਸ਼ਾਨਾਂ ਦੀ ਪੈਰਵੀ ਕਰੋ। ਹਰ ਰੋਜ਼ ਆਪਣੀ ਸਹੂਲਤ ਲਈ ਇਕੋ ਸਮੇਂ ਗੋਲੀ ਲੈਣ ਦਾ ਨਿਤਨੇਮ ਬਣਾ ਲਓ, ਮਿਸਾਲ ਵਜੋਂ ਸੌਣ ਦੇ ਸਮੇਂ।

4. ਜਦੋਂ ਤੁਸੀਂ ਪੈਕ ਖ਼ਤਮ ਕਰ ਲਓ, ਸੱਤ ਦਿਨ ਬੰਦ ਕਰਕੇ ਫਿਰ ਨਵਾਂ ਪੈਕ ਸ਼ੁਰੂ ਕਰੋ।

ਮਿਨੂਲੈਟ ਬਾਰੇ ਪੂਰੀ ਜਾਣਕਾਰੀ ਤੁਸੀਂ ਆਪਣੇ ਡਾਕਟਰ ਪਾਸੋਂ ਪ੍ਰਾਪਤ ਕਰ ਸਕਦੇ ਹੋ।

Punjabi

শুরুর দিন

কি ভাবে মিনুলেট খাবেন

সোম	১।	রক্তঃস্রাব বা মাসিকের প্রথম দিন থেকেই মিনুলেট খাওয়া শুরু করুন। ধরা যাক, আপনার রক্তঃস্রাব শুরু হল মংগলবার, আপনি 'মংগলবার' লেখা বড়ি খাবেন।
মংগল		
বুধ	২।	বড়ি যে বার থেকে খাওয়া শুরু করবেন, সেই বারের পাশে রূপালী চিহ্নিত অংশ ছিঁড়ে ফেলুন। এরপর প্রতিবার যখনই নতুন প্যাকেট শুরু করবেন – সেই দিনটিই আপনার শুরুর দিন বলে জানবেন।
বৃহস্পতি		
শুক্র	৩।	প্রতিদিন একটা করে বড়ি খাবেন এবং একটা নির্দিষ্ট সময়েই তা খাওয়ার অভ্যাস করুন – যেমন, বিছানায় যাওয়ার আগে।
শনি	৪।	এক সপ্তাহ বড়ি খাওয়ার পর নতুন প্যাকেট শুরু করার আগে এক সপ্তাহ অপেক্ষা করবেন।
রবি		'মিনুলেট' সম্পর্কে বিস্তারিত জানতে হলে অসুধের দোকানে জিজ্ঞাসা করুন।

Bengali

DIWRNOD DECHRAU

▶ Llun
▶ Maw
▶ Mer
▶ Iau
▶ Gwe
▶ Sad
▶ Sul

Sut mae cymryd Minulet®

1. Dechreuwch gymryd Minulet ar ddiwrnod cyntaf gwaedu'r mislif. Er enghraifft, os dydd Mawrth yw diwrnod cyntaf gwaedu'ch mislif, dechreuwch trwy gymryd y bilsen a nodwyd "Maw".

2. O dan "Diwrnod Dechrau", crafwch ymaith yr arwydd arian (▶) gyferbyn â'r diwrnod pryd y cymerwch eich pilsen gyntaf. Hwn fydd eich diwrnod dechrau i bob pecyn newydd a Minulet hefyd.

3. Cymerwch un bilsen bob dydd. Dilynwch y saethau i'r cyfeiriad a ddangosir. Er hwylustod i chi, trefnwch gymryd y bilsen yr un pryd bob dydd: er enghraifft, wrth fynd i'r gwely.

4. Ar ôl gorffen y pecyn, arhoswch saith diwrnod cyn dechrau'r pecyn nesaf.

Mae gwybodaeth lawn ar gael i chi oddi wrth eich meddyg.

Welsh

आरम्भ का दिन

(सोम)
(मंगल)
(बुध)
(गुरू)
(शुक्र)
(शनि)
(रवि)

मिनुलेट कैसे लें

1. मासिक धर्म के पहले दिन से मिनुलेट लेना शुरू करें। उदाहरण के लिए यदि आपके मासिक धर्म का पहला दिन मंगलवार है तो कोई भी गोली जिस पर 'Tue' लिखा है से लेना शुरू करें।

2. जिस दिन से आप पहली गोली लेती हैं उस के बाद 'Start Day' सम्बन्धी चान्दी रंगा निशान(▶)खुर्च दें। मिनुलेट के हर नए पैक का यह शुरू का दिन भी होगा।

3. प्रति दिन एक गोली लें। दिखाई गई दिशा में तीर के निशान का अनुसरण करें। अपनी सुविधा के लिए ऐसा नियम बनायें कि गोली प्रति दिन उसी समय ही लें। जैसे सोने से पहले।

4. एक पैकट समाप्त होने पर, अगला पैकट शुरू करने से पूर्व सात दिन ठहरिए।

मिनुलेट बारे पूरी जानकारी अपने डाक्टर से मिल सकती है।

Hindi

شروع کرنے کا دن

پیر
منگل
بدھ
جمعرات
جمعہ
ہفتہ
اتوار

مینولیٹ کو استعمال کرنے کا طریقہ

(۱) مینولیٹ کی پہلی گولی کا استعمال اس دن شروع کیجئے جو آپ کے ماہواری خون آنے کا پہلا دن ہو۔ مثال کے طور پر اگر آپ کے ماہواری خون آنے کا پہلا دن منگل ہے تو کوئی بھی گولی جس پر منگل لکھا ہوا استعمال کیجئے۔

(۲) "سٹارٹ ڈے" کے نیچے سلور کے تیر کے نشان (▶) کو مٹا دیجئے جو کہ اس دن کے ساتھ ہے جس دن آپ نے پہلی گولی استعمال کی ہے آپ یہی دن ہر بار نئے پیک کو استعمال کرنے کے لئے مقرر ہونے والا پہلا دن ہوگا۔

(۳) روزانہ صرف ایک گولی استعمال کیجئے اور تیر کے نشانات کا خیال رکھیئے۔ اپنی سہولت کے لئے روزانہ مقررہ وقت پر گولی کا استعمال کیجئے۔ مثلاً سونے سے پیشتر۔

(۴) جب آپ ایک پیک ختم کر لیں تو دوسرا شروع کرنے سے پہلے سات دن کا وقفہ ضرور دیجئے۔

مینولیٹ کے بارے میں مکمل معلومات آپ کے ڈاکٹر سے مل سکتی ہے۔

Urdu

Fig. 19.4
Multilingual leaflet.

For the pharmacist, often conscious of how time-consuming successful counselling may be, it must be recognised that to establish an initial pharmacist-patient relationship requires sufficient emphasis upon patient watching and listening.

Counselling may be described succinctly as helping people to help themselves. The importance of listening to and understanding the patient cannot be over-emphasised. Simple facts clearly expressed are fundamental to successful counselling.

With the advent of original pack dispensing, the pharmacist is likely to have the opportunity to devote even more time to communication and counselling, which should be recognised as a professional priority.

Pharmacists should not only advise prescribers and patients about medicines, but monitor adverse drug reactions, consult with prescribers about prescribing and dispensing procedures, advise members of the public about non-prescription medicines, and expand the primary health-care role of giving advice to patients in response to symptoms. Pharmacists may also contribute to health promotion, take part in diagnostic screening procedures, and provide domiciliary pharmaceutical services. Counselling is the cornerstone of all these facets of the pharmacists' role.

Pharmacists are being encouraged to maintain patient medication records for patients who regularly visit the same pharmacy. Records may be of benefit, particularly in the care of the elderly and patients on long-term medication, in the detection of adverse reactions and drug interactions.

One method of record keeping has been the use of the electronic 'smart-card'. The prescriber records the patient's medication on the card, and this is retained by the patient. Subsequently, the patient may elect to show it to the pharmacist when he hands in a prescription or purchases a non-prescription medicine. The pharmacist may then check and update the card as appropriate, providing an invaluable aid to the promotion of compliance and the more effective use of medicines.

It has yet to become commonplace to build up patient medication records. As a result, pharmacists must be particularly cautious when giving advice. A common enquiry concerns the use of a medicine, and such enquiries demand tact when responding. Pharmacists have no access to patient records, and are not aware of the prescriber's diagnosis. A further complication arises in the multitude of indications of many medicines, and this problem should be explained in lay terms to patients in response to their enquiries. Patients may describe the prescriber's diagnosis, in which case pharmacists should make a calculated decision as to the information which can be given. It may, however, be necessary to suggest that patients discuss their treatment more fully with the prescriber, particularly if patients are uncertain of the basis of treatment.

In addition, the opportunity may be provided to give further advice on how and when the medicine should be taken or used.

Most patients are only able to recall about a third of what they have been told, and it is recommended that, when counselling, the more important points should be stated at the beginning and repeated at the end of the interview. Among factors which have been found to decrease effective interaction between patients and prescribers, and which may equally handicap counselling by pharmacists, are:

- patients are too fearful or nervous to ask questions
- patients are unwilling to ask questions for fear of appearing ignorant
- patients are confused by medical terminology or jargon
- patients do not appreciate the importance of the information conveyed
- prescribers or pharmacists devote insufficient time to explain instructions adequately
- the consultation is inappropriately terminated (e.g. by prescribers writing a prescription, or pharmacists placing the medicine in a bag and handing it out without explanation).

Pharmacists have the opportunity and responsibility to ensure that patients understand all relevant information relating to the prescribed treatment. Pharmacists should use, as appropriate, suitable verbal, written, or audiovisual communication techniques (see Section 19.2) to inform, educate, or reinforce the knowledge of patients about their medicines.

Factors Influencing Effective Patient Counselling

Environment   Space, furnishing, privacy, and noise can be significant influences on effective counselling. Few community pharmacies in the UK have a separate counselling area, although more are now experimenting with counselling booths. These provide a measure of discreet confidentiality while still enabling the pharmacist to be readily available to supervise pharmacy medicine sales. In the absence of a specifically designated area, a greater impression of privacy may be conveyed around a quiet end of a medicine counter or prescription reception point, or even by a reduction in lighting at one end. Pharmacists should be aware of the potential security risks of using the dispensary as a counselling area. Pharmacies which have established counselling facilities engender and experience a heightened awareness by the public of the profession's contribution to primary health-care.

Personal factors   To most people, a clean white laboratory coat or uniform, or smart business-like clothing, conveys a professional image which helps to put the patient at ease and conveys confidence. It is important that pharmacists can be distinguished from dispensing technicians and assistants. Name badges which include the word 'Pharmacist' and the green cross symbol for pharmacy may be helpful.

Pharmacists' behaviour can also contribute to the ease and effectiveness of communication and counselling. An awareness of the non-verbal aspects of communication (*see* Section 19.2) is very important.

Time   The major limiting factor determining how much patient counselling actually happens in pharmacy practice is time. This may be unfortunate but applies to many similar professional situations involving counselling. The structure of UK community pharmacy (consisting mostly of single-pharmacist pharmacies), the informal access, and erratic workload often make it difficult for pharmacists to devote sufficient time to counselling.

In the last 30 years, NHS prescriptions dispensed annually in each pharmacy in Great Britain have nearly doubled to about 33 000. In order to devote adequate time to counselling, dispensing should ideally be performed by technicians under supervision, or a second pharmacist should be available, but in reality the erratic workload may make this difficult.

19.4 COMPLIANCE AND THE EXTENT OF NON-COMPLIANCE

It is only since the mid-1960s that compliance-rates have been studied in medical practice among groups of patients with various diseases (e.g. depression, acute infections, various chronic diseases, and in pregnancy). During this time, many papers have been published, reporting and reviewing many facets of compliance and non-compliance.

Compliance in keeping appointments for disease screening initiated by health professionals is often below 50%, but it rises markedly where children are involved. When an appointment is initiated by the patient for treatment, compliance again improves.

Patients on short-term medication tend to show greater compliance than those on long-term therapy, as might be expected. It is also apparent that the motivation for compliance is greater for the treatment of disease rather than its prevention. Many other factors may affect compliance (e.g. the age and intelligence of the patient, and whether any significant improvement may be noted by the patient as a result of continued treatment).

Compliance and Patient Perceptions

Research has not identified any one specific cause for non-compliance, nor does it seem possible to identify a special type of patient who lacks compliance. The active participation of patients in their treatment may be influenced by factors which limit or promote compliance.

Factors Contributing to Poor Compliance

(*see also* Table 19.4)

Among inhibiting factors are:

- anxiety
- lack of appropriate dosage aids
- length of illness
- personal characteristics (e.g. lack of independence, or despair)
- poverty
- social and cultural factors (e.g. illness as an excuse, or fatalism)
- social isolation
- wrong information.

TABLE 19.4
Factors contributing to poor patient compliance

• The patient does not take the prescription to the pharmacy or collect the dispensed medicine.
• The directions for use are not understood (e.g. due to inadequacy of directions, reading difficulty, language difficulty, or complexity of instructions).
• The purpose of the medicine, and the reasons for taking it, may not be understood. This may be due to omission by the prescriber or pharmacist, or a lack of comprehension.
• Physical difficulties (e.g. in opening the container or handling small tablets).
• Problems associated with administration of the drug (e.g. retention of a suppository, unpleasant taste, or difficulty in swallowing).
• The patient may consider there is no improvement in his condition after dosage.
• Real and imagined side-effects.
• Inconvenience of dosage regimen (e.g. difficulty in arranging administration in the working day).

The key factor in promoting patients' participation in their treatment is motivation. The way in which patients perceive their motivation for living and their resultant life-style are most important influences. The acceptance of being ill, handicapped, or disabled, former experience of illness, and attitude are characteristics which may encourage patients to take part actively in their treatment.

In practical terms, pharmacists may find that non-compliance is directly related to, or affected by, one or more of the following:

- difficulty in keeping to dosage regimen because of life-style (e.g. work routine)

  Some formulations may not be as easily administered at work as a tablet or a cream. Many patients find it easier to remember to take medicines at meal times than an hour beforehand. If remembered later, the patient may be inhibited from taking the missed dose. A common example is the administration of antacid preparations. These may need to be administered during the working day, and it may be easier for patients to carry tablets to work rather than a large mixture bottle.

  The act of swallowing solid oral dosage forms may also pose problems for some patients. Pharmacists may be made aware of this difficulty, whereas patients may be reluctant to discuss this 'minor' point with the prescriber. A brief telephone call from the pharmacist to the prescriber may help to overcome this problem.

- the treatment regimen is too complex and not properly understood (Fig. 19.5)

  What action might pharmacists take in such a situation? Pharmacists can design a chart to help the patient to understand the regimen. If the patient is not living alone, it may be possible to recruit a member of the family to help with the dosage schedule. Different types of container for different tablets or capsules may also be helpful.

However, in this particular case, it would be most sensible to refer to the prescriber and discuss how critical the reducing dose steps are likely to be. Some clinicians consider it satisfactory to reduce the dose of prednisolone by 5 mg every 5 to 7 days down to 5 mg daily, which should then be reduced slowly. This results in a much simpler reducing dosage schedule. The importance of active communication between pharmacists and prescribers, and pharmacists and patients should be obvious.

Another common contributor to non-compliance is polypharmacy. It has been frequently shown that patients receiving three or more drugs at the same time tend to have compliance problems.

- a lack of confidence in prescriber or medication

  Whatever the personal views of the pharmacist, it is imperative that the patient's confidence is maintained in both the medication and the prescriber. This may have the additional benefit of improving the prescriber/pharmacist relationship.

- the influence of incorrect and conflicting information or ideas derived from the patient's family and friends, and the popular press, about the medication or condition being treated.

  It is a source of concern that changes in the availability of medicines may be announced in the national press before health-care professionals are formally notified. Equally, patients may read an article in the press about the possible harmful effects of medicines they are taking, and not surprisingly, become reluctant to take them. In this situation, pharmacists should discuss the benefits and risks of treatment, and try to convince patients that, to the best of their knowledge, such claims should not cause them undue concern. It should also be stressed that it may be harmful to stop treatment abruptly. Professional judgment will determine whether patients require further reassurance from their prescribers.

A patient is presented with two containers of prednisolone tablets, bottle A containing 5 mg prednisolone tablets and bottle B containing 1 mg prednisolone tablets.

On days 1 to 5, take TWO tablets from bottle A morning and night, then from days 6 to 10, take TWO tablets in the morning and ONE at night from bottle A, then from days 11 to 15, take TWO in the morning from bottle A. Do not take any tablets from bottle B on days 1 to 5, then on day 6 take FOUR at night with tablet from bottle A, then on day 7 take THREE at night from bottle B, TWO at night on day 8 from bottle B, ONE at night on day 9, and no tablets from bottle B on day 10. On day 11 start again with FOUR tablets from bottle B, THREE tablets from bottle B on day 12, TWO tablets from bottle B on day 13, ONE tablet from bottle B on day 14 and no tablet from bottle B on day 15.

Thus on days 1 to 5, a total of 20 mg prednisolone is to be taken, 19 mg total on day 6, 18 mg total on day 7, 17 mg on day 8, 16 mg on day 9, 15 mg on day 10, 14 mg on day 11, 13 mg on day 12, 12 mg on day 13, 11 mg on day 14, and 10 mg on day 15.

Fig. 19.5
Prednisolone reducing dosage schedule.

Child-resistant Containers

Child-resistant closures and containers (British Standard 5321:1975) have been required for tablet and capsule formulations of aspirin and paracetamol since 1975 and certain liquid products since 1987 supplied without a prescription. Their original voluntary use became a requirement of professional practice in January 1989. However, patients who experience difficulty in the use of child-resistant containers may be supplied alternatives, but such patients should be counselled about the extra care needed in storage of such medicines. Users with potential problems (e.g. the elderly and patients with mild or moderate arthritis) benefit from counselling by pharmacists. Providing the technique in using child-resistant containers is demonstrated, and patients are convinced of their ability to use the closures by carrying out the procedure themselves, a significant majority subsequently experience few difficulties. It should be accepted that further counselling may be necessary to persuade some patients that such containers are desirable and have contributed significantly to decreased child mortality figures due to accidental poisoning.

The Pharmacist's Contribution to Compliance

It is generally considered that patient education is the most important variable affecting compliance. Information provided to patients concerning their medicine must be understood. Faulty comprehension has been reported to contribute to many compliance problems. If the medicine has been prescribed, information provided by pharmacists must reinforce and complement the prescriber's directions.

As the involvement of pharmacists in the primary health-care team is increasingly recognised, the importance of communication with patients cannot be overemphasised. The correct information at the appropriate level is the most important constructive influence on compliance that pharmacists can make. Information that pharmacists should consider important for patients includes the:

- action to be taken in the event of a missed dose
- action to be taken in the event of suspected or confirmed pregnancy
- aim of the treatment
- arrangement of further supplies
- discarding of unused medicine beyond a specific expiry date
- dosage or amount to be used
- duration of treatment

- excipients which may potentially produce adverse effects
- expected side-effects which may be reduced by appropriate action by the patient (e.g. reduction of gastric irritation caused by some non-steroidal anti-inflammatory drugs by administration after food)
- frequency and correct times of administration or use (administrative schedule)
- intended use and expected action, and advice in the event of no apparent effect
- maximum dose in 24 hours
- medicines, food, or activities the patient has to avoid during treatment
- method of use
- pharmaceutical form of the medicine and its identity
- side-effects to be referred to the prescriber
- storage of medication.

The aim of treatment is particularly relevant if pharmacists are responding to symptoms described by a patient, but should be considered with caution in regard to prescribed medicines as this is a professional matter between prescribers and patients. Patient confidentiality, as well as the patient's confidence in the prescriber, must be respected. Pharmacists must be selective with the range of the information conveyed. It would usually be inappropriate to counsel or advise patients on all the headings listed, as these can cover information as diverse as that in a product data sheet. The attention, understanding, and memory of most patients would soon be overstretched, unfounded anxieties might be aroused, and the time required would be considerable and impractical.

What is essential is for pharmacists to ensure that patients possess sufficient information for the effective and safe use of medicines. Pharmacists who are able to develop a rapport with patients who regularly visit the pharmacy, and who can establish confidence in the minds of patients in a familiar and unthreatening environment, have the opportunity to contribute increasingly to patients' confidence in the medicine.

Ways to Improve Compliance

Daily dose reminders   The design of special treatment packs, calendar packs, and medication dose compartment aids, suitably labelled, have all been aimed at stimulating patient compliance through a better understanding of their treatment.

For difficult cases of non-compliance often aggravated by forgetfulness, especially in the elderly, pharmacists may find it helpful to introduce patients to one of the special medicine packaging devices. These compliance aids vary considerably in sophistication, design, and cost.

Most daily dose reminders consist of a tray divided into compartments, which may be labelled with times during the day or days of the week. There may also be space for inclusion of a patient's individual label, and one device incorporates Braille markings to assist the blind and partially sighted.

Guidelines are laid down by the Royal Pharmaceutical Society for the use of daily dose reminders. Medicines should not be dispensed directly into these compliance aids unless the statutory labelling requirements can be fulfilled. If patients request that pharmacists load the daily dose reminder, this should be done using the dispensed medicine which carries the legally required label. An example of a widely used daily dose reminder is illustrated in Fig. 19.6.

A number of other devices may be more useful. If an elderly infirm patient is visited regularly by a community nurse, the patient's medication can be prepared on a labelled tray, which may include liquid medicines already measured out in dispensing cups. Such cups, complete with lids, are made in different colours and capacities and are available from several sources.

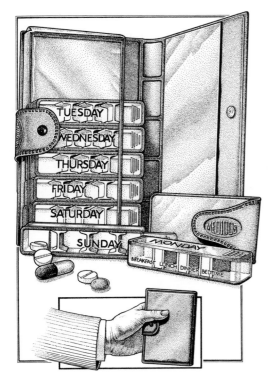

Fig. 19.6
An example of a daily dose reminder (Medidos).

However, such compliance aids are only available for limited distribution in special cases; in other cases, patients must purchase them.

Family support   Where it is possible to invoke the support of other members of a patient's family who can give encouragement, improve understanding and, if necessary, supervise the taking or using of the medicine, compliance will invariably improve, at least in the short term. Such involvement is most helpful and should be considered essential where compliance aids (e.g. those described above) require regular refilling.

Information   The information contained in the section describing pharmacists' contribution to compliance (*see above*) is a comprehensive list of the range of advice that pharmacists could provide for patients. In reality, however, the oral information conveyed may be considerably more succinct, and may be summarised by the following points:

• how and when to take/use the medicine
• how much to take/use
• how long to keep taking/using the medicine
• what to do in the event of a missed dose
• what to do if something goes wrong
• is it safe to drive?
• is it safe to take a small quantity of alcoholic drink?

19.5 DISCUSSION

Pharmacists have the opportunity to play an exceptionally important role in ensuring that patients obtain the maximum benefit from the use of prescribed medicines. It should not be considered acceptable that patients be given their medicines with no input from pharmacists regarding use, the potential benefits, and the action to be taken in the event of problems.

Communication plays a vital role in pharmacists' activities. Pharmacists must watch and listen carefully, paying particular attention to non-verbal signs (e.g. facial expression, posture, and body movements). They must be able to convey sympathy and yet confidence, confirming and enhancing patients' attitude towards their treatment. This may be especially difficult if patients appear unreceptive. It should always be remembered that a prescription is likely to be presented by individuals who are unwell themselves, or who may be concerned about a close relative or friend. If pharmacists can convey understanding, while at the same time maintaining professionalism, the attitude of patients may be correspondingly uplifted.

The type and range of information required for effective patient counselling is continually expanding, and pharmacists must be aware of the sources which can provide useful information. Guidance on the individual products for which there is a special need for counselling (e.g. because of well documented drug or food interactions) is provided in an appendix in the BNF. The listed products are annotated with a capital 'C', and the requirement is reiterated in the individual product monograph.

Conversely, the use of recommended cautionary and advisory labels may be deemed inappropriate by prescribers in certain circumstances. In such cases, prescribers may endorse the prescription NCL (no cautionary labels), and specify any alternative wording that is required.

In some instances, it is recommended that more than one cautionary label should be appended to a medicine. On occasions, however, pharmacists may use their professional knowledge and discretion to omit one or more of the labels. In this event, adequate counselling to compensate for the decision to delete an advisory label is required.

In addition to written aids to counselling, the organised use and availability of videotapes may provide a useful adjunct. Patients may watch a demonstration of the technique which should be used in administration of a drug (e.g. the use of a pressure inhaler), and pharmacists should be available to answer any questions. Whatever audio-visual aids are used, however, it is important that pharmacists consider them an accessory to adequate patient counselling, not a substitute.

In 1987, the cost to the taxpayer of medicines supplied through the NHS in Great Britain was £2.1 billion. The degree of non-compliance is notoriously difficult to assess accurately, but figures of up to 30% have been suggested. Notwithstanding the vast waste of resources which these estimates represent, it also indicates that up to one-third of all medicines may not be used satisfactorily. Clearly, there is considerable scope for improving compliance, and pharmacists must play a vital role in the education of patients to achieve this. Equally, the increasing proportion of elderly people in the population, and their increasing dependence on medicines (see Chapter 18) suggests that problems in compliance may get worse rather than better. Many patients are bewildered by the complexity of dosage schedules, and pharmacists must fulfil their professional responsibilities by devoting time and effort to improving understanding and compliance.

Pharmacists should be alert to any indicators of poor compliance. Patients on long-term continuous therapy (e.g. beta-adrenoceptor blocking drugs, non-steroidal anti-inflammatory drugs, or cardiac glycosides) may obtain repeat prescriptions from their surgery at regular intervals. Any indication by patients that they have sufficient tablets left not to require the full quantity on the prescription should prompt pharmacists to examine whether compliance has been satisfactory. This must obviously be approached sensitively, without appearing to criticise, and discreet questioning may highlight problems with side-effects or adverse reactions that may warrant referral.

At present it is not practically or economically feasible for community pharmacists to monitor compliance by the detection methods available for some drugs (e.g. penicillin, theophylline, digoxin, or phenytoin) in urine, blood, or saliva. Hospital pharmacists may be able to co-ordinate such analyses with procedures used for therapeutic drug monitoring. However, the range of drugs for which analysis may be easily carried out, and indeed the number of drugs for which monitoring would be cost-effective, is small. A far greater improvement in patient compliance may be achieved by effective communication and counselling.

Chapter 20

MINOR ILLNESS AND RESPONDING TO SYMPTOMS

20.1 INTRODUCTION

People's ability and willingness to cope with minor ailments without consulting a doctor is of vital importance and is potentially one of the most significant areas in which pharmacists can contribute to the maintenance of health. The primary health-care system would be totally unable to cope with the extra demand if all episodes of minor illness were referred to a doctor. More importantly, the public's willingness to deal with most problems themselves confirms their responsibility for their own health and can encourage a more sensible attitude to life-style to promote good health.

A patient's decision to seek medical advice is commonly based on a knowledge of health and health-related topics (e.g. obtained through experience or by reading articles in the press), perceptions of good health, and the advice given by others (e.g. relatives, friends, and members of the primary health-care team). It is essential that the information on which decisions are based is sound and factual. Pharmacists can play an important role in correcting misconceptions about health, ill health, and its treatment and are viewed as highly trained and easily accessible health-care professionals.

Many minor illnesses do not require any medical treatment. Reassurance or suggestions about life-style modifications (e.g. smoking, diet, or alcohol use) may be adequate. However, some conditions can benefit from the use of non-prescription medicines and patients may ask for these directly or purchase them after recommendation by the pharmacist.

Perceptions of Health

There is a wide diversity in people's perceptions of health, which is related to a complex range of factors (e.g. socio-economic status). The World Health Organization has defined health as a state of complete physical, mental, and social well-being. Health should not be considered as solely a biological or medical issue. For people whose health is reasonable, health is not a major concern but tends to be taken for granted. Family responsibilities, political issues, and economic and employment issues are commonly more dominant concerns than health. Happiness and quality of life may be greater considerations than health, although the inextricable link between these factors cannot be ignored.

Health is also the capacity to function as expected and being able to cope with life, and is associated with a cheerful positive approach to life. Conversely, unhappiness has been associated with reduced health and a greater susceptibility to illness.

Factors Influencing the Decision not to Seek Medical Advice

The decision to seek medical advice, to self-medicate, or to do nothing when symptoms occur is complex. Only a small proportion of symptoms are reported to a doctor and many people do nothing at all to treat minor symptoms. Factors which determine whether a doctor is consulted include the severity of the symptom and the anxiety it may be causing, the desire to appease members of the family, and a need for sickness certification. Medical advice is more commonly sought on behalf of the very young, by the elderly, women between 15 and 44 years of age, widows and widowers, and families with three or more children. However, symptoms are more commonly reported, but medical referral not sought, in those of an anxious or neurotic disposition or who are divorced or separated.

The greater proportion of minor illness for which medical advice is not sought has been called the 'iceberg' of illness. The reasons why people do not seek medical advice include the belief that their symptom cannot be altered through the use of drugs and must be accepted as part of their physical make-up, or concern that the symptom is too trivial to warrant the attention of the doctor (despite the anxiety the symptom may be causing the sufferer). Some patients may have experienced unpleasant side-effects through the former use of prescription medicines and be reluctant to take an unfamiliar drug. Some people may even prefer to take a non-prescription medicine that has been previously used with success, even if the reported symptoms are different. Other factors may include the relative inaccessibility of the doctor's surgery (e.g. the length of the walk or the availability of public transport), lack of access to a telephone (e.g. absence of a telephone in the home or of a nearby phonebox), the time spent in getting to the surgery and waiting for the consultation, and the potential loss in earnings of the visit.

20.2   MINOR ILLNESS AND ITS MANAGEMENT

There is no agreed definition of what constitutes a minor illness, although the following criteria can be used as a framework. The condition should be:

- of limited duration
- self-limiting
- something which is perceived as non-threatening.

The range of minor illness changes with age. Many of the problems of the elderly are considered in Chapter 18 and of children in Chapter 17. Common minor illnesses in adults and their treatment are described in detail in Section 20.3 below. The Royal Pharmaceutical Society has issued a list of minor ailments which can benefit from short-term symptomatic treatment. Equally importantly, the recommendations include a list of symptoms which are strongly suggestive of more serious disease and which should be referred to a doctor (Table 20.1).

Most symptoms reported by members of the public can be categorised into 7 main groups:

- ailments of the skin (e.g. minor cuts and grazes, and acne)
- digestive ailments (e.g. indigestion, heartburn, and upset stomach)
- female complaints (e.g. menstrual, premenstrual, and vaginal problems)
- pain (e.g. headache, muscle aches and pain, back problems, and arthritis/rheumatism)
- problems of well-being (e.g. tiredness, sleeping problems, stress, and anxiety)
- respiratory ailments (e.g. common cold)
- sensory complaints (e.g. eye, ear, and mouth complaints).

Pharmacists' Contribution to the Treatment of Minor Illness

The reluctance of patients to seek a doctor's advice for the treatment of many episodes of minor illness and the

TABLE 20.1
Symptoms suggestive of serious disease which should be referred for medical consultation

Ankle swelling	Persistent or recurrent pyrexia
Anorexia	Spontaneous bruising
Blood loss from any orifice	Swelling or lumps of any size
Difficulty in swallowing	Tenderness over the blood
History of severe and	vessels
particularly penetrating	Urinary symptoms
injury	Yellow or green discharge
Increasing breathlessness	from the penis
Loss of weight	or vagina
Menstrual abnormality	Yellow or green sputum
Pain in the chest, abdomen,	Yellow skin colour
head, or ears	

ready accessibility of the community pharmacy highlights the important contribution which pharmacists can make to maintaining health. Pharmacists can advise the public on all health-care matters.

Over 70% of medicines which are considered appropriate for treatment of minor illness are legally classified in the UK as pharmacy [P] medicines, i.e. they must be sold under the direct supervision of the pharmacist. Pharmacists can therefore influence the public's choice of medicines and can ensure that such medicines are appropriately used. Equally importantly, pharmacists can use their considerable background knowledge on health and related subjects to positively influence aspects of the public's life-style (health promotion).

One way of increasing the potential contribution of pharmacists' response to symptoms is to increase the range of medicines which are available for recommendation. This can be achieved in the UK by changing drugs from prescription-only medicine [POM] status to pharmacy medicine [P] status (POM to P). In the USA, the deregulation process has been actively underway since 1972 through the Food and Drug Administration's (FDA) OTC drug review. This was instigated to ensure that all non-prescription medicines contain ingredients which are of proven safety and efficacy, and are informatively labelled. Safety is judged by a low incidence of adverse reactions or significant side-effects when the product is used with adequate instructions. Warnings are also given against unsafe use. Due to its widespread availability, the drug must have a minimal potential to cause harm when subject to abuse. Effectiveness is more difficult to gauge, but is defined as producing clinically significant relief in a large proportion of the target population when correctly used. Since the review began in 1972, more than 15 drugs have been released from prescription-only classification, although some of these were already non-prescription products in other countries. Similar trends in France have made available a wide range of topical antifungals (clotrimazole, econazole, isoconazole, and miconazole) for the treatment of candidiasis.

In the UK, similar but less numerous conversions from POM to P status have taken place. These include loperamide, ibuprofen, and hydrocortisone cream and ointment of 1% or less. These conversions must be balanced against the fact that all new chemical entities (NCEs) to the UK are automatically included by the POM order. Five years after the product licence has been granted, the medicine must be reviewed as a prescription-only medicine or will automatically revert to pharmacy medicine status.

The Range of Products which can be Recommended for Minor Illness

There is a tremendous variety of non-prescription medicines which the public can purchase for minor illness. The average number of non-prescription medicines held in the home (more than 7 in the UK and as high as 17 in the USA) suggests that patients may resort to these rather than visit the pharmacy on each occasion that symptoms are experienced. Medicines are often purchased for future expected symptoms, and this makes it difficult to be confident that the patient will make the best use of the advice given by the pharmacist.

The indications for the range of non-prescription medicines available are listed in Table 20.2.

Problems Associated with the Use of Non-prescription Medicines

Many members of the public may need convincing that the misuse of non-prescription medicines has as great a potential for harm as misuse of prescription-only medicines. The purchaser may presume that, because the medicine is freely available and the pharmacist has been involved in its supply, there can be no problems associated with its use. In essence this is true, but only if the product is used for the purpose for which it was intended and at the correct dose and dosage interval. Consumers may ignore the contra-indications and other detailed

TABLE 20.2

Minor illnesses for which non-prescription medicines are available

Acne	Indigestion
Arthralgia	Infant colic
Athlete's foot	Insect stings and bites
Birth marks	Minor cuts and grazes
Bruises and sprains	Mouth ulcers
Chilblains and cramp	Nappy rash
Cold sore and chapped lips	Nasal congestion
Constipation	Pain
Corns and calluses	Pruritus
Coughs and colds	Psoriasis
Cradle cap	Rashes
Dandruff	Scabies
Diarrhoea	Sickness
Ear wax	Sore throat
Earache	Sunburn
Eczema	Tear deficiency
Eye infections and inflammation	Teething and toothache
Fungal infections	Tiredness
Haemorrhoids	Travel sickness
Halitosis	Verrucas
Hayfever	Warts
Headache	Worm infections
Head lice	

428 MINOR ILLNESS AND RESPONDING TO SYMPTOMS

information on the package and administer drugs to inappropriate groups (e.g. young children and the elderly). Even if all adequate safety and precautionary measures are taken, non-prescription medicines can still provoke adverse reactions, interact with prescribed or other non-prescription medicines, and interfere with biochemical tests. More importantly the patient may delay seeking medical advice or overdose deliberately or accidentally.

In self-treatment, people have to assess their own symptoms and their diagnosis may be incorrect. The importance of pharmacists helping patients come to the correct decision about their symptoms is paramount. Patients may overlook potentially more serious but less debilitating symptoms in preference to those which are more familiar. They may make a subconscious decision to ignore a symptom or its seriousness, and not seek professional advice because they cannot afford socially or financially to admit to its presence. In addition, in opting for self-medication patients presume that the symptom is self-limiting.

Patients who have previously used non-prescription medicines may visit their doctor but fail to inform him of the treatment they have already used or are still using. Many doctors do not ask their patients what, if any, non-prescription medicines they are taking.

Adverse reactions can occur with almost all non-prescription medicines, but some of the most common derive from the use of salicylates, paracetamol, iron preparations, and antihistamines. Acute overdosing with non-prescription medicines forms a significant proportion of poisoning cases. Aspirin and paracetamol contribute a large proportion of the deaths from poisoning in adults, while in children under 10 years of age aspirin is a common cause of death. Although it is acknowledged that these drugs are frequently supplied on prescription, their ready availability for purchase emphasises the public's responsibility to ensure the safe use and storage of drugs.

The inadequate storage of drugs in the home provides a potentially hazardous environment, especially for young children. Although there is a similar hazard with prescription medicines, a considerably larger number of non-prescription than prescription medicines are stored at home. The patient's perception that non-prescription medicines are less harmful than those which have been obtained from the doctor may lead to less care in their safe storage.

Educating the Public about Non-prescription Medicines

Pharmacists can be an invaluable source of information on the safe and appropriate use of non-prescription medicines. However pharmacists are by no means the sole source of information on medicines that can be bought or prescribed by doctors.

Consumer magazines (and in particular those targeted at women and mothers), television and radio, and home-doctor books are impersonal and popular sources of advice. Some professional organisations also produce compendia of non-prescription and prescription-only medicines, and are widely available. In the USA, the Physicians Desk Reference (covering prescription-only medicines) has sales of a similar order to the Bible. There are equivalent publications for non-prescription drugs produced in the USA and Australia. Self-care and health-care books abound in non-specialist bookshops, and contain detailed reference to drugs which can be bought and prescribed. A range of specialist publishers have also grown around the health-care market and these produce a broad range of inexpensive publications. Some pharmacies stock these publications, especially those concerned with 'alternative' forms of medication, and it is good practice for pharmacy staff to be able to counter in balanced and scientific terms some of the claims made for these products. They should also be capable of providing unbiased advice for consumers confused by the range of options.

One particularly worrying feature of this proliferation of information is that many articles and books are written by journalists with little, if any, training in health matters, and as a consequence are unable to provide balanced arguments for the claims they make. It is essential that professional bodies provide their members with enough information to enable them to promote the positive aspects of health-care, and for individual members to keep abreast of developments in the press and media.

Advertising pharmacy medicines in the UK is governed by the Medicines Act 1968 (SI 1978 No. 41). Product advertising is permitted for the prevention or treatment, or both, of most conditions which have been described as minor. Advertising is not allowed for products which claim to relieve chronic tiredness or fatigue, restore or enhance sexual potency or libido, rejuvenate or prevent ageing, or for the treatment of insomnia or sleeplessness other than by the secondary effect of relief of pain or other symptoms.

Summary

Responding to symptoms plays an important part in health-care. Most general-sales-list medicines and by definition all pharmacy medicines are sold through community pharmacies. The potential for pharmacists to further develop a counselling and advisory role in the treatment of minor illness is tremendous. Some members of the public may know exactly which non-prescription medicine they want and input from pharmacists may be unwanted or indeed, on occasions, unwelcome. Despite this, pharmacists have a legal responsibility to supervise all sales of pharmacy medicines, and a professional responsibility to help consumers choose the most appropriate medicine for their symptoms. Conversely, other members of the public can be reassured and extremely grateful for a positive caring attitude from the pharmacist who clearly wishes to help, who devotes time to find out about their condition, and recommends the most appropriate treatment. Not only does the public benefit from the development of this role, but the pharmacist gains confidence and satisfaction in a professional and personal capacity.

20.3 RESPONDING TO SYMPTOMS

Introduction

The AIM of responding to symptoms is:

- A – Assessment
- I – Interpretation
- M – Management

Members of the public seeking advice from pharmacists about symptoms and self-medication usually fall into one of three categories. Some patients may have already made their own diagnosis from their symptoms, and will seek advice on treatment only. Others may describe a symptom, or group of symptoms, which require interpretation and a recommendation of a course of action or treatment. Thirdly, patients may request a specific category of medicine (e.g. an analgesic) but require advice on item selection.

By observing and interviewing patients, pharmacists must confirm a patient's self-diagnosis, interpret any symptoms described, and select the most appropriate regimen.

It must be remembered that pharmacists' ability to respond to patients' symptoms is limited because pharmacists cannot effectively examine patients. However, the following guidelines will prompt pharmacists to ask relevant questions to distinguish major disorders from minor ailments.

Assessment and Interpretation

For an account of effective communication between pharmacists and patients, *see* Section 19.2.

- Establish who the patient is.

  Do not assume it is the person presenting the symptom.

- Evaluate appearance, demeanour, and manner. Does the patient appear ill?

  Remember to act sympathetically towards those who are either unwell themselves, or who may be worried about a sick relative or friend.

- Establish a profile of the patient's symptoms by considering the following questions:

  What is the primary symptom?
  What is the present location of the symptom (e.g. where is the pain)?
  What is the nature and severity of the symptom (e.g. is it a sharp or dull pain, or a dry or productive cough)?
  Are there any accompanying symptoms?
  Have any of these factors changed since their appearance (e.g. have the symptoms worsened, or has the pain moved or radiated elsewhere)?
  Did the symptom appear gradually or suddenly?
  How long has it been present?
  Can the presence of one symptom be linked to an associated event (e.g. alcohol consumption, emotional disturbances, diet, menstruation, injury, use of cosmetics, or time of day)?
  Does anything make the symptom worse or better (e.g. movement or food)?
  Is this an isolated occurrence of the symptom, or is it recurrent?
  Have any family or friends complained of similar symptoms?

- Establish a treatment history

  Has the doctor been consulted for this symptom? If so, was treatment given?
  Has self-medication already been tried? If so, what was the outcome?
  Are any other drugs (prescribed or purchased from a pharmacy) being taken for an unrelated condition?

- Establish, by observation or questioning, the existence of any risk factors.

  How old is the patient?
  Is the patient pregnant?
  Does the patient suffer from any chronic conditions (e.g. diabetes mellitus)?
  Does the patient have any known drug allergies (e.g. to aspirin or lanolin)?

Certain questions are particularly pertinent when considering specific symptoms, and these have been highlighted as Key Questions at the beginning of each of the following sections. The Key Questions are not, however, intended to be the only questions that might be asked, as all the above factors should always be considered when interviewing patients about their symptoms.

Management

The answers obtained from interviewing the patient should indicate one of the following courses of action:

- make a tentative diagnosis and give advice regarding the treatment

  Pharmacists should take the opportunity to suggest the best course of action if the symptoms persist after a few days treatment (e.g. medical referral or return to the pharmacy).

- refer the patient to a doctor either immediately if considered urgent, or by making an appointment for a consultation

- suggest no medicinal treatment, but counsel the patient (e.g. on diet)

  Often reassurance alone is an effective measure.

20.3.1 DIARRHOEA

Introduction

Diarrhoea is normally a self-limiting condition in which bowel frequency is increased and stool solidity is decreased. Patients usually recover quickly with or without the aid of dietary measures or medication.

An awareness of the usual pattern of bowel frequency and motion consistency is essential in assessing the symptom and its severity. The age of patients also influences the urgency with which remedial action or referral should be undertaken. Very young and very old patients are particularly susceptible to the effects of dehydration caused by diarrhoea.

Key Questions

- How old is the patient?
- How long has the diarrhoea been present?
- Has there been a change in frequency and consistency of bowel motions?
- Has the patient eaten anything which might have caused the diarrhoea?
- Has the patient got a raised temperature, or recently lost weight for no apparent reason?

Assessment and Interpretation

Onset and duration   The recent frequency and urgency of defaecation will indicate the severity of the problem. Usually, if bowel movements have occurred less than 2 or 3 times in the previous 8 hours, urgent medical referral is not necessary, providing no other symptoms give cause for concern. Some patients will report looser motions than normal without a change in frequency. In this case, the urgency of the situation is minimal, but it should be reviewed within 24 hours.

If diarrhoea has persisted for more than 48 hours, and there is no sign of abatement, it is wise to refer patients to the doctor. The presence of the accompanying symptoms described below will determine the urgency of referral.

Recurrence should be urgently referred, since this is abnormal. Possible diagnoses to be considered are ulcerative colitis, Crohn's disease, or irritable bowel syndrome. Typically, patients with inflammatory bowel disease will visit the toilet 10 to 20 times daily.

Accompanying symptoms   If *blood* is present in the stool, referral is essential since this could be a sign of a serious underlying condition (e.g. inflammatory bowel disease, dysentery, fissures or tears of the bowel mucosa, or colorectal cancer). The failure to report blood loss may not always indicate its absence, as it may be difficult for some patients to identify.

The appearance of *mucus* in the stool suggests that the integrity of the intestinal mucosa has been compromised, and requires referral. Small amounts may not be of clinical significance but merely a sign of mucosal inflammation and damage. However, the extent should be evaluated by doctors, not by pharmacists.

Diarrhoea accompanied by either severe *abdominal pain* that is persistent, or mild pain that has lasted for more than 48 hours, warrants urgent medical referral. Conversely, short-lasting mild episodes are usually self-limiting, and do not warrant immediate action.

A history of *alternating bouts of constipation and diarrhoea* with colicky abdominal pain, or a continuous dull ache in adolescents and young adults, is suggestive of irritable bowel syndrome. In elderly patients, a history of either *alternating or simultaneous diarrhoea and constipation* may be an indication of spurious diarrhoea. Such symptoms are usually caused by impacted faeces producing partial obstruction of the bowel, in addition to liquid faeces that may squeeze past the obstruction, causing diarrhoea. Referral is recommended to permit investigation and treatment of the primary obstruction.

Patients with diarrhoea accompanied by *vomiting* over a 24-hour period require medical referral to exclude the possibility of gastro-enteritis, or rarer conditions such as dysentery or cholera.

Any severe *weight loss* during a short period of time in the absence of dieting (e.g. weight loss of more than 3 kg in 2 to 3 weeks) requires referral. It may simply represent a loss of appetite through illness, but more serious pathology may exist (e.g. malabsorption or carcinoma), and any weight loss with diarrhoea should be medically investigated.

Causative and modifying factors   Changes to *diet* may affect bowel movements. Overindulgence in alcohol or foods with high-fibre content (e.g. fruit and vegetables) may cause diarrhoea. Likewise unaccustomed intake of spicy or unusual foods may irritate the intestine and stimulate peristalsis. Food poisoning may be suspected if other people who have eaten the same food are similarly affected.

If there is a recent history of European *travel*, gastro-enteritis of viral or bacterial origin should be suspected. If the symptoms last for 48 hours or more, medical referral is necessary. Patients returning from the Middle East, South-east Asia or Africa should be referred to exclude dysentery, cholera, and typhoid fever.

Diarrhoea may be caused by *drug administration* (e.g. laxatives, antibacterials, iron, an overdose of digoxin, antacids containing magnesium, and adrenergic neurone blocking drugs such as guanethidine).

A summary of the possible causes of diarrhoea is given in Part C.

Management

Non-drug treatment   If the diarrhoea does not represent any serious pathology, it will resolve within a few days without treatment. However, a regular intake of fluids should be ensured, particularly in young children, to replace excessive losses in the faeces. Patients should be advised to sip plenty of fluids throughout the day.

Drug treatment   Electrolyte replacement solutions (BNF 9.2.1) may be recommended. Glucose, present in these solutions, acts as a carrier for the transport of sodium and water from the intestine into the blood. The availability of these non-prescription preparations has rendered obsolete the use of traditional remedies containing sugar and salt in water or fruit juice. The use of these latter potentially harmful remedies should be discouraged.

Attempts to reduce diarrhoea may in some cases be counter-productive as it is an important means of flushing out toxins and irritants from the intestine. However, patients will request symptomatic relief for social

reasons and personal comfort. Non-prescription medicines available (BNF 1.4.2) contain either opiates (e.g. morphine or codeine) or loperamide, and act by reducing the contractibility of the colon. There is little evidence that adsorbent agents such as kaolin and chalk (BNF 1.4.1) give any reduction in diarrhoea, but their placebo effect may be considerable.

20.3.2 CONSTIPATION

Introduction

The normal frequency of bowel movement in the population varies from about three times per day to once every three days. This wide variation makes definition of constipation difficult, but it may be described as a diminished stool frequency associated with the forced passage of small hard faeces. As with the assessment of diarrhoea it is the change in bowel frequency which determines the severity of the condition.

Key Questions

- How long has the patient been constipated?
- How often does the patient normally go to the toilet?
- Can the symptoms be linked to any external factors?
- Does the patient have alternating diarrhoea and constipation?

Assessment and Interpretation

Nature and severity   If the condition is of recent origin, and is causing minor concern rather than significant discomfort, symptomatic relief may be suggested. A recurrent bout of constipation should be referred, as any underlying pathology may still be present.

Accompanying symptoms   *Blood* passed through the rectum may appear mixed in the faeces or as leakage coating the stool. Its appearance warrants referral to the doctor. Recurrent constipation may result in the development of haemorrhoids, caused presumably by straining at stool. Subsequent constipation and straining may cause these rectal varices to tear or burst, producing blood which coats the stool or stains underwear. Less frequently, blood will arise from other bowel disorders (e.g. anal fissures, obstructions, including tumours, and inflammatory bowel disease).

Any acute *distension of the abdomen* should be referred for medical examination.

The presence of severe *pain* warrants immediate referral. Mild or moderate pain of more than 48 hours' duration requires prompt medical investigation.

For a discussion of constipation accompanied by, or alternating with, diarrhoea, *see* Diarrhoea, Section 20.3.1.

Patients who are constipated and are *vomiting* require referral to eliminate the possibility of an obstruction.

A recent history of *weight loss* of greater than 3 kg should be medically investigated to exclude the possibility of carcinoma.

A summary of faecal characteristics in disease is given in Table 20.3.

Causative and modifying factors   A *diet* lacking in fibre will invariably result in constipation, particularly if patients lead a sedentary life-style. A reduced fluid intake will produce a similar effect since the colon will absorb the maximum volume of water possible in an attempt to conserve fluid.

A lack of *physical activity* (e.g. in immobile or bedridden patients) will be especially liable to cause constipation.

Drugs which may cause constipation include iron; antacids containing aluminium, calcium, or bismuth salts; opioids (e.g. in antidiarrhoeal medicines, cough suppressants, and analgesics); antimuscarinic drugs and drugs with antimuscarinic activity (e.g. anti-emetics, antihistamines, antipsychotics, and anti-parkinsonism agents).

Progesterone secreted in the latter stages of *pregnancy* has a spasmolytic action on most types of smooth muscle. The intestine therefore becomes atonic, causing stasis of the faeces. This is a natural physiological consequence of pregnancy, and patients should be appropriately advised and reassured.

Constipation may also be caused by reduced patient mobility, faddish diets, and prescription of iron supplements in the second and third trimesters.

A summary of the possible causes of constipation is given in Part C.

Management

Non-drug treatment   Whenever possible, drug use in the treatment of constipation should be avoided.

In mild constipation, dietary adjustment and an increased fluid intake may be sufficient. Fruit, vegetables, wholemeal bread, brown rice, and potatoes form the basis of a healthy non-constipating diet, together with avoidance of refined products (e.g. white bread and white sugar).

Adjustments to life-style to ensure adequate exercise, and that the urge to defaecate is not ignored, may be necessary. In particular, children should be taught to be regular and unhurried in their toilet habits.

Drug treatment   If laxatives are considered necessary, their use should be restricted to short courses of up to four days only. Referral should be advised if the condition has not resolved within one week.

Bulk-forming drugs (BNF 1.6.1) are recommended for simple constipation in the absence of impaction. When mixed with liquids, they swell in the colon, inducing peristalsis. Their action develops over several days, and so they are ineffective when a rapid effect is required. Care should be taken, particularly in the elderly, that sufficient fluid is taken with these products to prevent the risk of oesophageal obstruction.

TABLE 20.3
Faecal characteristics in disease

	Description	Possible causes
Quantity	Increased quantity and bulky	High-fibre diet Pancreatic disease (e.g. chronic pancreatitis) Malabsorption syndromes
Odour	Musty Rancid	Putrefaction of protein in pancreatic disease Carbohydrate fermentation
Colour	Canary yellow	Milk diet
	Dark	Meat diet, wines, fruit, beer, iron and bismuth preparations
	Green or yellowish-green	Presence of bile due to excessive peristalsis
	Clay coloured	Bile-duct obstruction
	Pale and yellow	Steatorrhoea
	Bright red	Haemorrhoids, cancer, polyps of the large intestine
	Dark, tarry	Peptic ulceration

Stimulant laxatives (BNF 1.6.2) irritate the bowel mucosa, or stimulate the nerve plexus of smooth muscle, both of which increase bowel motility. They exert an effect within 6 to 12 hours. Short-term use only is recommended as prolonged usage can cause griping pain, diarrhoea, and vomiting. Atrophy of bowel smooth muscle and adverse effects on the innervation of the colon can also occur.

Faecal softeners (BNF 1.6.3) are surfactant drugs. They increase the wetting efficiency of water, facilitating the mixing of fats and water to soften the faecal mass. Some agents are useful for patients with haemorrhoids and fissures where the passage of a hard stool is painful.

Laxatives with lubricating properties (e.g. liquid paraffin) coat the faecal mass and prevent water absorption from the colon. Liquid paraffin may seep from the anus; seepage from the oesophagus into the trachea when the patient is in a prone position may cause lipoid pneumonia, especially in the elderly. Under most circumstances, liquid paraffin should not be recommended.

Osmotic laxatives (BNF 1.6.4) are rapidly effective evacuants suitable only for short-term use. Their presence in the bowel leads to water retention due to an osmotic effect. This causes mechanical stimulation of the bowel and increased peristalsis.

20.3.3 NAUSEA AND VOMITING

Introduction

Nausea is a sensation of sickness accompanied by a loathing of food and often increased salivation.

Vomiting is the forceful ejection of the stomach contents caused by the diaphragm and abdominal wall being drawn in to press on the stomach.

Some patients may confuse vomiting with waterbrash, which is an effortless regurgitation of fluid into the mouth often accompanied by heartburn. Heartburn may be a normal event. However, it may accompany indigestion, particularly after meals or on lying down.

Key Questions

- Has the patient eaten anything which may have caused the symptoms?
- Is the patient taking, or been prescribed, any medicines?
- Does the patient experience any other symptoms at the same time?

Assessment and Interpretation

Nature and severity   Projectile vomiting may be caused by pyloric stenosis, especially in babies, and also in adults with a history of peptic ulceration (usually duodenal) with a more recent onset of vomiting. Projectile vomiting demands a medical referral.

Vomit which is particularly sour smelling also requires referral as it indicates obstruction (e.g. pyloric stenosis).

Blood-stained vomit (haematemesis) should be regarded as unusual and requires referral. Blood may appear fresh and bright red, or dark with a clotted appearance. If the blood originates in the stomach, it will have been degraded by gastric acid, producing a dark-coloured vomit with an appearance like coffee grounds ('coffee-ground' vomitus).

Onset and duration   Vomiting which has occurred frequently during a period of more than 24 hours requires referral. Similarly a deterioration in nausea or increased incidence of vomiting over a longer period of time requires investigation.

Vomiting which is preceded by nausea, even of short duration, usually indicates a gastro-intestinal cause and is the most common presentation. However, sudden vomiting without nausea is characteristic of a central cause (e.g. a cerebral tumour or injury), and although much rarer, it should be borne in mind (*see also* Accompanying symptoms below).

Accompanying symptoms   Episodic or chronic vomiting accompanied by *weight loss* requires referral for investigation of the cause.

Abdominal *pain* may cause reflex vomiting as in liver disease, appendicitis, biliary colic, renal colic, hernias, and genital disorders. Sometimes paroxysmal coughing can lead to vomiting (e.g. in pertussis). Other disorders that may lead to vomiting include Ménière's disease and acute pain in extra-abdominal body systems (e.g. in glaucoma).

Diarrhoea accompanying vomiting suggests gastro-enteritis as the most likely cause, usually due to ingestion of some insult or to infection. Recent travellers to hot countries should be referred to eliminate dysentery and food poisoning.

Central nervous system disorders (e.g. space-occupying lesions, meningitis, head injury, and subdural haemorrhage) may result in vomiting, dizziness, drowsiness, loss of balance, and personality changes. Migraine attacks frequently terminate with nausea and vomiting. The presence of headache and any other symptoms of the aura of migraine should be ascertained.

A history of nausea or vomiting related to anxiety or an emotional disturbance requires appropriate treatment of the underlying psychological component. Reassurance may be all that is required but, in more severe cases, a medical referral is advised.

Some other psychiatric disorders may present with vomiting (e.g. anorexia nervosa and bulimia). These commonly occur in teenage girls and the history, although generally of long duration, is usually very difficult to elicit from the patient herself, although it may be reported by friends and relatives.

A summary of the nature of vomitus in disease is given in Table 20.4.

Causative and modifying factors   If the cause can be elicited, the decision of whether to refer or not becomes easier.

Common *dietary causes* are hot or spicy foods, overindulgence in food or alcohol, and sensitivity to certain foods (e.g. seafoods and pork). Such cases will usually spontaneously resolve within 24 hours.

Many *drugs* can cause nausea and vomiting (e.g. nonsteroidal anti-inflammatory drugs, colchicine, digoxin in toxic doses, iron, levodopa, theophylline, oestrogens, and cytotoxic drugs).

Motion is a common cause of nausea and vomiting and, in severe cases, may persist for a day or two after the journey.

Infection may cause vomiting, especially otitis media in children and the early stages of various viral illnesses (e.g. measles). Conditions affecting the abdomen may result in reflex vomiting (*see* Accompanying symptoms above).

Heart failure, particularly right-sided heart failure, may result in congestion of the abdominal organs with blood, giving a sensation of nausea and sometimes vomiting.

Episodes of vomiting, which may sometimes be severe, in patients with *diabetes mellitus* require immediate referral to exclude loss of control of the diabetes. Alternatively, symptoms of increased frequency of urination,

thirst, weight loss, and persistent fungal infections (e.g. in the skin and in women particularly in the perivulval area) should be treated with suspicion and diabetes excluded by immediate referral.

Chronic *alcoholic patients* may suffer from early morning vomiting.

Two types of vomiting may occur in *pregnancy*. The familiar syndrome of morning sickness comprises regular bouts of short-lived nausea, vomiting, or both, during the first few weeks of pregnancy. It may occur at any time of the day but is mostly associated with mornings. It usually resolves spontaneously around the third month of pregnancy. Drugs should not be recommended, but reassurance, frequent small meals, rest, and bed rest in the mornings are sensible recommendations.

A more severe form of vomiting which may occur in early pregnancy is hyperemesis gravidarum. It may lead to dehydration and shock and requires medical referral.

The possible causes of nausea and vomiting are listed in Part C.

Risk factor   *Vomiting in children* is usually self-remitting but certain points should be remembered. Many babies regurgitate their milk after a meal (posseting) and mothers should be reassured that this is normal. However, in cases of projectile vomiting (even though the baby may be alert and apparently normal) and in babies who appear distressed, irritable, or very drowsy, referral is required as soon as possible. Children over two years of age require referral if they have vomited for more than 24 hours.

Management

If the cause of vomiting has been identified or is suspected, the underlying disorder should be attended to as a priority.

TABLE 20.4
The nature of vomitus

	Description	Possible causes
Colour	Bright red	Presence of blood immediately after haemorrhage
	Dark brown ('coffee-ground' vomitus)	Peptic ulceration
	Yellow or yellowish-green	Present in intestinal obstruction, but absent in pyloric stenosis
Consistency	Jelly-like	Presence of mucus due to chronic gastritis
Odour	Exceptionally offensive	Malignant disease of the pylorus
	Faeculent	Intestinal obstruction
Quantity	Copious	Pyloric obstruction (e.g. stenosis or carcinoma)

Non-drug treatment   As in any self-remitting gastro-intestinal disorder, vomiting should be treated by resting the stomach. Patients should be dissuaded from drinking milk or eating heavy or fatty meals for 24 hours, as these will exacerbate the situation. Sips of bland drinks, ideally water, should be taken regularly to prevent dehydration, although this is unlikely to occur in the cases of short duration commonly reported to pharmacies. Food should be avoided until the patient feels hungry, at which time items such as bread, toast, or plain biscuits should be given. If tolerated, intake may be gradually increased until a normal diet is resumed.

Drug treatment   There are few oral drugs available to treat vomiting attacks. Both antihistamines and antimuscarinic drugs may be useful to prevent attacks, especially of motion sickness. Hyoscine, and antihistamines such as cinnarizine, diphenhydramine, and promethazine (BNF 4.6) which also possess anticholinergic properties, may be useful, but should be used with caution in patients with glaucoma, prostatitis, constipation, and those who drive.

Babies and young children should be given oral rehydration fluids (BNF 9.2.1) that replace glucose, sodium, and potassium lost during vomiting. Glucose enhances the absorption of electrolytes across the inflamed mucosa. The use of proprietary formulations in children should be encouraged in preference to homemade remedies which may result in inappropriate loads of sodium and potassium.

20.3.4 INDIGESTION

Introduction

Indigestion (dyspepsia) is the term commonly used to describe epigastric discomfort, chest pain, or both, that may occur shortly after eating or drinking. Patients will often use the term to describe a variety of non-specific gastro-intestinal symptoms. It is important that pharmacists can evaluate the presenting symptoms in order to exclude any sinister pathology before recommending remedial action.

Key Questions

- Can the patient pinpoint exactly where the discomfort is?
- Does it occur after eating, or following a bowel movement?
- Has the patient eaten anything which may have caused the upset?
- Is it relieved by antacids or food?

Assessment and Interpretation

Onset and duration   If this is the first episode of indigestion, it may be treated with antacids except where the patient is over 40 years of age. New occurrences should be regarded with caution since ulceration, and cancer of the stomach, are more common in this age group. It would be wise therefore to refer patients in this category to their doctors.

If similar attacks of indigestion have occurred before, it may be treated with antacids for up to 7 days. If no improvement is felt, patients should be referred to the doctor for assessment. Attacks that are worse than in the past or are accompanied by new symptoms also require referral for assessment.

Symptoms of indigestion that are worse at night may be caused by duodenal lesions (e.g. an ulcer), which appear to be subject to exacerbation by night-time secretion of gastric acid into the duodenum.

Accompanying symptoms   A *bloated feeling* or a *sensation of fullness* is common in patients with peptic ulceration. Although such symptoms may transiently disappear along with indigestion after treatment with antacids, they may return and in such cases referral for a medical investigation is required.

A loss of appetite often occurs in patients with abdominal symptoms, especially in peptic ulceration, which may lead to a *loss in weight*. Significant weight changes require referral as they may be due to sinister pathology (e.g. cancer of the stomach), which must be excluded at an early stage.

Vomiting or constipation, or both, in the presence of indigestion demands immediate referral.

A patient with indigestion complaining of tiredness may have gastro-intestinal *blood loss* in the vomit or stool. This may lead to anaemia and requires referral.

Causative and modifying factors   *Drugs* (e.g. non-steroidal anti-inflammatory drugs, steroids, digoxin, and iron) may cause indigestion.

Common *dietary causative factors* to enquire after include overindulgence in food or drink, rushed meals, and unusual or spicy foods. Indigestion may be relieved by eating because food can act as a barrier between gastric acid and the mucosa. Alternatively, food may stimulate acid production and consequently aggravate the condition. This relationship with food merely reassures the patient that the origin of discomfort is in the gastro-intestinal tract. Small amounts of food eaten frequently will usually offer the best relief of symptoms. If treatment with antacids and dietary adjustment do not relieve the indigestion, then referral should be made to investigate for the presence of peptic ulceration. Coffee, tea, alcohol, and smoking are likely to exacerbate indigestion.

Bending over or *lying down* may aggravate acid reflux, leading to heartburn. Symptoms may be aggravated by obesity or hiatus hernia, again especially on bending down.

A summary of the possible causes of indigestion is given in Part C.

Isolated or recurrent factors   *Recurrent symptoms* of indigestion or heartburn require medical investigation, despite patients' assertions that the condition is normal for them. Nevertheless, many cases will show negative pathology.

If the patient has had indigestion in recent weeks and the symptoms are worse on this occasion, or other symptoms are present regardless of whether they respond to antacids, a referral should be advised.

In the second and third trimesters of *pregnancy*, the growing foetus and uterus may press against the bowel and stomach. This may cause indigestion, especially heartburn, which is aggravated on stooping or lying down. Oral iron preparations are a common cause of gastro-intestinal upset in pregnant women.

Various *chronic illnesses* can eventually cause indigestion. Patients with heart failure may suffer gastro-intestinal symptoms (e.g. indigestion, anorexia, and nausea) due to congestion and stasis of blood in the abdominal organs. Diabetic patients may have similar symptoms and require referral to check the control of their plasma-glucose concentration.

Management

Non-drug treatment   If there is an obvious benign cause of an acute attack of indigestion, reassurance may initially be sufficient. Counselling on the avoidance of stress, smoking, and coffee, and on the importance of small, regular, non-spicy meals and weight reduction, where appropriate, is important if the effects of drug therapy are not to be negated.

Drug treatment   Antacids are the primary, and very effective, non-prescription treatment for indigestion and the symptoms of peptic ulceration. Where reflux oesophagitis or heartburn is the problem, products containing alginates are useful to help suppress the movement of acid through the oesophageal sphincter.

Antacids containing sodium bicarbonate (e.g. magnesium trisilicate mixture) should be avoided in patients with heart failure or with renal dysfunction because of the risk of overloading with sodium and water. The fact that magnesium salts are osmotic laxatives and aluminium salts can be constipating may influence the choice of antacid for individual patients.

Aluminium salts are thought to bind and inactivate pepsin which, in association with gastric acid, may be a major cause of gastric mucosal breakdown. In addition, aluminium salts bind to bile acids. This may be a useful property as some gastric mucosal lesions may be caused by reflux of bile from the duodenum into the stomach. It has been suggested that food enhances the neutralising properties of magnesium but diminishes those of aluminium salts.

Antacids containing calcium carbonate may cause rebound indigestion by the direct stimulant effect of calcium on gastrin production, leading to increased secretion of gastric juice. A choice of an antacid containing a single magnesium or aluminium salt is recommended, depending on bowel habits. Antacids are best taken one hour after meals, at which time gastric emptying is slowed and contact time with the gastric contents is maximised.

Many proprietary antacids contain mixtures of magnesium and aluminium salts. The rationale for such mixtures may be to counteract the effects on the bowel habit of the individual agents, although these mixtures offer no advantages over single agents. Dimethicone, which may reduce flatulence by lowering the surface tension of bubbles of gas in the gastric fluid, is also present in many products.

In pregnancy, reassurance is often all that is required. However, a simple antacid (e.g. milk of magnesia) may be useful and is safe after the first trimester. Antacids interact with iron in the gastro-intestinal tract, and this type of reaction may be reduced by arranging the dosage times so that the two are not taken within two hours of each other.

20.3.5 COUGHS AND COLDS

Introduction

Upper respiratory-tract infection may be caused by bacterial or, more commonly, viral invasion, resulting in the common cold. Although the symptoms of a cough and head cold may present separately, they often occur together.

Key Questions

- When did the cough start?
- Is the cough productive or dry?
- Is the cough painful?
- Has the patient got a fever?

- Has there been a change in character of a persistent cough?
- What is the appearance of the sputum?
- Is it worse at a particular time of day?

Assessment and Interpretation

Nature and severity   Patients with a head cold may complain of nasal congestion or nasal discharge (rhinorrhoea). The colour of nasal secretions is not normally a helpful sign, except when other symptoms (e.g. headache or facial tenderness and aching over and under the eyes) suggest sinusitis. In such instances, if the mucus is green or brown and symptoms have persisted for one week without improvement, then referral should be made so that the doctor may assess whether antimicrobial treatment is necessary.

The type of cough should be ascertained. Coughs broadly fall into 1 of 3 categories. Firstly, a dry tickle felt in the throat may produce an irritating cough with no sputum. Secondly, the cough may be described as chesty, and sputum is produced. The third type is a chesty cough which does not produce sputum, and represents congestion in the bronchi.

Onset and duration   The onset of most respiratory-tract infections is often sudden, and the commonly described appearance of a sore throat, sneezing, and rhinorrhoea herald the well-known syndrome of the common cold.

A cough at night may be related to the presence of an allergen. However, the presence of night-time cough is not helpful in differentiating the cause, except in children where it may be a sign of asthma.

In an otherwise healthy person, the duration of symptoms is an important factor that will determine whether non-prescription medicines may be recommended by pharmacists or referral is appropriate. A cough that has not improved over 2 or 3 weeks should be investigated, and this time period should be shorter if symptoms are causing distress or becoming more severe.

Long-standing recurrent cough (e.g. since childhood) may indicate a chronic lung disorder (e.g. bronchiectasis), and the decision whether to refer will be based on the patient's past experience and the severity of the current symptoms.

Smokers, who normally disregard their cough, may suffer from chronic bronchitis which can occasionally flare up into an acute attack. The decision to refer again rests on the severity of symptoms, but with this type of patient some professional advice about the damage caused by cigarette smoke may be warranted.

Accompanying symptoms   If there is *sputum*, its nature may be helpful in deciding management. Clear white sputum is of little clinical significance, but copious, white, frothy sputum may be coughed up by chronic bronchitic patients and smokers. Brown or green sputum suggests the presence of a chest infection and patients should be referred if they feel ill. The presence of blood-stained sputum also requires referral. After a severe fit of coughing, it might be normal to pass 1 or 2 specks of blood in the sputum, but persistent blood specks or more obvious loss of blood requires referral as serious problems (e.g. carcinoma, tuberculosis, and pulmonary embolism) must be excluded.

A noticeably *raised temperature* is uncommon in adults suffering from the common cold. It may accompany more severe infections (e.g. influenza). If patients complain of night sweats and of feeling ill, or having a cough which has lasted for more than one week without improvement, referral is necessary to exclude serious conditions (e.g. tuberculosis).

General malaise, headache, and myalgia are common accompaniments to viral illnesses (e.g. influenza). Providing no other symptom is present that would suggest the need for medical referral, the patient should be reassured that the illness will begin to resolve in a few days.

A *sore throat* is a frequent early symptom of the common cold, which usually resolves spontaneously. Referral is not necessary providing it is not painful or causing difficulty with swallowing (*see* Sore Throat, Section 20.3.12).

Infected sinuses may cause *sinus pain* and headache. Sinus pain is characterised by a painful face, and tenderness to pressure below the eyes on the cheek bones and on the bony ridge above the eyes. Nasal mucus may be discoloured, indicating infection. Patients often complain of a long history of sinusitis, and a decision whether to refer will often depend on the benefit derived from previous treatment.

Patients may complain of persistent *catarrh* which exists for several days or weeks after other symptoms of a cold have disappeared. Providing they are otherwise well, symptomatic treatment is sufficient until the condition resolves.

Patients with rhinorrhoea or nasal congestion accompanied by *itchy red eyes* may be suffering from an allergy or infection. Allergy may represent a perennial rhinitis which may exist most of the year due to constant allergenic stimuli in the patient's environment (e.g. house-dust mite). More commonly, symptoms occur between April and July and are caused by seasonal allergies (e.g. hay fever). Under most circumstances, there are many symptomatic remedies which can be recommended before referral is necessary.

Wheezing represents an element of bronchoconstriction which, although more commonly associated by the layman with asthma, is not an uncommon component of other airways diseases (e.g. bronchitis and bronchiectasis). Wheezing in a child should be referred to the doctor. In adults, referral depends on the severity and whether patients are short of breath.

Patients who are *short of breath*, but have not normally been so in the past, require referral to exclude serious pathology and to obtain early treatment. It should be remembered that patients with cardiac problems (e.g. heart failure) may also report this symptom.

Severe *pain on coughing or on inspiration* requires referral to exclude conditions such as pleurisy and pulmonary embolism.

Patients with chronic chest symptoms should be questioned about *weight loss*. Severe weight loss may accompany lung cancer and tuberculosis. It should always be enquired after in smokers and chronic bronchitics.

Causative and modifying factors   It may be possible to relate the onset of symptoms to a particular causative factor (e.g. an allergen in hay fever or previous exposure to cold temperatures or people with the common cold).

Drugs may precipitate respiratory problems. Aspirin and other non-steroidal anti-inflammatory drugs may provoke an asthmatic attack in about 5% of asthmatic patients. Beta-adrenoceptor blocking drugs may also cause bronchoconstriction in asthmatics. A small proportion of patients (about 1%) undergoing treatment with angiotensin-converting enzyme (ACE) inhibitors may develop a persistent dry cough which disappears only when the treatment is withdrawn.

Some patients receiving antihypertensive therapy may develop nasal congestion.

Possible causes of cough are summarised in Part C.

Risk factors   Many risk factors (e.g. heart failure or smoking) may predispose patients to various pulmonary disorders.

In otherwise healthy people, *age* is the predominant risk factor for respiratory infections at both extremes of life. The elderly, especially the frail, the malnourished, and those who cannot keep warm are susceptible to chest infections. Such infections may make aged patients take to their beds where they may develop pneumonia. Infections may also result in confusion and a fall, perhaps causing fractured bones and leading to several weeks in hospital. The elderly should be encouraged to avail themselves of influenza vaccinations in the winter. If they become infected with the common cold virus, they need to take special care. If they feel ill, they should be advised to visit or call the doctor, who will assess their situation and decide suitable treatment.

At the other end of the age spectrum, young children, especially those under 9 months of age, require special attention. Infants who cannot feed because of nasal congestion, or who refuse to eat because they feel ill, require referral. Any vomiting, breathing difficulties, noisy breathing, or earache require referral. Similarly, those developing symptoms of a cold after immunisation should be referred. A night-time cough which persists needs assessment by a doctor, to exclude the presence of asthma.

Generally, children who are ill do not eat and it is this marker which will often give a clue as to whether it is necessary to refer.

Management

Non-drug treatment   Steam inhalations are effective in relieving nasal congestion. They are harmless and, although there is little evidence that additives do any harm, there is a suggestion that menthol may reduce the beating of the cilia which move the mucus layer along the upper respiratory-tract surface.

Steam inhalations or an increased fluid intake will also hydrate the inflamed pharyngeal mucosa and provide alleviation of dry coughs. Their use is also ideal in the treatment of productive coughs. Steam inhalations, or sitting a child in a bathroom with the hot water taps running, will hydrate the upper respiratory tree and encourage loosening of viscid sputum and secretion from mucous glands.

Drug treatment   The management of coughs and colds with no underlying pathology is symptomatic and, despite the belief or expectations of many visitors to the pharmacy, nothing will curtail the natural progression of the infection. Although many clinical authorities dismiss cough medicines as placebos, the general public regard them with the greatest esteem. They are, at the very least, powerful placebos and some may be considered to have some pharmacological efficacy.

Rhinorrhoea and nasal congestion may be alleviated by sympathomimetic agents. These vasoconstrictors shrink the inflamed tissues and reduce the activity of mucous glands in the nasal mucosa. They are available as systemic (BNF 3.10) or topical nasal (BNF 12.2.2) decongestants.

Oral products for the relief of coughs and colds are often combinations of a sympathomimetic agent, an antihistamine (to dry up secretions and to suppress any cough), and an analgesic with antipyretic properties. Sympathomimetic agents are contra-indicated in diabetic patients as they stimulate beta-receptors and can counteract the effects of hypoglycaemic agents. They are also contra-indicated in hypertension, hyperthyroidism, and angina. In such cases, if a decongestant is deemed absolutely necessary, a topical formulation may be preferable, as local vasoconstriction will inhibit its absorption from the nasal mucosa. Sympathomimetic agents should also be avoided in patients taking mono-amine-oxidase inhibitors and other antidepressant drugs.

Patients with glaucoma should not be given preparations containing antihistamines because of their intrinsic anticholinergic properties. These preparations may also cause a dry mouth, constipation, interference with accommodation, and sedation.

If an antihistamine alone is recommended (e.g. in allergic rhinitis), it may be logical to select one of the newer agents which reportedly cause less sedation than traditional products.

It is unlikely that nasal symptoms will persist. However, the use of topical decongestant sprays and drops for periods longer than 1 to 2 weeks may cause harmful effects and result in a rebound congestion (rhinitis medicamentosa).

Patients who are feverish, have aching limbs and muscles, headache, or general malaise may benefit from using a simple analgesic with antipyretic properties (e.g. paracetamol). A streaming rhinorrhoea results in appreciable fluid loss and requires plenty of drinks to replace that loss.

Cough suppressants are indicated for *dry, irritating, tickly coughs*. Not only will coughing cause further irritation and inflammation to the posterior surface of the oropharynx, but the cough may keep the patient awake at night or irritate others who live or work within close proximity.

The opioids are efficacious cough suppressants (BNF 3.9.1). Codeine, dextromethorphan, noscapine, or pholcodine are found in many proprietary cough products. Codeine may be abused and the use of pholcodine, which has similar cough suppressant activity, is preferred.

Antihistamines are also effective cough sedatives and may be used alone or combined with opioids. They may, however, cause drowsiness and, if this is the case, are best used at night.

Demulcents (e.g. glycerol, honey, and syrup) have been traditionally used to soothe the throat and tickly coughs. Solid dose forms (e.g. pastilles or lozenges) probably act more effectively than syrups.

For *chesty, but non-productive coughs*, a bronchodilator may encourage a clear airway and aid removal of sputum from the respiratory tree. Many products contain ephedrine and pseudoephedrine in combination with suppressants or expectorants. Contra-indications to these sympathomimetic drugs are listed under nasal congestion, (*see above*).

Productive coughs should be encouraged, not suppressed, to allow removal of sputum containing cell debris or irritating substances from the respiratory tract. It is in the use of expectorants that most doubt is cast upon the efficacy of cough products.

There are many expectorant drugs used in non-prescription cough products (e.g. ammonium salts, guaiphenesin, ipecacuanha, squill, and citric acid, *see* BNF 3.9.2). It is no coincidence that large doses of these drugs cause vomiting, because they are thought to stimulate the respiratory mucosa via an irritant effect on the gastric mucosa.

Polypharmacy is prevalent in cough products and many preparations marketed as expectorants contain mixtures of drugs which are pharmacologically antagonistic. These should be avoided. A combination of an expectorant and a cough suppressant cannot be justified, and the addition of an antihistamine to an expectorant is irrational on pharmacological grounds. Nevertheless, some combinations (e.g. an expectorant and a bronchodilator) are plausible and may be recommended with confidence.

20.3.6 HEADACHE

Introduction

Headache is possibly the most common symptom experienced and reported. It may usually be attributed to minor conditions (e.g. muscle tension), psychogenic causes, or dilatation of cranial blood vessels. Occasionally, serious causes (e.g. inflammation of the meninges, or tumours) are identified.

Key Questions

- Where is the headache?
- Did it come on suddenly for no apparent reason?
- Does anything aggravate its severity?

Assessment and Interpretation

Location   Headache at the *front of the head* may be idiopathic or due to sinusitis, nasal congestion, or migraine.

Pain in the back of the head (*occipital headache*) is frequently due to tension and anxiety, especially if the pain radiates over the top or sides. The patient will usually complain of a tight feeling around or over the head. This type of headache is one of the most commonly reported. Tension may be caused by neck injury or muscle spasm in the neck, back, or shoulder (e.g. torticollis or cervical spondylosis).

More serious causes include space-occupying lesions (e.g. tumours) and subarachnoid haemorrhage. Both may also produce headache which is either felt in other parts or radiates to them.

Pain originating on one side of the forehead and face (*unilateral headache*) frequently accompanies sinusitis, whilst the unilateral pain of classical migraine can originate in any area of the head. Unilateral pain of both conditions can become bilateral.

Herpes zoster virus infections of the nerves running over the top of the scalp and into the eye can cause shingles on one side of the face. A severe lancing pain may be felt before the characteristic rash is apparent.

Cluster headaches are a type of migraine headache, which may affect one side of the head or face.

Trigeminal neuralgia involves the cranial facial nerve. The slightest touch or pressure on this area of the face can provoke an extreme pain often described as sharp or lancing.

Pain felt in the *eye* should be referred as it may be due to glaucoma or trauma. Pain felt behind or around the eye can occur in sinusitis, migraine, or shingles.

Nature and severity   An extremely intense, possibly occipital, headache which comes on very suddenly without warning requires medical referral as it may indicate an emergency such as subarachnoid haemorrhage. If an equally intense pain has developed much more gradually, referral may be necessary to exclude the possibility of subdural haematoma. This possibility should be suspected following head injury, however trivial. Patients should be questioned about the occurrence of any possible trauma or incident.

Throbbing headache may be due to vascular changes (e.g. migraine or haemorrhage), or can accompany pyrexia of influenza or other viral infections.

Dull continuous headache may be due to tension, neck trauma, or a tumour.

Onset and duration   An early morning headache, which usually abates during the day, might, in some cases, be caused by space-occupying lesions. A clear-cut diagnosis is not possible, however, because benign idiopathic and tension headaches may also be present from the moment patients awaken.

Patients known to be hypertensive should be made aware that persistent severe early morning headache may be associated with uncontrolled hypertension. Referral should be recommended, especially if nausea, vomiting, nose bleeds, or bleeding from any other part of the body (e.g. haematuria) is noted. The nasal congestion of

sinusitis is often worsened by lying down. Early morning headache is often associated with this condition.

An intense pain lasting more than 48 hours which disrupts normal life-style requires referral.

Stress and tension headaches, and sinusitis, produce a continuous dull pain over several days. Migraine varies in duration from a few hours to more than a day, but rarely lasts more than two days. Cluster headaches last for 1 to 2 hours (usually at night-time), often recurring at the same time for weeks or months.

Brief pain, or a consistent pattern of pain which has existed for several years, is unlikely to have a serious cause. However, changes in its nature, reflected by increasing severity or duration, require medical attention.

Accompanying symptoms   Symptoms accompanying headache can be useful in evaluating the cause of some types of headache.

General malaise, aching, and fever may be indicative of a viral infection (e.g. the common cold, influenza, or mumps). A less frequently encountered cause is meningitis. More specific diagnosis is possible if additional symptoms are present, and include a rash (e.g. mumps or meningitis) or nasal congestion (e.g. sinusitis or common cold).

Meningitis should also be suspected if the patient complains of fever, together with *neck stiffness*, and extreme pain on both up-and-down and side-to-side movement of the head. Restriction of movement in a horizontal plane can occur in muscle spasm caused by cervical spondylosis, torticollis, or subarachnoid haemorrhage.

Headaches accompanied by *nausea or vomiting* may be characteristic of minor conditions (e.g. migraine) or serious illness (e.g. space-occupying lesions, haemorrhage, meningitis, and glaucoma).

Disturbed vision may accompany various forms of headache. Blurred vision can accompany classical migraine, while restricted field of vision and haloes around artificial lights may occur in glaucoma. By comparison, common migraine does not affect normal visual fields.

Emotional disturbances (e.g. tiredness and an inability to fall asleep) may accompany headache caused by depressive disorders, tension, and anxiety. Early morning awakening, poor appetite, and an inability to cope with worry are other indicators of emotional disturbances.

Patients reporting signs of *central nervous system involvement* in headache (e.g. drowsiness and irritability, numbness, paraesthesia, and unilateral muscle weakness) should be referred immediately. Serious pathology suggested by these symptoms include stroke, subarachnoid or subdural haemorrhage, or a tumour. The gradual development and intermittent appearance of slurred speech and personality changes with headache may indicate space-occupying lesions.

A cyclical pattern of headache immediately before or during *menstruation* suggests hormonal imbalance.

Causative and modifying factors   Pain on *movement* of the head or neck may indicate a neck injury or inflamed meninges. Bending down will exacerbate the headache of space-occupying lesions, sinusitis, and other causes. Sudden movements produced by coughing and sneezing will worsen the headache of space-occupying lesions. Exercise may also precipitate migraine. Conversely, migraine and many other types of headache may be relieved by lying down, particularly in a darkened room.

Diet can play an important role in causing headache. Migraine may be precipitated by various foods and drinks (e.g. chocolate, coffee, and alcohol) and by hunger. Diabetic patients may also suffer headaches when their condition becomes unstable.

Bright daylight and artificial light may aggravate migraine and the headache of meningitis. Conversely, entering a darkened room may worsen the headache caused by glaucoma through pupillary dilatation. The application of *heat* to the neck may alleviate pain due to local injury.

It is important to be aware of patients' *treatment history*. Patients should be asked about any current prescription or non-prescription medication and whether any link can be established between their symptoms and the use of drugs (e.g. oral contraceptives or indomethacin).

Possible causes of headache are summarised in Part C.

Management

Non-drug treatment   Any obvious causative factors such as food, alcohol, or eye strain should be eliminated.

Once other possible causes, and the possibility of serious underlying pathology, have been excluded, long-term headaches may normally be attributed to stress and tension. Despite the absence of obvious physical causes, such patients should be treated sympathetically. Counselling in relaxation techniques (e.g. lying down, gentle exercise, and massage) may be required to relieve the underlying cause. If the suggested measures show no improvement within 1 to 2 weeks, patients could reasonably be referred if they are anxious, or their life-style is being disrupted.

Drug treatment   Headaches are generally more responsive to treatment by analgesics if treatment is started promptly. This is particularly true for migraine head-

aches, in which an early loading dose of analgesic followed by regular maintenance doses throughout the attack, is essential.

Analgesics which may be purchased can be broadly classified into three categories:

- Those which exert a peripheral analgesic effect (e.g. aspirin or ibuprofen) by inhibiting the release of prostaglandins which mediate pain. By virtue of this action they also have anti-inflammatory properties which are useful when inflammation is the cause of pain.
- Those which are believed to act primarily on peripheral receptors, interrupting the pathways between the site of pain and the pain sensation areas in the brain (e.g. paracetamol).
- Those which act centrally to suppress pain pathways within the brain (e.g. codeine).

Different formulations of analgesics may be more appropriate for certain types of headache. Soluble formulations achieve peak plasma concentrations more rapidly than non-soluble forms. There is, however, no convincing evidence to suggest soluble forms relieve pain more quickly or effectively. Topical analgesics may be helpful in muscle tension or stiffness of the neck following trauma, or in tension headaches. The plethora of balms and rubs available may act through a counter-irritant effect, by local absorption of the analgesic, or both. The beneficial effects of local massage should also not be overlooked.

The choice of analgesic is empirical. Whenever possible, however, single-agent preparations are preferred to combination products.

Headache caused by minor neck injury, or tissue inflammation associated with nasal congestion or sinusitis, should theoretically benefit from the use of aspirin or ibuprofen rather than paracetamol. There is also some evidence to support the preferred use of ibuprofen in dental pain.

However, aspirin and ibuprofen are contra-indicated in several instances. Aspirin should not be recommended to children under 12 years of age because of its implication in Reye's syndrome. Aspirin and ibuprofen are also contra-indicated in the presence of a history of heartburn, indigestion, and peptic ulceration. Anyone with known hypersensitivity to aspirin should not be given ibuprofen.

Asthmatic patients may develop hypersensitivity to aspirin and other non-steroidal anti-inflammatory analgesics. Patients prescribed oral anticoagulant therapy (e.g. warfarin or phenindione) should not be given aspirin. Most patients will be aware of such interactions, but it is wise to ask all patients if they are taking other medication.

Women of child-bearing age might take analgesics (e.g. ibuprofen and aspirin) before they realise they are pregnant. Aspirin is potentially teratogenic, although evidence is inconclusive. Its main effects occur in the latter stages of pregnancy, causing prolonged term and an increased duration of labour. The incidence of minor bleeding in neonates, and internal bleeding at birth, are increased when aspirin is taken late in the pregnancy.

No teratogenic effects have been noted with ibuprofen use during pregnancy, but the data sheet recommends its avoidance during pregnancy if possible.

Paracetamol may be used in children and in other patients in whom aspirin is contra-indicated. If analgesia is required during pregnancy, the use of paracetamol is recognised as being safer than aspirin, due to the absence of clotting problems.

Codeine is only available in a non-prescription form as a combination product with aspirin or paracetamol. If taken regularly for prolonged periods, constipation may result.

20.3.7   ABDOMINAL PAIN

Introduction

In this section abdominal pain refers to pain below the rib cage, but also includes symptoms felt in the chest as a result of pathology associated with the oesophagus.

Key Questions

- Where exactly is the pain?
- Has the patient had a gastro-intestinal illness before?
- When did the pain start?
- Is it an intermittent or a constant pain?
- Has the pain spread to any other parts of the body?
- Is there anything that helps to reduce the pain?

Assessment and Interpretation

Location   Pain in the midline sections of the abdomen, i.e. epigastric, central, and suprapubic areas (*see* Fig. 1.1), is usually indicative of an intestinal or gastric cause. The pain of peptic ulceration is typically epigastric, central, or both. In duodenal ulceration, the pain may also be felt slightly to the right. In gastric ulceration, the pain may be to the left and higher in the abdomen than in duodenal ulceration. Appendicitis begins in the central area but radiates to the right iliac fossa. Pain in the right upper abdomen, just beneath the lower ribs, may be

caused by spasm in the bile duct/biliary system. However, this pain can sometimes be felt in the epigastrium.

The pain of irritable bowel syndrome is usually low down and typically occurs in the left iliac fossa, but may spread centrally or to the right iliac fossa. Diverticular disease similarly causes pain in the right or left iliac fossae.

Sometimes gastro-intestinal pain may be felt as a vague and generalised pain over most of the abdomen, as in gastro-enteritis.

Reflux oesophagitis may cause a burning pain in the epigastrium which may spread into the chest beneath the sternum.

Renal pain is felt in the loin area at the side or to the back of the abdomen. Infection or renal calculi affecting the ureters may cause pain radiating down from the loin to the iliac fossa on the affected side (ureteric or renal colic), and eventually the suprapubic area will be affected if the obstruction or infection affects the bladder and urethra.

Nature and severity   Pain in any hollow organ with a smooth muscular coat is usually colicky. Colic is a spasmodic pain that is griping, reaches a peak, and then eases before returning. This type of pain may reflect involvement of the stomach, large and small intestine, the ureters, urethra, and the bile ducts as well as genital organs (e.g. the uterus and Fallopian tubes). Sometimes abdominal pain is less severe and specific, presenting as a dull ache (as in irritable bowel syndrome).

The pain of peptic ulceration is often described by patients as a gnawing pain and this is a typical description of ulceration. However, the pain may also be of the burning or boring type.

If patients describe the pain as the worst they have ever felt or as unbearable, and it has been present as a continuous severe pain for more than one hour, drastically affecting normal activities, then immediate referral to a surgery or a hospital is necessary. Such symptoms are described as an acute abdomen, and in such cases, patients will be in obvious need of an urgent medical opinion. Possible causes of an acute abdomen include peritonitis, appendicitis, intestinal obstruction, biliary colic, bleeding or perforated peptic ulceration, renal colic, pancreatitis, strangulated hernia, occlusion of arteries in the abdomen, and gynaecological conditions.

Onset and duration   If the pain is described as moderate, mild, or occurring episodically with alternating periods of well-being, it is advisable to recommend medical referral after 7 days. However, if patients have had similar bouts in the past, referral should be made earlier as this would suggest recurrence of an unresolved complaint with underlying pathology that requires investigation.

Persistent abdominal pain reported by patients over 40 years of age who have never suffered from dyspepsia before requires referral to exclude peptic ulceration and cancer of the stomach. The latter, though relatively rare, occurs more frequently over this age.

Accompanying symptoms   Details of the *radiation of pain* are useful diagnostic features. The pain of appendicitis commences centrally and, after a few hours, spreads to the right iliac fossa, and requires immediate referral. Patients who complain of pain in the abdomen radiating to the tip of the shoulder are probably experiencing referred pain from the diaphragm, and should be reassured that this is normal. Pain in the upper abdomen, especially the right hypochondrium, which is referred to the back or shoulder blades is suggestive of biliary colic, and in acute episodes will be severe enough to warrant referral.

Pain originating from kidney disorders and renal colic initially presents with loin pain and may radiate to the back or spread downwards to the iliac fossa and supra-pubic area, and in males into the scrotum. It may also cause aching in the thighs.

Pain of ovarian and uterine disorders may also radiate to the thighs.

Pain can radiate from the stomach and spread into the chest as a result of acid reflux into the oesophagus. This may be caused by hiatus hernia, peptic or oesophageal ulceration, or milder forms of dyspepsia. If chest pain is severe, pharmacists should always refer patients immediately, unless patients can describe previous similar episodes and have no other signs of angina or myocardial infarction.

Recent *weight loss* of more than 3 kg over 2 to 3 weeks requires referral for investigation. It may represent the consequence of loss of appetite in someone with an abdominal complaint, but cancer of the stomach or large intestine requires exclusion in patients who are over 40 years of age.

Distension of the abdomen, described as a bloated feeling or sensation of fullness, may be caused by peptic ulceration. If it is persistent and accompanied by pain, referral should be recommended.

Vomiting, constipation, or both, in the presence of abdominal pain requires investigation to exclude the possibility of obstruction. Vomiting may also be a reflex action caused by intense pain. Difficulty in swallowing also requires referral.

The presence of *blood* in vomit, or in the stools, may be caused by a perforated ulcer or damaged inflamed areas in the gastro-intestinal tract, and requires immediate referral. Blood may appear as a characteristic red colour or may be black ('coffee-ground' vomitus) in either vomit or stool.

Colicky pain accompanied by *diarrhoea* may be suggestive of gastro-enteritis. Cases contracted in this country will normally resolve spontaneously, but if patients have recently returned from abroad, referral is advisable to exclude serious pathogens. Other possible diagnoses are ulcerative colitis, irritable bowel syndrome, and diverticular disease.

Complications of cardiovascular disease can cause abdominal pain. Abdominal pain with chronic back pain and occasionally fainting may be indicative of an aortic aneurysm, which may be fatal if it ruptures. Older patients with a history of myocardial infarction or atrial fibrillation may develop mesenteric ischaemia due to embolism. This produces severe pain and can lead to necrosis of the intestinal wall.

Causative and modifying factors   The pain of peptic inflammation or ulceration may usually be related to *food intake*. It may be relieved or aggravated by food, as food can buffer the effects of acid or stimulate acid production. Response to treatment with antacids suggests that the pain may be caused by a lesion in the gastro-intestinal tract rather than urinary, genital, or other abdominal organs.

Substances which stimulate gastric acid secretion (e.g. coffee, tea, alcohol, spicy foods, or smoking) aggravate the pain of peptic ulceration or inflammation of the gastro-intestinal tract.

Any aggravation of upper abdominal pain caused by *exercise or cold*, particularly if it radiates to the chest, requires referral to exclude angina. If the pain is severe and persists for an hour or more, immediate referral is required to exclude myocardial infarction.

Drugs can also provoke abdominal pain. Non-steroidal anti-inflammatory drugs may cause abdominal pain due to gastric or duodenal ulceration. Opioid drugs have a tendency to cause constipation, which may produce intestinal obstruction in some patients and result in abdominal pain. Some drugs can cause oesophageal ulceration (e.g. potassium chloride, amoxycillin, and doxycycline).

Possible causes of abdominal pain are summarised in Part C.

Risk factors   The *age* of the patient should be considered in assessing the symptom. A child complaining of abdominal pain for more than a few hours should be referred for a medical opinion. If the child does not appear ill, pharmacists can advise the parent to take the child to see the doctor the next day, as this allows time to judge whether the condition is self-limiting. Children may be judged to be ill, and therefore require immediate referral, if they show any of the following features:

- agitation
- behaviour significantly different from normal
- crying, due to pain
- distress
- drowsiness
- fever
- pallor
- unable to keep still because of the pain
- vomiting.

Possible causes of continual crying in babies are gastro-enteritis and obstruction. In gastro-enteritis, the presenting symptoms may include pain, vomiting, and diarrhoea. Obstruction may be caused by pyloric stenosis in which forceful projectile vomiting occurs. It may also be due to an intestinal obstruction, producing vomiting with or without constipation, and the baby will rapidly decline towards shock. Each of these conditions requires urgent referral.

Management

Management of abdominal pain depends on the cause. If a patient does not require medical referral, symptomatic remedies may be helpful. Antacids (BNF 1.1) and laxatives (BNF 1.6) may be tried in appropriate cases. Pain may be relieved by paracetamol or a mixture of codeine and paracetamol, although codeine may be constipating. Aspirin and ibuprofen should be avoided in disorders of the gastro-intestinal tract because of their tendency to irritate the abdominal mucosa.

Patients with diarrhoea, and especially children, require adequate hydration (*see* Section 20.3.1).

20.3.8 PAINFUL, FREQUENT, AND URGENT URINATION

Introduction

A syndrome of painful, frequent, and urgent urination (dysuria, frequency, and urgency) occurs in lower urinary-tract infection, although bacteriuria cannot be proved in many instances. The condition occurs in about 10 times as many women as men, and patients will often self-diagnose the symptoms as cystitis. However, the involvement of other parts of the urinary tract should always be borne in mind (e.g. the urethra causing urethritis, and the kidneys causing pyelonephritis).

Key Questions

- Is the patient male or female?
- How long has the patient had the symptoms?
- How old is the patient?
- Is there any itching or discharge?
- Does the urine appear normal?
- Did the symptoms begin slowly, over a period of time, or abruptly?
- Does the patient have to get up during the night to pass urine?

Assessment and Interpretation

Location The higher incidence of symptoms in females is thought to be due to the close proximity of the anus to the short urethra. This increases the likelihood of bacterial transmission to the bladder and urethra, which may result in cystitis and urethritis respectively.

When symptoms occur in men, the patient should be referred to exclude the possibility of prostatitis (particularly in older men), renal calculi, or other obstruction.

Nature and severity Many patients report symptoms without severe pain or general malaise. Some, particularly men, may complain of hesitancy or a weak flow of urine during micturition. If these are present together with frequency and chronic dribbling, the patient should be referred.

Onset and duration Dysuria, frequency, and urgency usually present suddenly. Accompanying symptoms (e.g. mild back pain or abdominal pain, possibly due to renal obstruction) may develop insidiously some time before the urinary symptoms.

Accompanying symptoms The presence of any accompanying symptoms requires medical referral.

Localised symptoms in women include urethral itching and a pricking or stabbing pain, which further suggest the presence of an infection. In men, pruritus and soreness due to inflammation of the tip of the penis, often involving the foreskin, may occur without any symptoms of cystitis. The most likely diagnosis is balanitis caused by bacterial or fungal infection, or contact with soaps, disinfectants, and other irritants. The presence of any penile discharge requires urgent referral either to the doctor or a specialist genito-urinary clinic at a local hospital.

Vomiting may occur either as a result of severe colicky pain in the ureters or urethra, or from infection. *Fever and rigors* also indicate the presence of infection.

Blood in the urine is not necessarily a serious sign as it may simply be due to inflamed tissue being sloughed off the urinary tract. The underlying pathology, however, may be serious (e.g. infection, bladder lesions, bladder and renal calculi, and kidney damage).

Vaginal symptoms (e.g. pruritus, discharge, or stinging when urine makes contact with an inflamed vaginal labia) indicate involvement of the genital tract.

Lower urinary-tract *pain* may radiate to the loins or back. Equally, back pain or colicky pain in the loins may radiate to the groin and thigh, and in men to the testicles. Such symptoms indicate spasm of the urinary tract due to infection, obstruction (e.g. renal calculi), or other lesions.

Thirst and excessive fluid intake can also accompany dysuria, frequency, and urgency. Fluid intake in excess of the normal 1 to 3 litres per day will cause frequency of micturition. If the patient is excessively thirsty as well as drinking large volumes, the possibility of diabetes mellitus should be considered.

Causative and modifying factors   *Diuretics* increase frequency of micturition. While most patients will realise their cause and effect relationship, their use should be enquired after.

Drinks (e.g. tea, coffee, or alcohol) also have a diuretic effect, and can precipitate nocturnal frequency. They should therefore be avoided in the evening in susceptible individuals.

Irritants (e.g. bubble baths, nylon underwear and tights, vaginal deodorants, or even over-zealous use of strongly perfumed soaps) may cause perineal and urethral symptoms similar to those produced by cystitis.

The incidence of frequency and urgency may increase at the *menopause*, and may be followed by the development of postmenopausal urinary incontinence. This is thought to be due to the lack of oestrogen to stimulate oestrogenic receptors on the urethra and bladder, producing atrophic changes. Women initially reporting frequency and urgency between 45 and 55 years of age should be referred for assessment.

Anxiety or agitation may cause patients to report urinary symptoms that can be partially ascribed to their mental state. Counselling and reassurance, or medical referral, may be required.

Pregnancy is a common cause. Increased pressure on the bladder from the growing uterus is a normal consequence of pregnancy. Unless the resultant frequency is accompanied by pain or fever, the patient should require reassurance only.

Sexual intercourse can precede initiation or worsening of symptoms in women, probably as a consequence of infection arising from damage to the perineal mucosa.

Possible causes of painful, frequent, and urgent uri-nation are summarised under Urination abnormalities, Part C.

Isolated or recurrent symptoms   It should be ascertained whether the symptoms are similar to a previous acute attack, or whether they are persistent. If they represent a chronic attack, the patient should be referred, particularly if treatment previously initiated by the doctor has been unsuccessful.

Management

In an acute outbreak of symptoms without complications, symptomatic treatment may be suggested for up to 48 hours. If no improvement is obvious by this time, referral should be recommended. Although non-drug or drug treatments are discussed separately, their use is not exclusive.

Non-drug treatment   Patients should be advised to drink large volumes of fluid to dilute the bacteria in the bladder, and they should avoid delays in emptying the bladder.

Elimination of bacteria is facilitated by 'double micturition'. This involves passing a second flow of urine by voluntary effort after the main stream has subsided. Bladder emptying is therefore more complete, and helps reduce the residual volume of infected urine.

Drug treatment   Nearly all the urinary symptoms may be attributed to the acidification of urine by pathogens such as *Escherichia coli*. The aim of treatment is therefore to render the urine alkaline, for which citric acid and its salts (e.g. potassium citrate and sodium citrate) are effective. However, care must be taken in the elderly, and patients with renal or heart disease, to prevent hyperkalaemia or hypernatraemia. Sodium bicarbonate powder may also be taken to alkalinise the urine, but similar precautions are required.

Hexamine is an antibacterial drug which produces its effect by conversion to formaldehyde at a low pH. However, due to the requirement for the urine to be acid, and the occurrence of side-effects (e.g. gastro-intestinal disturbances and bladder irritation), its use is no longer recommended.

A lubricating jelly may resolve any problems accompanying sexual intercourse.

The presence of pain or stinging on micturition may be relieved by paracetamol. The use of aspirin is not recommended as it will exacerbate symptoms by making the urine acidic.

20.3.9 MUSCULOSKELETAL DISORDERS

Introduction

Disorders of the skeleton and muscles result in symptoms which most commonly present to pharmacists as pain in the back or limbs. Such disorders may be of multifactorial origin, but those which pharmacists may commonly see will usually be due to ageing, injury, or inappropriate and excessive movement of joints. These and other associated problems are described below.

Key Questions

- Where is the pain?
- When did the pain start?
- Is there any stiffness, tenderness, swelling, numbness, or tingling?
- Is the pain worse at certain times or aggravated by any activity?
- Has the pain changed in nature or location?

Assessment and Interpretation

Location, nature, and severity   The principal causes of a stiff or painful *neck* are likely to be due to injury, torticollis, cervical spondylosis, and meningitis. These conditions can usually be differentiated by further history taking.

Pain or stiffness in the *shoulder* may be caused by injury to the joint or muscles (e.g. following overuse or excessive movement during exercise or sport). Stiffness in the shoulders and an inability to raise the arms may be caused by rheumatoid conditions in the older patient or by a frozen shoulder.

Pain at the *elbow* may be caused by strenuous overactivity of the muscles and their tendons which insert into the humerus at the elbow joint. Such pain is often due to sport or heavy manual work. It can cause golfer's elbow, which is characterised by pain on the inner side of the joint, and tennis elbow, which is more common and causes discomfort on the outer edge of the joint.

Gout predominantly affects men and may characteristically involve the *metatarsophalangeal joint of the great toe*, which becomes extremely painful and tender. Other joints may be similarly affected.

Apart from trauma, the two conditions most likely to present with pain in the *forearm* are tenosynovitis and carpal tunnel syndrome. The pain of tenosynovitis usually traces a line down the flexor surface of the forearm, wrist, thumb, and sometimes palm. The fingers become stiff and remain curled, and stretching causes pain. Sometimes numbness and tingling in the fingers is felt. Crackling or grating noises on movement may be heard or felt, especially in the wrist.

Carpal tunnel syndrome, caused by pressure on a nerve in the *wrist*, may present with symptoms similar to tenosynovitis. It is characterised by pain in the forearm, and numbness and tingling in the thumb and three fingers, the little finger rarely being affected. It is more common in women than men.

Rheumatoid arthritis commonly affects the wrist and *finger joints*, causing pain, swelling, and stiffness. Whereas osteoarthritis classically affects the distal and proximal interphalangeal joints, metacarpophalangeal joints, and the wrists, rheumatoid arthritis in adults rarely affects the distal interphalangeal joints.

A fracture of the wrist commonly occurs after a fall on an outstretched hand. There is pain and tenderness and the hand cannot be moved.

Pain in the upper back or thoracic spine is unusual. The ribs attach to the twelve thoracic vertebrae, and strains or tears of the muscles of the chest or upper back may cause pain on breathing after coughing, or lifting heavy weights.

Pain from internal organs may penetrate to the upper back (e.g. in gallstones). Shingles may present as a unilateral superficial pain in the back and chest.

The lower back, comprising the lumbar and sacral regions of the spine, is more commonly associated with back pain than is the upper back. *Low back pain* is often termed lumbago, but this is a very general term and gives no indication of the cause.

Ankylosing spondylitis can cause pain anywhere in the spine, but most often occurs in the neck and lumbar regions. Similarly, osteoarthritis affects the lumbar region. The most common cause of acute lumbar pain is a prolapsed intervertebral disc (slipped disc). This causes severe pain, particularly after a major strain, injury, or fall. Sometimes the muscles or ligaments surrounding the lumbar vertebrae may be torn or strained without significant prolapse of the disc, giving rise to milder symptoms.

Chronic back pain may indicate conditions such as osteitis deformans, osteoporosis (particularly in postmenopausal women), and rarely a tumour, or aortic aneurysm.

Any back pain that fails to resolve needs a medical assessment. Often the cause will not be sinister but merely poor posture or failure of an acute back injury to heal. Nevertheless, other causes require exclusion by the doctor.

Vascular disorders may present symptoms in the *lower limbs*. A common disorder that pharmacists encounter is chilblains, which may occur in the feet as a burning sensation. Other sites affected include the hands, earlobes, and nose.

A painful calf that is swollen, hot, red, and tender suggests the possibility of deep vein thrombosis. It may be particularly suspected in women taking combined oral contraceptives, those who have experienced previous episodes, and those with cardiovascular disease. It may also be seen in patients who have been bedridden for some time and, in all cases, requires immediate referral.

Blue painful *feet*, which may accompany similar symptoms in the fingers, can be caused by Raynaud's syndrome and be precipitated by cold, emotional disturbances, or non-selective beta-adrenoceptor blocking drugs.

Pain in the calf or foot may be due to cramp, especially at night and in pregnancy. Pain in the back of the thigh and lower leg, arising suddenly especially during physical exercise, may be caused by an Achilles tendon or hamstring injury.

Rheumatoid arthritis and osteoarthritis may affect the knees and feet, causing pain, swelling, stiffness, and difficulty in walking. A swollen knee may also arise as a result of bursitis (housemaid's knee).

Pain or stiffness in the legs accompanied by difficulty in movement should always be referred to exclude fractures and other causes.

Varicose veins are painful and unsightly and are usually easily recognisable, but any oedematous swelling or redness requires referral. Swollen legs, particularly involving the ankles and feet, may be symptomatic of heart failure and require referral.

Pain along the sole of the foot and heel bone may be a consequence of torn tendons causing plantar fasciitis, often arising through trauma or running.

Bunions occur predominantly in the elderly through deformed joints in the great toe caused by osteoarthritis. In the presence of ill-fitting shoes, this causes a painful toe and bony protrusion on the inside of the foot at the base of the great toe.

Accompanying symptoms   *General malaise* can accompany musculoskeletal symptoms. Inflammation or trauma may occur in various parts of the body. This is because some rheumatoid disorders are systemic diseases, and some bone disorders cause symptoms unrelated to the initial site of pain (e.g. weight loss or muscle wasting may occur in rheumatoid arthritis or polymyalgia rheumatica). Fever, fatigue, skin rashes, and general malaise may also be seen and should be referred for investigation, as anaemia is a common accompaniment of chronic diseases (e.g. rheumatoid arthritis). Headache with back pain or muscle weakness

require referral since they may accompany osteitis deformans or arteritis of polymyalgia in older patients.

Paraesthesia may commonly indicate a trapped nerve and can occur in patients with inflamed joints. Symptoms in the fingers, hands, or arms may occur in spondylitis, torn muscles, or strained ligaments around the cervical and upper thoracic spinal vertebrae. Pain and stiffness spreading from a frozen shoulder may reach the back, chest, and arms. Care must be taken to differentiate these symptoms from those which might occur after myocardial infarction, where typically pain in the chest radiates to the neck, jaw, and sometimes to the arms, often in the form of paraesthesia. It should be remembered that myocardial infarction does not always present with a classical chest pain. Symptoms of sudden onset in the jaw, neck, and arms accompanied by a feeling of being unwell or distressed should be referred immediately for a medical opinion, especially if a history of cardiac problems is reported.

A rare cause of tingling sensations in the extremities is a form of focal epilepsy, and persistent or recurring bouts of symptoms require referral.

The most common spread of symptoms in a musculoskeletal disorder is *sciatica*, which follows a prolapsed intervertebral lumbar disc. Pain and paraesthesia may spread from the lower back to the buttock, thigh, calf, or foot. A tear of a back muscle rarely radiates pain below the knee. Any back pain accompanied by bowel or bladder symptoms could indicate that there is pressure on sacral nerve roots and a referral is necessary in such cases.

Pain, either chronic back pain or abdominal pain, requires referral. In older patients the cause may be serious (e.g. an aortic aneurysm), although such cases will be rarely seen in the pharmacy. Chronic back pain, especially in the presence of fatigue, anaemia, infection, and weight loss should always be referred to exclude sinister pathology (e.g. myeloma).

Renal colic may be felt as pain in the lower back at the level of the kidneys, which often spreads to the loins, groin, and testes. Dysmenorrhoea causes lumbar pain that may radiate to the thighs and is experienced around and during the time of menstruation.

Causative and modifying factors   *Movement and extremes of temperature* can affect many musculoskeletal symptoms. Most are worsened by movement of the affected tissues, and serious injury (e.g. a fractured bone) results in immobility as a protective mechanism. Tennis and golfer's elbow are made worse by gripping, and by turning the forearm; tenosynovitis is worsened by stretching the forearm, wrist, or hand. Walking precipitates the painful symptoms of a deep vein thrombosis or of intermittent claudication, whilst cramp is likely to occur at rest or lying down. Back pain caused by a prolapsed disc is made worse by movement and even by apparently unrelated activity (e.g. coughing or sneezing).

Vascular disorders (e.g. Raynaud's syndrome or chilblains) are exacerbated by exposure of the affected extremities to low temperatures. Arthritic symptoms appear to be exacerbated by cold and wet conditions.

A wide variety of *additional factors* can influence symptoms. Many symptoms are worse at different times of the day. Rheumatoid arthritis produces a characteristic stiffness, and osteoarthritic joints are especially painful in the morning. The pain of tenosynovitis and of frozen shoulder is worse at night.

Varicose veins are most painful and troublesome during menstruation. Some disorders are more common in certain age groups and in one sex. Tenosynovitis, carpal tunnel syndrome, Raynaud's syndrome, and polymyalgia rheumatica are more common in women than men. The age of the patient may be helpful in differentiating some disorders. Osteoporosis and osteitis deformans rarely occur before 40 years of age and polymyalgia is more common over 50 years of age. Rheumatoid arthritis, however, may occur at any age.

Vascular problems (e.g. cold extremities and Raynaud's syndrome) may be precipitated by beta-adrenoceptor blocking drugs.

Back pain due to a strain or prolapsed disc will usually be alleviated if the patient rests for several days on a hard mattress (*see* Non-drug treatment below). If this is unhelpful, referral is necessary. If the primary disorder is in other organs (e.g. urinary tract, gastrointestinal tract, aorta, or reproductive organs), rest will not be helpful.

Risk factors   *Old age* is an important risk factor, and elderly patients presenting with musculoskeletal complaints should generally be referred. Many symptoms may be attributable to chronic inflammatory disease or may be the trigger for such disease processes to take a hold. Some of the causes of inflammatory conditions may be serious and warrant investigation. Many accompanying factors, which sometimes remain clinically silent for a long period (e.g. the anaemia of chronic disease), are potentially serious and will often only be revealed upon medical investigation.

Management

Non-drug treatment   The symptomatic management of painful and inflammatory conditions in the short term involves heat and rest. When systemic symptoms or other accompanying factors suggest a more serious disorder or trauma a medical referral is necessary. Similarly symptoms which persist for more than a few days without improvement require a medical evaluation. Although medical therapy cannot always alleviate painful conditions, the patient should be advised to see a doctor to confirm the absence of any chronic systemic disease.

Acute localised inflammatory disease may be alleviated by local application of hot-water bottles, heat pads, and counter-irritant agents (e.g. liniments and balms). Resting the affected part of the body is essential and is only effective if the rest is complete. Complete bed rest is essential for severe back pain caused by a prolapsed disc, with meals in bed, and only visits to the toilet allowed. The bed or mattress should be firm (a board should be placed beneath the mattress, if required) and the patient should lie flat, preferably without a pillow under the head, although one small pillow may be used if necessary. A pillow under the knees if the patient is lying on his back, or between the legs if the patient is lying on his side, will be helpful.

A simple back muscle strain may show improvement in a matter of days, but a prolapsed disc can take up to 6 weeks to completely resolve. The latter condition, or one not resolving in a few days, therefore requires medical supervision, although some input by pharmacists may also be appropriate.

In those who have recovered from a musculoskeletal disorder or who are prone to relapse, the importance of preventive measures (e.g. weight reduction if appropriate, gentle exercise, swimming, and good posture) should be emphasised. Posture may be improved by remembering to keep the back straight, to support it when sitting, and to bend the knees when lifting.

Drug treatment   Non-opioid analgesics (e.g. aspirin or ibuprofen) will be helpful because of their anti-inflammatory properties. Care should be taken to establish that there are no contra-indications to these drugs (e.g. a history of gastro-intestinal symptoms or allergy). Combination analgesic products may be helpful, and mixtures of aspirin and codeine or paracetamol and codeine can be beneficial.

20.3.10 EYE DISORDERS

Introduction

Ocular symptoms most likely to be encountered in the pharmacy are red eye, styes, swollen painful lids, and sore gritty eyes. Responding to such symptoms requires special care. The risk of confusing common symptoms of minor disorders and potentially serious conditions is significant, with potentially grave consequences for patients. Whenever advice on eye problems is sought, all available information must be obtained from patients before recommending a course of action.

Symptoms are discussed according to involvement of either the eyeball or eyelids. (For information on the structure of the eye, *see* Section 11.2.)

Key Questions

- Has vision been affected?
- Is pain present within the eye or is the irritation or discomfort on the surface?
- Is the eye watering?
- Has there been any trauma to or around the eye?
- How severe is the pain?

Assessment and Interpretation – Eyeball

Primary symptoms and location   Redness and inflammation of the eye commonly indicates conjunctivitis of bacterial, environmental, or allergic origin. Confirmation of inflammation may be observed by noting the increased redness of the conjunctiva when the lower lid is pulled down. The degree of redness may vary, being particularly marked in allergic conjunctivitis due to either pollen or cosmetics.

Similar symptoms may be caused by dry eye. More serious pathology (e.g. uveitis, including iritis, and glaucoma) may be suggested if the conjunctiva close to the pupil is more inflamed than the periphery, and in the presence of other symptoms.

Accompanying symptoms   The presence or absence of accompanying symptoms is the most important indicator of any underlying pathology.

Superficial discomfort (e.g. pruritus, and a feeling of soreness or grittiness) is characteristic of conjunctivitis. However, the presence of *pain*, especially within the eye, indicates a much more serious condition (e.g. glaucoma or uveitis) and requires immediate referral, preferably direct to a hospital.

Sticky eyes in the morning, or the daytime accumulation of pus in the corner of the eye, suggests the presence of infective conjunctivitis.

Disturbed vision is not a consequence of conjunctivitis as the inflammation does not affect the cornea. Pharmacists should therefore be alert to reports of visual disturbances, as these indicate more serious conditions. The appearance of haloes around lights, particularly when leaving a darkened room, suggests closed-angle glaucoma. Blurred vision, difficulty in focusing, and

tunnel vision may be caused by a thrombosed artery, intra-ocular haemorrhage, retinal detachment, optic nerve damage, and closed-angle glaucoma. Gradual loss of vision may be caused by chronic glaucoma, cataracts, and retinal or macular degeneration. Any such symptoms therefore require referral.

If there is *abnormal redness* of the facial or peri-orbital skin, eye symptoms may be secondary to another focus of infection (e.g. cellulitis and herpesvirus infection).

Hazy pupils can occur in certain eye disorders. In conjunctivitis, the pupils will be bright and normal. However, in uveitis and glaucoma, the iris and pupil may appear hazy or cloudy. Additional indications of uveitis include pupillary constriction due to a swollen iris, and a misshapen pupil caused by the adhesion of the iris to the lens.

In closed-angle glaucoma, the pupils appear partially dilated and do not respond to light. They may also be oval in shape. These effects are less pronounced in open-angle glaucoma.

Severe eye pain can produce *nausea and vomiting*. In this event, or in any associated change in visual acuity or appearance of the pupil, the patient should be referred immediately.

Subconjunctival haemorrhage, a red haemorrhagic area in the white of the eye, can appear spontaneously following sneezing or as a result of trauma to the head or eye. In the latter case, the patient should be referred to exclude underlying pathology.

Assessment and Interpretation – Eyelids

Primary symptoms and location   Inflammation, either on the margin or under the eyelid, is the most common symptom. A stye is due to inflammation of a hair follicle at the base of an eyelash on the eyelid margin. Glandular inflammation of the eyelid margin is termed blepharitis. Hard lumps which usually appear under the upper eyelid indicate a chalazion.

Accompanying symptoms   A stye may cause *pain*, whereas a chalazion and blepharitis are associated with *soreness*.

Skin changes around the eye and eyelid can develop. Some eyelashes may be lost in blepharitis and there is frequently scaling and crusting of the lid margins. Seborrhoea of the face and scalp, together with dandruff, is commonly present.

Outward (*ectropion*) and inward (*entropion*) turning of the eyelid is often associated with eye irritation.

Duration   Styes usually resolve spontaneously within a few days. Blepharitis and chalazion are chronic disorders which may subside temporarily, but frequently recur.

Risk factors for eye disorders   *Age* is an important risk factor. Many eye disorders (e.g. glaucoma, ectropion, and entropion) have a high incidence in the elderly. In the very young, symptoms suggesting an eye infection in a baby under two months of age may have derived from the delivery, and be particularly serious if the mother had a sexually-transmitted disease. All newborn babies with eye disorders should be referred.

Diabetes mellitus commonly causes reversible changes in lens shape or serious retinal pathology, especially if diabetic control is poor. All diabetic patients who complain of visual disturbances or eye infection should be referred for medical assessment.

Management

Non-drug treatment   Red inflamed eyes due to allergic conjunctivitis may be relieved by elimination of the allergen whenever possible. Styes will resolve spontaneously within 2 or 3 days, although healing can be facilitated by applying a clean piece of cotton wool or lint soaked in warm water for 15 minutes. This procedure should be repeated 2 or 3 times each day until the stye comes to a head. In blepharitis, the eyelid margins should be bathed in warm water or a dilute solution of a baby shampoo to assist de-scaling. The accompanying presence of dandruff should also be treated with a suitable shampoo. The use of a non-medicated moisturising base (e.g. emulsifying ointment or aqueous cream) will help prevent skin flaking and keep the eyelid margins soft and hydrated.

Despite its dramatic appearance, subconjunctival haemorrhage will disappear spontaneously within two weeks and requires only reassurance.

Drug treatment   Infective conjunctivitis may be treated with non-prescription antibacterial agents. Two related compounds available as eye-drops (propamidine) and an eye ointment (dibromopropamidine) have been shown to be active against common pathogens (e.g. streptococci and staphylococci). The eye-drops should be instilled hourly during the day, and the eye ointment applied at night, to give sustained action. If the symptoms show no sign of improvement within 48 hours, the patient should be referred. Allergic conjunctivitis may be treated with local application of an antihistamine (e.g. antazoline), usually in combination with a vasconstrictor (e.g. xylometazoline). Patients should be advised that this preparation may cause transient stinging when applied to a sore eye.

20.3.11   EAR DISORDERS

Introduction

The ear is closely associated anatomically with the upper respiratory tract. Many symptoms and disorders in the ear may present as features that may be identified with disorders in the respiratory system.

Key Questions

- Is there pain or discomfort?
- Is the patient's hearing affected?
- Is the patient feeling dizzy?
- Can the patient hear ringing or humming noises?
- Has there been any recent trauma or injury to the affected ear?

Assessment and Interpretation

Nature and severity   The most serious disorder affecting the *outer ear* is a tumour. The outer ear is exposed to the sun and it may be the site for solar keratosis, which is the precursor of malignant epithelioma. Any recently noticed sore area, which does not resolve and is growing in size, should be referred. Basal cell carcinoma (rodent ulcer) may arise on the pinna, often on its upper edge, in the form of an ulcer with a raised border.

Trauma to the pinna may result in profuse bleeding because of its abundant blood supply. Similarly, contusions may produce large haematomas between the skin and cartilage, eventually producing fibrous scarring which may result in the deformed 'cauliflower ear'. Bleeding points should be compressed with a clean gauze pad and patients referred to a hospital. Contusions require surgical drainage.

The pinna and auditory canal may sometimes appear red and inflamed due to eczema or infection. Various substances may cause obstruction of the auditory canal (e.g. wax or foreign bodies, including insects).

Pain within the ear may be due to inflammatory causes in the outer ear. However, if no lesions are visible, then the source of the pain or ache may be inflammation in the *middle ear* caused by infection (i.e. otitis media). It may affect one or both ears.

Severe injury (e.g. a blow to the head or directly on the ear) may rupture the tympanic membrane and cause pain. Similarly, the eardrum may rupture when the pressure inside the middle ear is less than on the outside (e.g. due to aircraft making a descent or divers descending below 10 metres). The Eustachian tube, which normally equalises the pressure, becomes occluded.

Deafness may be due to congenital or occupational causes as well as wax, otosclerosis, sero-mucinous otitis media (glue ear) and old age.

Disorders of the *inner ear* may affect hearing and balance, causing vertigo or dizziness.

Onset and duration   The cause of sudden deafness may be obvious (e.g. following poking of the ear with a variety of instruments from matchsticks to pencils). Noise damage may also cause sudden hearing loss.

Sudden dizziness may be caused by a viral infection of the inner ear, whereas a more chronic progressive onset may be due to Ménière's disease.

Causative and modifying factors   Previous episodes of inflammation may indicate *otitis externa*. There are two causes, infective and reactive, although both may be present at any one time. Reactive otitis externa represents a chronic tendency to eczema. The auditory canal may be sore and pruritic. Scaling and red skin may be present. The infective form may be caused by bacteria, viruses, or fungi and is usually acute. It may be recognised by the presence of a discharge, ranging from clear fluid to white or green exudate, together with soreness and irritation which, if untreated, may lead to painful ears.

Some patients may have an *aural fistula* (i.e. a congenital blind pit in front of the external canal) which is of no significance, except when it becomes infected.

An *insect sting* in the ear canal can produce oedema, causing occlusion of the canal. Immediate referral is necessary.

Deafness caused by *wax* in the auditory canal usually affects one ear, although eventually both ears may be involved if untreated. Excessive wax may also produce a feeling of numbness on the affected side of the face, and an uncomfortable feeling in the ear.

Environmental factors can also precipitate ear disorders. Patients subject to excessive noise in their occupation or domestic environment may suffer noise damage and deafness. Transient deafness may accompany the other symptoms of otitis media.

Otitis media classically presents as earache which may be accompanied by symptoms of an *upper respiratory-tract infection*, and occurs commonly in children. The pain may be intense and throbbing, affecting one or both ears. There may be fever and tenderness around the ear. Inflammation of the middle ear may cause the drum to bulge out and possibly burst, which is painful. A discharge of pus and blood may be found in the auditory canal after perforation of the drum.

Sero-mucinous otitis media also occurs in children and is similar to otitis media but produces a sticky effusion. It is a chronic form of otitis media.

Disorders of the inner ear are characterised by *vertigo or dizziness*, often with nausea and vomiting. Tinnitus may also be present. Repeated attacks with increasing deafness are characteristic of Ménière's disease. Dizziness without deafness, accompanied by upper respiratory-tract infection, may be caused by viral infection of the inner ear. It should be remembered that elderly people often have dizzy spells unrelated to the ear, and such patients require referral.

Risk factors   *Occupations and sports* can increase the risk of ear disorders. Swimmers should be especially careful to occlude the ears (e.g. by using ear plugs) if they are prone to otitis externa. This helps keep the ears clean and dry, excludes micro-organisms, and prevents a warm wet environment in which they would proliferate. High-speed water sports (e.g. water-skiing) may subject some people to ruptured eardrums due to barotrauma.

Workers in environments of excessive noise should be protected by the use of ear protectors.

Children are especially prone to ear disorders. They may be the victims of their own mischievous pastimes by lodging foreign bodies in their ear canals. Developmental changes (e.g. teething) may subject them to earache. The enlargement of the adenoids may cause obstruction of the Eustachian tube. Upper respiratory-tract infections in small children frequently cause earache and otitis media because of inflammation and blockage of the Eustachian tube, which is narrow in children.

Management

Ear wax is difficult to remove other than by syringing. However, softening the wax using cerumenolytic ear-drops (BNF 12.1.3) is recommended, with drops instilled regularly for a few days before syringing. Olive oil and sodium bicarbonate ear-drops are claimed to be effective, but there is little clinical evidence to support their use. If patients have a history of ear infections accompanied by perforation, or have a chronically discharging ear, then drops must not be instilled until a doctor has examined the eardrum to check for perforation.

The entry of flies and other insects into the auditory canal may cause great irritation and panic. Instillation of olive oil should kill the intruder and the ear should be syringed that day. If the insect has stung the ear, referral should be made as quickly as possible.

Otitis externa should be referred for antimicrobial treatment. However, pharmacists may advise patients that improved ear hygiene may be helpful and enhance antimicrobial therapy by leaving the canal clean and dry so that invading micro-organisms cannot colonise it. Ear plugs should not be used during infection as they serve only to retain the exudate and provoke further infection.

Pain in the ears and the presence of a discharge require referral. If no analgesics are prescribed, paracetamol may be suggested to give symptomatic benefit.

Any trauma to the outside of the ear, especially that resulting in bleeding, requires immediate referral.

20.3.12   SORE THROAT

Introduction

A sore throat is a common early accompaniment to the common cold and as such is unremarkable. However, certain causes of sore throats have potentially serious consequences and these should be enquired for where appropriate. (For a description of the relevant anatomy, see Section 3.4.)

Key Questions

- Is swallowing affected?
- Is breathing impaired?
- Has the patient lost his voice?

Assessment and Interpretation

Location and nature   The patient may complain of a dry irritating feeling at the back of the throat or oropharynx, and this is a common accompaniment to the common cold. If the throat is painful and the pain persists for more than two days, whether or not accompanied by symptoms of the common cold, it is possible that a bacterial infection, usually streptococcal, is the cause.

Examination in a well-lit area and asking the patient to say 'Ah' with the mouth open as wide as possible may reveal a red inflamed throat, and tonsils if present. White pus-filled spots on the tonsils will confirm tonsillitis and require referral for assessment and treatment. White spots elsewhere in the mouth (e.g. on the tongue and on the buccal mucosa) are likely to be due to candidiasis. However, aphthous ulcers, which are white patches on the mucosa, are more likely to be painful, especially when eating. Another disorder, lichen planus, may present with a lace-like pattern on the buccal mucosa, which may resemble candidiasis.

A sore throat causing a hoarse voice is likely to be due to laryngitis caused by bacterial infection. However, hoarseness in the presence of other symptoms may have different causes. Persistent hoarseness requires referral, as the possibility of sinister pathology (e.g. carcinoma of the respiratory tract) exists in a small number of cases.

Difficulty in swallowing may be a complication of a sore throat or may be due to obstruction from another source, and needs investigation to eliminate sinister causes.

Accompanying symptoms   If the sore throat is mild and symptoms of the *common cold* develop within 48 hours, the sore throat will normally resolve spontaneously within a short period.

Pain and general malaise may accompany a sore throat. If the throat is painful and there are large tender lymph nodes in the neck, a bacterial infection, possibly of the tonsils is likely. In such a case, referral for assessment of the value of antibacterial treatment is necessary. Alternatively, in young adults, the possibility of glandular fever should be borne in mind. Although a rash is associated with glandular fever, it may be late in appearing, and is often brought on by a course of ampicillin. If the patient feels ill apart from symptoms of a cold, referral is advisable. Fever, night sweats, or persistent aching muscles or joints accompanying a painful throat also demand referral.

Because of its proximity via the Eustachian tube, the ear often becomes infected from the throat. *Ear pain* is a sign of spread of infection and requires referral.

A *rash* accompanying a sore throat suggests a systemic disease (e.g. glandular fever, meningitis, or one of the childhood infectious diseases). Cases should always be referred for a medical opinion, unless pharmacists are aware of local outbreaks of measles, mumps, or chickenpox.

Awareness of a *lump in the throat* is a rare symptom, causing patients to complain of not being able to swallow or breathe normally. This may represent a quinsy-like illness and is characterised by ulceration of the tonsils in which inflammation interferes with the aperture of the trachea. If the patient cannot swallow normally or complains of an awareness of a lump in the throat, referral should be made.

Marked *mouth ulceration* is a painful condition. If patients have a history of ulceration, the decision to refer is based on the severity and the experience of the outcome of previous attacks. However, mouth ulceration which spreads to the outside of the lips and is accompanied by malaise or fever requires urgent referral to exclude serious disorders, especially when patients are taking immunosuppressant drugs (e.g. corticosteroids or cytotoxic agents), drugs capable of causing bone-marrow suppression (e.g. antiepileptics, procainamide, or tricyclic and tetracyclic antidepressants), or drugs causing the Stevens-Johnson syndrome (e.g. co-trimoxazole and sulphonamides).

Causative and modifying factors   The most common cause of a sore throat is a bacterial or viral infection, although acid reflux and environmental influences (e.g. smoke or vapours) may also be implicated. Treatment with antibacterials can suppress the normal flora of the buccal cavity and allow an overgrowth of candida. Similarly, corticosteroid inhalations can cause a local immunosuppressive effect, resulting in candidiasis. Diabetics are particularly prone to recurrent infections, including oral thrush or candidiasis.

Rarer, but more serious, causes of a sore throat that are accompanied by infective lesions around the mouth are aplastic anaemia or agranulocytosis caused by drugs. These are rare adverse effects but should be borne in mind with certain drugs (e.g. chloramphenicol).

A summary of the possible causes of a sore throat is given under Throat discomfort, Part C.

Management

Non-drug treatment   Apart from medication, patients should avoid smoky or dusty atmospheres and reduce or stop smoking.

Drug treatment   Although it is difficult to distinguish between viral and bacterial throat infections, a rule of thumb may be applied that involvement of the tonsils or the ears should be referred for assessment of treatment with antibacterials. Patients with heart-valve disease should be referred to prevent secondary spread of streptococci to the endocardium. Other throat infections will usually be viral, for which antibacterial agents are of no use.

Infection presumed to be viral should be treated with a high fluid intake. If patients find swallowing painful, a light fluid diet should be taken. Lozenges may offer symptomatic relief. Hard lozenges (like hard-boiled sweets) have a longer lasting effect than soft lozenges. Their use is probably nothing more than placebo, but the flow of saliva which is stimulated by sucking may have a soothing effect. When adults suffer from painful sore throat and symptomatic relief is required until the doctor can be visited, gargling with 2 or 3 soluble aspirin tablets may provide adequate local relief of pain and inflammation. If pain spreads to the ears, non-opioid analgesics may be recommended as an interim measure until the doctor is seen.

20.3.13   SKIN DISORDERS

Introduction

Skin lesions are often difficult to diagnose because of the wide variability in appearance, location, and severity of signs and symptoms. Although there is an important visual aspect to examination of skin disorders, questioning patients is as important as with other illnesses and minor symptoms. Nevertheless, those with skin complaints in which the skin surface is intact (i.e. there is no break in the skin surface and no ulceration) will rarely be in a life-threatening situation, providing there are no accompanying systemic symptoms. Thus self-medication for a short time will usually be appropriate.

Key Questions

- What is the nature and distribution of the lesion?
- When did it appear?
- Is the patient aware of having been in contact with an infected person?
- What food has the patient recently eaten?
- What medicines, if any, is the patient taking?
- What chemicals or household cleaners has the patient been using?
- Has the patient been in contact with any animals?

Assessment and Interpretation

Nature of lesion   (A diagrammatic representation of common skin lesions is illustrated in Fig. 13.1.) A *rash* may be defined as a raised or flat patch of skin, of a colour which is different from the normal surrounding skin. This definition covers the majority of skin lesions, but the more popular lay description is of an area of redness. An erythematous rash may be seen in the various types of eczema, urticaria, psoriasis, tinea infections, photosensitivity, sunburn, cellulitis, rosacea, acne, and lichen planus.

Eczematous rashes will often produce *scales* and appear erythematous. In time they become dry and the scales become more obvious. A greasy or shiny rash with scaling may indicate seborrhoeic dermatitis. In young babies this scaling can be profuse on the scalp and face, producing areas of adherent white to yellow scales, called cradle cap. Extensive scaling also typifies psoriasis, in which thick, silvery white, scaly *plaques* may totally or partially overlie a pink or red lesion.

Small *blisters* containing clear fluid are termed vesicles, whereas larger versions are referred to as bullae. If the fluid is purulent, the blisters are described as pustules.

Pustular lesions are typically seen on the face in acne, impetigo, and herpes simplex virus infection; vesicles occur on the trunk and limbs in chickenpox and shingles, and on hands and feet in pompholyx and psoriasis. Bullae are seen in some drug rashes, sunburn, and atopic dermatitis.

Characteristics of shape are important features of identification. Psoriatic lesions usually occur as patches with well defined edges, distinguishing them from the normal skin. Small, red, discrete patches may be seen in tinea infections and eczema, and in particular discoid or nummular eczema. (Nummular eczema derives its name from the latin word *nummus*, meaning a coin, which describes its red, round, or oval appearance.) Tinea lesions have better delineated edges to the red patches, whereas eczematous patches blend into normal skin. Tinea lesions have redder margins compared to the centre of the lesion, giving the impression of spreading from the centre outwards.

Sometimes erythema may present as streaks or lines, especially on the arms or face. This is characteristic of contact dermatitis (e.g. caused by handling plants such as the primula, and hair dyes and other scalp preparations).

Confluent erythematous patches with irregular but well demarcated outlines can occur, especially on the trunk and limbs. They have white centres caused by oedema, and are characteristic of urticaria.

Pigmentation can occur. Eczematous spots may eventually change to a brown colour after a few weeks, especially after chronic scratching. Brown spots are also typical of a resolving lichen planus. Psoriatic lesions may present on close examination as brown spots on an erythematous background.

Changes in pigmentation (e.g. variability in the colour seen in a mole or an increase in its size) require referral for a medical opinion to exclude malignancy (e.g. melanoma). This is also true if bleeding, ulceration, or pain occurs in a pigmented mole. However, melanoma may develop as a new lesion and not necessarily as an extension of a pre-existing mole.

An *ulcer* is a cavity or pit which most commonly occurs on the skin at sites of pressure sores on the sacrum, buttocks, legs, and feet. In diabetic patients, ulceration may develop because of poor circulation in the lower leg, feet, and toes.

Neoplasms of the skin are usually raised lesions, but they may be described as ulcers by the lay public if they are inflamed. The most common benign tumour of the skin is the *wart*, which is a raised papular lesion usually of normal skin tone or greyish colour. Warts are self-limiting lesions (although facial and genital warts require medical referral) and most people will develop them at some time. Sometimes warts may appear pedunculated, resembling a cauliflower or bunch of grapes (mosaic warts).

The two most common skin cancers are the slow-growing basal cell carcinoma (rodent ulcer) and the faster growing squamous cell carcinoma. These are located on exposed areas.

Basal cell carcinoma may present initially as a small nodule with telangiectases over the surface (i.e. discrete dilated capillaries can be seen). The nodule may ulcerate or bleed, and its edges are usually raised or 'rolled' so that the lesion has the appearance of a volcano with the ulcer in the middle. Cystic forms may appear like raw warty lesions. It is sound policy to refer any chronic ulcerated or sinister looking lesions on sun-exposed areas. Sometimes, however, basal cell carcinoma presents as a flat slowly spreading area, and location and duration are the clues to diagnosis.

Squamous cell carcinoma may appear as a nodule or an ulcer and often the edges are rolled, as in basal cell carcinomas.

Location   The distribution of a rash or other skin lesions can be very helpful in determining the type of skin disorder. A useful guide is that if an imaginary vertical line is drawn down the body to split it in two, a symmetrical distribution of lesions on both sides generally points to an endogenous skin disorder (e.g. atopic dermatitis). Conversely, asymetrical lesions indicate an exogenous type caused by contact or infection (e.g. contact dermatitis, tinea, or cellulitis).

An area of erythema appearing on skin areas exposed to sunlight (e.g. face, neck, and arms) suggests photosensitivity caused by applied or ingested chemicals, usually drugs (Table 20.5). This type of lesion will have a defined edge corresponding to the limits of coverage by clothing. It should be remembered that photosensitivity can occur at any time of year, not just summer. If the palms of the hands are involved, photosensitivity can be excluded as these are not light-sensitive areas. Small lesions on sun-exposed areas which do not resolve require a medical opinion to exclude malignancy.

Conversely, a rash appearing on skin which has been, or is, covered by an article of clothing, jewellery, or

TABLE 20.5
Examples of photosensitising drugs

Oral:	Amiodarone
	Azapropazone and other non-steroidal anti-inflammatory drugs
	Chlorpromazine
	Hydrochlorothiazide
	Nalidixic acid
	Protriptyline
	Sulphonamides (especially co-trimoxazole)
Topical:	Antihistamines
	Sunscreen agents

cosmetics should alert pharmacists to the possibility of a contact dermatitis.

Atopic dermatitis is characteristically located on the cheeks of babies and on the flexures of the neck, front of wrists and elbows, and behind the knees in young children. The distribution is usually symmetrical on each side of the body. Seborrhoeic dermatitis, seen more commonly in children than adults, may occur on the scalp, ears, and eyebrows but may be more widespread on the axillae and groin, and in babies in the napkin area.

Psoriasis is commonly seen on the backs of the elbows, the front of the knees, the scalp, and anywhere on the trunk. It may also appear on the groins and axillae, but the face is rarely affected. The nails may be affected in psoriasis, giving a pitted appearance.

Acne vulgaris is a common problem in adolescents and young adults and may occur on the face, neck, upper back, and shoulders. Rosacea occurs on the forehead and cheeks of older people.

Certain skin areas are invaded by ringworm. Tinea pedis attacks the spaces between the toes and the sole of the foot. This should be easily distinguishable from contact dermatitis caused by leather shoes or sandals, which has a wider distribution over the foot. The groin area may become infected with tinea pedis, producing highly inflamed skin with a pronounced border. The napkin area of babies may become inflamed due to primary irritant dermatitis, usually caused by the formation of ammonia in the urine. The dermatitis may sometimes be contaminated (e.g. by *Candida*) in the area where the skin folds in the legs become erythematous. In a simple napkin rash these areas are normally spared.

Isolated, red, small discrete, round lesions of 1 or 2 centimetres diameter on the trunk and limbs may represent tinea corporis, but a similar appearance can be seen in nummular eczema, contact dermatitis, and small plaques of psoriasis.

Isolated, small, red spots commencing at the wrists or between the fingers and spreading to the arms and trunk may indicate scabies. Larger red lumps occurring anywhere on the limbs or trunk may be due to insect bites. The legs or arms are particularly affected after walking in grass or working in the garden in the summer. Bed bugs will cause lesions noted particularly on awaking.

An erythematous rash covering a large proportion of the body is likely to be an allergic reaction to ingested food or drugs, or in a child, an infectious disease (*see* Management of special cases below).

Other typically located lesions seen on the face are impetigo around the mouth (in children), herpes simplex virus infections (cold sore), varicella-zoster virus infections (on the scalp, around the eye, the trunk, usually unilaterally). Perianal lesions may be caused by ringworm (although anal irritation may also be due to haemorrhoids or threadworm) and genital lesions may be caused by warts or lice.

Infections of the skin (e.g. cellulitis) may be seen as an erythematous patch usually about five centimetres wide. The patch may occur anywhere on the body but commonly appears on the face or limbs. A red area on the lower leg might also be caused by thrombophlebitis or deep vein thrombosis. Such lesions require early medical attention, especially if they are painful. An erythematous rash over the inside of the ankles and shins may be due to stasis eczema, caused by poor circulation, especially in patients with ankle oedema.

Onset, spread, and duration The initial lesion of most skin disorders usually occurs suddenly and this may allow its relationship to a possible allergen or irritant in eczema to be identified. Sometimes an infective event may herald a skin condition (e.g. a sore throat before guttate psoriasis or the upper respiratory symptoms seen before the common infectious diseases of children, *see* Management of special cases below).

Scabies presents, initially, with a few isolated, itching, red spots on the back of the hands, wrist, or forearm before spreading to other parts of the limbs and trunk, but not the face and scalp.

In babies, a rash in the napkin area may be a simple contact dermatitis, but if it spreads to the rest of the trunk it may indicate seborrhoeic dermatitis.

The duration of a skin lesion may be the determinant of whether to recommend treatment or refer the patient to a doctor. Any rash which has not resolved after one week and is causing symptomatic distress should be referred. Similarly individual lesions which are slow growing or insidiously changing in shape or colour and can represent malignancy (e.g. melanomas, or basal and squamous cell carcinomas) should be referred.

Accompanying symptoms and family history Any systemic symptoms (especially of malaise) experienced by patients with an undiagnosed skin lesion require referral to exclude serious pathology.

Patients with psoriasis may also have arthritis, as the two are often seen together as part of a disease complex.

Conjunctivitis and blepharitis may be associated with facial rashes (e.g. rosacea) and phototoxic reactions. If the rash is florid and the conjunctivitis severe, referral is advised.

The symptom mostly associated with skin lesions is pruritus. This is not a very discriminating symptom. Severe pain, however, demands referral, and the distribution of a painful rash on the face, scalp, trunk, or arm may suggest varicella-zoster virus infection (e.g. shingles).

Sometimes symptoms may develop in the skin without the appearance of a visible lesion (Table 20.6). Pain without a rash requires referral, but pruritus is common in these circumstances on the scalp (pediculosis capitis), on the skin (lice and fibre-glass dermatitis), and more rarely in systemic disease (e.g. kidney or liver disease). Referral is necessary except in patients with known disease who may need educating about the condition. Some drugs can cause pruritus with or without an eruption on the skin.

Bleeding from skin lesions is generally regarded as serious, especially if melanoma or other skin cancer is a possibility. Warts, however, often bleed with little consequence, usually as a result of the patient paring down the lesion with a file or blade.

An enquiry about any family history of the suspected disorder may help diagnosis of skin disorders. Patients with atopic dermatitis will usually report hay fever, asthma, or atopic dermatitis in another member of the family. Psoriatic patients (except babies with napkin psoriasis) often have relatives who suffer from the disorder.

Causative and modifying factors   Because most skin lesions itch, patients will scratch, although the temporary relief afforded by this is outweighed by the harmful consequences of scratching. Deleterious effects can include exacerbation of erythema (as in urticaria), spread of infected lesions to other parts of the body (e.g. tinea), infection through scratching with dirty nails or fingers (infective eczema), or delayed healing.

A variety of factors may exacerbate or relieve skin lesions and symptoms. Exposure to sunlight may initiate or exacerbate photosensitive reactions (e.g. those due to drugs) and rosacea, while other conditions (e.g. acne vulgaris and psoriasis) will often improve on exposure to ultraviolet light. Acne tends to be worse in the winter months. Exposure to irritants or allergens will initiate or

cause recurrences of contact dermatitis (Table 20.7), and several topical agents (e.g. coal tar, industrial cutting oils, and cosmetics) or ingested drugs (e.g. corticosteroids and antiepileptics) may exacerbate acne. There is no convincing evidence that dietary constituents (e.g. fats, chocolate, nuts, or coffee) cause or aggravate acne, despite the claims of many patients to the contrary.

Trauma to the skin may initiate or worsen psoriasis. Less obvious trauma may allow viruses or fungi to penetrate the stratum corneum. This is thought to occur particularly when the soles of the feet are wet and the skin becomes macerated.

Conversely a dry skin, which can result from a chronic skin disorder (e.g. eczema or ichthyosis), will aggravate the condition with which it presents, causing further itching, scratching, and general worsening of the condition.

Drugs may cause erythematous skin eruptions. Aspirin and the penicillins may cause acute urticaria, recognised by its rapid onset after administration to a sensitised patient.

Finally, it should be remembered that failure to find the cause of a rash is often a signal to claim it to be of nervous origin, particularly by patients. Indeed, stress is thought to aggravate psoriasis and endogenous eczemas.

Management

The general principles of the treatment of skin disorders follow the same rules of treatment of other disorders. If the condition has not resolved by the end of one week (or earlier if patients are feeling ill), referral should be considered.

TABLE 20.6
Conditions causing generalised pruritus with no visible lesion

Diabetes mellitus
Dry skin (especially in the elderly)
Gallstones
Hodgkin's disease
Iron-deficiency anaemia
Kidney failure
Liver failure
Pregnancy
Thyroid disorders

TABLE 20.7
Common primary irritants and contact allergens causing contact dermatitis

A. Primary irritants	
Acids	Detergents
Alkalis	Mineral oils
Antiseptic solutions	Soaps
Bleach	Shampoos
Degreasing solvents	Washing powders

B. Contact allergens	
Adhesive plaster	Leather
Cement	Ointments and creams containing lanolin, local anaesthetics, antihistamines, sulphonamides, and preservatives
Clothing	
Cosmetics	
Deodorants	Plants (e.g. primula and chrysanthemum)
Elastic	
Glues and resins	Rubber gloves
Hair colourants	Watch strap
Jewellery	Wood resins

Pruritus   Pruritus can be alleviated by cooling (e.g. with cold compresses), calamine lotion, by oral antihistamines, or topical hydrocortisone (if pruritus is caused by allergic contact or primary irritant dermatitis, or insect bites and stings). Dry skin which itches should be hydrated by regular long term application of emulsifying ointment or aqueous cream.

Eczema   If eczema is of exogenous origin, avoidance of, or protection from, the offending causative agent, if known, is the first line of treatment. Rubber gloves should be worn to prevent contact with detergents, and barrier creams used to protect hands from irritant oils or chemicals in the workplace. Factors which exacerbate eczema (e.g. exposure to cold winds, wool, and man-made fibres) should also be avoided.

Napkin rash requires frequent nappy changes to keep the skin dry and to prevent contact with irritant ammonia in the urine. Plastic occlusive pants should be avoided. If it is suspected that residual detergent after washing nappies is the cause of irritation, extra care in rinsing should be taken.

There are a number of proprietary creams available for napkin rash. It should be remembered that creams are used for treatment to allow evaporation of water from the skin, preventing further maceration and damage. Barrier silicone creams or zinc and castor oil cream are suitable as preventive measures as they form a barrier to prevent irritants gaining contact with the skin. On tender skin where a rash is already present, this type of product will only exacerbate the problem.

Dry eczematous patches due to contact dermatitis or atopy require hydration with emulsifying ointment, aqueous cream, or a proprietary product. Perfumed soap often acts as an irritant and the use of emulsifying ointment as a soap replacement or as a soak (100 g added to the bath) in eczematous conditions can be helpful. Emollients are also useful.

Wet or weeping eczematous lesions are usually treated with potassium permanganate soaks or compresses for about 15 minutes three times each day.

Stasis eczema on the ankles and shins is best referred to elicit and treat the cause. Graduated compression hosiery, hydrocortisone cream, or coal tar-impregnated bandages may be prescribed.

In babies and children, atopic dermatitis can be treated with emulsifying ointment, but recurrences require referral.

Infantile seborrhoeic dermatitis (cradle cap) may respond to shampoos containing cetrimide or to gentle rubbing with olive oil to soften the scales before washing the hair. More resistant cases may require keratolytic agents (e.g. 1% salicylic acid in aqueous cream, with or without resorcinol or sulphur). If the rash has spread to the trunk, referral is advisable to assess the value of a topical corticosteroid. In adults, scaling of the scalp may be relieved by compound coconut ointment, creams containing 5% salicylic acid, or by referral for corticosteroid lotions.

Psoriasis   Psoriasis should be referred when lesions recur. They require potent corticosteroid preparations, dithranol, and attendance at hospital clinics for treatment with PUVA. Psoriasis of the scalp may be treated with coal tar lotions, and liquid coal tar is often added to bath water.

Infections and infestations   Candida and tinea infections may be treated topically with imidazole derivatives (e.g. clotrimazole, miconazole, or econazole) as they are effective against both fungi and some staphylococci. In the presence of a moist environment, which encourages growth of micro-organisms (e.g. in skin folds or between digits), the liberal use of talc will also promote healing by drying the skin. When the feet (tinea pedis) or groin (tinea cruris) are involved, daily washing to promote hygiene is also recommended. Tinea corporis, tinea capitis, and nail infections are more resistant to treatment and should be referred to allow consideration of the use of griseofulvin. If treatment is recommended, patients should be advised to continue for at least two weeks, to prevent relapses, even if resolution of the rash is rapid.

Impetigo is a staphyloccocal infection which should in all cases be referred to the doctor.

Warts are extremely difficult to cure. Success depends on the ability of the immune system to counter the virus rather than the use of non-prescription products. However, caustic solutions containing salicylic acid abound on the market. They dissolve the keratin layers on the epidermis and, together with abrasion using an emery board or pumice stone, allow a pleasing cosmetic appearance by paring the wart so that it is less prominent. Care must be taken that surrounding normal skin is not exposed to the keratolytic agent. A solution of formalin 4% is traditionally prescribed for plantar warts. The affected part of the foot is soaked for 15 minutes each day in the solution, ideally in a saucer or other suitable shallow container.

Head lice (pediculosis capitis) are ideally treated by applying an alcoholic lotion of malathion or carbaryl, drying, and leaving on overnight, followed by shampooing the next morning. Preparations of these two agents are also available which can be washed off after only two hours. All members of the household should be treated.

Body lice (pediculosis corporis) may be treated in a similar way after bathing, and 1% gamma benzene hexachloride solution may be used instead of carbaryl or malathion. Bedding and clothes should be washed. Pubic lice (pediculosis pubis) will respond to the above agents, but gamma benzene hexachloride is likely to be less irritant. Oral antihistamines, crotamiton cream, or both may relieve the associated itch. Scabies may also respond to 1% gamma benzene hexachloride solution or to application of benzyl benzoate. After bathing, the skin should be covered from neck to toe (not head) with the application. It should be washed off 24 hours later. Patients should be warned that itching may persist after the mite has been cleared from the skin, and can be relieved by oral antihistamines.

Acne vulgaris   A wide range of products are available for the treatment of acne. Non-prescription products may be classed as keratolytics (e.g. benzoyl peroxide, potassium hydroxyquinoline sulphate, and salicylic acid) and antibacterials, although some are claimed to have a combination of properties. The keratolytic agents break down the keratin plugs in the hair follicles and allow sebum to drain to the skin surface. They should be used cautiously, initially using the lowest concentration products and increasing as necessary. Patients should be warned that the face may become red and sore after the initial application of a keratolytic agent and that this may be alleviated by initially applying less frequently. Antibacterial agents allegedly act by reducing the population of *Propionibacterium acnes*, one of the bacteria that splits the triglycerides of sebum into fatty acids.

Patients should be warned that the treatment of acne vulgaris is prolonged and at times unrewarding. Difficult cases, especially those associated with emotional disturbances, may benefit from a referral. It may be helpful to raise morale when patients complain that treatments are not working by recommending alcohol-based cleansing lotions or surgical spirit. These may be used for short periods to degrease the skin and give a temporary respite.

The effects of sunlight   Sunburn and photosensitivity reactions are more difficult to treat than to avoid. Patients should be educated about the effects of sunlight, with recommendations to use sunscreens with high protection factors, particularly for the fair skinned and those going on summer holidays to a hot climate. Despite the apparently healthy look of a suntan, overexposure can be painful and in the long term damaging.

Management of Special Cases

Diabetes   Diabetic patients are susceptible to recur-

rent infections of the skin, especially with candida and tinea. They are also prone to ulceration arising from injuries to the skin of the foot, and to ischaemia in the feet. Foot ulcers may become serious before they are brought to the attention of health-care personnel, because diabetes can interfere with the sensory nervous pathways from the skin and make many skin disorders painless.

Infectious diseases of childhood   Although the infectious diseases of childhood are dealt with in this separate section, it should be remembered that these disorders may also occur in adulthood in a minority of cases.

Measles is becoming less common as vaccination (*see* Section 17.5) becomes more widespread in infants. It is hoped that triple vaccination with MMR vaccine in infants will reduce the incidence of rubella, although chickenpox and scarlet fever may still be seen. Since these diseases usually occur only once in a lifetime and often occur in epidemics, especially amongst schoolchildren and playgroups, it should be enquired whether the child has had the suspected illness before, if they have had any vaccinations, and whether any of the child's friends have had similar symptoms recently.

Distinguishing the *type of rash* is important. Measles is a flat blotchy rash, whereas that of rubella is less well defined with smaller erythematous marks. The rash of chickenpox consists of pustules surrounded by small reddened areas. The pustules eventually burst and dry to form crusts. Scarlet fever appears as a bright red flush of the face and as a gooseflesh appearance around the neck.

The *location and spread of the rash* is also diagnostic. The rash of measles begins usually on the face and neck, and spreads downwards to the trunk and limbs. Rubella also begins on the face or back of the neck and spreads down over the trunk, but it can be extremely variable and transitory in appearance. Chickenpox and scarlet fever do not spread in the same way as measles and rubella. Spots occur on the trunk and face in chickenpox and then increase in number, whereas the flush of scarlet fever is limited to the face and gooseflesh to the neck and upper half of the trunk.

A summary of the *onset and accompanying symptoms* is given in Table 17.7.

Advice from pharmacists is often sought on *treatment of infectious disorders of childhood*. Measles is a notifiable disease (i.e. doctors are obliged to notify the local authority of any incidence). Parents of children with suspected measles should be advised to telephone the surgery to relate their suspicions, and the doctor can decide whether the child should be brought to see him or warrants a home visit. Unless otitis media is suspected or the child appears otherwise unwell, symptomatic treatment only of the upper respiratory symptoms and of the rash (with calamine lotion or an oral antihistamine) is required.

Rubella rarely requires treatment, but advice about avoiding contact with pregnant or suspected pregnant women should be given.

Chickenpox causes intense pruritus, for which oral antihistamines and calamine lotion are useful. Scratching should be discouraged.

Since scarlet fever is caused by a streptococcal infection, referral is necessary so that treatment with an antibacterial can be instituted.

20.3.14 ITCHING AROUND THE ANUS AND VULVA

Introduction

Itching of the skin around the anus (pruritus ani) and vulva (pruritus vulvae) is often a source of embarassment to patients, many of whom will request advertised products rather than seek advice about its cause or the most appropriate form of treatment. Tactful and discreet questioning may be required to identify the precise site of the symptoms, especially if reported by women.

Symptoms of pruritus ani are primarily presented by middle-aged men, whilst it is those middle-aged women who have previously undergone gynaecological operations who commonly complain of pruritus vulvae.

The conditions most commonly associated with pruritus ani are haemorrhoids and anal fissure in adults, and nematode infections (e.g. threadworm) in children. Pruritus vulvae commonly accompanies trichomoniasis, candidiasis, and bacterial infections.

Key Questions

Pruritus ani

- Can the patient identify the precise location of the discomfort?
- Is there any blood or mucus associated with the stools?

Pruritus vulvae

- Can the patient identify the precise location of the discomfort?
- Is there a discharge?
- What is the appearance of the discharge?
- What is the patient's age?

Assessment and Interpretation

Nature and severity   The mild itching associated with haemorrhoids, anal fissure, and threadworms often wor-

sens within 2 to 3 days. Threadworm infection may be accompanied by severe burning sensations at night. Pruritus vulvae frequently arises through the irritant effect of vaginal discharge on the vulva, which may be severe enough to cause sleep and emotional disturbances.

Onset and duration   Pruritus caused by threadworm infection appears suddenly and, within 48 hours, may become excruciating at night-time due to severe excoriation of the anal region. Other forms of pruritus may develop insidiously and be exceptionally difficult to eradicate.

Accompanying symptoms   The presence of any accompanying symptoms requires referral.

Blood in the stool is an important symptom. Fresh blood coating the stool commonly derives from the rectum or anus, and usually indicates haemorrhoids or anal fissure. Blood mixed in the stool will have a higher origin in the gastro-intestinal tract and may suggest ulcerative colitis, peptic ulceration, or carcinoma. Blood spots on toilet paper following defaecation indicate an external fissure or external haemorrhoids. Both may resolve spontaneously.

Perineal *rash*, sometimes spreading to the groin, may indicate candidal or ringworm infection.

Threadworm infection is a common cause of *abdominal pain* in children, especially if it is associated with irritability and tiredness caused by lack of sleep. In adults, vomiting and constipation accompanying abdominal pain may suggest intestinal obstruction.

Blisters and sores can result from intense pruritus. Pruritus of the genitalia may be an early sign of genital herpes infection. Itching is quickly followed by the production of a cluster of small blisters around the anus or buttocks, or in the rectum or cervix. These can break down to form tender ulcers.

The presence of *white threadworms* on the buttocks at night-time is caused by the migration of females to the anus from the intestinal mucosa to lay their eggs. Their presence will provoke intense irritation.

Recurrent attacks of pruritus may be associated with *symptoms of diabetes mellitus*. The highly vascularised anal and vulval region are vulnerable to bacterial and fungal infection, especially in the presence of high plasma-glucose concentrations. Recurrent pruritus in known diabetic patients suggests poor disease control. If diabetes has not been diagnosed, enquiries should be made about the presence of associated symptoms (e.g. polyuria, nocturia, thirst, and weight loss).

Perineal inflammation, and in particular pruritus vulvae, may produce *painful urination*. Equally the presence of a urinary-tract infection may produce pruritus by the presence of proteolytic enzymes and ammoniacal metabolites in the urine.

Internal genital infections may produce a *vaginal discharge* which irritates the perineum. A foul smelling yellowish-green discharge results from trichomoniasis, while the discharge of candidiasis is creamy white. Bacterial infection produces a greyish-white discharge which, if due to anaerobes, often has a fishy smell.

Causative factors   *Poor hygiene* can be a factor in pruritus ani. It is a common misconception that haemorrhoids themselves produce pruritus. However, pruritus ani is most commonly due to faecal contamination, which itself can arise from haemorrhoids. Similarly, anal fissures produce extreme pain on defaecation, impairing toilet hygiene. Excessive perspiration and poor ventilation due to obesity are other contributory factors. Following identification, excessive use of soaps may aggravate the symptoms, particularly if applied with vigorous rubbing.

Constipation may give rise to excessive straining at stool which will aggravate pruritus and the severity of haemorrhoids.

Broad-spectrum antibacterials (especially tetracyclines) are a frequent cause of pruritus.

Miscellaneous causative agents include inappropriate clothing (e.g. close fitting underwear and tights), vaginal deodorants and perfumed talcum powder, and other locally applied irritants. Their continued use in the presence of symptoms will exacerbate the condition.

A summary of the possible causes of pruritus ani and pruritus vulvae is given under Itch, Part C.

Risk factor   *Pregnancy* is a common risk factor. Vulval engorgement of pregnancy can produce perineal pruritus. Other common accompaniments to pregnancy may also contribute to its occurrence (e.g. constipation, dysuria, and urinary-tract infection).

Management

If identified, the underlying cause of pruritus should be eliminated.

Non-drug treatment   One of the most important aspects of treatment is the attention to hygiene. Daily washing of the perineum will remove both faeces and perspiration; overfrequent washing, however, should be avoided. It is preferable to use soft washing materials rather than coarse flannels. Build-up of moisture may be reduced by the application of non-perfumed talcum powder. Loose underwear, preferably cotton rather than nylon, should be recommended.

Non-drug hygienic measures are necessary in order to facilitate eradication of threadworm infection. After anthelmintic treatment has been started, a shower or bath should be taken each morning to remove the eggs. Hands should be washed thoroughly after going to the toilet and before meals, and fingernails kept trim and clean. Underwear and nightclothes should be washed daily for 2 to 3 days following the initial anthelminthic dose. Bedding should be changed on the same day. Each member of the household should be given a separate towel which should be washed daily for 2 to 3 days. Bedrooms should be thoroughly dusted or cleaned following dosage to prevent re-infection from eggs shed on skin scales.

Drug treatment   A multitude of wipes, ointments, and suppositories exist for the relief of symptoms. Great care, however, should be taken in their use, as the medication incorporated may aggravate the condition through sensitisation and irritation. They should not be used continuously for more than 2 or 3 days. A weak corticosteroid preparation may be prescribed by the doctor, but the use of non-prescription hydrocortisone in the anogenital region is not licensed in the UK.

If the presence of candidiasis or another fungal infection is suspected, interim treatment (e.g. over a weekend) by local application of an antifungal such as clotrimazole, miconazole, or econazole (BNF 5.2) may be suggested. However, patients should be advised to seek medical advice at the earliest opportunity.

If the cause of itching is threadworm, treatment may be initiated by pharmacists. The aims of treatment are to remove the worms from the gastro-intestinal tract, and to prevent re-infection. All members of a household must therefore be treated with a suitable anthelmintic such as mebendazole (BNF 5.5.1).

Chapter 21

PROFESSIONAL AND SELF-HELP ORGANISATIONS

21.1 INTRODUCTION

Pharmacists are often approached by patients for information about self-help groups, and it is important to be aware of the basis of their existence. The importance of the concept of self help in preventing the available health services from being overwhelmed has been explained in Section 20.1. Many people, and in particular those suffering from chronic illness or those who have gone through a traumatic experience (e.g. the loss of a child through a 'cot death'), benefit from contact with others who have had similar experiences. This fact should not be taken as a failure on the part of professionals to be of any assistance, but should be recognised as an important means of helping individuals to overcome their health problems themselves.

Other important functions of self-help organisations include the provision of literature for patients, which reinforces the advice given by medical and pharmacy staff, and innovation of new forms of care (e.g. the hospice movement). The publication of literature promotes self-reliance and self-determination, and, equally importantly, can help in raising funds for the group, many of which are run on a shoestring budget. Self-help organisations can act as a stimulus for government to introduce innovations in patient care, especially in 'less attractive' areas of health-care (e.g. for the mentally handicapped).

This Chapter provides background details and addresses of a wide range of health organisations located in the UK. It includes organisations of the pharmaceutical and medical professions, and organisations which have been established to provide help for patients suffering from particular conditions or in certain predicaments (e.g. disability). Although only British details have been provided, sister or comparable organisations with the same or similar titles frequently exist in other countries; readers in other countries should therefore seek local addresses.

For ease of use, the information has been divided in two Sections. Section 21.2 lists the conditions with which particular organisations are associated; with some self-help groups, this is obvious from the title of the organisation, but others aim to help a broader range of patients with differing conditions. Section 21.3 provides a directory of organisations, with current details of addresses and telephone numbers. Only those self-help organisations which have been considered as non-ephemeral and based at a relatively fixed address have been included. Details of the organisations have been included in other dedicated directories, where many details have been constant in two or more editions. Although all addresses and telephone numbers have been checked immediately before going to press, certain minor changes are inevitable during the expected life of this book. One major change from May 1990 is the alteration of London (01–) telephone numbers to 071– for central London and 081– for outer London.

It must be stressed, however, that inclusion in this listing should not be taken as a statement of approval of that organisation by the RPSGB; equally, non-inclusion should not be interpreted as non-approval.

One final point is of particular importance. If self-help organisations are recommended to patients, remember that, in addition to giving details of the address and telephone number, it would be beneficial to ask patients to enclose a stamped addressed envelope when they write to the organisation, to help offset administrative costs.

21.2 CATEGORIES OF ORGANISATIONS

Abortion
Birth Control Trust
British Pregnancy Advisory Service
Family Planning Association
Marie Stopes House
Pregnancy Advisory Service

Adoption and fostering
British Agencies for Adoption and Fostering

AIDS
Haemophilia Society
Terrence Higgins Trust

Alcohol dependence
Alcoholics Anonymous

Allergy
Action Against Allergy
Medic-Alert Foundation
Migraine Trust
National Eczema Society

Alternative therapy
British Herbal Medicine Association
British Holistic Medical Association
British Homoeopathic Association
British Osteopathic Association
Centre for the Study of Alternative Therapies
Council for Complementary and Alternative Medicine
General Council and Register of Osteopaths
Institute for Complementary Medicines
National Institute of Medical Herbalists

Alzheimer's disease
Alzheimer's Disease Society

Angina pectoris
British Heart Foundation
Chest Heart and Stroke Association
Coronary Prevention Group

Ankylosing spondylitis
Arthritis Care
Arthritis and Rheumatism Council
National Ankylosing Spondylitis Society

Arthritis and related conditions
Arthritis Care
Arthritis and Rheumatism Council
Leonard Cheshire Foundation
National Ankylosing Spondylitis Society

Asthma
Action Against Allergy
Asthma Society and Friends of the Asthma Research Council
Chest Heart and Stroke Association

Back pain
National Back Pain Association

Bereavement
Age Concern England
CRUSE
Foundation for the Study of Infant Deaths
National Association of Widows

Blindness
Guide Dogs for the Blind Association
Royal National Institute for the Blind

Breastfeeding
Association of Breastfeeding Mothers
National Childbirth Trust
Twins and Multiple Births Association

Bronchitis
Age Concern England
Chest Heart and Stroke Association

Cancer
British Association of Cancer United Patients
British Colostomy Association
Cancer Relief Macmillan Fund
Cancer Research Campaign
CRUSE
Halley Stewart Library
Hospice Information Service
Imperial Cancer Research Fund
Leukaemia Research Fund
Marie Curie Memorial Foundation
Womens National Cancer Control Campaign

Cerebral palsy
Leonard Cheshire Foundation
Spastics Society

Coeliac disease
Coeliac Society of the United Kingdom

Contraception and birth control
Birth Control Trust
British Pregnancy Advisory Service
Family Planning Association
Marie Stopes House
Pregnancy Advisory Service

Crohn's disease
Ileostomy Association of Great Britain and Northern
Ireland
National Association for Colitis and Crohn's Disease

Cystic fibrosis
Cystic Fibrosis Research Trust

Deafness and hard of hearing
British Association for the Hard of Hearing
National Deaf Children's Society
Royal National Institute for the Deaf

Dermatitis herpetiformis
Coeliac Society of the United Kingdom

Diabetes mellitus
British Diabetic Association
Diabetes Foundation
Medic-Alert Foundation

Disability, physical
Disabled Living Foundation
Equipment for the Disabled
Leonard Cheshire Foundation
Royal Association for Disability and Rehabilitation
(RADAR)

Down's syndrome
Down's Syndrome Association

Drug dependence and abuse
Alcoholics Anonymous
Institute for the Study of Drug Dependence
National Campaign against Solvent Abuse
Standing Conference on Drug Abuse
Terrence Higgins Trust
Re-Solv

Dyslexia
British Dyslexia Association
Dyslexia Institute

Eczema
National Eczema Society

Elderly, care of the
Age Concern England
Alzheimer's Disease Society
Help the Aged

Emphysema
Chest Heart and Stroke Association

Epilepsy
British Epilepsy Association
National Society for Epilepsy

Eye care
Eye Care Information Bureau
Optical Information Council

Glaucoma
International Glaucoma Association

Gout
Arthritis Care
Arthritis and Rheumatism Council

Haemophilia
Haemophilia Society

Heart disease
British Heart Foundation
Chest Heart and Stroke Association
Coronary Prevention Group

Herpes simplex virus infection
Herpes Association

Hydrocephalus
Association for Spina Bifida and Hydrocephalus

Hypertension
Action Against Allergy
British Heart Foundation
British Kidney Patient Association
Chest Heart and Stroke Association

Incontinence, urinary
Disabled Living Foundation
Equipment for the Disabled

Infertility
British Pregnancy Advisory Service
Family Planning Association
Infertility Advisory Centre
Marie Stopes House
National Association for the Childless

Kidney disease
British Kidney Patient Association

Medical and other professional organisations (non-pharmacy)
British Red Cross Society
British Dental Association
British Dietetic Association
British Medical Association
British Nutrition Foundation
Consumers' Association
General Medical Council
Health Education Authority
Intractable Pain Society of Great Britain and Ireland
National Consumer Council
Office of Fair Trading
Office of Health Economics
Optical Information Council
Royal Society of Health
St John Ambulance
Society of Chiropodists

Menopause
Marie Stopes House

Mental health/illness
Age Concern England
Leonard Cheshire Foundation
MIND (National Association for Mental Health)

Mental retardation/handicap
Down's Syndrome Association
Leonard Cheshire Foundation
MENCAP
National Autistic Society
Spastics Society

Migraine
Action Against Allergy
British Migraine Association
Migraine Trust

Motor neurone disease
Motor Neurone Disease Association

Multiple sclerosis
Action for Research into Multiple Sclerosis
Leonard Cheshire Foundation
Multiple Sclerosis Society of Great Britain and Northern Ireland

Muscular dystrophy
Muscular Dystrophy Group of Great Britain and Northern Ireland

Myocardial infarction
British Heart Foundation
Chest Heart and Stroke Association
Coronary Prevention Group

Pain
National Back Pain Association

Parkinsonism
Age Concern England
Leonard Cheshire Foundation
Parkinson's Disease Society of the United Kingdom

Pharmacy organisations
Association of the British Pharmaceutical Industry
Association of Pharmacy Technicians
Association of Teaching Hospital Pharmacists
British Pharmaceutical Students' Association
Clinical Pharmacokinetics Society
College of Pharmacy Practice
Committee of Regional Pharmaceutical Officers
Community Services Pharmacists' Group
Drug Information Pharmacists' Group
Guild of Hospital Pharmacists
Institute of Pharmacy Management International
National Association of Women Pharmacists
National Pharmaceutical Association
Pain Interest Group
Pharmaceutical Services Negotiating Committee
Proprietary Articles Trade Association
Proprietary Association of Great Britain
Radiopharmacy Group
Rural Pharmacists Association
Scottish Pharmaceutical Sciences Group
Society of Apothecaries of London
Society for Drug Research
United Kingdom Clinical Pharmacy Association

Phenylketonuria
National Society for Phenylketonuria and Allied Disorders

Pituitary dwarfism
  Association for Research into Restricted Growth

Poliomyelitis
  Disabled Living Foundation
  Equipment for the Disabled

Pregnancy and childbirth
  Association of Breastfeeding Mothers
  British Pregnancy Advisory Service
  Family Planning Association
  National Association for the Childless
  National Childbirth Trust
  Pregnancy Advisory Service
  Twins and Multiple Births Association

Psoriasis
  Psoriasis Association

Rubella
  National Rubella Council

Schizophrenia
  Schizophrenia Association of Great Britain

Sexually-transmitted diseases
  Family Planning Association
  Herpes Association

Sickle-cell anaemia
  Sickle Cell and Thalassaemia Information Centre

Speech disorders
  Action for Dysphasic Adults
  Association for Stammerers
  British Dyslexia Association
  Chest Heart and Stroke Association
  Dyslexia Institute
  Motor Neurone Disease Association

Spina bifida
  Association for Spina Bifida and Hydrocephalus
  Urostomy Association

Stoma therapy
  British Colostomy Association
  Ileostomy Association of Great Britain and Northern
    Ireland
  Urostomy Association

Stroke
  Action for Dysphasic Adults
  British Heart Foundation
  Chest Heart and Stroke Association

Sudden infant death syndrome
  Foundation for the Study of Infant Deaths

Systemic lupus erythematosus
  Arthritis Care
  Arthritis and Rheumatism Council

Thalassaemia
  Sickle Cell and Thalassaemia Information Centre

Ulcerative colitis
  Ileostomy Association of Great Britain and Northern
    Ireland
  National Association for Colitis and Crohn's Disease

Valvular heart disease
  British Heart Foundation
  Chest Heart and Stroke Foundation

21.3 DIRECTORY OF ORGANISATIONS

A

ACTION AGAINST ALLERGY (AAA)
43 The Downs
London SW20 8HG
Tel: 081-947 5082

Action Against Allergy is a registered charity which aims to promote an understanding of clinical ecology, the causative role of foods and chemicals in chronic illness (e.g. migraine, asthma, catarrh, skin rashes, and hypertension). It provides members with a personal information service, a postal book service, and arranges films and lectures. It also provides details to people of other sufferers in the same area so that local groups may be formed.

ACTION FOR DYSPHASIC ADULTS (ADA)
Northcote House
37a Royal Street
London SE1 7LL
Tel: 071-261 9572

Action for Dysphasic Adults is a registered charity which provides information and advice to dysphasics and their carers, and aims to create greater awareness among professionals and the general public of the nature of the condition and needs of dysphasic adults. Long-term and, where possible, intensive rehabilitation for dysphasic adults is encouraged in association with speech therapy services.

ACTION FOR RESEARCH INTO MULTIPLE SCLEROSIS (ARMS)

4a Chapel Hill
Stansted
Essex CM24 8AG
Tel: (0279) 815553

The Action for Research into Multiple Sclerosis is a registered charity which promotes patient-managed research and therapy programmes into the cause, diagnosis, treatment, cure, and prevention of multiple sclerosis (MS). It publishes research papers and articles; and offers advice on therapy, a 24-hour counselling service, and membership of a network of therapy groups throughout the UK.

AGE CONCERN ENGLAND

Bernard Sunley House
60 Pitcairn Road
Mitcham
Surrey CR4 3LL
Tel: 081-640 5431

Age Concern England is the national centre for approximately 950 independent local Age Concern groups serving the needs of elderly people with help from over 120 000 volunteers. Age Concern Engand's governing body also includes representatives of 70 national organisations, and works closely with Age Concern Scotland, Wales, and Northern Ireland. Age Concern groups provide a wide range of services, including visiting, day care, clubs, and specialist services for physically and mentally frail elderly people. Age Concern England supports and advises groups through national field officers, and a variety of grant schemes. Other work includes training, research, information, campaigning, and publishing.

ALCOHOLICS ANONYMOUS (AA)

General Service Office
PO Box 1
Stonebow House
Stonebow
York YO1 2NJ
Tel: (0904) 644026/7/8/9

Alcoholics Anonymous is a fellowship of men and women who share their experience, strength, and hope with each other that they may solve their common problem and help others to recover from alcoholism. The only requirement for membership is a desire to stop drinking. There are no dues or fees for AA membership; it is self-supporting through its own contributions. AA is not allied with any sect, denomination, politics, organisation, or institution; does not wish to engage in any controversy; and neither endorses nor opposes any causes. Its primary purpose is to help other alcoholics achieve sobriety.

ALZHEIMER'S DISEASE SOCIETY

158-160 Balham High Road
London SW12
Tel: 081-675 6557

The Alzheimer's Disease Society is a registered charity which supports professionals and relatives of those suffering from Alzheimers's disease. It also promotes, funds, and disseminates information on research. Local branches organise relative support groups, day centres, sitting services, and resource and information centres. The Society also has central Caring and Research Funds.

ARTHRITIS CARE

6 Grosvenor Crescent
London SW1X 7ER
Tel: 071-235 0902

Arthritis Care is a registered charity and a national welfare organisation for sufferers from arthritic diseases. Membership of the charity is open to all sufferers, and all those interested in their welfare. It provides practical help for those with special needs, as well as information about facilities and aids available. There are over 370 local branches in the UK, a residential home for the severely disabled, specially-adapted holiday centres, and self-catering units.

ARTHRITIS AND RHEUMATISM COUNCIL

41 Eagle Street
London WC1R 4AR
Tel: 071-405 8572

The Arthritis and Rheumatism Council aims primarily to support research to find the causes of rheumatic disease. It also stimulates teaching in rheumatology in medical schools, and aims to make the general public more aware of arthritis and rheumatism. The organisation is divided into 30 regions with a total of 1100 branches.

ASSOCIATION OF BREASTFEEDING MOTHERS

131 Mayow Road
London SE26 4HZ
Tel: 081-659 5151

The Association of Breastfeeding Mothers is a registered charity and aims to educate parents about the means and advantages of breastfeeding. This is achieved by local meetings countrywide, training counsellors, and the encouragement of local support groups. Publications and seminars help to educate health professionals to advise mothers on breastfeeding, and on twins, insufficient milk, and other topics. A books-by-post service is also operated.

ASSOCIATION OF THE BRITISH PHARMACEUTICAL INDUSTRY (ABPI)

12 Whitehall
London SW1A 2DY
Tel: 071-930 3477

The Association of the British Pharmaceutical Industry is the trade association representing manufacturers of prescription medicines. The Association was formed in 1930 and now represents 152 companies which produce nearly 99% of medicines supplied to the NHS. The main functions of the Association are to maintain and improve the reputation of the industry and its contribution to the health and economic welfare of the nation; to assist contact between member companies and government departments, professional, scientific and trade organisations and other similar bodies; and to act as a channel of communication and to act on collective decisions made by its members.

ASSOCIATION OF PHARMACY TECHNICIANS

c/o Bramley Cottage
Allenend
Middleton
Nr Tamworth
Staffordshire B78 2BW
Tel: 021-378 2211 Ext. 3326

The Association of Pharmacy Technicians was founded in 1952 to enhance and further the status of pharmacy technicians. The Association consists of a national executive, with branches and groups nationwide. An annual conference and study day is organised by the Association, and all members receive a journal.

ASSOCIATION FOR RESEARCH INTO RESTRICTED GROWTH (ARRG)

61 Lady Walk
Maple Cross
Rickmansworth
Herts WD3 2YZ
Tel: (0923) 770759

The Association for Research into Restricted Growth is a national voluntary organisation which is concerned with all aspects of the health and social welfare of people of unusually short stature. It acts as a forum for the exchange of information, support, and practical advice. It provides family counselling and contacts for parents of affected children, and an advisory panel for medical problems. Its publications include ARRG News, a quarterly magazine, and information on coping with restricted growth.

ASSOCIATION FOR SPINA BIFIDA AND HYDROCEPHALUS (ASBAH)

22 Upper Woburn Place
London WC1H 0EP
Tel: 071-388 1382

The Association for Spina Bifida and Hydrocephalus is a welfare and research organisation which provides information, advisory and welfare services, and practical assistance in all aspects of life with spina bifida and hydrocephalus. It also supports and promotes research into the prevention, treatment, and management of spina bifida and hydrocephalus. There is a regular magazine, LINK, and a group for young people, LIFT. A national organisation supports the work of approximately 80 local associations. Specialist field workers and counsellors are also provided.

ASSOCIATION FOR STAMMERERS (AFS)

c/o The Finsbury Health Centre
Pine Street
London EC1R 0JH

The Association for Stammerers is a nationwide organisation registered as a charity. It advises stammerers about therapy and supports local self-help groups where members can socialise, practise fluency techniques, and discuss their problems. It produces information leaflets and a quarterly magazine, and informs the public of the problems of stammerers.

ASSOCIATION OF TEACHING HOSPITAL PHARMACISTS

c/o P Sharrott, Hon. Secretary
Brandenburgh House
Charing Cross Hospital
Fulham Palace Road
London W6 8RF
Tel: 081-741 2761

The Association of Teaching Hospital Pharmacists is for pharmacists who have a direct professional responsibility for pharmaceutical services in major teaching hospitals, with membership limited to one pharmacist from each teaching district/health board in the UK. The Association has several aims, amongst which are the furtherance of pharmaceutical education to medical undergraduates, and the development of pharmaceutical research in teaching hospitals.

ASTHMA SOCIETY AND FRIENDS OF THE ASTHMA RESEARCH COUNCIL

300 Upper Street
London N1 2XX
Tel: 071-226 2260

The Asthma Society and Friends of the Asthma Research Council is a national registered charity which raises funds for medical research into asthma, disseminates information about asthma, and supports sufferers and their families. A network of approximately 150 branches exists throughout the country and these hold regular meetings, provide a library of books on asthma and related subjects, and encourage the normal integration of asthma sufferers at school, work, and play. The Society also provides many leaflets on all aspects of asthma, its prevention, treatment, and management.

—————————— B ——————————

BRITISH ASSOCIATION OF CANCER UNITED PATIENTS (BACUP)

121–123 Charterhouse Street
London EC1M 6AA
Information Service, Tel: 071-608 1661

The British Association of Cancer United Patients is a registered charity which was set up to provide information and support to cancer patients, their families and friends, health professionals, and the general public. A team of experienced cancer nurses answer telephone and written enquiries on all aspects of cancer care. It has a comprehensive directory of both local and national resources (e.g. support groups, counselling services, home care services, insurance brokers, and transport services). BACUP produces leaflets and booklets on the main types of cancer and on the emotional and practical problems of coping with the disease. Publications are sent free of charge to patients and their relatives. BACUP News, published three times a year, is sent regularly on request. The Cancer Information Service is available Monday to Friday 10 am to 5.30 pm, extended to 7 pm Tuesdays and Thursdays.

BIRTH CONTROL TRUST

27-35 Mortimer Street
London W1N 7RJ
Tel: 071-580 9360

The Birth Control Trust, together with its sister organisation the Birth Control Campaign, aims to advance medical and sociological research into contraception, sterilisation, and legal abortion. It operates from a national office in London, and produces leaflets and booklets, which may be obtained by post.

BRITISH AGENCIES FOR ADOPTION AND FOSTERING (BAAF)

11 Southwark Street
London SE1 1RQ
Tel: 071-407 8800

The British Agencies for Adoption and Fostering is a registered charity and the professional association for all those concerned with adoption, fostering, and social work with children and families. It aims to promote good standards of professional practice; to increase public understanding of the issues involved; and to bring children with special needs improved opportunities for family life. It provides training and consultancy, gives advice and information, and publishes books, leaflets, and a journal.

BRITISH ASSOCIATION FOR THE HARD OF HEARING (BAHOH)

7-11 Armstrong Road
London W3 7JL
Tel: 081-743 1110/1353

The British Association for the Hard of Hearing is a registered charity and the national organisation for those who have lost all or part of their hearing after acquiring normal speech and language, and who communicate via a hearing aid and/or lipreading. It has 230 social clubs in the UK at which lipreading may be practised. It also publishes a magazine, and leaflets and aids are available.

BRITISH COLOSTOMY ASSOCIATION

38-39 Eccleston Square
London SW1V 1PB
Tel: 071-828 5175

The British Colostomy Association is a registered charity which exists to provide help, advice, and reassurance to colostomy patients in the UK, and to represent their interests. Members of the group involved in patient care themselves have a colostomy. There is a national headquarters, with area officers throughout the UK and Eire. The group is also a member of the International Ostomy Association.

BRITISH DENTAL ASSOCIATION (BDA)

64 Wimpole Street
London W1M 8AL
Tel: 071-935 0875

The British Dental Association is the professional body which represents dentists in a trade union and scientific role, and holds the initiative on all key issues which affect them. It aims to protect and promote the image of dentistry. Activities include an annual conference; national and local meetings of the different standing committees; and the publication of the British Dental Journal and BDA News which are circulated free to members. The BDA has 21 branches, and 120 sections, with regional offices in both Scotland and Northern Ireland.

BRITISH DIABETIC ASSOCIATION (BDA)

10 Queen Anne Street
London W1M 0BD
Tel: 071-323 1531

The British Diabetic Association is a registered charity which was formed to provide advice and information for all diabetics and their families, to promote greater public understanding about diabetes, and to support research into the prevention, treatment, and cure of the disease and its complications. There are over 350 local groups and branches throughout the UK, which arrange regular meetings and social events. BDA also publishes a wide range of literature, provides videos and posters, and arranges educational activity weekends for diabetics and their families.

THE BRITISH DIETETIC ASSOCIATION

Daimler House
Paradise Circus Queensway
Birmingham B1 2BJ
Tel: 021-643 5483

The British Dietetic Association is a registered charity which aims to advance the science and practice of dietetics through promotion of training and education of dieticians; spreading the knowledge and further understanding of dietetics; and to facilitate the exchange of information amongst members, other professionals, and the general public. Groups within the association with special interests include parenteral and enteral nutrition, renal disease, community nutrition, paediatric nutrition, and the elderly. Pharmacists may obtain advice on the use of therapeutic dietary products from their local dietitian.

BRITISH DYSLEXIA ASSOCIATION
98 London Road
Reading
Berks RG1 5AU
Tel: (0734) 668271/2

The British Dyslexia Association is a registered charity committed to encouraging the early identification of children handicapped by specific learning difficulties. It offers a comprehensive counselling, information, and referral service for dyslexic children and their parents, dyslexic adults, and teachers. It organises courses, conferences, produces leaflets, and seeks to provide professional expertise to both parents and children. There are 68 local associations, and 57 corporate members (e.g. independent schools, and university and hospital departments).

BRITISH EPILEPSY ASSOCIATION
Anstey House
40 Hanover Street
Leeds LS3 1BE
Tel: (0532) 439393

The British Epilepsy Association is a registered charity concerned with the interests of people with epilepsy, their families, and professionals working with them. It produces a comprehensive range of literature giving information and practical advice on coping with epilepsy and investigates, through the British Epilepsy Research Foundation, medical and social aspects of the condition. Services are provided by a headquarters and 6 regional offices.

BRITISH HEART FOUNDATION
102 Gloucester Place
London W1H 4DH
Tel: 071-935 0185

The British Heart Foundation is a registered charity which supports research projects into cardiovascular disease; informs doctors throughout the country of advances in the field through the issue of a Factfile; and provides the public with proven risk factors related to heart diseases. It also strives to improve facilities for cardiac care by providing life-saving equipment for hospitals and ambulance services.

BRITISH HERBAL MEDICINE ASSOCIATION
PO Box 304
Bournemouth
Dorset BH7 6JZ
Tel: (0202) 433691

The British Herbal Medicine Association aims to encourage the availability of herbal medicine, and to promote a wider knowledge and recognition of its value. It seeks to advance the science and practice of herbal medicine by modern techniques, and to promote high standards of quality and safety in herbal products. It also fosters research into phytotherapy. The Association publishes the British Herbal Pharmacopoeia.

BRITISH HOLISTIC MEDICAL ASSOCIATION
179 Gloucester Place
London NW1 6DX
Tel: 071-262 5299

The British Holistic Medical Association was set up by a group of doctors and medical students interested in the whole-person approach to health-care. It publishes books, tapes, and a journal, and has a nationwide network of local groups run by professional members for personal growth, education, and support.

BRITISH HOMOEOPATHIC ASSOCIATION
27a Devonshire Street
London W1N 1RJ
Tel: 071-935 2163

The British Homoeopathic Association is a registered charity which works to widen the availability of homoeopathy by doctors both within and outside the NHS. It acts as an advice centre, dealing with many enquiries annually. It holds first aid and self-help seminars for the general public, and special meetings to encourage pharmacists and veterinarians. It is a national organisation with a Council, of whom two members are pharmacists.

BRITISH KIDNEY PATIENT ASSOCIATION
Bordon
Hants GU35 9JP
Tel: (04203) 2021/2

The British Kidney Patient Association is a national registered charity concerned with the welfare of kidney patients (both dialysis and transplant patients), and the provision of kidney machines and holiday dialysis centres. It also aims to create a greater awareness of the needs for kidney donors, and the problems caused by their lack of availability.

BRITISH MEDICAL ASSOCIATION (BMA)
BMA House
Tavistock Square
London WC1H 9JP
Tel: 071-387 4499

The British Medical Association was founded in 1832 to promote the medical and allied sciences, and to maintain the honour and interests of the medical profession. Five autonomous committees represent and negotiate on behalf of doctors in general practice, hospitals (consultant and junior staff), community medicine, and universities. Publications include the British Medical Journal, BMA News Review, scientific medical journals, abstracts of medicine and surgery, and special reports.

BRITISH MIGRAINE ASSOCIATION
178a High Road
Byfleet
Weybridge
Surrey KT14 7ED
Tel: (09323) 52468

The British Migraine Association is a registered charity run for migraine sufferers by migraine sufferers, their families, and friends. It encourages and supports research into its causes and treatment, and provides information on all aspects of the condition to sufferers, all branches of the medical profession, and the media. It also aims to provide friendly, cheerful reassurance and understanding to sufferers.

THE BRITISH NUTRITION FOUNDATION
15 Belgrave Square
London SW1X 8PS
Tel: 071-235 4904

The British Nutrition Foundation is a charity, supported by contributions from its member companies, which aims to provide sound, impartial, and objective information about food and nutrition. It aims to help individuals understand how they may best match their diet with their life-style, and sets out to achieve these aims through education, information, and research. Its resources are available to health-care professionals, educators, the media, MPs and government departments, industry, and the public.

BRITISH OSTEOPATHIC ASSOCIATION
8–10 Boston Place
London NW1 6QH
Tel: 071-262 5250

The British Osteopathic Association is an association of osteopathic physicians. Members of the Association are either doctors of osteopathy, trained at one of the osteopathic colleges of medicine and surgery in the USA, or medical practitioners who have undertaken postgraduate studies at the London College of Osteopathic Medicine. The Association produces a directory of its practising members.

THE BRITISH PHARMACEUTICAL STUDENTS' ASSOCIATION (BPSA)
c/o 1 Lambeth High Street
London SE1 7JN
Tel: 071-735 9141

The British Pharmaceutical Students' Association is the only organisation to cater solely for the needs of pharmacy students, and especially preregistration graduates. The organisation encourages and facilitates interchange of ideas and opinions between its members, and provides a platform for communication to other pharmaceutical organisations. The BPSA tries to achieve its aims by organising national and regional events to which both students and graduates are invited. Local conferences, sports matches, and social events have been commonplace in past years.

BRITISH PREGNANCY ADVISORY SERVICE (bpas)
Austy Manor
Wootton Wawen
Solihull
West Midlands B95 6BX
Tel: (05642) 3225

The British Pregnancy Advisory Service is a registered charity

providing education, research, and a range of services, including counselling and treatment of problems connected with fertility and infertility. It carries out pregnancy tests, vasectomies, female sterilisation, and sterilisation reversals at its five nursing homes.

BRITISH RED CROSS SOCIETY
9 Grosvenor Crescent
London SW1X 7EJ
Tel: 071-245 5454

The British Red Cross Society offers training in first aid and related skills to its members and the general public. Welfare duties are carried out for home-bound patients, and elderly and disabled people. It also raises funds and provides relief supplies internationally.

C

CANCER RELIEF MACMILLAN FUND
Anchor House
15-19 Britten Street
London SW3 3TZ
Tel: 071-351 7811

The Cancer Relief Macmillan Fund is a registered charity (as The National Society for Cancer Relief) and was founded by Douglas Macmillan in 1911 to bring care and support to cancer patients. Specially trained nurses are provided to look after cancer patients in their own homes. The Fund also provides help to cancer patients by building continuing care homes which provide in-patient and day care; giving cash grants to patients and families in financial need; and funding an education programme in the new skills of pain relief.

CANCER RESEARCH CAMPAIGN
2 Carlton House Terrace
London SW1Y 5AR
Tel: 071-930 8972

The Cancer Research Campaign is a registered charity aiming to defeat cancer. To achieve this, it supports research at centres throughout the UK, providing funds for projects on the recommendation of its Scientific and Education Committees. A field staff of 22 area appeals organisers provides the link between about 1000 voluntary local committees and the headquarters.

CENTRE FOR THE STUDY OF ALTERNATIVE THERAPIES
51 Bedford Place
Southampton
Hants SO1 2DG
Tel: (0703) 334752

The Centre for the Study of Alternative Therapies was set up by medically qualified practitioners who work at the centre and offer skills in a wide range of complementary medical techniques. Clinical services are offered in acupuncture, manipulative medicine, homoeopathy, and clinical ecology. The techniques are also taught, largely at postgraduate level, and research is also carried out.

THE CHEST HEART AND STROKE ASSOCIATION

Tavistock House North
Tavistock Square
London WC1H 9JE
Tel: 071-387 3012

The Chest, Heart, and Stroke Association is a registered charity which works to prevent chest, heart, and stroke illnesses, and helps people who suffer from them. It offers advice and welfare services, publishes leaflets and booklets, funds research, and organises conferences. Its headquarters in London are supplemented by branches in Edinburgh and Belfast, and there is a nationwide network of stroke clubs and schemes.

CLINICAL PHARMACOKINETICS SOCIETY

c/o RPSGB
1 Lambeth High Street
London SE1 7JN
Tel: 071-735 9141

The Clinical Pharmacokinetics Society aims to establish and develop pharmacy involvement in drug level monitoring and pharmacokinetic interpretation services. A wide range of objectives include the evaluation of therapeutic drug monitoring (TDM) services; education and training in TDM; and an extension of databases for the evaluation of population pharmacokinetic parameters.

COELIAC SOCIETY OF THE UNITED KINGDOM

PO Box 220
High Wycombe
Bucks HP11 2HY
Tel: (0494) 37278

The Coeliac Society is a registered charity which exists to help those who have been medically diagnosed as having coeliac disease or dermatitis herpetiformis. It is a national organisation with 57 local groups. The Society publishes the Coeliac Handbook, a list of gluten-free manufactured products, and other aids for patients.

COLLEGE OF PHARMACY PRACTICE

111 Lambeth Road
London SE1 7JL
Tel: 071-735 0418

The College of Pharmacy Practice was established by the Council of the PSGB as a company, limited by guarantee, and with charitable status. The principle purposes of the College are to promote and maintain a high standard of practice; to advance education and training in all pharmaceutical disciplines and at all levels; to establish standards of vocational training; to advance knowledge of the application of pharmacy in total health care; and to conduct, promote, and facilitate research into the practice of pharmacy, and to publish the results of those endeavours. All pharmacists registered in Great Britain are eligible to become student members and can take the College's two part Practitioner Membership Examination after being registered for three years and being a College member for one year.

COMMITTEE OF REGIONAL PHARMACEUTICAL OFFICERS

c/o Mr T H Furber
Trent Regional Health Authority
Fulwood House
Old Fulwood Road
Sheffield S10 3TH
Tel: (0742) 306511

The Committee of Regional Pharmaceutical Officers comprises all Regional Pharmaceutical Officers in England and exists to co-ordinate all aspects of hospital pharmacy in England.

COMMUNITY SERVICES PHARMACISTS' GROUP

c/o RPSGB
1 Lambeth High Street
London SE1 7JN
Tel: 071-735 9141

The Community Services Pharmacists' Group aims to co-ordinate the activities of pharmacists involved in priority care services whilst being employed in the managed service. These pharmacists provide a service to community units, priority care groups, and residential care units which consists of a supply function, together with a role in policy formation, implementation, and monitoring.

CONSUMERS' ASSOCIATION

2 Marylebone Road
London NW1 4DX
Tel: 071-486 5544

The Association for Consumer Research (ACRE) is a registered charity which undertakes research and comparative testing of goods and services. Its trading subsidiary, the Consumers' Association, publishes a range of Which? magazines, and also Self Health and the Drug and Therapeutics Bulletin. The Research Institute for Consumer Affairs (RICA) is a sister organisation to ACRE which carries out projects aimed at helping elderly and disabled people.

CORONARY PREVENTION GROUP

60 Great Ormond Street
London WC1N 3HR
Tel: 071-833 3687

The Coronary Prevention Group is a registered charity devoted to the prevention of coronary heart disease. It provides information and practical advice on the major causes of the disease. The group is run by the country's leading experts on heart disease and deals with issues ranging from nutrition, farming, smoking, and exercise to recovering from a heart attack. The group also publishes a range of information on the subjects.

COUNCIL FOR COMPLEMENTARY AND ALTERNATIVE MEDICINE (CCAM)
Suite 1
19a Cavendish Square
London W1M 9AD
Tel: 071-409 1440

The Council for Complementary and Alternative Medicine provides a forum for communication and co-operation between professional bodies representing acupuncture, chiropractic, homoeopathy, medical herbalism, naturopathy, and osteopathy. It also aims to promote and maintain the highest standards of training, qualification, and treatment in these therapies, and to facilitate the dissemination of information about them. A register of CCAM member practitioners is held at the headquarters.

CRUSE, THE NATIONAL ORGANISATION FOR THE WIDOWED AND THEIR CHILDREN
126 Sheen Road
Richmond
Surrey TW9 1UR
Tel: 081-940 4818/9047

CRUSE is a registered charity which offers help, advice, and information on practical problems, and opportunities for social contacts, to all bereaved people. It also runs training courses in bereavement counselling, and a number of fact sheets and other literature are available through either the national organisation or from its 130 branches in the UK.

CYSTIC FIBROSIS RESEARCH TRUST
Alexandra House
5 Blyth Road
Bromley
Kent BR1 3RS
Tel: 081-464 7211

The Cystic Fibrosis Research Trust is a registered charity which finances research into a cure for cystic fibrosis and to improve current methods of treatment. Branches throughout the UK help and advise parents with the everyday problems of caring for children with cystic fibrosis. The Trust also aims to educate the public about the disease and to promote its earlier diagnosis in children.

———————— D ————————

DIABETES FOUNDATION
177a Tennison Road
London SE25 5NF
Tel: 081-656 5467

The Diabetes Foundation supports research into the causes and

complications of diabetes with the primary objective of finding the cure for the disease. It provides a programme of public awareness and education, and represents the interests of diabetics in the UK. A free copy of the educational magazine Diabetic Life is available on request to diabetics and to the parents of diabetic children.

DISABLED LIVING FOUNDATION (DLF)
380-384 Harrow Road
London W9 2HU
Tel: 071-289 6111

The Disabled Living Foundation provides information on all non-medical aspects of living with a disability (including mental, physical, and sensory, together with multiple handicaps and the infirmities of age). It provides a general information service on aids and equipment (including a subscription service for updated information and enquiry service), and advisory services on incontinence, visual handicap, clothing, and music. There is a demonstration centre in which equipment may be viewed and tried out. The DLF also organises publications and seminars.

DOWN'S SYNDROME ASSOCIATION
First Floor
12-13 Clapham Common Southside
London SW4 7AA
Tel: 071-720 0008

The Down's Syndrome Association is a registered charity which aims to create and develop the environment in which people with the condition may realise their full potential. It provides information about health, education, teenage problems, and life after school. The Association promotes research into ways of improving life of people of all ages with Down's syndrome. The Association has a national administrative office and resource centre based in London, and a network of branches throughout the UK.

DRUG INFORMATION PHARMACISTS' GROUP
c/o Mrs J Blake
Northwick Park Hospital
Watford Road
Harrow
Middlesex HA1 3UJ
Tel: 081-423 4535

The Drug Information Pharmacists' Group comprises the regional principal pharmacists in drug information from England, together with representatives from Wales and Northern Ireland.

THE DYSLEXIA INSTITUTE
133 Gresham Road
Staines
Middlesex TW18 2AJ
Tel: (0784) 59498/63851/63852

The Dyslexia Institute aims to provide a teaching, teacher-training, assessment, and advisory service for dyslexics and those working with them. It also hopes to increase general awareness of the difficulties encountered by dyslexics at school and at home. In order to ensure that more teachers nationally are informed and skilled in dealing with the problem, the Institute aims to increase the provision made for it at teacher-training level. It is a national organisation with assessment and teaching centres around the country.

─────────── E ───────────

EQUIPMENT FOR THE DISABLED
Mary Marlborough Lodge
Nuffield Orthopaedic Centre
Headington
Oxford OX3 7LD
Tel: (0865) 750103

The DHSS-sponsored Equipment for the Disabled publishes a series of reference books giving details of the range of equipment and aids available to help disabled people. These include specially manufactured equipment, everyday consumer goods, and DIY ideas. Practical advice, and points to consider before purchase, are also given. All items are tested and assessed by disabled people either at home or in the hospital prior to their inclusion.

EYE CARE INFORMATION BUREAU
4 Ching Court
Shelton Street
London WC2H 9DG
Tel: 071-836 1765

The Eye Care Information Bureau supplies the public with information on general eye care. Advice may also be obtained by telephone. Any detailed questions are answered by an ophthalmic optician (optometrist).

─────────── F ───────────

THE FAMILY PLANNING ASSOCIATION (FPA)
27-35 Mortimer Street
London W1N 7RJ
Tel: 071-636 7866

The Family Planning Association is a registered charity which provides information, advice, and education on birth control, fertility, reproductive health, sex education, sexuality, and relationships. It aims to preserve and protect the good health, physical and mental, of individuals, couples, and families, and prevent the hardship and distress caused by unwanted conceptions. It is a national organisation, with regional offices around the UK. It runs an information service for health professionals and consumers, and organises courses for professionals in education and health.

FOUNDATION FOR THE STUDY OF INFANT DEATHS
15 Belgrave Square
London SW1X 8PS
Tel: 071-235 1721/0965

The Foundation for the Study of Infant Deaths is a registered charity which raises funds for research into the causes and prevention of cot death (sudden infant death syndrome). It gives personal support to bereaved families by letter, telephone, and leaflets, and puts parents in touch with previously bereaved parents (Friends of the Foundation) who offer an individual befriending service. It also acts as a centre of information on cot death for parents and professionals, and for the exchange of knowledge within the UK and abroad.

─────────── G ───────────

GENERAL COUNCIL AND REGISTER OF OSTEOPATHS
21 Suffolk Street
London SW1Y 4HG
Tel: 071-839 2060

The General Council and Register of Osteopaths exists to protect the public by insisting for its membership on a standard of excellence in osteopathic training, practice, and behaviour. This is achieved by accrediting four-year full-time courses at certain educational establishments approved by Council, and by maintaining a strict Code of Ethics. Only graduates of accredited courses are entitled to membership of the Register and to use the abbreviation of MRO. Details of local registered osteopaths may be obtained by contacting the secretary at the above address.

GENERAL MEDICAL COUNCIL (GMC)
44 Hallam Stret
London W1N GAE
Tel: 071-580 7642

The General Medical Council is the statutory body for the regulation of the medical profession. Its duties include the promotion of high standards and co-ordination of all stages of medical education; keeping and publishing a register of duly qualified doctors; providing advice for doctors on standards of professional conduct and on medical ethics; and taking action in cases of serious professional misconduct or where a doctor's fitness to practice appears to be seriously impaired by reason of a mental or physical condition. Its membership comprises representatives nominated by the Crown, appointed by the universities having medical faculties, and by the medical corporations, and elected directly by members of the profession.

THE GUIDE DOGS FOR THE BLIND ASSOCIATION
Alexandra House
9–11 Park Street
Windsor
Berks SL4 1JR
Tel: (0753) 855711

The Guide Dogs for the Blind Association is a registered charity responsible for the breeding and training of guide dogs, and training blind people (and associated aftercare services) to work with them. The Association has approximately 420 branches throughout England, Scotland, and Wales whose members operate on a voluntary basis.

GUILD OF HOSPITAL PHARMACISTS
ASTMS Divisional Officer
79 Camden Road
London NW1 9ES
Tel: 071-267 4422

The Guild of Hospital Pharmacists represents the interests of hospital pharmacists in professional matters and in negotiations on salaries and conditions of employment. The Guild merged with the Association of Scientific, Technical and Managerial Staff (ASTMS) in order to provide the professional negotiating skills needed within the Pharmaceutical Whitley Council where salaries and conditions of service are decided. Membership of the Guild is open to all practising hospital pharmacists, who participate in the work of the Guild through local groups, which conduct professional, business, and social meetings throughout the year. Policies at national level on professional and non-professional matters are decided by a Council of 24 members, who are elected by the membership.

──────────── H ────────────

HAEMOPHILIA SOCIETY
123 Westminster Bridge Road
London SE1 7HR
Tel: 071-928 2020

The Haemophilia Society is a registered charity which represents the interests of people with haemophilia, and provides them, their families, and health-care professionals with help, advice, and assistance as appropriate. The problems of HIV and AIDS are particularly important with respect to the safety of blood products. It is a national society, with a number of locally run groups.

HALLEY STEWART LIBRARY
St Christopher's Hospice
51 Lawrie Park Road
Sydenham
London SE26 6DZ
Tel: 081-778 9252

The library contains a small specialised collection of books and journal articles on all aspects of terminal care and bereavement, and lists of references on specific topics can be sent to enquirers. Books and reprints are also available through a mail order service.

HEALTH EDUCATION AUTHORITY
Hamilton House,
Mabledon Place
London WC1H 9TX
Tel: 071-631 0930

The Health Education Authority was formed in 1987 to replace the Health Education Council. The Authority advises the Government on, and undertakes, health education. It plans and carries out national, regional, or local programmes in co-operation with health authorities, Family Practitioner Committees, local authorities and education authorities, and voluntary organisations. It sponsors research and evaluation in relation to health education, and assists in the provision of appropriate training. It produces leaflets and material promoting health education, and provides a national centre of information and advice.

HELP THE AGED
St James's Walk
London EC1R 0BE
Tel: 071-253 0253

Help the Aged is a registered charity which works to improve the quality of life of all elderly people in the UK and overseas, especially those who are frail, neglected, and forgotten. It provides food and clothing, supports day centres, and self-help projects. Through its publications, it advises on the welfare of elderly people, including safety, health, mobility, and finance.

THE HERPES ASSOCIATION
41 North Road
London N7 9DP
Helpline: 071-609 9061

The Herpes Association is a registered charity which provides information and advice to those who have outbreaks of herpes, and aims to promote an accurate public awareness of the condition. It supports and encourages local self-help groups and publishes a quarterly newsletter.

HOSPICE INFORMATION SERVICE
St Christopher's Hospice
51–59 Lawrie Park Road
Sydenham
London SE26 6DZ
Tel: 081-778 9252

The Hospice Information Service provides a resource and link for members of the public and health-care professionals. A directory of Hospice Services in the UK and Eire is published annually. A list of overseas organisations is also available. A varied educational programme is offered by the teaching hospice, including courses for pharmacists.

──────────── I ────────────

ILEOSTOMY ASSOCIATION OF GREAT BRITAIN AND NORTHERN IRELAND (IA)
Central Office
Amblehurst House
Black Scotch Lane
Mansfield
Notts NG18 4PF
Tel: (0623) 28099

The Ileostomy Association is a registered charity whose primary aim is to help anyone who has undergone, or is about to undergo, ileostomy surgery to return to a full and active life. There are about 70 local volunteer support groups which are each backed by its own medical president. The IA actively promotes and supports research both into the cause of inflammatory bowel diseases, and ways of improving the quality of care and management of ileostomies.

IMPERIAL CANCER RESEARCH FUND (ICRF)
PO Box 123
Lincoln's Inn Fields
London WC2A 3PX
Tel: 071-242 0200

The Imperial Cancer Research Fund is a registered charity which aims to carry out research into the causes, prevention, and treatment of cancer. It runs the largest cancer research institute in Europe and supports laboratories in London and throughout the UK. It has 9 regional appeals' centres covering England, Wales, and Scotland.

INFERTILITY ADVISORY CENTRE
2nd Floor
London Independent Hospital
1 Beaumont Square
London E1 4NL
Tel: 071-790 9616

The private Infertility Advisory Centre investigates and treats both male and female infertility. It performs active *in vitro* fertilisation and gamete intrafallopian tube transfer (GIFT), as well as artificial insemination.

INSTITUTE FOR COMPLEMENTARY MEDICINE
21 Portland Place
London W1N 3AF
Tel: 071-636 9543

The Institute for Complementary Medicine is a registered charity which aims to increase public awareness of natural therapies through education and research. It is concerned with the establishment of national standards of professional training for natural therapy practitioners, and can provide members of the public with information on practitioners, research documents, and books. It also has begun a programme of research into the workings of complementary treatment. It runs special courses introducing natural therapies. Some of the therapies covered are acupuncture, osteopathy, chiropractic therapy, herbal medicine, and homoeopathy. A directory of registered practitioners is held by the Institute.

INSTITUTE OF PHARMACY MANAGEMENT INTERNATIONAL
c/o Mr G S Knowles
Seaways Cottage
Marine Road
Hoylake
Merseyside L47 2AS

The Institute of Pharmacy Management International initiates fundamental and practical research programmes and promotes up-to-date teaching of pharmaceutical administration relevant to all branches of the profession. A journal is published quar-terly, and an annual conference permits members to present original work concerning pharmacy practice. The college of the Institute enables members to qualify for a diploma of the Institute through attendance of study modules during a residential course.

INSTITUTE FOR THE STUDY OF DRUG DEPENDENCE (isdd)
1-4 Hatton Place
London EC1N 8ND
Tel: 071-430 1991

The Institute for the Study of Drug Dependence is a registered charity which provides a centre for the study of drug misuse, and aims to advance public understanding of the subject through collation, interpretation, and dissemination of information. It provides a reference library, enquiry service, and current awareness bulletins for use by interested individuals or organisations.

INTERNATIONAL GLAUCOMA ASSOCIATION (IGA)
c/o King's College Hospital
Denmark Hill
London SE5 9RS
Tel: 071-274 6222 Ext. 2466 (Mon. and Thurs. only)

The International Glaucoma Association is a registered charity which offers all those interested in preventing blindness from glaucoma a forum for the exchange of ideas, and aims to increase awareness of the problems of the disease. It sends out information booklets free on receipt of a large SAE. It also supports research into the causes and treatment of glaucoma from donations received.

INTRACTABLE PAIN SOCIETY OF GREAT BRITAIN & IRELAND
The Association of Anaesthetists
9 Bedford Square
London WC1B 3RA
Tel: 071-631 1650

The Intractable Pain Society is open for membership to all persons of consultant or equivalent status with a direct input into the control of intractable pain. The Society aims to raise the standards of treatment of intractable pain, to provide facilities for the exchange of information, opinions, and experience between active workers in the field, and to increase awareness of the facilities available for the treatment of intractable pain. Research and teaching in the relief of pain is also encouraged.

L

THE LEONARD CHESHIRE FOUNDATION
Leonard Cheshire House
26-29 Maunsel Street
London SW1P 2QN
Tel: 071-828 1822

The Leonard Cheshire Foundation is a charitable trust presiding over 75 Cheshire Homes in the UK and overseas, and is affiliated to a further 147. The homes accomodate predominantly the physically handicapped, although several homes cater for mentally handicapped children and adults. The common aim of all homes is to provide shelter and care in an atmosphere as close as possible to that of a family home. Family support services are also offered for handicapped people who prefer to remain in their own homes.

LEUKAEMIA RESEARCH FUND

43 Great Ormond Street
London WC1N 3JJ
Tel: 071-405 0101

The Leukaemia Research Fund is the national charity for the support of research into leukaemia and allied blood disorders. It is advised by a medical and scientific panel. The fund is currently supporting research at more than 60 hospitals and university medical centres in the UK. It promotes international symposia, research meetings, and workshops. It also provides patient support through an information service.

M

MARIE CURIE MEMORIAL FOUNDATION

28 Belgrave Square
London SW1X 8QG
Tel: 071-235 3325

The Marie Curie Memorial Foundation is a registered charity which provides nursing care for cancer patients through its 11 Marie Curie Homes throughout the UK, and through its nationwide Community Nursing Service. This service is administered on behalf of the Foundation through the local health authority, and is completely free of charge. The Foundation also runs its own Cancer Research Institute in Surrey, and training courses for health professionals involved in cancer care.

MARIE STOPES HOUSE

108 Whitfield Street
London W1P 6BE
Tel: 071-388 0662/2585

The Marie Stopes House is run by a registered charity and offers a comprehensive birth control service on a private, fee-paying basis. It advises on all aspects of contraception, gynaecological advice, full health checks for women, menopause and PMS consultations, male and female sterilisation, abortion advice and referral, and an advisory service for slimmers. There are three centres in England, and 12 regional vasectomy centres.

MEDIC-ALERT FOUNDATION

11-13 Clifton Terrace
London N4 3JP
Tel: 071-263 8596/7

The Medic-Alert Foundation is a registered charity whose services are funded by a once-only life-membership fee, and

voluntary contributions from friends, members, and companies. The Medic-Alert emblem is worn as a bracelet or necklet, and is engraved with the wearer's special medical condition and a 24-hour emergency telephone number, which may be contacted by emergency service personnel.

MENCAP (THE ROYAL SOCIETY FOR MENTALLY HANDICAPPED CHILDREN AND ADULTS)

MENCAP National Centre
123 Golden Lane
London EC1Y 0RT
Tel: 071-253 9433

MENCAP is a registered charity with 55 000 members, most of whom are parents and friends of people with a mental handicap. A constantly expanding service is provided through 8 divisional offices, with approximately 550 local affiliated groups. Services include: welfare and legal advice, and counselling families with a mentally-handicapped member; holiday services; trustee visitors service; education, training, and pathway employment service; Gateway leisure clubs; and residential services and training establishments. MENCAP National Centre can provide local contacts for new parents, to meet other families with mentally-handicapped children, and a wide range of literature outlining MENCAP's services is available from the information department.

THE MIGRAINE TRUST

45 Great Ormond Street
London WC1N 3HD
Tel: 071-278 2676

The Migraine Trust aims to provide assistance for furthering research into the causes, alleviation, and treatment of migraine. It promotes, assists, and encourages schemes for research, education, technical training, and treatment, and promotes the exchange of information relating to the condition. It makes grants for research into the causes and treatment of migraine at universities and research institutions throughout the world. It is a national organisation, with local groups, and also funds the Princess Margaret Migraine Clinic in London.

MIND (NATIONAL ASSOCIATION FOR MENTAL HEALTH)

22 Harley Street
London W1N 2ED
Tel: 071-637 0741

MIND is a registered charity which aims to uphold the rights and represent interests of people with mental health problems. It provides advice and information, a legal casework service, and training courses and conferences. MIND is also a specialist publisher on mental health subjects. There is a national headquarters, 7 regional offices, and approximately 200 local associations which provide a range of services (e.g. employment schemes, accommodation projects, day centres, advice, and information).

MOTOR NEURONE DISEASE ASSOCIATION

61 Derngate
Northampton NN1 1UE
Tel: (0604) 250505/22269

The Motor Neurone Disease Association is a registered charity which aims to promote and encourage research into the disease, and to improve the provision of care of patients in liaison with the statutory services. The organisation covers the UK with 43 local branches around the country.

THE MULTIPLE SCLEROSIS SOCIETY OF GREAT BRITAIN AND NORTHERN IRELAND

25 Effie Road
Fulham
London SW6 1EE
Tel: 071-736 6267

The Multiple Sclerosis Society is a registered charity which exists to promote and encourage research into finding the cause and cure of multiple sclerosis (MS), and to provide a welfare and support service for families with a sufferer. Headquarters are based in London, supporting 390 local branches which provide practical assistance and support to those with MS. It also supports hospital and university research into the disease, and there are short-stay and holiday centres for those more severely affected.

MUSCULAR DYSTROPHY GROUP OF GREAT BRITAIN AND NORTHERN IRELAND

35 Macaulay Road
Clapham
London SW4 0QP
Tel: 071-720 8055

The Muscular Dystrophy Group is a registered charity with the prime aim of funding research to find the cause, an effective treatment, and a cure for all neuromuscular diseases. It is an entirely voluntary organisation, with 9 professional regional organisers and 450 local branches and representatives. It is also concerned with patient welfare and medical services.

--- N ---

NATIONAL ANKYLOSING SPONDYLITIS SOCIETY (NASS)

6 Grosvenor Crescent
London SW1X 7ER
Tel: 071-235 9585

The National Ankylosing Spondylitis Society is a registered charity concerned with sufferers from the disease, their families, friends, and doctors. It is also involved in promotion of research into the disease. The Society aims to provide a forum for sufferers and to educate patients, professions, and the public in the problems of the disease. The Society is managed by an elected council which is advised by a Medical Advisory Council, who also provide medical information and articles for the NASS Newsletter.

NATIONAL ASSOCIATION FOR THE CHILDLESS

318 Summer Lane
Birmingham B19 3RL
Tel: 021-359 4887

The National Association for the Childless is a self-help support group offering advice and information to people with infertility problems. A quarterly newsletter is produced and, on joining the association, members can obtain literature on a wide range of subjects relating to infertility.

NATIONAL ASSOCIATION FOR COLITIS AND CROHN'S DISEASE (NACC)

98a London Road
St Albans
Herts AL1 1NX

The National Association for Colitis and Crohn's Disease is a registered charity and gives general support to sufferers from inflammatory bowel diseases, their families, and others concerned. It publishes information and raises funds for research into causes and the cure of inflammatory bowel disease. The Association consists of a national executive and 40 area groups, which arrange meetings (e.g. medical information lectures and social events). It publishes 6 booklets and a biannual newsletter is sent free to members.

NATIONAL ASSOCIATION OF WIDOWS (NAW)

Chell Road
Stafford ST16 2QA
Tel: (0785) 45465

The National Association of Widows is a registered charity and offers advice, information, and friendly support to all widows. There are branches throughout the country which provide the basis for a social life for widows; a specialist advice and information service is available from the head office.

NATIONAL ASSOCIATION OF WOMEN PHARMACISTS (NAWP)

c/o RPSGB
1 Lambeth High Street
London SE1 7JN
Tel: 071-735 9141

The National Association of Women Pharmacists was founded to provide a service designed to keep women pharmacists well-informed. NAWP organises an annual national weekend refresher course which is especially designed for those women who have stopped working to raise a family and wish to re-enter the profession. The Association produces a quarterly newsletter supplemented by fact sheets on specific subjects. Local branches of the NAWP hold informal meetings with guest speakers, covering a variety of subjects. Some branches help organise locums in their area. The affairs of the Association are administered by an executive elected from membership.

THE NATIONAL AUTISTIC SOCIETY
276 Willesden Lane
London NW2 5RB
Tel: 081-451 3844

The National Autistic Society is a registered charity and the only organisation working specifically for autistic people. It aims to provide and promote day and residential centres for the care, education, and training of autistic children and adults. It encourages research into the problems of the autistic and aims to stimulate greater understanding among doctors, teachers, and the general public. It provides an advisory service for parents and interested professionals on the nature of childhood autism, and publishes and distributes literature on the management and education of autistic children.

NATIONAL BACK PAIN ASSOCIATION
31-33 Park Road
Teddington
Middlesex TW11 0AB
Tel: 081-977 5474/5

The National Back Pain Association is a registered charity which supports research and education into the causes, prevention, and treatment of back pain. It organises local branches, which are supported by a regional organisation, in which information on back pain is disseminated, and exercise classes carried out.

NATIONAL CAMPAIGN AGAINST SOLVENT ABUSE
245a Coldharbour Lane
London SW9 8RR
Tel: 071-733 7330

The National Campaign against Solvent Abuse is a registered charity which provides information, counselling, and support to solvent abusers and their families. It provides lectures for schools, parent groups, and professional organisations on aspects of solvent abuse, and supports an international information service. Constantly updated information is always available covering all aspects of solvent abuse. The help-line (telephone number above) is operated by ex-solvent abusers.

THE NATIONAL CHILDBIRTH TRUST (NCT)
9 Queensborough Terrace
London W2 3TB
Tel: 071-221 3833

The National Childbirth Trust is a registered charity concerned with education for pregnancy, birth, and parenthood. It aims to help parents achieve greater enjoyment and satisfaction before, during, and following childbirth through antenatal classes, support with breastfeeding, and friendly encouragement after the baby is born. The Trust publishes a wide range of leaflets, and maternity goods are also supplied through its offices. There are 7 NCT regions, with over 300 local branches.

NATIONAL CONSUMER COUNCIL (NCC)
20 Grosvenor Gardens
London SW1W 0DH
Tel: 071-730 3469

The National Consumer Council represents the interests of consumers when they buy or use goods and services (including health services). It particularly watches over the interests of inarticulate and disadvantaged consumers; promotes advice services for consumers nationwide; and encourages consumer representation in nationalised industries. Scottish and Welsh Consumer Councils also exist, and there is a General Consumer Council in Northern Ireland. It does not deal directly with individual consumer enquiries, but does monitor problems taken to other agencies (e.g. citizens advice bureaux).

NATIONAL DEAF CHILDREN'S SOCIETY
45 Hereford Road
London W2 5AH
Tel: 071-229 9272/4 (VOICE)
Tel: 071-229 1891 (VISTEL)

The National Deaf Children's Society is a registered national charity concerned with the needs of parents and families of deaf children. It specialises in advice and information on education, health, and social services. The Society gives grants to parents and families for equipment, holidays, and education. It also operates a lending library of radio hearing aids and other equipment. There are 140 local groups run by parents and interested professionals.

NATIONAL ECZEMA SOCIETY
Tavistock House North
Tavistock Square
London WC1H 9SR
Tel: 071-388 4097

The National Eczema Society is a registered charity which aims to help people with eczema and their families. It has a research fund and also has established an NES Research Fellowship at the Hospital for Sick Children, Great Ormond Street, London. The NES has branches and local support groups throughout the country, and organises an annual holiday scheme for children and for young people.

NATIONAL INSTITUTE OF MEDICAL HERBALISTS
41 Hatherley Road
Winchester
Hants SO22 6RR
Tel: (0962) 68776

The National Institute of Medical Herbalists is the professional body of practising herbalists. It supplies information on herbal medicine, and a list of qualified practitioners may be obtained by sending a SAE. All members of the Institute are graduates of the School of Herbal Medicine at Tunbridge Wells.

NATIONAL PHARMACEUTICAL ASSOCIATION (NPA)

Mallinson House
40-42 St Peter's Street
St Albans
Herts AL1 3NP
Tel: (0727) 32161

The National Pharmaceutical Association is the trade association and parent body of a group of organisations serving pharmacy proprietors. Membership, which is voluntary, comprises 96% of all retail pharmacies in the UK (excluding those of Boots and the Co-operative Societies). As the Retail Pharmacists Union and later the National Pharmaceutical Union (NPU), the NPA was formed in 1921 to champion the interests of pharmacy proprietors and to serve as an organisation for the promotion, improvement, and protection of its members. Soon after its foundation, it joined forces with the Chemists' Defence Association, thus conferring on NPA members automatic insurance against claims for which they are liable as retail pharmacists, entitlement to legal defence against certain prosecutions, legal representation before industrial and other tribunals, and legal defence.

THE NATIONAL RUBELLA COUNCIL

105 Gower Street
London WC1E 6AH
Tel: 071-631 5344

The National Rubella Council has the prime objectives of increasing immunisation against rubella, and preventing the birth of infants with the congenital rubella syndrome. Equally, advice and support is given to families with handicapped children, and to ensure that they receive the services and benefits to which they are entitled. Information is given as leaflets, videos, and a newsletter. The Council consists of 11 voluntary organisations concerned with the effects of congenital rubella syndrome.

THE NATIONAL SOCIETY FOR EPILEPSY (NSE)

Chalfont Centre for Epilepsy
Chalfont St Peter
Gerrards Cross
Bucks SL9 0RJ
Tel: (02407) 3991

The National Society for Epilepsy is a registered charity which caters for the needs of people suffering from epilepsy, offering assessment, treatment, rehabilitation, and long-term care. Research is also carried out into new drugs at the centre. The assessment centre is run in conjunction with the National Hospital for Nervous Diseases. An education department produces a range of leaflets and videos for teaching purposes.

NATIONAL SOCIETY FOR PHENYLKETONURIA AND ALLIED DISORDERS

26 Towngate Grove
Mirfield
West Yorkshire

The National Society for Phenylketonuria and Allied Disorders is an organisation which aims to assist the parents of children born with phenylketonuria (PKU) to manage the problems of the condition. It achieves this by arranging meetings with parents of other children similarly affected, producing and distributing booklets and leaflets, and publishing a comprehensive cookery book to allow the use of a varied and interesting diet in the management of PKU. It also explores holiday opportunities for families with particular dietary needs.

O

OFFICE OF FAIR TRADING

Field House
Bream's Buildings
London EC4 1PR
Tel: 071-242 2858

The Office of Fair Trading is a government department which keeps a watch on trading matters in the UK and protects both consumers and businessmen against unfair practices. This is achieved through the publication of information to help people get to know their rights and obligations; and the encouragement of Codes of Practice drawn up by trade organisations.

OFFICE OF HEALTH ECONOMICS

12 Whitehall
London SW1A 2DY
Tel: 071-930 9203

The Office of Health Economics was founded by the Association of the British Pharmaceutical Industry in 1962. It exists to undertake research on the economic aspects of medical care, and to investigate health and social problems. It also collects data from other countries, and publishes its findings, data, and conclusions.

OPTICAL INFORMATION COUNCIL (OIC)

19-24 Temple Chambers
Temple Avenue
London EC4Y 0DT
Tel: 071-353 3556

The Optical Information Council is an impartial body responsible for the promotion of information on eye care services and products available from registered opticians. It produces a range of public information leaflets and posters.

P

PAIN INTEREST GROUP

c/o RPSGB
1 Lambeth High Street
London SE1 7JN
Tel: 071-735 9141

The Pain Interest Group aims to promote pharmaceutical involvement in pain control and to increase the knowledge base of the RPSGB membership. It does this by organising meetings with top level speakers and by disseminating the experience of other pharmacists to the rest of the membership. This is mainly achieved by case history presentations at meetings and via the newsletter, which is circulated at irregular intervals.

PARKINSON'S DISEASE SOCIETY OF THE UNITED KINGDOM (PDS)
36 Portland Place
London W1N 3DG
Tel: 071-323 1174

The Parkinson's Disease Society is a registered charity which helps patients and their relatives with the problems arising from Parkinson's disease. It also collects and disseminates information, and encourages and provides funds for research into the disease. The national headquarters are in London, with approximately 150 local voluntary branches. Medical and welfare advisory panels exist to help patients in the management of their condition.

THE PATIENTS ASSOCIATION
Room 33
18 Charing Cross Road
London WC2H 0HR
Tel: 071-240 0671

The Patients Association is a registered charity and provides an advice service and collective voice for patients, independent of Government, the health professions, and the drug industry. It is financed by members' subscriptions, donations, and a Government grant. The Association promotes and protects the interests of patients. It gives information and advice to individuals, and aims to promote understanding and goodwill between patients and those in medical and paramedical activities. Information leaflets are distributed free to members.

PHARMACEUTICAL SERVICES NEGOTIATING COMMITTEE (PSNC)
59 Buckingham Street
Aylesbury
Bucks HP20 2PJ
Tel: (0296) 32823

The Pharmaceutical Services Negotiating Committee is a statutory body representing the interests of pharmacy contractors who dispense NHS prescriptions. Pharmacists' fees and other payments are negotiated with the Department of Health, and cover, in addition to dispensing, a number of other services (e.g. appliance fitting and the oxygen therapy service). It is independent of the Royal Pharmaceutical Society of Great Britain and the National Pharmaceutical Association.

PREGNANCY ADVISORY SERVICE
11-13 Charlotte Street
London W1P 1HD
Tel: 071-637 8962

The Pregnancy Advisory Service is a registered charity which provides counselling, support, and termination of pregnancy. It also offers pregnancy testing, post-coital contraception, sterilisation, cervical smears, and artificial insemination by donors.

PROPRIETARY ARTICLES TRADE ASSOCIATION (PATA)
4 Margaret Street
London W1N 7LG
Tel: 071-580 4511

The Proprietary Articles Trade Association was formed to ensure that pharmacists received a fair remuneration for their services through the operation of resale price maintenance. It does this through the support of the majority of manufacturers, wholesalers, and community pharmacists.

PROPRIETARY ASSOCIATION OF GREAT BRITAIN (PAGB)
Vernon House
Sicilian Avenue
London WC1A 2QH
Tel: 071-242 8331

The Proprietary Association of Great Britain represents the manufacturers of medicines intended for use without a medical prescription, and is involved in all matters which affect the marketing and use of non-prescription medicines. It represents its members' interests in negotiations with all Government departments over legislation or other requirements which could influence these products. It administers Codes of Standards which require all labels, leaflets, and advertising be accepted by the Association before publishing.

THE PSORIASIS ASSOCIATION
7 Milton Street
Northampton NN2 7JG
Tel: (0604) 711129

The Psoriasis Association is a registered charity which provides support and mutual aid for those affected with psoriasis. It provides information on all aspects of the condition, and supports research into its causes, treatment, and cure. Through a network of over 60 branches and groups, it supports individuals and provides a point of social contact. The Association also publishes a journal three times a year.

— R —

THE RADIOPHARMACY GROUP
c/o RPSGB
1 Lambeth High Street
London SE1 7JN
Tel: 071-735 9141

The Radiopharmacy Group brings together practising radiopharmacists and aims to develop close contact with colleagues in medical physics and nuclear medicine. This has been formally acknowledged by incorporation of the group into the British Nuclear Medicine Society (BNMS) as the Radiopharmacy Group. The President of the group is a member of the Council of the BNMS.

RE-SOLV

St Mary's Chambers
19 Station Road
Stone
Staffs ST15 8JP
Tel: (0785) 817885/46097

Re-Solv (The Society for the Prevention of Solvent and Volatile Substance Abuse) provides information and education on all aspects of solvent abuse.

ROYAL ASSOCIATION FOR DISABILITY AND REHABILITATION (RADAR)

25 Mortimer Street
London W1N 8AB
Tel: 071-637 5400

RADAR is an umbrella organisation with more than 400 local associations in membership. It provides advice and information concerning access, holidays, housing, and mobility. It also gives welfare advice and help, and provides skill and disability training.

ROYAL NATIONAL INSTITUTE FOR THE BLIND (RNIB)

224 Great Portland Street
London W1N 6AA
Tel: 071-388 1266

The Royal National Institute for the Blind is a registered charity and works for all Britain's 135 000 blind people. It provides an education advisory service, schools, and colleges; further education for school leavers, commercial college, and a school of physiotherapy; a rehabilitation centre; residential care homes for the elderly; hotels and a hostel; a conference centre; shops; careers advice and employment services; advice services on social security benefits and monitors developments in legislation affecting the interests of visually handicapped people; Braille and tape libraries for students; and the talking-book library. It gives advice and practical help to blind people and their families, and to teachers, social workers, health-care staff, and others. It also supports research into the prevention of blindness, and into the needs of the visually handicapped.

ROYAL NATIONAL INSTITUTE FOR THE DEAF (RNID)

105 Gower Street
London WC1E 6AH
Tel: 071-387 8033

The Royal National Institute for the Deaf is a voluntary organisation concerned with all aspects of deafness and hearing impairment, in all age groups. It provides a wide range of services to hearing-impaired people, their families, and to professional people working with them. Services include education and employment information, a library, medical research, rehabilitative and longer-term residential care services, and scientific and technical services.

THE ROYAL SOCIETY OF HEALTH (RSH)

RSH House
38a St George's Drive
London SW1V 4BH
Tel: 071-630 0121

The Royal Society of Health is a registered charity and its aims are to promote the protection and preservation of health and to advance health-related sciences. Members are recruited from all health and health-related professions (including pharmacy), and the level of entry is based upon the qualifications held. The Society holds examinations in a wide range of health subjects, and promotes conferences, lectures, and visits. A bi-monthly journal containing papers on health matters, nutrition, and environmental and social services is published by the Society.

RURAL PHARMACISTS' ASSOCIATION

1 The Square
Wiveliscombe
Somerset TA4 2JT
Tel: (0984) 23284

The Rural Pharmacists' Association exists to ensure that all rural patients receive the same professional standards of pharmaceutical supervision and care as patients in urban areas, to protect and improve the position of the rural pharmacist by all legal means, and to advance the profession of pharmacy in rural areas. It also gives counsel and advice to rural pharmacists, and advises the Council of the Royal Pharmaceutical Society on matters affecting rural pharmacy. Membership is open to any pharmacist who is engaged in, or actively considering engaging in, rural pharmacy, or pharmacists who show interest in and work for the benefit of rural pharmacy.

—————————— S ——————————

ST JOHN AMBULANCE

1 Grosvenor Crescent
London SW1X 7EF
Tel: 071-234 5231

St John Ambulance is a charitable foundation of the Order of St John. Uniformed members attend public events, providing first-aid cover, and first-aid training is given to industry, in schools, and to the general public. The St John Ambulance Air Wing provides emergency transport of donor organs for transplant, and the Aeromedical Service provides fully trained staff to accompany those taken ill while abroad on their journey to Britain. Cadets and Badgers are organisations which give young people the chance to pursue a wide variety of activities, and also learn about first-aid and nursing.

SCHIZOPHRENIA ASSOCIATION OF GREAT BRITAIN (SAGB)
Bryn Hyfryd
The Crescent
Bangor
Gwynedd LL57 2AG
Tel: (0248) 354048

The Schizophrenia Association of Great Britain is a registered charity and aims to help patients suffering from mental illness and their families in every possible way; and to promote research into the biochemical and nutritional factors involved in producing psychiatric symptoms in the genetically-inherited form. It aims to educate the public about schizophrenia through newsletters, conferences, symposia, and lectures. Grants are also made available for research work.

SCOTTISH PHARMACEUTICAL SCIENCES GROUP
36 York Place
Edinburgh EH1 3HU
Tel: 031-556 4386

The Scottish Pharmaceutical Sciences Group aims to provide a forum for the advancement of the pharmaceutical sciences in Scotland, and to enable academic, administrative, community, hospital, and industrial pharmacists and all others interested in the pharmaceutical sciences to meet regularly for the reading and discussion of topics of current interest. It also provides facilities for meetings in Scotland at an economic cost and liaises with other scientific bodies.

SICKLE CELL AND THALASSAEMIA INFORMATION CENTRE
St Leonard's Hospital
Nuttall Street
London N1 5LZ
Tel: 071-739 8484 Ext. 4646

The Sickle Cell and Thalassaemia Information Centre provides a screening service and a counselling service for carriers and their partners. It also counsels, supports, and advises people with the condition, and provides information to the public, community groups, the local City and Hackney Health Authority, and the NHS.

SOCIETY OF APOTHECARIES OF LONDON
Blackfriars Lane
London EC4V 6EJ
Tel: 071-236 1189

The Society of Apothecaries was founded in 1617 by Royal Charter as a Guild for Apothecaries in London. In 1815, under the Apothecaries Act, the Society was empowered to set up the first non-university licensing board to examine candidates who wished to practice medicine in England and Wales. The Act also made the Society responsible for running a register of those who were qualified to practice, and was the earliest legislation requiring a candidate to show that he had clinical experience. In the Act, the Society was also made responsible for examining assistants who worked with doctors in dispensing. The Society still conducts examinations 11 times a year for a registerable licence to practice medicine in the UK, and examines candidates for Diplomas in Medical Jurisprudence, Venereology, the History of Medicine, and the Philosophy of Medicine.

THE SOCIETY OF CHIROPODISTS
53 Welbeck Street
London W1M 7HE
Tel: 071-486 3381

The Society of Chiropodists is the recognised examining body for the state registration of chiropodists, and represents its members on the Whitley Council. Annual and one-day conferences are held, concerned with postgraduate education of its members. Foot-health leaflets and posters, and careers guidance on chiropody, are also offered. There are 50 local branches throughout the UK, with 7 area branch committees. Its journal, The Chiropodist, is published weekly.

SOCIETY FOR DRUG RESEARCH (SDR)
c/o Institute of Biology
20 Queensberry Place
London SW7 2DZ

The Society for Drug Research was founded in 1966 with the aid of the Pharmaceutical Society to provide a common meeting ground for all who are interested or involved in drug research. The SDR has become recognised as the British representative body for medicinal chemistry and has representatives on the National Committee for Pharmacology and other national committees. The SDR has about 1000 members, mostly from pharmaceutical industry, hospitals, and academic institutions. The members elect a committee to conduct its business. Membership is open to any person interested in furthering the aims of the Society and the annual subscription provides free entry to the meetings.

THE SPASTICS SOCIETY
12 Park Crescent
London W1N 4EQ
Tel: 071-636 5020

The Spastics Society is a national organisation which supports services, information, and advice for children and adults with cerebral palsy, and their families. Eight regional offices coordinate activities run by 184 local groups.

THE STANDING CONFERENCE ON DRUG ABUSE (SCODA)
1-4 Hatton Place
Hatton Garden
London EC1N 8ND
Tel: 071-430 2341/2

The Standing Conference on Drug Abuse is a registered charity co-ordinating voluntary organisations and agencies working in the drugs field. Regional workers keep in touch with developments, and a bi-monthly newsletter is published. A Freephone drug problem service gives recorded telephone contact numbers. A national directory of drug services is also published.

T

TERRENCE HIGGINS TRUST/BM AIDS

London WC1N 3XX
or 52-54 Grays Inn Road
London WC1X 8LT
Tel: 071-831 0330

The Terrence Higgins Trust is a registered charity which provides information and support for people with AIDS and AIDS-related complex (ARC), and those who are HIV-positive. This is carried out through various groups within the Trust (e.g. Buddies, telephone help line, legal services, health education, drugs education group, families support group, and partners support group). Health education to the community at large is also promoted. The drugs education group provides support to IV-drug users who are either HIV-positive or who have AIDS/ARC. A mobile health education display attends conferences, seminars, pubs, and discos.

TWINS AND MULTIPLE BIRTHS ASSOCIATION (TAMBA)

Pooh Corner
54 Broad Lane
Hampton
Middlesex TW12 3BG
Tel: 081-941 0641

The Twins and Multiple Births Association is a registered charity which gives encouragement and support to parents of twins and multiple births; and aims to educate the public and medical profession of the incidence, effects, and problems of multiple births. It provides information and literature for parents of multiple births. It also promotes the establishment of twins clubs, and maintains a national register of such clubs (currently nearly 200). A medical and education subgroup exists for professionals involved in health, education, social care, or research.

U

UNITED KINGDOM CLINICAL PHARMACY ASSOCIATION

c/o M J S Burden
73 Aylestone Road
Leicester LE2 7LL
Tel: (0533) 549849

The United Kingdom Clinical Pharmacy Association was established in 1981 to further the interests of all pharmacists whose activities are directed towards the patient. The main objectives of the Association are to improve the quality of patient care by encouraging the rational and effective use of medicines and the promotion of an interdisciplinary approach to drug therapy; to stimulate the development of clinical pharmacy in the UK; and to develop means to evaluate the pharmacist's contribution to overall patient care. Student membership is open to all pharmacy students and preregistration graduates. Ordinary membership is open to all pharmacists working in the UK.

UROSTOMY ASSOCIATION

Buckland
Beaumont Park
Danbury
Essex CM3 4DE
Tel: (024541) 4294

The Urostomy Association is a registered charity which aims to assist patients, both before and following the formation of a urinary stoma, through counselling. It also supports them in returning to lead a full life. There are 22 branches nationwide, and a postal branch covers areas not serviced by a local branch and for those unable to attend meetings.

W

WOMEN'S NATIONAL CANCER CONTROL CAMPAIGN (WNCCC)

1 South Audley Street
London W1Y 5DQ
Tel: 071-499 7532/3/4

The Women's National Cancer Control Campaign is a registered charity and was formed to help women overcome their fears about cancer, and to take simple precautions which could save their lives, through education and early detection. A wide range of literature is produced to educate and inform women about cervical smears and breast self-examination. The Campaign also has several mobile clinics and organises screening for women at their place of work and in local shopping centres. It can also provide enquirers with details of screening facilities throughout the country.

PART C
SYMPTOM AND DISEASE
IDENTIFICATION

Introduction

Although pharmacists are not expected to diagnose disease, it is important that they are aware of the diverse range of conditions which can cause many of the more common symptoms. It will be readily apparent from the descriptions given in the disease monographs which comprise Chapters 1 to 13 that individual diseases can cause many different symptoms. Some symptoms may be considered characteristic of a particular disease and provide a valuable clue to the correct diagnosis. Other symptoms, however, are non-specific and may manifest in a wide variety of conditions; in such cases, the symptom may occur as a consequence of generalised ill-health. Pharmacists who are presented with one or more symptoms by members of the public must be aware of the possible causes and, even in the absence of diagnosis, must be able to differentiate between the symptoms of minor illness and those which forebode a more serious condition. The means by which this can be satisfactorily achieved for a wide range of common symptoms has been discussed in **Chapter 20**.

Part C of this book has been written to provide pharmacists with a quick reference guide to the possible causes of certain symptoms. The information has been derived by extracting the symptoms recorded in the disease monographs, and tabulating the causative conditions under the disease classifications used in this volume. It must be stressed, however, that by virtue of its method of preparation, the disease list stated under each symptom cannot be comprehensive. Other diseases may cause the symptom, and this listing is intended to provide a perspective of the diversity of causative conditions. Equally, no attempt has been made in this reference guide to quantify or qualify the nature of the symptom; if pharmacists are confronted with a patient reporting a particular symptom, use of this guide will indicate many of the possible causes of the symptom and may suggest a suitable course for further questioning. The guide will also enable pharmacists to consult the appropriate monographs to gain a detailed description of the clinical picture in which the reported symptom can occur. It will also be apparent that the description of one symptom does not diagnose a disease; almost all diseases can only be characterised by recognition of two or more symptoms.

To make the guide concise, many individual symptoms have been grouped under a single heading. The list of symptoms incorporated under this umbrella term immediately follows the symptom heading.

———————— A ————————

Abdominal distension
[*abdominal mass; abdominal swelling; ascites; hepatomegaly; hepatosplenomegaly; splenomegaly*]
Blood and lymph disorders
  amyloidosis
  haemolytic anaemias
  haemolytic disease of the newborn
  polycythaemia vera
  splenomegaly
Cardiovascular system disorders
  cor pulmonale
  right heart failure
  tricuspid regurgitation
  tricuspid stenosis
Gastro-intestinal and related disorders
  acute hepatitis
  acute pancreatitis
  ascites
  chronic cholecystitis
  chronic hepatitis
  cirrhosis of the liver
  coeliac disease
  congenital megacolon
  dyspepsia
  focal ischaemia of the small intestine
  haemolytic jaundice
  ileus
  irritable bowel syndrome
  toxic megacolon
  tropical sprue
  tuberculous peritonitis
Gynaecological disorders
  dysmenorrhoea
  premenstrual syndrome
Infections
  American trypanosomiasis
  brucellosis
  chronic fulminating meningococcaemia
  cytomegalovirus infection
  giardiasis
  infectious mononucleosis
  infective endocarditis
  toxocariasis
  toxoplasmosis (congenital)
  trematode infections
  visceral leishmaniasis
  Weil's disease
Malignant disease
  cancer of the liver
  cancer of the stomach
  Hodgkin's disease
  leukaemias
  ovarian tumours
  pancreatic (exocrine) cancer
Metabolic disorders
  galactosaemia
  glycogen storage diseases
  hepatolenticular degeneration
  hereditary fructose intolerance
Musculoskeletal and connective tissue disorders
  systemic lupus erythematosus

Nervous system disorders
  Reye's syndrome
Nutritional disorders
  lactose intolerance

Abdominal pain and discomfort

[*abdominal ache; abdominal colic; abdominal fullness; abdominal tenderness; biliary colic; epigastric pain; griping pain; hepatic tenderness; pelvic pain; renal colic; suprapubic pain*]

Non-specific causes
  drugs
  hernia
  insect bites
  intestinal obstruction
  ovarian cyst
  psychosomatic causes
  rupture (e.g. of the liver or spleen)
Blood and lymph disorders
  anaphylactoid purpura
  polycythaemia vera
  sickle-cell anaemia
  splenomegaly
Cardiovascular system disorders
  aortic aneurysm
  myocardial infarction
  right heart failure
  tricuspid regurgitation
Endocrine disorders
  Addison's disease
  adrenocortical insufficiency, acute
Gastro-intestinal and related disorders
  appendicitis
  ascites
  cholangitis
  cholecystitis
  choledocholithiasis
  chronic persistent hepatitis
  cirrhosis of the liver
  Crohn's disease
  diverticular disease
  dyspepsia
  gallstones
  gastritis
  gastro-enteritis
  ileus
  irritable bowel syndrome
  ischaemic gastro-intestinal disorders
  pancreatitis
  peptic ulceration
  peritonitis
  toxic megacolon
  tropical sprue
  ulcerative colitis
  Whipple's disease
Gynaecological disorders
  dysmenorrhoea
  endometriosis
Infections
  ascariasis
  botulism
  cestode infections
  cystitis
  dysentery
  epididymitis
  giardiasis

hookworm infection
Legionnaire's disease
leptospirosis
mumps
pelvic actinomycosis
pneumonia
prostatitis
pseudomembranous colitis
pyelonephritis
salmonellal infections
salpingitis
shigellosis
strongyloidiasis
trematode infections
trichiniasis
trichuriasis
urinary-tract infections
Malignant disease
  bladder cancer
  cancer of the gall bladder
  cancer of the liver
  cancer of the stomach
  carcinoid syndrome
  cervical cancer
  chronic leukaemias
  colorectal cancer
  ovarian tumours
  pancreatic (exocrine) cancer
  phaeochromocytoma
  renal cancer
  spinal cord tumours
  Zollinger-Ellison syndrome
Metabolic disorders
  hypercalcaemia
  porphyrias
Musculoskeletal and connective tissue disorders
  polyarteritis nodosa
Nervous system disorders
  partial seizures
Nutritional disorders
  lactose intolerance
Obstetric disorders
  ectopic pregnancy
  pre-eclampsia and eclampsia
Renal disorders
  acute glomerulonephritis
  polycystic kidney disease
  renal calculi and colic
Skin disorders
  hereditary angioedema

Abscess formation *see also* Eye abscess

Ear disorders
  mastoiditis
Infections
  osteomyelitis
Skin disorders
  pilonidal disease

Accident-prone

Nervous system disorders
  amphetamine-type drug dependence
  barbiturate-type drug dependence
  volatile solvent-type drug dependence

Acne *see* Skin lesions

Altered bowel habit *see also* Constipation, Diarrhoea, *and*
Constipation and diarrhoea
[*increased difficulty in bowel evacuation; increased frequency of
bowel evacuation; reduced frequency of bowel evacuation*]
Endocrine disorders
 hyperthyroidism
Gastro-intestinal and related disorders
 constipation
 diarrhoea
 diverticular disease
 irritable bowel syndrome
 proctitis

Amnesia *see also* Memory impairment
Infections
 infective endocarditis
 Legionnaire's disease
Malignant disease
 intracranial tumours
Nervous system disorders
 dialysis encephalopathy
 partial seizures

Anaemia
Blood and lymph disorders
 thrombotic thrombocytopenic purpura
Gastro-intestinal and related disorders
 coeliac disease
 peptic ulceration
 polyps
 short-bowel syndrome
 ulcerative colitis
Infections
 abdominal actinomycosis
 African trypanosomiasis
 hookworm infection
 trichuriasis
 visceral leishmaniasis
Malignant disease
 cancer of the stomach
 leukaemias
 non-Hodgkin's lymphoma
 oesophageal cancer
 ovarian tumours
Musculoskeletal and connective tissue disorders
 giant cell arteritis
 osteopetrosis
 rheumatoid arthritis
 systemic lupus erythematosus
Nutritional disorders
 pyridoxine deficiency
 vitamin A deficiency
Renal disorders
 interstitial nephritis
 renal failure

Anal and rectal bleeding
Gastro-intestinal and related disorders
 anal fissure
 anorectal fistula
 Crohn's disease
 haemorrhoids

 polyps
 proctitis

Anal discomfort *see also* Anogenital lesions
Gastro-intestinal and related disorders
 anal fissure
 anorectal fistula
 haemorrhoids
 proctitis

Anal skin tag
Gastro-intestinal and related disorders
 anal fissure
 haemorrhoids

Anginal pain *see* Chest pain

Anogenital lesions *see also* Anal discomfort *and* Vaginal
discomfort
Infections
 herpesvirus infections (HSV 2)
Skin disorders
 lichen planus

Anorexia *see* Loss of appetite

Appetite, loss of *see* Loss of appetite

Arthralgia *see* Joint pain and tenderness

Aura
Nervous system disorders
 epilepsy
 migraine

—————————— B ——————————

Back pain and tenderness
[*back ache; loin pain; loin tenderness; lumbago*]
Cardiovascular system disorders
 aortic aneurysm
Gynaecological disorders
 dysmenorrhoea
 endometriosis
Infections
 African trypanosomiasis
 brucellosis
 chickenpox
 herpes zoster
 influenza
 lymphatic filariasis
 Marburg disease and Ebola fever
 prostatitis
 pyelonephritis
 salpingitis
 tetanus
 viral meningitis
 yellow fever
Malignant disease
 cervical cancer
 renal cell carcinoma

Musculoskeletal and connective tissue disorders
  ankylosing spondylitis
  fibrositis
  osteoporosis
  sciatica
Nervous system disorders
  anxiety
Renal disorders
  acute glomerulonephritis
  acute renal failure
  polycystic kidney disease
  renal calculi and colic

Bad breath *see* Breath, abnormal odour

Behaviour disturbances *see also* Emotional disturbances *and*
Perception disturbances
[*aggression; agitation; confusion; delirium; delirium tremens; exhibitionism; hyperactivity; intolerance of noise; involuntary
noises; irrationality; loss of concentration; loss of self control;
obsession; personality disorders; promiscuity; psychoses;
resistance to change; restlessness; self-neglect; temper tantrums;
unreliability; violence; wild and illogical speech; withdrawn*]
Blood and lymph disorders
  thrombotic thrombocytopenic purpura
Cardiovascular system disorders
  atherosclerosis in cerebral arteries
Endocrine disorders
  hypoglycaemia
  hypopituitarism
  primary aldosteronism
  type I diabetes mellitus
Infections
  African trypanosomiasis
  cryptococcal meningitis
  cysticercosis
  encephalitis
  infective endocarditis
  paratyphoid fever
  Pontiac fever
  postviral fatigue syndrome
  psittacosis
  pyogenic meningitis
  rabies
  typhoid fever
  typhus fevers
Malignant disease
  insulinoma
  intracranial tumours
Metabolic disorders
  hepatolenticular degeneration
  hypercalcaemia
  hypernatraemia
  hypocalcaemia
  hyponatraemia
  porphyrias
Musculoskeletal and connective tissue disorders
  polyarteritis nodosa
  systemic lupus erythematosus
Nervous system disorders
  anxiety
  autism
  cerebral palsy
  chorea

  dementia
  depressive disorders
  dialysis encephalopathy
  drug dependence
  extradural haemorrhage
  Gilles de la Tourette syndrome
  hepatic encephalopathy
  mania and manic-depressive illness
  mental retardation
  post-tonic-clonic epileptic seizures
  schizophrenia
  subarachnoid haemorrhage
  subdural haemorrhage
  tardive dyskinesia
Nutritional disorders
  anorexia nervosa
  beri-beri
  bulimia nervosa
Renal disorders
  renal failure

Blinking *see also* Eyelid fluttering
Eye disorders
  corneal ulceration
Nervous system disorders
  Gilles de la Tourette syndrome

Blister *see* Skin lesions

Blood from the anus *see* Anal and rectal bleeding

Blood from the nipple *see* Breast abnormalities

Blood in saliva *see* Saliva, blood in

Blood in sputum *see* Sputum

Blood in stools *see* Faeces, changes in

Blood in urine *see* Urine abnormalities

Blood in vomit *see* Nausea and/or vomiting

Body odour
Metabolic disorders
  phenylketonuria
Skin disorders
  bromhidrosis

Bone pain and tenderness *see also* Joint pain and tenderness
Blood and lymph disorders
  sickle-cell anaemia
Endocrine disorders
  hyperparathyroidism
Gastro-intestinal and related disorders
  coeliac disease
Infections
  osteomyelitis
Malignant disease
  acute leukaemias
  Hodgkin's disease

myeloma
prostatic cancer
Musculoskeletal and connective tissue disorders
osteitis deformans
osteoporosis
Nutritional disorders
osteomalacia
Renal disorders
renal osteodystrophy

Bone structure abnormalities *see also* Joint abnormalities *and* Skeletal deformity
[*bone destruction; bone weakness; brittle bones; fracture*]
Endocrine disorders
hyperparathyroidism
Gynaecological disorders
Turner's syndrome
Infections
osteomyelitis
Malignant disease
myeloma
Musculoskeletal and connective tissue disorders
osteitis deformans
osteopetrosis
osteoporosis
Renal disorders
renal osteodystrophy

Bony projections on fingers
[*Heberden's nodes*]
Musculoskeletal and connective tissue disorders
osteoarthritis

Breast abnormalities
[*blood from the nipple; breast cancer; breast discomfort; breast distortion; breast size, decreased; breast tenderness; gynaecomastia; lump in the breast; retracted nipple*]
Endocrine disorders
adrenal virilisation
hyperthyroidism
hypogonadism
Gastro-intestinal and related disorders
cirrhosis of the liver
Gynaecological disorders
premenstrual syndrome
Male genital disorders
Klinefelter's syndrome
Malignant disease
breast cancer

Breath, abnormal odour
[*halitosis; ketones on the breath*]
Endocrine disorders
type I diabetes mellitus
Infections
herpesvirus infections (HSV 1)
Vincent's infection

Breathing difficulties
[*apnoea; breathlessness; dyspnoea; hypercapnia; hyperpnoea; hyperventilation; inspiratory 'whoop'; orthopnoea; reduced exercise tolerance; respiratory distress; respiratory failure; sensation of suffocation; stridor; tachypnoea; wheezing*]

Blood and lymph disorders
anaemias
pulmonary embolism and infarction
sickle-cell anaemia
Cardiovascular system disorders
angina pectoris
cardiac arrest
cardiomyopathy
circulatory failure, acute
congestive heart failure
cor pulmonale
hypertension
left heart failure
myocardial infarction
myocarditis
pericarditis
pulmonary hypertension
pulmonary oedema
valvular heart disease
Endocrine disorders
hypothyroidism (neonatal)
Gastro-intestinal and related disorders
acute intestinal ischaemia
ascites
cystic fibrosis
Infections
ascariasis
aspergillosis
botulism
epiglottitis
laryngeal diphtheria
Legionnaire's disease
malaria
pertussis
Pneumocystis carinii pneumonia
pneumonia
pulmonary anthrax
psittacosis
septicaemia
tonsillar diphtheria
trematode infections
trichiniasis
tuberculosis
visceral leishmaniasis
Malignant disease
cancer of the hypopharynx
cancer of the larynx
cancer of the pleura and peritoneum
carcinoid syndrome
chronic lymphoid leukaemia
lung cancer
Metabolic disorders
acidosis
alkalosis
hypocalcaemia
hypokalaemia
Musculoskeletal and connective tissue disorders
muscular dystrophy
polymyositis and dermatomyositis
rheumatoid arthritis
sarcoidosis
systemic juvenile chronic arthritis
systemic sclerosis
Nervous system disorders
anxiety

cerebral oedema
myasthenia gravis
tonic-clonic epileptic seizures
Nose disorders
rhinitis
Nutritional disorders
beri-beri
Renal disorders
glomerulonephritis
Respiratory system disorders
acute bronchitis
alveolitis
asthma
bronchiectasis
chronic bronchitis and emphysema
croup
pleurisy and pleural effusion
pneumoconioses
pneumothorax
respiratory distress syndrome
sudden infant death syndrome
Skin disorders
angioedema
hereditary angioedema

Bruising *see* Skin haemorrhage

Buboes *see* Swelling, glandular

Bullae *see* Skin lesions

──────── C ────────

Chest pain
[*anginal pain; pain around the ribs; tightness in the chest*]
Blood and lymph disorders
anaemias
polycythaemia vera
pulmonary embolism and infarction
Cardiovascular system disorders
angina pectoris
aortic aneurysm
aortic regurgitation
aortic stenosis
atherosclerosis in coronary vessels
atrial fibrillation
cardiomyopathy
mitral stenosis
myocardial infarction
myocarditis
pericarditis
pulmonary hypertension
tricuspid stenosis
Endocrine disorders
hyperthyroidism
Gastro-intestinal and related disorders
achalasia
acute gastritis
dyspepsia
hiatus hernia
reflux oesophagitis

Infections
cryptococcosis
Lassa fever
legionellosis
Marburg disease and Ebola fever
plague
pneumonia
post-primary pulmonary tuberculosis
trematode infections
Malignant disease
cancer of the pleura and peritoneum
lung cancer
oesophageal cancer
phaeochromocytoma
Musculoskeletal and connective tissue disorders
ankylosing spondylitis
sarcoidosis
Nervous system disorders
anxiety
Respiratory system disorders
asthma
extrinsic allergic alveolitis
pleurisy and pleural effusion
pneumothorax

Chills and sensation of intense cold *see also* Shivering
Gastro-intestinal and related disorders
cholangitis
choledocholithiasis
Infections
chickenpox
cutaneous anthrax
Lassa fever
leptospirosis
malaria
mumps
plague
pseudomembranous colitis
psittacosis
salmonellosis
scarlet fever
septicaemia
Obstetric disorders
septic abortion

Clubbing of the fingers
Gastro-intestinal and related disorders
cirrhosis of the liver
Whipple's disease

Cold extremities *see also* Cyanosis
Infections
postviral fatigue syndrome
Nutritional disorders
anorexia nervosa

Cold intolerance
Endocrine disorders
hypopituitarism
hypothyroidism

Cold skin *see* Cyanosis

Colic *see* Abdominal pain and discomfort

Coma *see* Consciousness, loss of

Consciousness, impaired *see also* Consciousness, loss of
[*stupor*]
Infections
  cholera
  encephalitis
  psittacosis
  septicaemia
  tuberculous meningitis
  typhus fevers
Malignant disease
  intracranial tumours
Metabolic disorders
  hypercalcaemia
  respiratory acidosis
Nervous system disorders
  cerebral oedema
  hepatic encephalopathy
  hypertensive encephalopathy
  subarachnoid haemorrhage
  subdural haemorrhage
  tonic-clonic epileptic seizures

Consciousness, loss of *see also* Consciousness, impaired
[*coma*]
Cardiovascular system disorders
  cardiac arrest
  heart block
Endocrine disorders
  hypoglycaemia
  hypothyroidism
  type I diabetes mellitus
Gastro-intestinal and related disorders
  cirrhosis of the liver
Infections
  acquired immunodeficiency syndrome
  African trypanosomiasis
  cholera
  encephalitis
  paratyphoid fever
  pyogenic meningitis
  rabies
  tuberculous meningitis
  typhoid fever
Malignant disease
  insulinoma
Metabolic disorders
  hepatolenticular degeneration
  hypercalcaemia
  hypernatraemia
  respiratory acidosis
Nervous system disorders
  absence seizures
  cerebral oedema
  hepatic encephalopathy
  hypertensive encephalopathy
  Reye's syndrome
  stroke
  subarachnoid haemorrhage
  tonic-clonic epileptic seizures

Nutritional disorders
  beri-beri
Obstetric disorders
  pre-eclampsia and eclampsia
Renal disorders
  renal failure

Constipation *see also* Altered bowel habit, Diarrhoea, *and*
Constipation and diarrhoea
Non-specific causes
  change from breast to bottle feeding
  drugs
  inadequate dietary fibre
  incomplete bowel emptying
  insufficient exercise
  lack of response to defaecation stimulus
  painful anal conditions
Blood and lymph disorders
  anaemias
Endocrine disorders
  hypothyroidism
  type I diabetes mellitus
Gastro-intestinal and related disorders
  anal fissure
  appendicitis
  diverticular disease
  haemorrhoids
  ileus
  pyloric stenosis
Infections
  botulism
Malignant disease
  cancer of the bile ducts
Metabolic disorders
  hypercalcaemia
  porphyrias
Nervous system disorders
  parkinsonism
Nutritional disorders
  anorexia nervosa

Constipation and diarrhoea *see also* Altered bowel habit,
Constipation, *and* Diarrhoea
Gastro-intestinal and related disorders
  congenital megacolon
  diverticular disease
  irritable bowel syndrome
Infections
  paratyphoid fever
  typhoid fever

Convulsions *see also* Seizures
Blood and lymph disorders
  thrombotic thrombocytopenic purpura
Endocrine disorders
  hypoglycaemia
Gastro-intestinal and related disorders
  kernicterus
Infections
  acquired immunodeficiency syndrome
  African trypanosomiasis
  cholera
  encephalitis
  listeriosis

meningococcal infections
mumps
pertussis
rabies
toxoplasmosis (congenital)
tuberculous meningitis
Malignant disease
insulinoma
Metabolic disorders
hepatolenticular degeneration
hypocalcaemia
hyponatraemia
maple-syrup urine disease
phenylketonuria
porphyrias
respiratory alkalosis
Musculoskeletal and connective tissue disorders
systemic lupus erythematosus
Nervous system disorders
alcohol withdrawal
barbiturate withdrawal
dementia
dialysis encephalopathy
hydrocephalus
hypertensive encephalopathy
mental retardation
Reye's syndrome
subarachnoid haemorrhage
Nutritional disorders
bulimia nervosa
pyridoxine deficiency
Obstetric disorders
pre-eclampsia and eclampsia
Renal disorders
renal failure

Co-ordination impaired *see also* Movement difficulties

Endocrine disorders
hypoglycaemia
Infections
encephalitis
Malignant disease
intracranial tumours
Nervous system disorders
alcohol-type drug dependence
cannabis-type drug dependence
chorea
Guillain-Barré syndrome
multiple sclerosis
parkinsonism
volatile solvent-type drug dependence

Corneal changes *see also* Eye pain and discomfort

[*corneal thickening; corneal ulceration; dry cornea; kerato-malacia*]
Eye disorders
dry eye
ectropion and entropion
exophthalmos
Infections
ophthalmia neonatorum
trachoma
Nutritional disorders
vitamin A deficiency

Cough
[*dry cough; productive cough*]
Non-specific causes
inhalation of irritants (e.g. tobacco smoke)
Cardiovascular system disorders
aortic aneurysm
heart failure
mitral stenosis
Infections
ascariasis
aspergillosis
common cold
cryptococcosis
influenza
laryngeal diphtheria
Lassa fever
legionellosis
leptospirosis
Marburg disease and Ebola fever
measles
paratyphoid fever
pertussis
plague
Pneumocystis carinii pneumonia
pneumonia
psittacosis
pulmonary actinomycosis
pulmonary anthrax
strongyloidiasis
toxocariasis
trematode infections
tuberculosis
typhoid fever
visceral leishmaniasis
Malignant disease
cancer of the pleura and peritoneum
lung cancer
Musculoskeletal and connective tissue disorders
sarcoidosis
Nose disorders
rhinitis
Oropharyngeal disorders
laryngitis
Respiratory system disorders
acute bronchitis
alveolitis
asthma
bronchiectasis
chronic bronchitis and emphysema
croup
pleurisy
pneumoconioses
pulmonary oedema

Cramp *see* Muscle spasm

Cyanosis *see also* Cold extremities
Blood and lymph disorders
pulmonary embolism and infarction
Cardiovascular system disorders
acrocyanosis
left heart failure
pulmonary hypertension
Raynaud's syndrome

right heart failure
shock
Gastro-intestinal and related disorders
acute intestinal ischaemia
Infections
cholera
laryngeal diphtheria
Pneumocystis carinii pneumonia
psittacosis
Malignant disease
carcinoid syndrome
phaeochromocytoma
Nervous system disorders
tonic-clonic epileptic seizures
Respiratory system disorders
pneumothorax
pulmonary oedema
respiratory distress syndrome

Cyst

Endocrine disorders
hyperparathyroidism
Gynaecological disorders
benign mammary dysplasia
Skin disorders
acne vulgaris
pilonidal disease

——————— D ———————

Dehydration

Endocrine disorders
diabetes insipidus
type I diabetes mellitus
Gastro-intestinal and related disorders
ascites
gastro-enteritis
ileus
peritonitis
pyloric stenosis
toxic megacolon
ulcerative colitis
Infections
cholera
dysentery
shigellosis
Metabolic disorders
galactosaemia
Nervous system disorders
motion sickness
Renal disorders
renal failure
Skin disorders
exfoliative dermatitis

Dental abnormalities

Endocrine disorders
hypoparathyroidism
Nutritional disorders
scurvy

Developmental abnormalities *see also* Failure to thrive
[*growth rate accelerated; growth rate slowed; impaired intellectual
development; impaired physical development; impaired sexual development; late onset of walking and crawling; latent development;
premature sexual development; retarded development*]
Blood and lymph disorders
beta thalassaemia
Endocrine disorders
adrenal virilisation
Cushing's syndrome
growth hormone deficiency
hypogonadism
hypopituitarism
precocious puberty
Gynaecological disorders
Turner's syndrome
Infections
ascariasis
cytomegalovirus infection
(congenital)
hookworm infection
Lyme disease
Metabolic disorders
glycogen storage diseases
pseudohypoparathyroidism
Musculoskeletal and connective tissue disorders
muscular dystrophy
osteopetrosis
Nutritional disorders
acrodermatitis enteropathica
rickets
vitamin A deficiency
zinc deficiency
Renal disorders
renal osteodystrophy

Diarrhoea *see also* Altered bowel habit, Constipation, *and*
Constipation and diarrhoea
Non-specific causes
allergic reaction to food or drugs
drugs (e.g. antibacterials)
excessive dietary sugar
excessive use of laxatives
excessive use of sugar substitutes
Blood and lymph disorders
amyloidosis
anaemias
lymphangiectasia
Endocrine disorders
Addison's disease
adrenocortical insufficiency, acute
hyperthyroidism
Gastro-intestinal and related disorders
acute intestinal ischaemia
chronic pancreatitis
coeliac disease
Crohn's disease
cystic fibrosis
diverticular disease
gastro-enteritis
short-bowel syndrome
toxic megacolon
tropical sprue
ulcerative colitis

Gynaecological disorders
  endometriosis
  primary dysmenorrhoea
Infections
  acquired immunodeficiency syndrome
  acute fulminating meningococcaemia
  amoebiasis
  ascariasis
  botulism
  cestode infections
  cholera
  dracontiasis
  dysentery
  giardiasis
  Lassa fever
  legionellosis
  listeriosis
  malaria
  Marburg disease and Ebola fever
  measles
  poliomyelitis
  pseudomembranous colitis
  septicaemia
  shigellosis
  strongyloidiasis
  toxic shock syndrome
  trematode infections
  trichiniasis
  trichuriasis
  upper respiratory-tract infections
  urinary-tract infections
  visceral leishmaniasis
Malignant disease
  cancer of the bile ducts
  carcinoid syndrome
  colorectal cancer
  glucagonoma
  Zollinger-Ellison syndrome
Metabolic disorders
  galactosaemia
  porphyrias
Nervous system disorders
  anxiety
  diabetic neuropathy
  opiate withdrawal
Nutritional disorders
  acrodermatitis enteropathica
  lactose intolerance
  pellagra
Renal disorders
  renal failure

Dizziness

Blood and lymph disorders
  anaemias
  polycythaemia vera
Cardiovascular system disorders
  atrial fibrillation
  hypertension
  orthostatic hypotension
Ear disorders
  labyrinthitis
  Ménière's disease
  otosclerosis

Infections
  botulism
  cestode infections
  influenza
  Lassa fever
Malignant disease
  intracranial tumours
Nervous system disorders
  anxiety
  motion sickness
  multiple sclerosis
  partial seizures
  syringobulbia
  transient ischaemic attacks
  vertigo

Dribbling, persistent
Metabolic disorders
  hepatolenticular degeneration
Nervous system disorders
  Bell's palsy
  cerebral palsy
  parkinsonism

Dry cough *see* Cough

──────────────── E ────────────────

Ear discharge
Ear disorders
  acute otitis media
  chronic otitis media
  otitis externa
Infections
  myiasis

Ear pain
Non-specific causes
  hard wax
  injury
  referred pain (e.g. in herpes zoster)
  unerupted lower molars
Ear disorders
  acute otitis media
  chronic otitis media
  mastoiditis
  otitis externa
Infections
  myiasis
  tonsillitis
  upper respiratory-tract infections
Malignant disease
  cancer of the pharynx
  cancer of the tongue

Eczema
Cardiovascular system disorders
  varicose veins
Infections
  scabies
Metabolic disorders
  phenylketonuria

Nutritional disorders
  acrodermatitis enteropathica

Emotional disturbances *see also* Behaviour disturbances *and*
Perception disturbances
[*anxiety; apathy; apprehension; depression; elation; excitement;
insomnia; irritability; loss of interest; monotonous and slowed
speech; nervousness; neurosis; panic reactions; sensation of fear;
sleep disturbance; stress; waking early*]
Blood and lymph disorders
  anaemias
Cardiovascular system disorders
  myocardial infarction
Endocrine disorders
  adrenocortical insufficiency, acute
  Cushing's syndrome
  hyperparathyroidism
  hyperthyroidism
  hypoglycaemia
  hypoparathyroidism
  type I diabetes mellitus
Gastro-intestinal and related disorders
  acute intestinal ischaemia
Gynaecological disorders
  menopause
  premenstrual syndrome
Infections
  cestode infections
  enterobiasis
  poliomyelitis
  pneumonia
  post-primary pulmonary tuberculosis
  postviral fatigue syndrome
  rabies
Malignant disease
  intracranial tumours
  myeloma
  phaeochromocytoma
Metabolic disorders
  metabolic alkalosis
  porphyrias
Musculoskeletal and connective tissue disorders
  systemic lupus erythematosus
Nervous system disorders
  anxiety
  chorea
  dementia
  depressive disorders
  dialysis encephalopathy
  drug dependence
  hepatic encephalopathy
  mania and manic-depressive illness
  parkinsonism
  partial seizures
  Reye's syndrome
  schizophrenia
  subarachnoid haemorrhage
Nutritional disorders
  anorexia nervosa
  bulimia nervosa
Renal disorders
  renal failure
Respiratory system disorders
  pulmonary oedema

Eructation *see* Flatulence and eructation

Erythema *see* Skin redness

Eye abscess
Eye disorders
  dacryocystitis

Eye closure, inability
Nervous system disorders
  Bell's palsy

Eye discharge
Eye disorders
  conjunctivitis
Infections
  ophthalmia neonatorum
  trachoma

Eye discoloration
Eye disorders
  chalazion
  scleritis and episcleritis

Eye inflammation and congestion
Eye disorders
  conjunctivitis
  entropion
  uveitis
Infections
  herpesvirus infections
  Lassa fever
  leptospirosis
  measles
  myiasis
  ophthalmia neonatorum
  rubella
  toxic shock syndrome
  trachoma
  yellow fever
Nervous system disorders
  cluster headache

Eye movement restricted
Eye disorders
  exophthalmos
Infections
  tuberculous meningitis

Eye pain and discomfort *see also* Corneal changes
[*dry eye; eye irritation; eye movement, painful; retro-orbital pain*]
Non-specific causes
  eyelid defects
  local infection
  reduced tear flow caused by:
    ageing
    inflammation of the lachrymal glands
Eye disorders
  closed-angle glaucoma
  corneal ulceration
  dacryocystitis
  dry eye

ectropion and entropion
optic neuropathies
scleritis and episcleritis
uveitis
Infections
common cold
trachoma
viral meningitis
Musculoskeletal and connective tissue disorders
rheumatoid arthritis
systemic lupus erythematosus
Nervous system disorders
Bell's palsy

Eye swelling

Endocrine disorders
hypothyroidism
Infections
infectious mononucleosis
ophthalmia neonatorum

Eye, watery

[*epiphora; lachrymation*]
Non-specific causes
foreign body
irritants
obstruction of the lachrymal duct
Eye disorders
blepharitis
corneal ulceration
dacryocystitis
ectropion and entropion
scleritis and episcleritis
uveitis
Infections
trachoma
Nervous system disorders
Bell's palsy
opiate withdrawal
Nose disorders
rhinitis

Eyelid discharge

Infections
stye

Eyelid fluttering *see also* Blinking

[*blepharospasm*]
Eye disorders
dry eye
Nervous system disorders
absence seizures

Eyelid lag and retraction

Endocrine disorders
hyperthyroidism

Eyelid pain

Infections
stye

Eyelid scaling and crusting

Eye disorders
blepharitis

Eyelid swelling
Eye disorders
blepharitis
chalazion
conjunctivitis
Infections
myiasis
stye
trachoma
Nervous system disorders
cluster headache
Skin disorders
seborrhoeic dermatitis

Eyelid ulceration
Eye disorders
blepharitis

———————————— F ————————————

Facial expression, abnormal changes in
Nervous system disorders
absence seizures

Facial features, changed

[*blank expression; bloated face; coarsening of facial features; facial distortion; facial mass; facial mooning; facial palsy; facial paralysis and sagging; hollow cheeks; mask-like expression; swelling around the eye*]
Endocrine disorders
acromegaly
Cushing's syndrome
hypothyroidism
Infections
lepromatous leprosy
mucocutaneous leishmaniasis
pyogenic meningitis
tuberculous meningitis
Malignant disease
cancer of the salivary glands
Nervous system disorders
Bell's palsy
parkinsonism

Facial flushing *see also* Hot flushes *and* Skin redness
Endocrine disorders
Cushing's syndrome
Infections
scarlet fever
typhus fevers
yellow fever
Malignant disease
carcinoid syndrome

Facial pain and discomfort

[*sinus pain; pain around one eye*]
Malignant disease
cancer of the pharynx
cancer of the salivary glands
Nervous system disorders
Bell's palsy

cluster headache
trigeminal neuralgia
Nose disorders
sinusitis

Faeces, changes in

[*blood in the stools; bloody diarrhoea; faecal mucus; faeces, discoloration; melaena; steatorrhoea; stools, unusual*]
Blood and lymph disorders
lymphangiectasia
Cardiovascular system disorders
oesophageal varices
Gastro-intestinal and related disorders
acute gastritis
acute hepatitis
acute intestinal ischaemia
cholangitis
cholestatic jaundice
chronic pancreatitis
coeliac disease
cystic fibrosis
haemolytic jaundice
irritable bowel syndrome
ischaemic colitis
peptic ulceration
short-bowel syndrome
tropical sprue
ulcerative colitis
Whipple's disease
Infections
amoebiasis
ascariasis
dysentery
giardiasis
Marburg disease and Ebola fever
salmonellal infections
schistosomiasis
shigellosis
trichuriasis
yellow fever
Malignant disease
cancer of the bile ducts
colorectal cancer
Zollinger-Ellison syndrome

Failure to thrive *see also* Developmental abnormalities *and*
Feeding and swallowing difficulties
Blood and lymph disorders
beta thalassaemia
Gastro-intestinal and related disorders
congenital megacolon
cystic fibrosis
Infections
giardiasis
Metabolic disorders
galactosaemia
hereditary fructose intolerance
Nervous system disorders
mental retardation
Nutritional disorders
lactose intolerance

Fainting

[*syncope*]

Blood and lymph disorders
pulmonary embolism and infarction
Cardiovascular system disorders
aortic stenosis
atrial fibrillation
cardiomyopathy
heart block
orthostatic hypotension
pulmonary hypertension
shock
tricuspid stenosis
Infections
salmonellosis
Obstetric disorders
ectopic pregnancy

Fatigue *see also* Prostration

[*debilitation; drowsiness; exhaustion; lassitude; lethargy; physical depression; somnolence; tiredness; weakness*]
Blood and lymph disorders
anaemias
polycythaemia vera
Cardiovascular system disorders
heart failure
mitral regurgitation
myocarditis
pulmonary hypertension
shock
Endocrine disorders
Addison's disease
adrenocortical insufficiency, acute
hyperthyroidism
hypoglycaemia
hypopituitarism
hypothyroidism
subacute thyroiditis
type I diabetes mellitus
Gastro-intestinal and related disorders
chronic hepatitis
coeliac disease
Crohn's disease
gastro-enteritis
irritable bowel syndrome
kernicterus
ulcerative colitis
Whipple's disease
Gynaecological disorders
premenstrual syndrome
Infections
acquired immunodeficiency syndrome
cestode infections
cholera
cryptococcal meningitis
dysentery
encephalitis
giardiasis
infectious mononucleosis
Legionnaire's disease
Lyme disease
plague
pneumonia
poliomyelitis
pyelonephritis
rabies

septicaemia
syphilis
tonsillar diphtheria
toxic shock syndrome
toxoplasmosis
trypanosomiasis
viral meningitis
visceral leishmaniasis
Malignant disease
acute leukaemias
cancer of the pleura and peritoneum
cancer of the stomach
colorectal cancer
insulinoma
intracranial tumours
lung cancer
pancreatic (exocrine) cancer
renal cell carcinoma
Metabolic disorders
acidosis
hypercalcaemia
hypernatraemia
maple-syrup urine disease
Nervous system disorders
amphetamine withdrawal
anxiety
dialysis encephalopathy
hepatic encephalopathy
Huntington's chorea
mania and manic-depressive illness
mental retardation
opiate-type drug dependence
parkinsonism
Reye's syndrome
subarachnoid haemorrhage
Nutritional disorders
scurvy
Renal disorders
chronic glomerulonephritis
interstitial nephritis
renal failure
Respiratory system disorders
asthma
chronic bronchitis and emphysema

Feeding and swallowing difficulties *see also* Failure to thrive
and Swallowing difficulties
[*difficulty in chewing, eating, and speaking; regurgitation of food*]
Endocrine disorders
hypothyroidism (neonatal)
Gastro-intestinal and related disorders
achalasia
congenital megacolon
hiatus hernia
reflux oesophagitis
Infections
meningococcal infections
Malignant disease
cancer of the mouth
Metabolic disorders
maple-syrup urine disease
Nervous system disorders
Bell's palsy
myasthenia gravis

Oropharyngeal disorders
glossitis

Feeling of satiety
[*abdominal fullness*]
Blood and lymph disorders
splenomegaly
Gastro-intestinal and related disorders
dyspepsia
Malignant disease
cancer of the stomach

Fever
[*pyrexia*]
Blood and lymph disorders
agranulocytosis
anaphylactoid purpura
thrombotic thrombocytopenic purpura
Cardiovascular system disorders
myocarditis
Ear disorders
acute otitis media
mastoiditis
Endocrine disorders
subacute thyroiditis
Gastro-intestinal and related disorders
acute cholecystitis
acute pancreatitis
appendicitis
cholangitis
choledocholithiasis
cirrhosis of the liver
Crohn's disease
diverticular disease
gastro-enteritis
peritonitis
toxic megacolon
tropical sprue
ulcerative colitis
Whipple's disease
Infections
amoebiasis
ascariasis
bacterial infections, many
chronic pulmonary aspergillosis
cryptococcosis
filariasis
malaria
Pneumocystis carinii pneumonia
primary amoebic meningo-encephalitis
schistosomiasis
toxocariasis
toxoplasmosis
trichiniasis
trypanosomiasis
viral infections, many
visceral leishmaniasis
Male genital disorders
torsion of the testis
Malignant disease
cancer of the liver
cancer of the pleura and peritoneum
chronic lymphoid leukaemia
lymphomas
renal cancer

Metabolic disorders
  gout
Musculoskeletal and connective tissue disorders
  giant cell arteritis
  polyarteritis nodosa
  polymyalgia rheumatica
  rheumatoid arthritis
  sarcoidosis
  systemic juvenile chronic arthritis
Nervous system disorders
  malignant hyperthermia
Nose disorders
  sinusitis
Obstetric disorders
  septic abortion
Oropharyngeal disorders
  aphthous stomatitis
  pharyngitis
  sialadenitis
Renal disorders
  acute glomerulonephritis
  interstitial nephritis
Respiratory system disorders
  croup
  extrinsic allergic alveolitis
Skin disorders
  erythema nodosum
  exfoliative dermatitis
  pityriasis lichenoides
  Stevens-Johnson syndrome
  toxic epidermal necrolysis

Flatulence and eructation
Gastro-intestinal and related disorders
  cholecystitis
  irritable bowel syndrome
  dyspepsia
Infections
  giardiasis

Foot discomfort
Blood and lymph disorders
  sickle-cell anaemia
Endocrine disorders
  acromegaly
Musculoskeletal and connective tissue disorders
  ankylosing spondylitis
Skin disorders
  callosities and corns

—————————— G ——————————

Gangrene
Blood and lymph disorders
  embolism
Cardiovascular system disorders
  atherosclerosis in leg arteries
Gastro-intestinal and related disorders
  acute intestinal ischaemia

Gum disorders *see* Oropharyngeal lesions

—————————— H ——————————

Hair loss
[*alopecia*]
Endocrine disorders
  hyperthyroidism
  hypoparathyroidism
  hypopituitarism
Infections
  tinea capitis
Musculoskeletal and connective tissue disorders
  systemic lupus erythematosus
Nutritional disorders
  acrodermatitis enteropathica
Skin disorders
  alopecia
  exfoliative dermatitis

Hand discomfort
Blood and lymph disorders
  sickle-cell anaemia
Endocrine disorders
  acromegaly
Musculoskeletal and connective tissue disorders
  systemic sclerosis
Skin disorders
  callosities

Headache
Non-specific causes
  neck stiffness
  prolonged car driving
  psychogenic causes
Blood and lymph disorders
  anaemias
  polycythaemia vera
Cardiovascular system disorders
  cerebral aneurysm
  hypertension (severe)
Endocrine disorders
  acromegaly
Eye disorders
  glaucoma
Gastro-intestinal and related disorders
  irritable bowel syndrome
Gynaecological disorders
  menopause
  premenstrual syndrome
  primary dysmenorrhoea
Infections
  acquired immunodeficiency syndrome
  African trypanosomiasis
  brucellosis
  cellulitis
  chickenpox
  cryptococcal meningitis
  cutaneous anthrax
  encephalitis
  erysipelas
  infectious mononucleosis
  influenza
  Lassa fever
  legionellosis

leptospirosis
Lyme disease
lymphangitis
malaria
Marburg disease and Ebola fever
meningitis
meningococcal infections
mumps
plague
pneumonia
poliomyelitis
postviral fatigue syndrome
psittacosis
rabies
rubella
salmonellal infections
shigellosis
syphilis
tonsillar diphtheria
tonsillitis
toxic shock syndrome
typhus fevers
yellow fever
Malignant disease
insulinoma
intracranial tumours
myeloma
phaeochromocytoma
Metabolic disorders
respiratory acidosis
Musculoskeletal and connective tissue disorders
arthritis
cervical spondylosis
fibrositis
giant cell arteritis
osteitis deformans
osteomyelitis
Nervous system disorders
anxiety
barbiturate withdrawal
hydrocephalus
hypertensive encephalopathy
migraine
post-tonic-clonic epileptic seizures
stroke
subarachnoid haemorrhage
subdural haemorrhage
trigeminal neuralgia
Nose disorders
sinusitis
Obstetric disorders
pre-eclampsia and eclampsia
Renal disorders
acute glomerulonephritis
Respiratory system disorders
chronic bronchitis and emphysema
Skin disorders
pityriasis lichenoides

Hearing impairment *see also* Sensory derangement
Non-specific causes
drugs (e.g. gentamicin and other aminoglycosides)
foreign body
occlusion of the Eustachian tube
wax

Ear disorders
labyrinthitis
mastoiditis
Ménière's disease
otitis externa
otitis media
otosclerosis
Infections
cytomegalovirus infection (congenital)
Lassa fever
pyogenic meningitis
toxoplasmosis (congenital)
tuberculous meningitis
typhus fevers
Malignant disease
cancer of the nasopharynx
Musculoskeletal and connective tissue disorders
osteitis deformans
osteopetrosis
Nervous system disorders
cerebral palsy
syringobulbia
transient ischaemic attacks
Nose disorders
rhinitis

Heart beat abnormalities

[*arrhythmias; atrial fibrillation; bradycardia; ECG changes; heart block; heart conduction defects; heart murmurs; palpitations; tachycardia*]
Blood and lymph disorders
amyloidosis
anaemias
Cardiovascular system disorders
arrhythmias
atherosclerosis in coronary vessels
cardiomyopathy
congestive heart failure
cor pulmonale
left heart failure
myocardial infarction
myocarditis
pericarditis
valvular heart disease
Endocrine disorders
hyperthyroidism
hypoglycaemia
Gastro-intestinal and related disorders
peritonitis
toxic megacolon
Infections
brucellosis
cholera
gas gangrene
hookworm infection
infective endocarditis
lymphangitis
malaria
psittacosis
scarlet fever
tetanus
trichiniasis
Malignant disease
carcinoid syndrome

insulinoma
phaeochromocytoma
Metabolic disorders
hyperkalaemia
hypokalaemia
porphyrias
Musculoskeletal and connective tissue disorders
polyarteritis nodosa
systemic sclerosis
Nervous system disorders
anxiety
barbiturate withdrawal
Respiratory system disorders
asthma

Heat intolerance
Endocrine disorders
hyperthyroidism

Hiccup
Renal disorders
renal failure

Hirsutism
[*excessive facial and body hair*]
Endocrine disorders
acromegaly
adrenal virilisation
Cushing's syndrome
hyperprolactinaemia
Gynaecological disorders
polycystic ovary syndrome

Hot flushes *see also* Facial flushing *and* Skin redness
Gynaecological disorders
menopause
Infections
malaria
Malignant disease
carcinoid syndrome

Hunger
Endocrine disorders
hyperthyroidism
hypoglycaemia
Gastro-intestinal and related disorders
pyloric stenosis
Malignant disease
insulinoma

——————— I ———————

Incontinence
[*faecal incontinence; urinary incontinence*]
Gastro-intestinal and related disorders
acquired megacolon
Infections
typhus fevers
Malignant disease
spinal cord tumours
Nervous system disorders
dementia

multiple sclerosis
spina bifida
tonic-clonic epileptic seizures

Indigestion
[*dyspepsia; heartburn*]
Non-specific causes
dental:
ill-fitting dentures
deficient teeth
dental caries
overindulgence in food or alcohol
Cardiovascular system disorders
ischaemic heart disease
Endocrine disorders
hyperparathyroidism
Gastro-intestinal and related disorders
cholecystitis
chronic gastritis
hiatus hernia
peptic ulceration
reflux oesophagitis
Malignant disease
cancer of the gall bladder
cancer of the stomach
pancreatic cancer

Infection, increased susceptibility to
Blood and lymph disorders
agranulocytosis
aplastic anaemia
haemolytic anaemias
Gastro-intestinal and related disorders
cystic fibrosis
Infections
prostatitis
Malignant disease
most types
Musculoskeletal and connective tissue disorders
muscular dystrophy
osteopetrosis
Nervous system disorders
opiate-type drug dependence
Nutritional disorders
vitamin A deficiency
Renal disorders
nephrotic syndrome
polycystic kidney disease
renal calculi and colic
Respiratory system disorders
bronchiectasis
Skin disorders
exfoliative dermatitis

Infertility *see also* Sexual disturbances
Endocrine disorders
hyperprolactinaemia
hypogonadism
hypopituitarism
Gynaecological disorders
endometriosis
polycystic ovary syndrome
Male genital disorders
Klinefelter's syndrome

Itch
[*pruritus; pruritus ani; pruritus vulvae*]
Non-specific causes
  allergy
  drugs (e.g. antibacterials)
  dry skin (especially in the elderly)
  hyperhidrosis
  irritants
  poor hygiene
  pregnancy
  psychosexual disorders
  rectal prolapse
Blood and lymph disorders
  iron-deficiency anaemia
  polycythaemia vera
Cardiovascular system disorders
  chilblains
  varicose veins
Ear disorders
  otitis externa
Endocrine disorders
  diabetes mellitus
  thyroid disorders
Eye disorders
  blepharitis
  conjunctivitis
Gastro-intestinal and related disorders
  anal fissure
  anorectal fistula
  cholangitis
  choledocholithiasis
  cholestatic jaundice
  cirrhosis of the liver
  colitis
  Crohn's disease
  diarrhoea
  haemorrhoids
  proctitis
Gynaecological disorders
  vaginitis
  vulvitis
Infections
  African trypanosomiasis
  cestode infections
  chickenpox
  cystitis
  enterobiasis
  filariasis
  herpes labialis
  hookworm infection
  impetigo
  Lyme disease
  pediculosis capitis
  pediculosis corporis
  pityriasis versicolor
  salpingitis
  scabies
  schistosomiasis
  skin candidiasis
  strongyloidiasis
  tinea infections
  trichomoniasis
  vaginal candidiasis
Malignant disease
  cancer of the bile ducts
  colorectal cancer
  Hodgkin's disease
  melanoma
  vulval neoplasm
Nose disorders
  rhinitis
Renal disorders
  chronic glomerulonephritis
  renal failure
Skin disorders
  eczema
  lichen planus
  pityriasis rosea
  urticaria
Urinary-tract disorders
  incontinence

———————————— J ————————————

Jaw pain
Musculoskeletal and connective tissue disorders
  giant cell arteritis

Joint abnormalities *see also* Bone structure abnormalities,
Joint pain and tenderness, Movement difficulties, *and* Skeletal
deformity
[*ankylosis; joint destruction; joint disease; joint haemorrhages;
joint weakness*]
Blood and lymph disorders
  haemophilia
Infections
  infective arthritis
Musculoskeletal and connective tissue disorders
  ankylosing spondylitis
Nervous system disorders
  diabetic neuropathy
Renal disorders
  renal osteodystrophy

Joint inflammation
Infections
  infective arthritis
  rheumatic fever
Malignant disease
  cancer of the bone
Metabolic disorders
  gout
Musculoskeletal and connective tissue disorders
  ankylosing spondylitis
  frozen shoulder
  juvenile chronic arthritis
  rheumatoid arthritis

Joint pain and tenderness *see also* Bone pain and tenderness
and Joint abnormalities
[*arthralgia*]
Blood and lymph disorders
  anaphylactoid purpura
Endocrine disorders
  acromegaly
Gastro-intestinal and related disorders
  acute hepatitis
  chronic active hepatitis

Infections
  chronic fulminating meningococcaemia
  disseminated gonococcal infection
  infective arthritis
  infective endocarditis
  Lyme disease
  rheumatic fever
  syphilis
  tonsillitis
Malignant disease
  cancer of the bone
Metabolic disorders
  gout
Musculoskeletal and connective tissue disorders
  ankylosing spondylitis
  bursitis
  frozen shoulder
  osteoarthritis
  polyarteritis nodosa
  rheumatoid arthritis
  sarcoidosis
  systemic lupus erythematosus
  systemic sclerosis
  tendinitis and tenosynovitis
Renal disorders
  interstitial nephritis
Respiratory system disorders
  fibrosing alveolitis
Skin disorders
  erythema nodosum
  Stevens-Johnson syndrome

─────────── L ───────────

Limb discomfort *see also* Muscle spasm
Blood and lymph disorders
  deep vein thrombosis
  embolism
Cardiovascular system disorders
  Raynaud's syndrome
  varicose veins
Gynaecological disorders
  primary dysmenorrhoea
Metabolic disorders
  porphyrias
Nervous system disorders
  restless leg syndrome
Nutritional disorders
  scurvy

Limping
[*intermittent claudication*]
Blood and lymph disorders
  embolism
Cardiovascular system disorders
  atherosclerosis in leg arteries

Lip lesions *see also* Oropharyngeal lesions
[*angular stomatitis; cheilitis; cracked lips; swelling of the lips*]
Endocrine disorders
  type I diabetes mellitus

Infections
  anterior nasal diphtheria
  yellow fever
Malignant disease
  glucagonoma
Nutritional disorders
  pyridoxine deficiency
  riboflavine deficiency

Loss of appetite
[*anorexia*]
Blood and lymph disorders
  anaemias
Endocrine disorders
  Addison's disease
Gastro-intestinal and related disorders
  appendicitis
  congenital megacolon
  dyspepsia
  gastric ulceration
  gastritis
  gastro-enteritis
  hepatitis
  ileus
  kernicterus
  tropical sprue
  tuberculous peritonitis
  ulcerative colitis
Infections
  acquired immunodeficiency syndrome
  actinomycosis
  amoebiasis
  anthrax
  chickenpox
  dysentery
  enterobiasis
  giardiasis
  herpesvirus infections (HSV 2)
  influenza
  legionellosis
  malaria
  meningitis
  psittacosis
  pyelonephritis
  rabies
  salmonellal infections
  schistosomiasis
  secondary syphilis
  shigellosis
  tuberculosis
Malignant disease
  cancer of the hypopharynx
  cancer of the stomach
  chronic leukaemias
  metastatic carcinoma of the liver
  myeloma
  oesophageal cancer
  pancreatic (exocrine) cancer
  Wilms' tumour
Metabolic disorders
  hereditary fructose intolerance
  hypercalcaemia
  hyponatraemia

Nervous system disorders
depressive disorders
motion sickness
Nutritional disorders
scurvy
zinc deficiency
Renal disorders
interstitial nephritis
renal failure
Skin disorders
toxic epidermal necrolysis

—————— M ——————

Memory impairment *see also* Amnesia
Cardiovascular system disorders
atherosclerosis in cerebral arteries
Nervous system disorders
anxiety
dementia
partial seizures

Menstrual disturbances
[*amenorrhoea; dysmenorrhoea; menorrhagia; oligomenorrhoea*]
Blood and lymph disorders
anaemias
thrombocytopenia
Endocrine disorders
adrenal virilisation
Cushing's syndrome
hyperprolactinaemia
hyperthyroidism
hypogonadism
hypothyroidism
Gastro-intestinal and related disorders
chronic active hepatitis
Gynaecological disorders
endometriosis
polycystic ovary syndrome
Turner's syndrome
Infections
gonorrhoea
pelvic actinomycosis
Metabolic disorders
pseudohypoparathyroidism
Nervous system disorders
depressive disorders
Nutritional disorders
anorexia nervosa

Mouth symptoms *see* Oropharyngeal lesions

Movement difficulties *see also* Co-ordination impaired *and*
Joint abnormalities
[*akinesia; apraxia; arm jerking; ataxia; body rocking; chorea;
hemiparesis; hemiplegia; hyperkinesia; immobility; inability to
walk; joint stiffness; lip smacking; neuromuscular disturbances;
paralysis; persistent chewing; 'ram-rod' posture; repetitive nodding; rigidity; spastic syndromes*]
Blood and lymph disorders
haemophilia

Endocrine disorders
primary aldosteronism
Infections
botulism
herpes zoster
Legionnaire's disease
leprosy
osteomyelitis
poliomyelitis
rabies
subacute sclerosing panencephalitis
tetanus
toxoplasmosis (congenital)
Malignant disease
spinal cord tumours
Metabolic disorders
hepatolenticular degeneration
hyperkalaemia
hypokalaemia
phenylketonuria
porphyrias
Musculoskeletal and connective tissue disorders
many disorders
Nervous system disorders
absence seizures
cerebral palsy
chorea
dementia
epilepsy
extradural haemorrhage
Guillain-Barré syndrome
hepatic encephalopathy
hydrocephalus
motor neurone disease
multiple sclerosis
myasthenia gravis
parkinsonism
spina bifida
stroke
subarachnoid haemorrhage
subdural haemorrhage
syringomyelia
tardive dyskinesia
tics
transient ischaemic attacks
Nutritional disorders
beri-beri

Mucus in stools *see* Faeces, changes in

Muscle pain and tenderness *see also* Muscle spasm
[*myalgia*]
Blood and lymph disorders
anaphylactoid purpura
Endocrine disorders
adrenocortical insufficiency, acute
hypothyroidism
Infections
acquired immunodeficiency syndrome
brucellosis
chickenpox
chronic fulminating meningococcaemia
gas gangrene
influenza

Lassa fever
legionellosis
leptospirosis
Lyme disease
malaria
measles
psittacosis
pulmonary anthrax
rabies
secondary syphilis
tonsillitis
toxic shock syndrome
toxoplasmosis
typhus fevers
viral meningitis
yellow fever
Musculoskeletal and connective tissue disorders
fibrositis
polyarteritis nodosa
polymyalgia rheumatica
systemic lupus erythematosus
systemic sclerosis
Nervous system disorders
diabetic neuropathy
motor neurone disease
post-tonic-clonic epileptic seizures

Muscle spasm *see also* Limb discomfort *and* Muscle pain and
tenderness
[*cramp; facial twitching; reflex spasms; tetany; unnatural head
posture*]
Endocrine disorders
primary aldosteronism
type I diabetes mellitus
Infections
cholera
salmonellosis
tetanus
Metabolic disorders
alkalosis
glycogen storage diseases
hypernatraemia
hypocalcaemia
hypokalaemia
Musculoskeletal and connective tissue disorders
many disorders
Nervous system disorders
motor neurone disease
multiple sclerosis
Nutritional disorders
beri-beri
bulimia nervosa
Renal disorders
renal failure

Muscle stiffness *see also* Muscular rigidity
Infections
tetanus
Musculoskeletal and connective tissue disorders
fibrositis
polymyalgia rheumatica

Muscle wasting
[*emaciation; muscle atrophy*]

Endocrine disorders
Cushing's syndrome
hypogonadism (male)
Gastro-intestinal and related disorders
ascites
cirrhosis of the liver
Infections
actinomycosis
dysentery
visceral leishmaniasis
Malignant disease
spinal cord tumours
Metabolic disorders
hepatolenticular degeneration
Musculoskeletal and connective tissue disorders
cervical spondylosis
polymyositis and dermatomyositis
Nervous system disorders
carpal tunnel syndrome
motor neurone disease
syringomyelia
Nutritional disorders
anorexia nervosa

Muscle weakness
Endocrine disorders
acromegaly
Cushing's syndrome
hyperthyroidism
primary aldosteronism
Infections
botulism
postviral fatigue syndrome
Malignant disease
spinal cord tumours
Metabolic disorders
glycogen storage diseases
hepatolenticular degeneration
hypercalcaemia
hypokalaemia
hyponatraemia
Musculoskeletal and connective tissue disorders
muscular dystrophy
polymyositis and dermatomyositis
Nervous system disorders
carpal tunnel syndrome
motor neurone disease
multiple sclerosis
myasthenia gravis
subdural haemorrhage
Sydenham's chorea
Nutritional disorders
bulimia nervosa
rickets and osteomalacia

Muscular rigidity *see also* Muscle stiffness
Infections
subacute sclerosing panencephalitis
tetanus
Nervous system disorders
malignant hyperthermia
parkinsonism
tonic-clonic epileptic seizures

—————— N ——————

Nail lesions

[*crumbling nails; deformed and/or discoloured nail body; nail pitting and ridging; swelling of the nail fold*]

Endocrine disorders
  hypoparathyroidism
Gastro-intestinal and related disorders
  cirrhosis of the liver
Infections
  paronychia
  tinea unguium
Malignant disease
  glucagonoma
Musculoskeletal and connective tissue disorders
  psoriatic arthritis
Skin disorders
  lichen planus

Nail loss

Skin disorders
  exfoliative dermatitis

Nasal congestion

Infections
  common cold
  influenza
  lepromatous leprosy
Malignant disease
  cancer of the nasopharynx
Nervous system disorders
  cluster headache
Nose disorders
  rhinitis
  sinusitis

Nasal discharge

[*rhinorrhoea*]

Infections
  anterior nasal diphtheria
  common cold
  lepromatous leprosy
  measles
Nervous system disorders
  opiate withdrawal
Nose disorders
  rhinitis
  sinusitis

Nasal irritation *see also* Sneezing

Infections
  anterior nasal diphtheria
  common cold
Nose disorders
  rhinitis

Nausea and/or vomiting

Non-specific causes
  diet
  drugs
  intestinal obstruction
  pregnancy

  psychological factors
  unpleasant smells or sights
Blood and lymph disorders
  anaemias
Cardiovascular system disorders
  angina pectoris
  myocardial infarction
  oesophageal varices
  syncope
  tricuspid regurgitation
Ear disorders
  acute otitis media
  labyrinthitis
  Ménière's disease
Endocrine disorders
  Addison's disease
  adrenocortical insufficiency, acute
  hyperthyroidism
Eye disorders
  closed-angle glaucoma
Gastro-intestinal and related disorders
  acute hepatitis
  acute intestinal ischaemia
  appendicitis
  cholangitis
  cholecystitis
  choledocholithiasis
  cirrhosis of the liver
  congenital megacolon
  dyspepsia
  focal ischaemia of the small intestine
  gastritis
  gastro-enteritis
  ileus
  ischaemic colitis
  kernicterus
  pancreatitis
  peptic ulceration
  peritonitis
  pyloric stenosis
Gynaecological disorders
  dysmenorrhoea
Infections
  acquired immunodeficiency syndrome
  acute fulminating meningococcaemia
  botulism
  cestode infections
  chickenpox
  cholera
  cryptococcal meningitis
  cutaneous anthrax
  dracontiasis
  dysentery
  erysipelas
  giardiasis
  influenza
  Lassa fever
  leptospirosis
  liver fluke disease
  Lyme disease
  malaria
  Marburg disease and Ebola fever
  meningitis
  pelvic actinomycosis
  pertussis

poliomyelitis
Pontiac fever
psittacosis
salpingitis
scarlet fever
secondary syphilis
septicaemia
shigellosis
tonsillar diphtheria
toxic shock syndrome
trichiniasis
urinary-tract infections
yellow fever
Male genital disorders
    torsion of the testis
Malignant disease
    cancer of the bile ducts
    cancer of the stomach
    carcinoid syndrome
    intracranial tumours
    myeloma
    Wilms' tumour
Metabolic disorders
    galactosaemia
    hypercalcaemia
    metabolic acidosis
    porphyrias
Nervous system disorders
    barbiturate withdrawal
    hypertensive encephalopathy
    migraine
    motion sickness
    Reye's syndrome
    subarachnoid haemorrhage
    transient ischaemic attacks
    vertigo
Nutritional disorders
    lactose intolerance
Obstetric disorders
    hydatidiform mole
    pre-eclampsia and eclampsia
Renal disorders
    glomerulonephritis
    interstitial nephritis
    renal calculi and colic
    renal failure
Skin disorders
    hereditary angioedema

Neck pain

Infections
    postviral fatigue syndrome
    tetanus
Musculoskeletal and connective tissue disorders
    cervical spondylosis
    torticollis

Neck stiffness

Infections
    encephalitis
    Lyme disease
    poliomyelitis
    pyogenic meningitis
    tetanus
    viral meningitis

Musculoskeletal and connective tissue disorders
    cervical spondylosis
    torticollis
Nervous system disorders
    subarachnoid haemorrhage

Neck swelling

[*bull neck; goitre; neck oedema*]
Endocrine disorders
    hyperthyroidism
    hypothyroidism
    thyroiditis
Infections
    epiglottitis
    tonsillar diphtheria

Nodules *see also* Skin lesions

Infections
    African trypanosomiasis
    cutaneous leishmaniasis
    rheumatic fever
    sporotrichosis
    tinea capitis
    tinea corporis
Malignant disease
    basal cell carcinoma
    Kaposi's sarcoma
    melanoma
Musculoskeletal and connective tissue disorders
    polyarteritis nodosa
    rheumatoid arthritis
Skin disorders
    erythema nodosum
    keloid
    pyoderma gangrenosum

Nosebleed

[*epistaxis*]
Blood and lymph disorders
    thrombocytopenia
Infections
    Marburg disease and Ebola fever
    paratyphoid fever
    typhoid fever
    yellow fever
Malignant disease
    acute leukaemias
Nutritional disorders
    scurvy

———————————— O ————————————

Odour, body *see* Body odour

Oedema *see* Swelling, oedematous

Oral pain

Infections
    oral candidiasis
Skin disorders
    lichen planus
    pemphigus

Oropharyngeal exudate
Infections
   cervicofacial actinomycosis
   diphtheria
   tonsillitis
Oropharyngeal disorders
   pharyngitis

Oropharyngeal lesions *see also* Lip lesions, Throat discomfort,
Tongue changes, *and* Tongue pain
*[aphthous stomatitis; gingival bleeding; gingival infection; gingival
inflammation; gingival patches; mouth ulcers; oral bleeding; oral
candidiasis; oral hairy leucoplakia; plaques; throat ulcers; tongue
patches]*
Blood and lymph disorders
   agranulocytosis
Gastro-intestinal and related disorders
   coeliac disease
   tropical sprue
Infections
   acquired immunodeficiency syndrome
   cervicofacial actinomycosis
   diphtheria
   herpesvirus infections (HSV 1)
   measles
   oral candidiasis
   syphilis
   Vincent's infection
   yellow fever
Malignant disease
   cancer of the mouth
Musculoskeletal and connective tissue disorders
   systemic lupus erythematosus
Nutritional disorders
   scurvy
Oropharyngeal disorders
   aphthous stomatitis
   gingivitis
   oral leucoplakia
   pharyngitis
Skin disorders
   lichen planus
   pemphigus

P

Pain during defaecation
[tenesmus]
Gastro-intestinal and related disorders
   anal fissure
   haemorrhoids
   ulcerative colitis
Gynaecological disorders
   endometriosis
Infections
   dysentery
   shigellosis

Palpitations *see* Heart beat abnormalities

Perception disturbances *see also* Behaviour disturbances *and*
Emotional disturbances
*[delusions; disorientation; distorted perception of time; halluci-
nations; nightmares; psychoses; sense of déjà-vu; sense of
unreality; sensitivity to light or noise]*
Blood and lymph system disorders
   thrombotic thrombocytopenic purpura
Infections
   African trypanosomiasis
   cysticercosis
   Legionnaire's disease
   rabies
Metabolic disorders
   hypocalcaemia
   porphyrias
Musculoskeletal and connective tissue disorders
   polyarteritis nodosa
   systemic lupus erythematosus
Nervous system disorders
   depressive disorders
   drug dependence
   mania and manic-depressive illness
   partial seizures
   Reye's syndrome
   schizophrenia

Productive cough *see* Cough

Prostration *see also* Fatigue
Blood and lymph disorders
   agranulocytosis
Eye disorders
   closed-angle glaucoma
Gastro-intestinal and related disorders
   gastro-enteritis
Infections
   brucellosis
   disseminated gonococcal infection
   malaria
   Marburg disease and Ebola fever
   typhus fevers

Pupillary changes
Cardiovascular system disorders
   cardiac arrest
Eye disorders
   uveitis
Nervous system disorders
   cerebral oedema
   cluster headache
   subdural and extradural haemorrhage

R

Rash *see* Skin lesions

Rectal pain, cyclic
Gynaecological disorders
   endometriosis

—————————— S ——————————

Saliva, blood in

Malignant disease
oropharyngeal cancer

Salivation, excessive

Gastro-intestinal and related disorders
gastric ulceration
Infections
epiglottitis
herpesvirus infections (HSV 1)
Vincent's infection
Malignant disease
cancer of the mouth
Nervous system disorders
motion sickness

Scrotal changes

[*orchitis; scrotal discoloration; scrotal inflammation; scrotal mass; testicular mass*]
Infections
epididymitis
lymphatic filariasis
Marburg disease and Ebola fever
mumps
Male genital disorders
Klinefelter's syndrome
torsion of the testis
varicocoele
Malignant disease
choriocarcinoma
testicular cancer

Scrotal pain

[*testicular pain and tenderness*]
Malignant disease
choriocarcinoma
testicular cancer

Seizures *see also* Convulsions

Nervous system disorders
epilepsy

Sensory derangement *see also* Hearing impairment

[*acroparaesthesia; agnosia; burning sensations; dysaesthesia; neuralgia; numbness; 'pins and needles'; prickling sensation; taste impairment*]
Cardiovascular system disorders
Raynaud's syndrome
Endocrine disorders
acromegaly
primary aldosteronism
type I diabetes mellitus
Gastro-intestinal and related disorders
acute hepatitis
cirrhosis of the liver
Infections
encephalitis
herpes zoster
leprosy
loiasis
postviral fatigue syndrome

Malignant disease
spinal cord tumours
Metabolic disorders
hypocalcaemia
respiratory alkalosis
Musculoskeletal and connective tissue disorders
cervical spondylosis
Nervous system disorders
Bell's palsy
carpal tunnel syndrome
dementia
diabetic neuropathy
Guillain-Barré syndrome
migraine
multiple sclerosis
restless leg syndrome
spina bifida
stroke
syringomyelia
tardive dyskinesia
transient ischaemic attacks
Nutritional disorders
beri-beri

Sexual disturbances *see also* Infertility

[*absence of erection or ejaculation; dyspareunia; impotence; loss of libido*]
Blood and lymph disorders
anaemias
Endocrine disorders
hyperprolactinaemia
hypogonadism
hypopituitarism
Gynaecological disorders
endometriosis
menopause
vaginitis
vulvitis
Infections
trichomoniasis
Malignant disease
cervical cancer
Nervous system disorders
depressive disorders
diabetic neuropathy
multiple sclerosis
Nutritional disorders
anorexia nervosa

Shivering *see also* Chills and sensation of intense cold

[*rigors*]
Blood and lymph disorders
agranulocytosis
Infections
brucellosis
infective arthritis
influenza
lymphangitis
malaria
pneumonia
pyelonephritis
pyogenic meningitis
typhus fevers
yellow fever

Metabolic disorders
   gout
Respiratory system disorders
   extrinsic allergic alveolitis
Skin disorders
   exfoliative dermatitis

Skeletal deformity *see also* Bone structure abnormalities *and* Joint abnormalities
[*bowing of the long bones; cubitus valgus; enlargement of the hands and feet; excessive growth of long bones; increased stature; kyphosis; reduced stature; scoliosis; spinal rigidity; vertebral collapse*]
Blood and lymph disorders
   haemophilia
Endocrine disorders
   acromegaly
   hyperparathyroidism
   hypogonadism
Gynaecological disorders
   Turner's syndrome
Male genital disorders
   Klinefelter's syndrome
Musculoskeletal and connective tissue disorders
   ankylosing spondylitis
   cervical spondylosis
   juvenile chronic arthritis
   muscular dystrophy
   psoriatic arthritis
   rheumatoid arthritis
   osteitis deformans
   osteoarthritis
   osteopetrosis
   osteoporosis
Nutritional disorders
   rickets
Renal disorders
   renal osteodystrophy

Skin depigmentation
Infections
   onchocerciasis
Metabolic disorders
   phenylketonuria
Skin disorders
   albinism
   ischaemic ulcers
   pityriasis alba
   pityriasis lichenoides
   vitiligo

Skin desquamation
[*exfoliating lesions*]
Infections
   Marburg disease and Ebola fever
   measles
   scarlet fever
   toxic shock syndrome
Malignant disease
   glucagonoma
Skin disorders
   exfoliative dermatitis
   toxic epidermal necrolysis

Skin haemorrhage
[*bruising; ecchymoses; petechiae*]
Blood and lymph disorders
   haemophilia
   thrombocytopenia
Endocrine disorders
   Cushing's syndrome
Infections
   infectious mononucleosis
   infective endocarditis
   Marburg disease and Ebola fever
   scabies
   scarlet fever
   typhus fevers
   yellow fever
Malignant disease
   leukaemias
   superficial spreading melanoma
Skin disorders
   pityriasis lichenoides
   strawberry naevus

Skin healing, impaired
Nutritional disorders
   scurvy
   zinc deficiency

Skin inflammation *see also* Skin pain and discomfort *and* Skin redness
Infections
   myiasis
   tinea infections
Malignant disease
   superficial spreading melanoma
Skin disorders
   acne vulgaris
   eczema
   erythema nodosum
   folliculitis
   lichen planus
   sunburn

Skin lesions *see also* Skin, non-specific changes in characteristics, Skin ulcers, *and* Nodules
[*blackheads; bullae; blisters; comedones; livid striae; macules; naevi; papules; rash; vesicles; wheals; whiteheads*]
Cardiovascular system disorders
   chilblains
   varicose veins
Endocrine disorders
   adrenal virilisation
   Cushing's syndrome
Gastro-intestinal and related disorders
   acute hepatitis
   chronic active hepatitis
Gynaecological disorders
   Turner's syndrome
Infections
   acquired immunodeficiency syndrome
   cellulitis
   chancroid
   chickenpox
   condylomata acuminata
   cutaneous anthrax

cutaneous leishmaniasis
erysipelas
filariasis
furunculosis
gas gangrene
herpes zoster
impetigo
infectious mononucleosis
leprosy
listeriosis
Lyme disease
lymphangitis
Marburg disease and Ebola fever
measles
meningococcal infections
myiasis
paratyphoid fever
pediculosis corporis
pediculosis pubis
pityriasis versicolor
rheumatic fever
rubella
scabies
scarlet fever
schistosomiasis
skin candidiasis
sycosis barbae
syphilis
tinea infections
toxic shock syndrome
toxoplasmosis
typhoid fever
typhus fevers
Malignant disease
chronic lymphoid leukaemia
glucagonoma
Kaposi's sarcoma
melanoma
Musculoskeletal and connective tissue disorders
dermatomyositis
juvenile chronic arthritis
polyarteritis nodosa
systemic lupus erythematosus
Nutritional disorders
pellagra
Oropharyngeal disorders
pharyngitis
Skin disorders
acne vulgaris
angioedema
decubitus ulcer
eczema
erythema multiforme
folliculitis
lichen planus
pemphigus
photosensitivity
pityriasis alba
pityriasis lichenoides
pityriasis rosea
psoriasis
pyoderma gangrenosum
sebaceous cyst
Stevens-Johnson syndrome
sunburn

telangiectasia
toxic epidermal necrolysis
ulcers
urticaria

Skin, non-specific changes in characteristics *see also* Skin lesions
[*cracked skin; dry skin; greasy skin; lichenification; reduced skin turgor; scaling; shiny skin; skin atrophy; skin coarsening; skin crusting; skin growth; skin maceration; skin necrosis; skin thickening*]
Cardiovascular system disorders
chilblains
Raynaud's syndrome
Ear disorders
otitis externa
Endocrine disorders
acromegaly
Cushing's syndrome
hypoparathyroidism
hypothyroidism
Infections
cholera
gas gangrene
impetigo
lepromatous leprosy
pityriasis versicolor
scabies
scarlet fever
skin candidiasis
tinea infections
Metabolic disorders
hypernatraemia
hyponatraemia
Musculoskeletal and connective tissue disorders
dermatomyositis
systemic sclerosis
Nutritional disorders
anorexia nervosa
pellagra
Skin disorders
callosities
eczema
haemangiomas
hyperhidrosis
ichthyosis
mole
photosensitivity
pityriasis
psoriasis
sunburn

Skin pain and discomfort *see also* Skin inflammation *and* Skin redness
Infections
erysipelas
furunculosis
gas gangrene
myiasis
warts
Musculoskeletal and connective tissue disorders
giant cell arteritis
Skin disorders
acne vulgaris
angioedema

callosities and corns
decubitus ulcer
eczema
erythema multiforme
erythema nodosum
folliculitis
hereditary angioedema
lichen planus
pemphigus
photosensitivity
pityriasis alba
pityriasis lichenoides
pityriasis rosea
pruritus
psoriasis
pyoderma gangrenosum
sunburn
toxic epidermal necrolysis
ulcers
urticaria

Skin pigmentation

Cardiovascular system disorders
varicose veins
Endocrine disorders
Addison's disease
Gastro-intestinal and related disorders
tropical sprue
Whipple's disease
Infections
gas gangrene
Musculoskeletal and connective tissue disorders
dermatomyositis
systemic sclerosis
Renal disorders
chronic renal failure
Skin disorders
lichen planus
mole
pilonidal disease
sunburn
telangiectasia

Skin redness *see also* Facial flushing, Hot flushes, Skin inflammation *and* Skin pain and discomfort [*erythema*]
Blood and lymph disorders
deep vein thrombosis
superficial thrombophlebitis
Cardiovascular system disorders
Raynaud's syndrome
Gastro-intestinal and related disorders
cirrhosis of the liver
Infections
cellulitis
erysipelas
impetigo
Lyme disease
paratyphoid fever
rheumatic fever
skin candidiasis
sycosis barbae
typhoid fever
Metabolic disorders
respiratory acidosis

Musculoskeletal and connective tissue disorders
bursitis
dermatomyositis
giant cell arteritis
systemic lupus erythematosus
Nervous system disorders
cluster headache
Nutritional disorders
pellagra
Skin disorders
angioedema
decubitus ulcer
eczema
erythema multiforme
erythema nodosum
photosensitivity
pityriasis alba
pruritus
sunburn
toxic epidermal necrolysis
ulcers
urticaria

Skin ulcers *see also* Skin lesions

Blood and lymph disorders
embolism
Cardiovascular system disorders
chilblains
Raynaud's syndrome
varicose veins
Infections
carbuncles
chancroid
cutaneous anthrax
cutaneous diphtheria
cutaneous leishmaniasis
sporotrichosis
syphilis
Malignant disease
basal cell carcinoma
breast cancer
nodular melanoma
Musculoskeletal and connective tissue disorders
polyarteritis nodosa
Skin disorders
decubitus ulcer
napkin rash
strawberry naevus
ulcers

Skin yellowing

Gastro-intestinal and related disorders
jaundice
Metabolic disorders
hyperlipidaemias

Sneezing *see also* Nasal irritation

Non-specific causes
dust
smoking
Infections
common cold
influenza
measles

Nervous system disorders
  opiate withdrawal
Nose disorders
  rhinitis

Speech disturbances *see also* Voice abnormalities

[*aphasia; aphonia; difficulty in eating and speaking; dysarthria; hoarseness; loss of voice; stuttering*]
Infections
  botulism
  epiglottitis
  laryngeal diphtheria
  Legionnaire's disease
  trichiniasis
Malignant disease
  cancer of the hypopharynx
  cancer of the larynx
  cancer of the mouth
  oropharyngeal cancer
Metabolic disorders
  hepatolenticular degeneration
Nervous system disorders
  autism
  Bell's palsy
  cerebral palsy
  dementia
  dialysis encephalopathy
  Gilles de la Tourette syndrome
  hepatic encephalopathy
  motor neurone disease
  multiple sclerosis
  parkinsonism
  stroke
  Sydenham's chorea
  syringobulbia
  transient ischaemic attacks
Nutritional disorders
  beri-beri
Oropharyngeal disorders
  glossitis
  laryngitis
  pharyngitis

Spots, facial *see* Skin lesions

Sputum
Blood and lymph disorders
  pulmonary embolism and infarction
Cardiovascular system disorders
  left heart failure
  mitral stenosis
  pulmonary hypertension
  tricuspid stenosis
Infections
  aspergillosis
  cryptococcosis
  leptospirosis
  lung fluke disease
  plague
  pneumonia
  post-primary pulmonary tuberculosis
  psittacosis
  pulmonary actinomycosis
Malignant disease
  lung cancer

Respiratory system disorders
  bronchiectasis
  chronic bronchitis and emphysema
  productive cough

Stools, unusual *see* Faeces, changes in

Swallowing difficulties *see also* Feeding and swallowing difficulties *and* Throat discomfort
[*dysphagia*]
Blood and lymph disorders
  agranulocytosis
Cardiovascular system disorders
  thoracic aortic aneurysm
Endocrine disorders
  subacute thyroiditis
Gastro-intestinal and related disorders
  achalasia
  reflux oesophagitis
Infections
  botulism
  epiglottitis
  infectious mononucleosis
  Lassa fever
  scarlet fever
  tetanus
  tonsillar diphtheria
  tonsillitis
Malignant disease
  cancer of the hypopharynx
  cancer of the larynx
  oesophageal cancer
  oropharyngeal cancer
  thyroid cancer
Metabolic disorders
  hepatolenticular degeneration
Musculoskeletal and connective tissue disorders
  polymyositis and dermatomyositis
  systemic sclerosis
Nervous system disorders
  cerebral palsy
  motor neurone disease
  myasthenia gravis
  parkinsonism
  syringobulbia
  transient ischaemic attacks
Oropharyngeal disorders
  glossitis
  laryngitis
  pharyngitis

Sweating abnormalities
[*hyperhidrosis; night sweats; sweating, loss of*]
Cardiovascular system disorders
  acrocyanosis
  angina pectoris
  circulatory failure, acute
  myocardial infarction
Endocrine disorders
  acromegaly
  hyperthyroidism
  hypoglycaemia
  subacute thyroiditis
Gastro-intestinal and related disorders
  acute intestinal ischaemia

Gynaecological disorders
  menopause
Infections
  acquired immunodeficiency syndrome
  brucellosis
  gas gangrene
  malaria
  post-primary pulmonary tuberculosis
  visceral leishmaniasis
Malignant disease
  chronic myeloid leukaemia
  insulinoma
  lymphomas
  phaeochromocytoma
Nervous system disorders
  cluster headache
  diabetic neuropathy
  motion sickness
  parkinsonism

Swelling, glandular *see also* Swelling, oedematous
[*adenopathy; buboes; lymphadenopathy*]
Gastro-intestinal and related disorders
  cirrhosis of the liver
  Whipple's disease
Infections
  acquired immunodeficiency syndrome
  American trypanosomiasis
  cellulitis
  chancroid
  cutaneous anthrax
  herpesvirus infections
  Lyme disease
  lymphangitis
  lymphatic filariasis
  mumps
  pediculosis capitis
  plague
  rubella
  syphilis
  tonsillar diphtheria
  toxoplasmosis
  trypanosomiasis
Malignant disease
  breast cancer
  cancer of the nasopharynx
  chronic lymphoid leukaemia
  lymphomas
Musculoskeletal and connective tissue disorders
  juvenile chronic arthritis
  rheumatoid arthritis
  sarcoidosis
  systemic lupus erythematosus
Oropharyngeal disorders
  sialadenitis
  sialolithiasis

Swelling, oedematous *see also* Swelling, glandular
[*oedema*]
Blood and lymph disorders
  anaemias
  anaphylactoid purpura
  lymphangiectasia
  superficial thrombophlebitis

Cardiovascular system disorders
  cardiomyopathy
  cor pulmonale
  heart failure
  myocarditis
  tricuspid stenosis
  varicose veins
Endocrine disorders
  Cushing's syndrome
  hypothyroidism
Gastro-intestinal and related disorders
  cirrhosis of the liver
  coeliac disease
  tropical sprue
Gynaecological disorders
  premenstrual syndrome
Infections
  American trypanosomiasis
  cellulitis
  cutaneous anthrax
  erysipelas
  gas gangrene
  hookworm infection
  trichiniasis
  yellow fever
Malignant disease
  breast cancer
  Hodgkin's disease
Metabolic disorders
  hyponatraemia
Musculoskeletal and connective tissue disorders
  dermatomyositis
  systemic lupus erythematosus
Nutritional disorders
  beri-beri
Obstetric disorders
  pre-eclampsia and eclampsia
Renal disorders
  glomerulonephritis
  nephrotic syndrome
  oedema
  renal failure
Respiratory system disorders
  chronic bronchitis and emphysema
Skin disorders
  angioedema
  decubitus ulcer
  eczema
  photosensitivity
  pityriasis lichenoides
  sunburn
  urticaria

——————————— T ———————————

Thirst
[*polydipsia*]
Endocrine disorders
  diabetes insipidus
  primary aldosteronism
  type I diabetes mellitus
Infections
  cholera

Metabolic disorders
hypercalcaemia
Renal disorders
renal failure

Throat discomfort *see also* Oropharyngeal lesions *and* Swallowing difficulties
[*dry throat; laryngeal spasm; lump in the throat; oedema of the throat; sore throat; tonsillar enlargement*]
Non-specific causes
irritants
Gastro-intestinal and related disorders
neurotic dysphagia
Infections
common cold
diphtheria
herpes simplex virus infections
infectious mononucleosis
influenza
Lassa fever
legionellosis
Marburg disease and Ebola fever
measles
poliomyelitis
rabies
scarlet fever
tonsillitis
toxic shock syndrome
Malignant disease
oropharyngeal cancer
Metabolic disorders
hypocalcaemia
Oropharyngeal disorders
laryngitis
pharyngitis
Respiratory system disorders
dry cough

Tongue changes *see also* Oropharyngeal lesions *and* Tongue pain
[*dry tongue; furred tongue; glossitis; macroglossia; red tongue; tongue atrophy*]
Blood and lymph disorders
amyloidosis
megaloblastic anaemias
Endocrine disorders
acromegaly
hypothyroidism
type I diabetes mellitus
Gastro-intestinal and related disorders
cirrhosis of the liver
tropical sprue
Infections
paratyphoid fever
scarlet fever
typhoid fever
Malignant disease
glucagonoma
Nervous system disorders
syringobulbia
Nutritional disorders
pyridoxine deficiency
riboflavine deficiency
Oropharyngeal disorders
glossitis

Tongue pain *see also* Oropharyngeal lesions *and* Tongue changes
Oropharyngeal disorders
glossitis

Tremor
Endocrine disorders
hyperthyroidism
hypoglycaemia
Metabolic disorders
hepatolenticular degeneration
Nervous system disorders
anxiety
opiate withdrawal

——————————— U ———————————

Urethral discharge
Infections
gonorrhoea
prostatitis
urethritis

Urination abnormalities
[*anuria; dysuria; nocturia; oliguria; polyuria; strangury; tenesmus; urinary frequency; urinary hesitancy; urinary obstruction; urinary retention; urinary urgency*]
Non-specific causes
irritants
urethral trauma
uterovaginal prolapse
Blood and lymph disorders
haemolytic anaemias
Cardiovascular system disorders
hypertension
shock
Endocrine disorders
adrenocortical insufficiency, acute
diabetes insipidus
hyperparathyroidism
hypopituitarism
primary aldosteronism
type I diabetes mellitus
Gastro-intestinal and related disorders
acute intestinal ischaemia
appendicitis
Gynaecological disorders
dysmenorrhoea
endometriosis
vaginitis
vulvitis
Infections
botulism
gonorrhoea
herpesvirus infections (HSV 2)
prostatitis
schistosomiasis
urinary-tract infections
Male genital disorders
benign prostatic hypertrophy
torsion of the testis

Malignant disease
  bladder cancer
  prostatic cancer
  urothelial tumours
Metabolic disorders
  hypercalcaemia
Musculoskeletal and connective tissue disorders
  cervical spondylosis
Nervous system disorders
  anxiety
  diabetic neuropathy
  multiple sclerosis
Renal disorders
  interstitial nephritis
  renal calculi and colic
  renal failure
Skin disorders
  napkin rash

Urine abnormalities

[*blood in urine; chyluria; haematuria; pyuria*]
Blood and lymph disorders
  anaphylactoid purpura
Gastro-intestinal and related disorders
  acute hepatitis
  cholangitis
  cholestatic jaundice
Infections
  infective endocarditis
  lymphatic filariasis
  urinary-tract infections
  Weil's disease
Malignant disease
  bladder cancer
  cancer of the bile ducts
  prostatic cancer
  renal cancer
Metabolic disorders
  maple-syrup urine disease
  porphyrias
Nutritional disorders
  scurvy
Renal disorders
  glomerulonephritis
  polycystic kidney disease
  renal calculi and colic

Uterine abnormalities

[*uterine bleeding, abnormal; uterine contractions; uterine enlargement; uterine prolapse*]
Gynaecological disorders
  menopause
Malignant disease
  choriocarcinoma
  endometrial cancer
Obstetric disorders
  abortion
  hydatidiform mole

—————————— V ——————————

Vaginal bleeding, abnormal
Malignant disease
  cervical cancer

Obstetric disorders
  abortion
  ectopic pregnancy
  hydatidiform mole
  postpartum haemorrhage

Vaginal discharge
Gynaecological disorders
  vaginitis
Infections
  gonorrhoea
  pelvic actinomycosis
  salpingitis
  trichomoniasis
  urethritis
  vaginal candidiasis
Malignant disease
  cervical cancer
  endometrial cancer

Vaginal discomfort *see also* Anogenital lesions
Gynaecological disorders
  menopause
  vaginitis

Visual disturbances

[*astigmatism; blindness, temporary; blurred vision; diminished acuity; diplopia; flashes of light; 'floaters' in the field of vision; haloes around lights; loss of accomodation; loss of central vision; loss of peripheral vision; night blindness; photophobia; photosensitivity; retinopathy; sensitivity to light*]
Blood and lymph disorders
  polycythaemia vera
Cardiovascular system disorders
  hypertension
  orthostatic hypotension
Endocrine disorders
  acromegaly
  hypoglycaemia
  diabetes mellitus
Eye disorders
  blepharitis
  cataract
  corneal ulceration
  dry eye
  exophthalmos
  glaucoma
  keratitis
  macular degeneration
  optic neuropathies
  papilloedema
  retinal detachment
  scleritis and episcleritis
  strabismus
  uveitis
Infections
  acquired immunodeficiency syndrome
  botulism
  cryptococcal meningitis
  measles
  myiasis
  postviral fatigue syndrome
  subacute sclerosing panencephalitis
  trachoma
  viral meningitis

Malignant disease
   intracranial tumours
   myeloma
Musculoskeletal and connective tissue disorders
   giant cell arteritis
Nervous system disorders
   cerebral palsy
   hydrocephalus
   migraine
   multiple sclerosis
   myasthenia gravis
   stroke
   transient ischaemic attacks
Nutritional disorders
   vitamin A deficiency
   zinc deficiency
Obstetric disorders
   pre-eclampsia and eclampsia
Skin disorders
   albinism

Voice abnormalities *see also* Speech disturbances
[*deepening of the voice; failure of the voice to break*]
Endocrine disorders
   acromegaly
   adrenal virilisation (in females)
   hypogonadism (in males)

Vomiting *see* Nausea and/or vomiting

Vulval changes
[*vulval atrophy; vulval swelling*]
Gynaecological disorders
   menopause
   vulvitis
Infections
   trichomoniasis

──────────── W ────────────

Weight changes
[*obesity; weight gain; weight loss*]
Endocrine disorders
   Addison's disease
   Cushing's syndrome
   hyperthyroidism
   hypogonadism (in adult males)
   hypothyroidism
   type I diabetes mellitus

Gastro-intestinal and related disorders
   chronic intestinal ischaemia
   cirrhosis of the liver
   coeliac disease
   Crohn's disease
   gastric ulceration
   pyloric stenosis
   tropical sprue
   tuberculous peritonitis
   ulcerative colitis
   Whipple's disease
Gynaecological disorders
   polycystic ovary syndrome
   premenstrual syndrome
Infections
   acquired immunodeficiency syndrome
   brucellosis
   cestode infections
   dysentery
   enterobiasis
   shigellosis
   trichuriasis
   tuberculosis
   visceral leishmaniasis
Malignant disease
   many diseases
Musculoskeletal and connective tissue disorders
   giant cell arteritis
   muscular dystrophy
   polyarteritis nodosa
   polymyalgia rheumatica
   rheumatoid arthritis
   sarcoidosis
Nervous system disorders
   depressive disorders
   mania and manic-depressive illness
Nutritional disorders
   anorexia nervosa
Obstetric disorders
   pre-eclampsia and eclampsia
Renal disorders
   interstitial nephritis
   oedema
Respiratory system disorders
   chronic bronchitis and emphysema
   fibrosing alveolitis

Wind *see* Flatulence and eructation

Wrist pain
Nervous system disorders
   carpal tunnel syndrome

PART D
GLOSSARY
OF
MEDICAL TERMS

GLOSSARY

Introduction

The glossary provides information on terms that have been used without explanation in the text. It is not intended to act as a comprehensive medical dictionary.

Where appropriate, the combining forms, prefixes, and suffixes that make up a word have been listed in brackets after the term itself; the hyphens appended to these forms illustrate their position within that particular term. An explanation of the meaning of the combining forms, prefixes, and suffixes is appended as a separate list after the main glossary.

The reader's attention has been drawn to terms that are related, by the use of cross-references. The relationship may be that the terms are antonyms, or that they represent varying degrees or stages of the same concept. Synonymous terms have been defined under one term only, and all other synonyms are referred to that term.

For those terms that have more than one definition, any cross-reference follows immediately after the definition to which it applies. If the cross-reference applies to all of the stated definitions, it starts on a new line after the last definition.

The reader should consult the index for a term encountered in the text that has not been included in the glossary, as it will usually be explained elsewhere.

─────────── A ───────────

Aberrance (ab-) An abnormal course.

Abrasion (ab-) An area where skin or mucous membrane has been removed by a mechanical process (e.g. rubbing).

Abscess A pus-filled cavity formed by tissue disintegration. *See also* COLD ABSCESS *and* MICRO-ABSCESS.

Accommodation Adaptation (e.g. the changing focus of the lens of the eye).

Acetaldehyde Acetaldehyde (ethanal) is an intermediate in the metabolic oxidation of ethanol. It is converted to acetyl-coenzyme A.

Acetylcholine A neurotransmitter released at nerve terminals of the parasympathetic nervous system, at neuromuscular junctions, and in autonomic ganglia. It is also present in brain tissue.

Acetyl-coenzyme A The principal precursor in the formation of lipids, and an intermediate in the Krebs' cycle.

Achilles tendon A tendon connecting the calf muscles to the heel.

Achlorhydria (a-) Absence of hydrochloric acid in gastric juice.

Acholuria (a-, -chol-, -uria) Absence of bile pigment in the urine.

Acid A substance that can combine with a base to form a salt; a proton donor; a liberator of hydrogen ions (H^+) in water. *See also* BASE(2).

Acid-base balance The ratio of acids to bases in body fluids, maintained homoeostatically with the aid of buffering systems. It ensures that the concentration of hydrogen ions (H^+) in body fluids remains within defined limits.

Acquired Refers to conditions that develop under the influence of external factors, and which are not of genetic or congenital origin.

Acroparaesthesia (acro-, -aesthesi-) Numbness, tingling, or other abnormal sensations (e.g. 'pins and needles') in the extremities, usually affecting the fingers, hands, and forearms. *See also* ANAESTHESIA, DYSAESTHESIA, *and* PARAESTHESIA.

Active immunisation The process of antibody formation, which may occur naturally following recovery from an infection, or may be induced by inoculation with a vaccine or toxoid. *See also* PASSIVE IMMUNISATION *and* VACCINATION(1).

Acuity Clarity, acuteness, sharpness; used especially to refer to vision.

Acute Refers to a disorder with a relatively severe course and of short duration. *See also* CHRONIC *and* SUBACUTE.

Adenitis (aden-, -itis) Inflammation of a gland.

Adenocarcinoma (aden-, -carcin-, -oma) A malignant neoplasm composed of glandular tissue. *See also* ADENOMA.

Adenoid (aden-, -oid) 1. Similar to a gland. 2. The term adenoids refers to lymphoid tissue in the nasopharynx; the pharyngeal tonsil.

Adenoma (aden-, -oma) A benign neoplasm composed of glandular tissue. *See also* ADENOCARCINOMA.

Adenomatous (aden-, -oma-) Refers to an adenoma or glandular hyperplasia.

Adenopathy (adeno-, -pathy) Enlargement of glands, particularly lymph nodes.

Adenosine triphosphate (tri-)   Adenosine triphosphate (ATP) is found in all cells where it acts as an energy store. The energy is released by hydrolysis of the high-energy phosphate bonds.

Adenosis (aden-, -osis)   1. Any disorder of a gland. 2. The abnormal development of glandular tissue.

Adhesion (ad-)   The joining of neighbouring surfaces of organs and tissues that are normally separate.

Adjunct (ad-, -junct)   A substance that is administered to assist or aid another in its actions or to provide a supportive measure.

Adrenalectomy (adren-, -ectomy)   The removal of an adrenal gland by surgery.

Adrenergic   Refers to sympathetic nerves or to the characteristics of adrenaline and substances producing similar effects (e.g. catecholamines). *See also* CHOLINERGIC *and* SYMPATHOMIMETIC.

Adrenoceptor (-ceptor)   A receptor on an effector organ innervated by postganglionic fibres of the sympathetic nervous system. There are two types of adrenoceptor, classified according to their reaction to noradrenaline and adrenaline, and to other excitatory or inhibitory drugs that interact with these receptors. Alpha-adrenoceptors generally produce excitatory responses while beta-adrenoceptors generally produce inhibitory responses.

Adrenocortical (adreno-, -cortic-)   Refers to the adrenal cortex.

Adventitia   The external layer of connective tissue surrounding an organ, often applied to the tunica externa of an artery.

Adynamic (a-, -dynami-)   Refers to loss of, or reduction in, normal function.

Aerobic (aer-)   Occurring in, or requiring the presence of, oxygen. *See also* ANAEROBIC.

Aerophagia (aer-, -phagia)   The excessive swallowing of air.

Aetiology (-logy)   The study of the cause(s) of a disease.

Affect   Feelings, mood, or emotions.

Affective disorder (dis-)   A disorder characterised by disturbances of affect.

Afferent (af-, -ferent)   Carrying inwards to a centre. *See also* EFFERENT.

Agenesis (a-, -gen-, -sis)   Absence of an organ or part as a result of complete failure of embryonic development. *See also* APLASIA, DYSPLASIA, *and* HYPOPLASIA.

Agnosia (a-, -gno-, -ia)   The inability to recognise or interpret sensory stimuli (e.g. auditory, visual, and olfactory).

Agonist   1. An agent that stimulates activity at cell receptors. 2. A muscle that causes movement on contraction while its opposing muscle remains relaxed. *See also* ANTAGONIST.

Airway   1. The passage from the nose or mouth to the alveoli, through which air passes during respiration. 2. A device placed in the nose or mouth to ensure the clear passage of air into, and out of, the lungs.

Akinesia (a-, -kine-, -ia)   Difficulty in initiating movement or an inability to move. *See also* BRADYKINESIA, DYSKINESIA, *and* HYPOKINESIA.

Albumin (alb-)   A water-soluble protein synthesised in the liver, and the major protein of blood plasma. Its principal functions are to maintain the intravascular colloid osmotic pressure and to transport water-insoluble substances.

Albuminuria (alb-, -uria)   The presence of albumin in the urine.

Alcohol dehydrogenase (-ol, de-, -hydro-, -ase)   An enzyme responsible for the dehydrogenation (oxidation) of alcohols to form an aldehyde or a ketone.

Alkaline phosphatase (-ase)   An hydrolytic enzyme that liberates inorganic phosphate. It is found in many body tissues, and is active at a high pH.

Allele (all-)   One of two or more different forms of a gene located at a given site on homologous chromosomes, and responsible for specific characteristics of an organism.

Allergy (all-)   A state of hypersensitivity to certain substances (allergens) that is mediated by the immune system. *See also* ATOPY.

Allograft (allo-)   Tissue transplant between two genetically different individuals of the same species.

Alpha-1-antitrypsin (anti-)   A plasma protein synthesised in the liver, which inhibits the action of proteolytic enzymes (e.g. trypsin and chymotrypsin).

Ambulant   Able to walk and not confined to bed.

Amino acid   An organic acid containing an amino group ($-NH_2$) and a carboxyl group ($-COOH$). Amino acids comprise the basic unit in the structure of proteins.

Amniocentesis (-centesis)   Aspiration of amniotic fluid, via the transabdominal route, for analysis.

Amputation   The complete or partial removal of an appendage or outgrowth of a body (e.g. limb or breast) by surgery.

Anabolism (ana-)   A form of metabolism in which living cells synthesise complex compounds from simpler substances. *See also* CATABOLISM.

Anaerobic (an-, -aer-)   Occurring in, or requiring the absence of, oxygen. *See also* AEROBIC.

Anaesthesia (an-, -aesthesi-)   Complete or partial loss of sensation. It may be caused by a lesion of the nervous system, or it may be artificially induced to perform painful procedures. *See also* ACROPARAESTHESIA, DYSAESTHESIA, *and* PARAESTHESIA.

Anaphylatoxin   A substance liberated during activation of the complement system. It induces degranulation of mast cells and the release of histamine.

Anaplasia (ana-, -plasia)   Retrogression of cells to a less differentiated, more primitive form, characteristic of neoplasms.

Anastomosis (-stomo-, -sis)   1. A connection between normally separate ducts, vessels, or cavities which may be formed by surgery, disease, or as a result of trauma. 2. A natural confluence of similar, usually tubular, structures.

Androgen (andro-, -gen)   Any substance capable of producing masculine characteristics in either sex.

Angioblast (angio-, -blast)   Embryonic tissue from which blood cells and vessels differentiate.

Angioplasty (angio-, -plasty)   Reconstruction of a blood vessel by surgery or by other methods (e.g. balloon dilatation).

Angular stomatitis (stomat-, -itis)   Superficial inflammation and erosion at one or more corners of the mouth.

Ankylosis (ankylo-, -sis)   Joint immobility caused by pathological changes of the joint or associated structures as a result of trauma, disease, or surgery.

Anogenital (-genit-)   Refers to the anus and genitalia.

Anorectal (-rect-)   Refers to the anus and rectum.

Anorexia (an-, -ia)   Loss of appetite.

Antagonist (ant-)   1. An agent that binds to cell receptors without eliciting a pharmacological response, and which can cancel or reverse the action of another. 2. A muscle that cancels or reverses the action of another. *See also* AGONIST.

Antenatal (ante-)   Refers to the period between conception and delivery. *See also* POSTNATAL.

Anterior horn (ante-)   The ventral portion of grey matter within the spinal cord containing motor cells. *See also* POSTERIOR HORN.

Antibiotic (anti-, -bio-)   An organic compound, produced by micro-organisms, that kills or inhibits the growth of other micro-organisms, and is used to treat infections. The term may also be applied to synthetic derivatives. *See also* ANTIMICROBIAL.

Antibody (anti-)   A specific immunoglobulin produced by the immune system in response to stimulation by an antigen, and which reacts only with that antigen or one that is closely related. *See also* ANTINUCLEAR ANTIBODY *and* AUTO-ANTIBODY.

Anticholinergic (anti-)   1. A substance that antagonises the action of acetylcholine at muscarinic and nicotinic receptors of the parasympathetic nervous system. 2. Inhibition of the passage of impulses through parasympathetic nerves. *See also* ANTIMUSCARINIC.

Antifibrinolytic (anti-, -ly-)   A substance that inhibits the enzymatic dissolution of fibrin.

Antigen (anti-, -gen)   An agent that, under suitable conditions, induces a specific immune response. It also interacts with antibodies or sensitised T-cells specific to it, or both.

Antigen determinant (anti-, -gen)   The chemical structure on the surface of an antigen responsible for the specific interaction with an antibody.

Antimicrobial (anti-, -micro-)   An agent that kills or inhibits the growth of micro-organisms. *See also* ANTIBIOTIC.

Antimicrobial resistance (anti-, -micro-)   A micro-organism may be naturally insensitive to an antimicrobial agent. Alternatively, a micro-organism may acquire resistance during use of an antimicrobial by natural selection of a resistant strain or by random mutation. Resistance may also be transferred from one micro-organism to another.

Antimuscarinic (anti-)   An agent that antagonises the action of acetylcholine at muscarinic receptors of the parasympathetic nervous system.

Antinuclear antibody (anti-, -nucle-)   An auto-antibody that interacts with specific components of cell nuclei (e.g. DNA).

Antiseptic (anti-, -sep-)   A chemical agent used to kill or inhibit the growth of micro-organisms on living tissue, in order to prevent or reduce the harmful effects of infection. *See also* DISINFECTANT.

Antiserum (anti-, -ser-)   A human or animal serum preparation containing antibodies, whose production is induced by the administration of an antigen or by natural infection. Antisera are used for passive immunisation. *See also* VACCINE.

Antitoxin (anti-, -toxi-)   An antibody that acts against a toxin, especially a bacterial exotoxin.

Anuria (an-, -uria)   Complete cessation of urine formation by the kidneys, and hence excretion.

Apathy   Indifference or lack of concern, interest, or emotion.

Aphasia (a-, -pha-, -ia)   A reduction in, or loss of, comprehension of spoken or written language, or the ability to speak or write. It is usually caused by a lesion of the speech centre of the brain.

Aphonia (a-, -phon-, -ia)   Loss of voice.

Aphtha   Small, shallow, and painful ulcer, usually of the oral mucosa.

Aplasia (a-, -plasia)   1. Incomplete development of an organ, tissue, or part, although the basic structure may be present. 2. Incomplete or absent formation of cellular products from an organ or tissue.
See also AGENESIS, DYSGENESIS, DYSPLASIA, *and* HYPOPLASIA.

Apnoea (a-, -pnoea)   Cessation of breathing. *See also* DYSPNOEA, HYPERPNOEA, ORTHOPNOEA, *and* TACHYPNOEA.

Appendage (ap-, -pend-)   An outgrowth from a body or organ.

Appendectomy (-ectomy)   The removal of the appendix by surgery.

Apposed (ap-)   Two surfaces in contact with each other. *See also* CONTIGUOUS.

Apraxia (a-, -prax-, -ia)   Impairment of voluntary muscular movement in the absence of paralysis or other impairment of motor or sensory pathways. *See also* ATAXIA.

Arachidonic acid   An essential unsaturated fatty acid found in animal fats, and a precursor of prostaglandins.

Arterial tension (arteri-, tens-)   The pressure provoked by blood within an artery.

Arterionecrosis (arterio-, -necro-, -sis)   Necrosis of arteries.

Arteritis (arter-, -itis)   Inflammation of an artery. *See also* VASCULITIS.

Arthralgia (arthr-, -algia)   Joint pain.

Arthropathy (arthro-, -pathy)   Any disease of the joints.

Articular (articul-)   Refers to a joint.

Artificial respiration (-spirat-)   A technique employed to produce respiratory movements when natural movements have ceased. *See also* ASSISTED VENTILATION.

Aschoff nodule   A granulomatous lesion with a central necrotic core.

Aseptic (a-, -sep-)   Refers to the complete absence of micro-organisms.

Asexual reproduction Production of offspring without gametes and fusion. Asexual methods include budding and fission. *See also* SEXUAL REPRODUCTION.

Asphyxia (a-, -ia) Impaired or absent ventilation caused by airway obstruction or lack of oxygen in inspired air. *See also* SUFFOCATION.

Aspiration (-spirat-) 1. To remove fluid from body cavities by applying suction. 2. Inhalation.

Assisted ventilation Respiratory support by mechanical means. *See also* ARTIFICIAL RESPIRATION.

Astigmatism (a-, -stig-, -ism) A focusing abnormality of the eye caused by irregular surfaces of the cornea or lens, resulting in blurred or distorted vision.

Astringent (-stringent) An agent that causes constriction of tissues to lessen secretion or discharge.

Astrocyte (astro-, -cyte) A cell found in the grey and white matter of the central nervous system, and forming part of the supporting network for neurones.

Astrocytoma (astro-, -cyt-, -oma) A malignant neoplasm composed of astrocytes.

Asymptomatic (a-) Symptom-free.

Ataxia (a-, -tax-, -ia) Impaired co-ordination of muscular movements. *See also* APRAXIA.

Atheroma (-oma) Plaques on arterial walls, initially of cholesterol deposits, which may become fibrous or calcified.

Athetosis (-osis) Repetitive, involuntary, slow, writhing movements of the limbs, usually most severe in the hands and feet.

Atony (a-, -ton-) Decreased tone of a tissue, resulting in weakness or loss of normal strength.

Atopic (a-, -top-) 1. Refers to atopy. 2. ECTOPIC(2).

Atopy (a-, -top-) A hypersensitivity to common allergens, involving immunoglobulin E (IgE). It is thought to be familial. *See also* ALLERGY.

ATP ADENOSINE TRIPHOSPHATE.

Atresia (a-, -ia) Abnormal closure of a channel in the body (e.g. bile duct) or an external orifice (e.g. anus).

Atrophy (a-, -trophy) The decrease in size of a cell, organ, tissue, or part of an organism. *See also* HYPERTROPHY *and* INVOLUTION.

Aura The sensations preceding the onset of any paroxysmal attack. The aura may be affective, sensory, or motor. *See also* PRODROMAL.

Auto-antibody (auto-, -anti-) An antibody produced in autoimmune diseases as a result of immunological intolerance of the body's own tissues. Auto-antibodies may be organ-specific or antinuclear.

Auto-immunity (auto-) The immune response directed towards the body's own tissues, which results in the production of auto-antibodies.

Auto-infection (auto-) Infection caused by micro-organisms already present in the body, and commonly, but not exclusively, transferred from one site to another.

Autolysis (auto-, -lysis) Destruction of cells or tissues by the action of the organism's own intracellar enzymes. It occurs after death, or it may be pathological.

Autonomous (auto-) Functionally independent.

Autosome (auto-, -some) Any of the chromosomes in a cell, excluding the sex chromosomes. In a human somatic cell there are 44 autosomes (22 pairs) and 2 sex chromosomes (1 pair).

Autotrophic (auto-, -trophic) A type of nutrition in which carbon dioxide is the sole source of carbon for synthesis of organic compounds. *See also* HETEROTROPHIC.

Avascular (a-, -vas-) Lack of blood supply to a tissue. *See also* VASCULAR.

Avirulent (a-) Not pathogenic.

Axon The long specialised process of a neurone along which impulses travel away from the cell body to other neurones and tissues.

Azoospermia (a-, -zoo-, -sperm-, -ia) Absence of spermatozoa in the semen.

B

Bacteraemia (bacter-, -aemia) The presence of bacteria in the blood.

Bacteriophage (bacterio-, -phag-) A virus that causes lysis of bacteria, usually specific for a particular strain or species.

Bacteriuria (bacteri-, -uria) The presence of bacteria in the urine.

Balanitis (balan-, -itis) Inflammation of the glans penis and the prepuce in the male, or the clitoris in the female.

Barrier nursing The nursing techniques applied to prevent the spread of infection from the affected patient to others. Reverse barrier nursing comprises the nursing techniques applied to infection-prone patients who are kept in isolation to prevent the acquisition of infection.

Basal (bas-) Refers to, or situated near, the base.

Base (bas-) 1. The lowest part of a structure or organ. 2. A non-acid that can combine with an acid to form a salt; a proton acceptor; a liberator of hydroxyl ions (OH^-) in water. *See also* ACID.

Behaviour disorder (dis-) A disorder of behaviour often associated with psychoses and related disorders, characterised by abnormal actions (e.g. disinhibition, hyperactivity, or mannerisms).

Behaviour therapy (therap-) Psychological treatment to alleviate the symptoms of abnormal behaviour produced by certain stimuli.

Benign A condition that is mild, favouring recovery, and not recurrent or malignant.

Betacarotene A provitamin found in some vegetables (e.g. carrots) and converted to vitamin A by the liver.

Betz's cells Large pyramidal neurones of the Betz cell area in the motor cortex. They form part of the pyramidal tract and control voluntary movement.

Bicarbonate   A salt of carbonic acid in which the anionic portion is HCO_3^-. Administered as sodium bicarbonate infusion to correct acid-base imbalance.

Biliary (bili-)   Refers to the gall bladder, bile ducts, or bile.

Biopsy (bio-)   The removal of living tissue, diseased or normal, for examination, used as an aid in diagnosis.

Biosynthesis (bio-, -syn-, -sis)   The formation of substances within a living organism by the process of synthesis, often under the control of enzymes.

Bipolar (bi-)   1. Possessing two poles, or processes at both ends. 2. At both ends of a cell. 3. Used to describe affective disorders characterised by both manic and depressive periods. *See also* UNIPOLAR.

Birth asphyxia (a-, -ia)   Birth asphyxia (neonatal asphyxia) occurs at, or during, birth, usually due to disorders *in utero*.

Birth canal   Comprises the cervix, vagina, and vulva, and through which the foetus passes during birth.

Blepharospasm (blepharo-, -spas-)   Tonic muscular spasm of the eyelid, resulting in complete or partial closure of the eye.

Blind antimicrobial treatment (anti-, -micro-)   Antimicrobial therapy administered to a patient with pyrexia of unknown origin (PUO), before microbiological confirmation of infection and antimicrobial sensitivity. *See also* BROAD-SPECTRUM ANTIMICROBIAL DRUG.

Bone marrow   Specialised tissue found in the cavity of long bones and the spongy tissue of all bones. It consists of a network of reticular fibres and cells, including blood cells at different stages of development, fat cells, and macrophages. Its functions include the production of erythrocytes, leucocytes, and platelets.

Bone reabsorption (re-)   Loss of bone tissue mediated by osteoclasts, which may be physiological or pathological.

Boss   A round protruding part of a structure or tissue.

Bradykinesia (brady-, -kine-, -ia)   Abnormally slow movement, and physical and mental response. *See also* AKINESIA, DYSKINESIA, *and* HYPOKINESIA.

Bradykinin   A polypeptide, and one of a group of kinins.

Broad-spectrum antimicrobial drug (anti-, -micro-)   Describes the activity of an antimicrobial drug to which a wide range of micro-organisms are sensitive. *See also* BLIND ANTIMICROBIAL TREATMENT.

Bronchopulmonary (broncho-, -pulmon-)   Refers to the lungs and the airways into them (i.e. the bronchi and bronchioles).

Bronchoscopy (broncho-, -scopy)   Examination of the bronchi using a fibre-optic bronchoscope, which is also a tool for biopsy.

Bronchospasm (broncho-, -spas-)   Spasmodic smooth muscle contraction of the bronchi.

Bunion   A swelling of the first metatarsophalangeal joint caused by a bursa. It results in displacement of the great toe.

—————— C ——————

Cachexia (cac-, -ia)   Severe generalised ill-health caused by chronic disorders or malnutrition, and marked by emaciation and general weakness.

Cadaver   A corpse. The term usually refers to a human body used for medical study or other procedures (e.g. transplantation).

Caesarean section (sect-)   Surgical delivery of a foetus by incision through the abdominal and uterine walls.

Calcification (calci-)   The physiological or pathological deposition of calcium salts in tissues, resulting in hardening.

Calculus (calc-)   A hard stone-like deposit of mineral salts or other material, found in certain body cavities and tissues (e.g. kidney, bladder, and gall bladder).

Cancer   A malignant neoplasm.

Cannabis   Part of any plant of the genus *Cannabis*. Its various forms are known by many names, including bhang, ganja, hashish, and marijuana.

Capsule (caps-)   1. Outer covering of an organ or structure. 2. A shell, usually made from a gelatin basis, containing glycerol in proportions that may be varied to regulate the degree of hardness. Capsules are used to enclose one or more drugs and excipients.

Capsulitis (caps-, -itis)   Inflammation of a capsule.

Carbohydrate (carbo-, -hydrat-)   A member of a large and diverse group of organic compounds containing carbon, hydrogen, and oxygen. Carbohydrates include sugars, starches, celluloses, and gums, and are classified as monosaccharides (e.g. glucose), disaccharides (e.g. sucrose), and polysaccharides (e.g. glycogen). They act as the principal source of metabolic energy in living cells.

Carbonic anhydrase (carbo-, -an-, -hydr-, -ase)   An enzyme that catalyses the conversion of carbon dioxide and water to carbonic acid, which further dissociates into hydrogen ions (H^+) and bicarbonate ions (HCO_3^-).

Carcinogen (carcino-, -gen)   An agent capable of inducing a malignant neoplasm.

Carcinoid (carcin-, -oid)   Histologically similar to a malignant neoplasm but clinically benign.

Cardiac (cardi-)   1. Refers to the heart. 2. Refers to the opening between the oesophagus and the stomach.

Cardiac massage, external (cardi-)   Rhythmic manual compression of the heart to maintain the circulation by applying pressure over the sternum.

Cardiac output (cardi-)   The amount of blood expelled per minute into the aorta from the left ventricle. It is equal to the stroke volume multiplied by the number of beats per minute.

Cardiac reserve (cardi-)   The capacity of the heart for increased function in response to greater demands, expressed as the maximum percentage that the cardiac output can increase above normal.

Cardiac tamponade (cardi-)   Compression of the heart as a result of the accumulation of fluid or blood within the pericardium.

Cardiogenic (cardio-, -genic) 1. Arising from the heart or as a result of its abnormal function. 2. Refers to the embryonic development of the heart.

Cardiomyocyte (cardio-, -myo-, -cyte) A cell of the myocardium.

Cardiomyotomy (cardio-, -myo-, -tomy) Incision through the muscle layer at the junction of the oesophagus and the stomach, but excluding the mucous membrane.

Cardioversion (cardio-, -vers-) Synchronised transthoracic electric shock applied under general anaesthesia to restore sinus rhythm of the heart.

Carditis (card-, -itis) Inflammation of the heart.

Carotid artery (arter-) An artery supplying the head and neck. There are two common carotid arteries, designated left and right. Each passes upwards through the neck, where they divide to form the internal and external carotid arteries.

Carotid sinus (sinu-) The small dilated region in the internal carotid artery. It contains baroreceptors that are sensitive to blood pressure fluctuations, and which are involved in the reflex control of blood pressure and heart-rate.

Carpal tunnel (carp-) The passage in the wrist between the carpal bones and ligaments, through which the median nerve passes.

Carrier 1. An individual who harbours (and is thus capable of transmitting) the micro-organisms capable of causing an infection, without showing any signs or symptoms of illness. *See also* RESERVOIR OF INFECTION. 2. An individual capable of transmitting an hereditary disease to offspring. 3. A substance used to transport a drug as an aid to efficacy.

Caseation 1. The precipitation of casein during the coagulation of milk. 2. A degeneration or necrosis in which morbid tissues are changed into a dry cheese-like mass.

Catabolism (cata-) A form of metabolism in which complex compounds are broken down by living cells to form simpler substances. *See also* ANABOLISM *and* FERMENTATION.

Catalase (cata-, -ase) An enzyme present in most cells, except some anaerobic bacteria, and responsible for the breakdown of hydrogen peroxide to water and oxygen.

Catarrh Inflammation of a mucous membrane (particularly one in the upper respiratory tract) causing an increased flow of mucus.

Catecholamine A sympathomimetic compound containing a catechol and an amine group. Physiological examples include adrenaline, noradrenaline, and dopamine.

Catheter A flexible tube inserted into a body cavity to withdraw or introduce fluids. *See also* INDWELLING CATHETER.

Cauda equina (caud-) The nerve roots arising from the lower part of the spinal cord and forming a tail-like structure.

Cauterisation The therapeutic destruction of tissue using heat, an electric current, or caustic agents. *See also* CRYOSURGERY.

Cavernous (cav-, -ous) Refers to a structure or tissue containing hollow spaces.

Cavitation (cav-) 1. The formation of hollow spaces within tissues. 2. A cavity.

Central vision Vision produced through stimulation of the macula lutea by light. *See also* PERIPHERAL VISION.

Cercaria The final free-swimming larval stage of flukes.

Cerebellum A motor area of the brain involved in the involuntary control of co-ordination, posture, and balance.

Cerebral (cerebr-) Refers to the cerebrum.

Cerebrovascular (cerebro-, -vas-) Refers to the blood vessels that supply the brain, and especially the cerebral hemispheres.

Cervical smear (cervic-) A cervical smear (Pap test) is the microscopic examination of cells obtained from the cervix of the uterus, and used to detect cervical cell abnormalities.

Cervicitis (cervic-, -itis) Inflammation of the cervix of the uterus.

Cervicofacial (cervic-, -faci-) Refers to the face and neck.

Cervix The neck of an organ or body, but generally refers to the neck of the uterus.

Chalone 1. A hormone that exerts an inhibitory effect. 2. A tissue-specific reversible inhibitor of mitosis produced by the tissue itself.

Chancre A primary ulcer-like lesion at the point of entry of an infection, usually applied to the primary lesion seen in syphilis.

Cheilitis (cheil-, -itis) Inflammation of the lips.

Chelate To form a complex with a metal ion, incorporating it into a ring and rendering it inactive.

Chemoprophylaxis (chemo-) The use of a chemotherapeutic agent as a preventive measure against disease.

Chemosurgery (chemo-) 1. The combined use of surgery and chemical agents to remove diseased tissue. 2. The therapeutic destruction of tissue using chemical agents.

Chemotaxis (chemo-, -tax-) The directional movement of a cell or organism in response to a chemical stimulus.

Chemotherapy (chemo-, -therap-) The treatment of disease using drugs.

Cheyne-Stokes respiration (-spirat-) An abnormal respiratory rhythm characterised by alternating periods of hyperpnoea and apnoea.

Chiasma The crossing of two elements or structures in an X-formation.

Cholecystectomy (chole-, -cyst-, -ectomy) The removal of the gall bladder by surgery.

Choledochotomy (choledocho-, -tomy) Surgical incision of the bile duct for investigation or the removal of gallstones.

Cholestasis (chole-, -stasis) The complete or partial inhibition of the flow of bile.

Cholesterol (chole-, -ster-, -ol) A steroid alcohol synthesised in the liver and used in the formation of bile acids and steroid hormones (e.g. oestrogens). Cholesterol may also be ingested in the diet (e.g. in animal fats, milk, egg-yolk, liver, and kidneys).

Cholinergic Refers to parasympathetic nerves or to the characteristics of acetylcholine and substances producing similar effects. *See also* ADRENERGIC.

Chondritis (chondr-, -itis) Inflammation of cartilage.

Chordae tendineae (chord-, ten-) The tendinous cords connecting each cusp of the tricuspid and mitral valves to the papillary muscles in the heart.

Chorionic gonadotrophin (gon-, -trophin) A hormone produced by placental tissue, and which stimulates the gonads. It is also found in the urine of pregnant females.

Chromaffin cell (chrom-) A specialised cell that readily stains with chromium salts, and is found in the adrenal medulla and other parts of the sympathetic nervous system. It is responsible for the storage and secretion of catecholamines.

Chromatolysis (chromato-, -lysis) The disintegration of the Nissl granules within a nerve cell body, caused by injury or cell fatigue.

Chromophobe cell (chromo-, -phobe) A cell that does not stain easily, if at all. In particular, it refers to some agranular cells in the anterior lobe of the pituitary gland.

Chromosome (chromo-, -some) A structure present in all cell nuclei, formed of chromatin and containing DNA. Animals have a characteristic number of chromosomes present in all somatic cells. In man, this number is 46 (23 pairs). *See also* AUTOSOME.

Chronic (chron-) Refers to a disorder which persists. *See also* ACUTE *and* SUBACUTE.

Chyluria (-uria) The presence of chyle in the urine.

Cicatrix The new tissue formed on healing of a wound; a scar.

Cilia (cili-) 1. Hair-like projections from a cell that facilitate movement. 2. Eyelashes. 3. Eyelids.

Circadian rhythm (circa-) The cycle of about 24 hours that marks repetitive biological activities and functions in living organisms. *See also* DIURNAL *and* NOCTURNAL.

Claudication Limping.

Clitoris A part of the female external genitalia situated at the anterior end of the vulva and corresponding to the male penis in structure, position, and origin. The clitoris is normally less than 2 cm long.

Clonus Muscular contraction and relaxation occurring in rapid succession. *See also* MYOCLONUS.

Clubbing Enlargement of the soft tissue of the fingers and toes, resulting in a characteristic deformity. The nails are curved and have a shiny appearance.

Coarctation Narrowing or stricture. *See also* STENOSIS.

Coccidioidomycosis (-myco-, -sis) A fungal infection caused by *Coccidioides immitis*, and affecting the skin, bone, viscera, or respiratory tract.

Codon A set of three nucleotides in one strand of DNA or RNA, and which carries the code for one amino acid.

Coenocytic (coeno-, -cyt-) Refers to a cell or mass of cytoplasm in which there is more than one nucleus.

Coenzyme (co-, -zym-) A non-protein organic substance that activates an enzyme.

Coitus Sexual intercourse between a male and a female.

Cold abscess An abscess that is not inflamed and warm, and develops slowly.

Colectomy (col-, -ectomy) The complete or partial removal of the colon by surgery.

Colitis (col-, -itis) Inflammation of the colon.

Collagen The constituent protein of the white fibres of connective tissue.

Collagenase (-ase) An enzyme that catalyses collagen degradation.

Collateral (col-) Secondary, subordinate, or alternative.

Colloid cyst A cyst containing material that resembles jelly, and which is sometimes found in the brain.

Colonoscopy (col-, -scopy) Examination of the colon using a fibre-optic colonoscope, which is also a tool for biopsy.

Colorectal (col-, -rect-) Refers to the colon and the rectum.

Colostomy (col-, -stomy) A surgical procedure to establish an opening (stoma) from the colon to the surface of the abdomen, and through which faeces may be eliminated. It may be temporary or permanent. The term may also be applied to the opening itself. *See also* ILEOSTOMY *and* UROSTOMY.

Coma A state of deep unconsciousness with no voluntary response to external stimuli. Some reflex actions may also be impaired. *See also* STUPOR.

Common bile duct The duct that transports bile to the duodenum. It is formed by the merging of the cystic duct from the gall bladder and the common hepatic duct from the liver.

Complement A series of 9 components (C1 to C9) activated in a specific sequence (cascade) by certain antigen-antibody complexes. Activated complement binds to the complex and destroys the antigen by several possible mechanisms (e.g. chemotaxis and inflammation, cell lysis, and phagocytosis). The system is regulated by inhibitory factors (e.g. C1-esterase inhibitor).

Compliance 1. A measure of the ability of an organ (e.g. heart, bladder, or lungs) to alter shape and size in response to varying demands. 2. Agreement, consent, or yielding to the wishes of another.

Computerised tomography Computerised tomography (CT) is a technique which uses X-rays and detectors to scan the body in cross-section. Visual images are produced by computer processing of the data.

Conception The start of pregnancy, marked by the fertilisation of an ovum.

Concretion 1. The formation of a solid mass. 2. CALCULUS.

Congenital (-gen-) Refers to any condition existing before or at birth. *See also* HEREDITARY.

Conidium An asexual spore formed at the tip of a conidiophore (a specialised branch of a mycelium). The conidium is non-motile and is produced by some species of fungi and filamentous bacteria.

Conjugated hyperbilirubinaemia *See* HYPERBILIRUBINAEMIA.

Consolidation The process of becoming firm or solid. *See also* CONCRETION.

Contagious May be transmitted from one individual to another.

Contiguous (con-) Two parts that are adjacent or in contact. *See also* APPOSED.

Contraction (-tract-) A shortening or reduction in overall size that is usually temporary, or an increase in tension (e.g. muscle contraction to facilitate movement).

Contracture (-tract-) A sustained shortening or contraction of muscle(s), caused by pathological changes in muscle tissue.

Contra-indication (contra-) A condition or disease that renders an otherwise acceptable treatment completely unsuitable.

Contusion A bruise; an injury that does not break the skin.

Convulsion An involuntary, violent, and spasmodic or prolonged contraction of skeletal muscles. *See also* SEIZURE.

Coralline Similar to, or branching like, coral.

Coronary Refers to vessels, nerves, or ligaments that encircle a structure, although usually applied to the arteries that lie over the outer surface of cardiac muscle.

Coronary bypass A surgical procedure to bypass an obstruction in a coronary artery. A vein (usually taken from the leg) or other suitable conduit is grafted between the aorta and coronary arteries and distal to the obstruction.

Cowpox A skin infection affecting the udders and teats of cows, caused by cowpox virus (vaccinia). It may be transmitted to man. *See also* VACCINATION(2).

Cramp An involuntary and painful spasmodic muscle contraction.

Craniotomy (cranio-, -tomy) A surgical procedure on the cranium.

Creatinine The end-product of metabolism in muscle tissue, excreted by the kidneys.

Creatinine clearance The volume of plasma cleared of creatinine, expressed as mL per minute.

Cribriform plate The bony plate at the top of the nasal cavity, which is perforated to allow the passage of the olfactory nerves. *See also* ETHMOID BONE.

Cross tolerance Tolerance acquired to one drug which is exhibited towards other, usually similar, agents.

Cryosurgery (cryo-) The therapeutic destruction of tissue using extremely low temperatures.

Cryotherapy (cryo-, -therap-) The use of low temperatures for therapeutic purposes. *See also* CAUTERISATION.

Crypt A small pocket or recess found on the surface of some tissues.

Cryptogenic (crypto-, -genic) Of unknown origin. *See also* IDIOPATHIC.

Crystalluria (-uria) The presence of crystals in the urine.

Cubitus valgus Deformity of the elbow, marked by a deviation away from the body when the arm is placed by the side.

Curettage The removal of material from a surface or cavity wall using a spoon-shaped instrument (curette).

Cutaneous (cut-) Refers to the skin.

Cuticle (cut-) 1. The epidermis. 2. The epidermis that surrounds the base of the nail. 3. A layer covering the free surface of epithelial cells.

Cyst 1. An enclosed cavity or sac with an epithelial lining, and often containing fluid. 2. A stage in the life-cycle of some parasites, marked by enclosure within a protective covering.

Cystadenoma (cyst-, -aden-, -oma) An adenoma in which fluid-filled cysts form.

Cystectomy (cyst-, -ectomy) 1. The removal of a cyst. 2. The complete or partial removal of the urinary bladder by surgery.

Cystic (cysti-) 1. Refers to a cyst. 2. Refers to the urinary bladder or to the gall bladder.

Cystic duct (cysti-) The duct passing from the gall bladder to the common bile duct, and through which bile passes.

Cystinuria (-uria) An hereditary disorder that results in excessive urinary excretion of cystine, arginine, lysine, and ornithine and results in the formation of urinary cystine calculi.

Cytoplasm (cyto-, -plas-) The protoplasm of a cell located outside the nucleus. *See also* NUCLEOPLASM.

Cytoplasmic membrane (cyto-, -plas-) The membrane enclosing the cytoplasm of a cell, composed of phospholipids and proteins.

Cytostatic (cyto-, -stat-) 1. Refers to the suppression of cell growth and multiplication. 2. Refers to the blockage of capillaries by leucocytes in the early stages of inflammation.

Cytotoxic (cyto-, -toxi-) Refers to agents that have an adverse effect on cells.

D

Dacryocystorhinostomy (dacryo-, -cysto-, -rhino-, -stomy) Surgical procedure to create a passage from the lachrymal sac to the nasal cavity.

Danders Scales from animal hair or bird feathers.

Dark adaptation Adjustment by the eye for night vision.

Dead space 1. The regions within the respiratory tract through which air passes, but exchange of oxygen and carbon dioxide does not take place. 2. A cavity that remains after incomplete closure of a wound.

Debility (de-) 1. Generalised weakness and loss of strength. 2. Loss of muscle tone due to illness.

Debridement (de-) The removal of dead, injured, or infected tissue, or foreign material from a wound.

Decerebrate (de-, -cerebr-) Loss of cerebral function as a result of brain damage.

Decerebrate posture A position characteristic of damage to the upper part of the brain stem. The patient's legs are rigidly extended with flexed ankles and toes, the arms are internally rotated, and the elbows are extended.

Decompression (de-) A procedure to relieve pressure exerted on or within tissues.

Defaecation (de-) The elimination of faeces from the rectum.

Definitive host The host within which a parasite reaches sexual maturity or its adult stage. *See also* INTERMEDIATE HOST.

Dehydration (de-, -hydrat-) The removal or loss of water from a substance or from body tissues.

Delirium A mental disorder of varying severity characterised by hallucinations, delusions, impaired perception, excitement, restlessness, and disorientation.

Delirium tremens Delirium caused by alcohol withdrawal in alcohol-dependent subjects.

Delusion A false belief that is firmly held, even in the presence of irrefutable evidence to the contrary. *See also* HALLUCINATION.

Demyelination (de-, -myel-) Loss of the myelin sheath surrounding nerves.

Denature (de-) To alter the nature of a substance; often applied to proteins that are physically changed by the action of heat or chemical agents. Also applied to the adulteration of alcohol to render it unfit for consumption.

Dendritic (dendr-) 1. Branching, like a tree. 2. Refers to the cytoplasmic thread-like extensions (dendrites) of neurones.

Dentition (denti-) The teeth; usually refers to natural teeth and their position.

Deoxyribonucleic acid (-nucle-) Deoxyribonucleic acid (DNA) is found in the nucleus of all living cells and is the store of genetic information. The molecular structure is a double helix, in which each of the two strands is composed of a deoxyribose-phosphate backbone with attached nitrogenous bases (adenine, cytosine, guanine, and thymine). The two strands are held together by hydrogen bonds between the bases, which pair in a specific sequence to determine the genetic information. *See also* RIBONUCLEIC ACID.

Dermabrasion (derma-) Skin abrasion using wire brushes or sandpaper, under local anaesthesia, to remove superficial lesions.

Dermatitis herpetiformis (derma-, -itis, herpet-, -form-) A chronic skin disorder with remissions and relapses, which is frequently associated with coeliac disease. It is characterised by intense pruritus and the presence of symmetrical groups of erythematous lesions (e.g. bullae, papules, and vesicles) on the buttocks, elbows, knees, scalp, and shoulders. Hyperpigmentation is a common feature, although hypopigmentation and scarring may also occur.

Dermatographism (dermato-, -graph-, -ism) Urticaria caused by firm stroking of the skin.

Desquamation (de-, -squam-) The shedding of an outer layer (e.g. epithelial cells of the skin) in the form of scales.

Dialysis (dia-, -lysis) The separation of small non-colloidal molecules from larger colloidal molecules in solution, across a semipermeable membrane. *See also* HAEMODIALYSIS *and* PERITONEAL DIALYSIS.

Diaphragm (dia-, -phrag-) A structure separating one area from another. It usually refers to the muscular structure that separates the thoracic cavity from the abdominal cavity.

Diaphysis The shaft of a long bone. *See also* EPIPHYSIS.

Diarthroidal joint (-arthr-) A joint that is freely movable (e.g. hip, elbow, or wrist).

Diastole The period during which the chambers of the heart dilate and fill with blood. *See also* SYSTOLE.

Diastolic pressure The minimum arterial blood pressure, which occurs during ventricular diastole. *See also* SYSTOLIC PRESSURE.

Diathermy (-therm-) The heat treatment of tissues using an electric current, ultrasonic waves, or electromagnetic radiation. It may be used to warm tissues or destroy them. *See also* CRYOSURGERY.

Differentiation Applied to cells and tissues as they mature into specialised forms and acquire specificity.

Diffusion (di-, -fus-) The spontaneous movement of molecules, ions, or particles in order to reach a uniform concentration throughout the solvent.

Dilatation The increase in volume or enlargement of orifices and hollow organs and structures (e.g. colon, arteries, and heart). *See also* DISTENSION.

Diphtheroid (-oid) Similar to diphtheria or the causative microorganism, *Corynebacterium diphtheriae*.

Diplegia (di-, -plegia) Paralysis affecting corresponding parts on both sides of the body. *See also* HEMIPLEGIA, PARAPLEGIA, *and* QUADRIPLEGIA.

Diploid (di-, -ploid) Having two sets of chromosomes.

Diplopia (dipl-, -opia) Double vision, in which two images of a single object are seen.

Disinfectant (dis-) A chemical agent used to destroy microorganisms, but not necessarily bacterial spores; it may reduce the number to a level below that which is harmful rather than kill all the micro-organisms present. The term may be applied to treatment of inanimate objects, as well as body surfaces and cavities. *See also* ANTISEPTIC.

Disseminated (dis-) Dispersed or spread throughout.

Disseminated intravascular coagulation (dis-, intra-, -vas-) A condition in which there is widespread activation of tissue factor, which leads to blood clotting within vessels. A generalised depletion of clotting factors eventually causes haemorrhage. A variety of disorders may allow elements that activate tissue factor to enter the blood. These include obstetric complications, Gram-negative endotoxins, adenocarcinomas, snake-bites, and major trauma.

Distension Enlargement due to internal pressure. *See also* DILATATION.

Diuresis (-ur-, -sis) An increase in urine production. *See also* ENURESIS *and* INCONTINENCE.

Diurnal Refers to activities that occur during the hours of daylight. *See also* CIRCADIAN RHYTHM *and* NOCTURNAL.

DNA DEOXYRIBONUCLEIC ACID.

Duodenal bulb The first part of the duodenum, adjacent to the pylorus.

Dynamic (dynami-) Refers to force and motion; active.

Dysaesthesia (dys-, -aesthesi-) Impairment of sensory function, particularly touch. *See also* ACROPARAESTHESIA, ANAESTHESIA, *and* PARAESTHESIA.

Dyscrasia (dys-) A general term for any abnormal condition, particularly developmental or metabolic disorders.

Dysfunction (dys-, -funct-) Functional abnormality of an organ.

Dysgenesis (dys-, -gen-, -sis) Defective development, often applied to embryonic development. *See also* AGENESIS, APLASIA, DYSPLASIA, *and* HYPOPLASIA.

Dyskinesia (dys-, -kine-, -ia) Difficulty in voluntary movement such that movements are partial, incomplete, or fragmentary. *See also* AKINESIA, BRADYKINESIA, *and* HYPOKINESIA.

Dyslexia (dys-, -ia) A reading abnormality in the presence of normal intellect, which may be caused by a brain lesion. There may also be spelling and handwriting impairment.

Dyspareunia (dys-, -ia) Difficult or painful sexual intercourse.

Dysplasia (dys-, -plasia) Abnormal development of an organ or part. *See also* AGENESIS, APLASIA, DYSGENESIS, *and* HYPOPLASIA.

Dyspnoea (dys-, -pnoea) Difficulty in breathing. *See also* APNOEA, HYPERPNOEA, ORTHOPNOEA, *and* TACHYPNOEA.

Dysuria (dys-, -uria) Difficult or painful urination. *See also* STRANGURY.

E

ECT ELECTROCONVULSIVE THERAPY

Ectopia (ecto-, -ia) Malposition or displacement of an organ or part. It is usually congenital.

Ectopic (ecto-) 1. Refers to ectopia. 2. Not in its normal location, or originating from an abnormal site.

Eczematous Refers to, or has the characteristics of, eczema.

EEG ELECTROENCEPHALOGRAM.

Efferent (e-, -ferent) Carrying outwards from a centre. *See also* AFFERENT.

Efficacy The capacity to produce a desired effect.

Effusion (e-, -fus-) The discharge or spread of fluid (e.g. blood), usually into parts of the body.

Elastase (-ase) An enzyme that catalyses the hydrolysis of peptide bonds (e.g. of elastin in connective tissue).

Electroconvulsive therapy (electro-, therap-) Electroconvulsive therapy (ECT) involves the passage of an electric current between two electrodes, usually at the anterior temporal regions of the scalp. It is performed under general anaesthesia and muscle relaxation, and a convulsion is induced. Adverse effects include amnesia and learning difficulties, but these are usually temporary. Serious adverse effects are rare.

Electrodesiccation (electro-) Destruction of tissue using an electric current applied with a small electrode. It results in dehydration and charring of tissue. *See also* ELECTROLYSIS.

Electroencephalogram (electro-, -encephalo-, -gram) An electroencephalogram (EEG) is a record of the brain's electrical activity. Characteristic distortion of normal wave patterns is associated with disorders of brain function.

Electrolysis (electro-, -lysis) Destruction of tissue using an electric current. It results in a focal inflammatory reaction. *See also* ELECTRODESICCATION.

Electrolyte balance (electro-) The concentration of plasma electrolytes within normal limits, and maintained by homoeostasis.

Emaciation Extreme leanness or wasting of the body with loss of subcutaneous fat, and caused by illness or starvation.

Embolectomy (-ectomy) The removal of an embolus by surgery.

Embolisation 1. Pathological occlusion of a blood vessel by a blood clot, bubble of air, foreign body, or fat (i.e. an embolus). 2. Formation of an embolus. 3. Therapeutic occlusion of a blood vessel.

Embryo The stage following fertilisation, usually characterised by the period of most rapid development. In man, this stage is the first 8 weeks of gestation. *See also* FOETUS *and* NEONATE.

Embryogenesis (-gen-, -sis) The process of embryo formation and development.

Empyema (em-, -py-) The collection of pus within a body cavity.

Encysted (en-, -cyst-) Enclosed in a resistant capsule. *See also* CYST.

Endarterectomy (end-, -arter-, -ectomy) The removal of the tunica intima of an artery by surgery.

Endemic (end-) Refers to a disease caused by factors constantly present in an affected region or community, but producing clinical symptoms in very few. *See also* EPIDEMIC.

Endocervix (endo-) The inner lining of the neck of the uterus, or the opening of the cervix into the uterus.

Endocrine (endo-) Refers to the functions of endocrine glands, which secrete hormones directly into the blood or lymph and not into a duct. *See also* EXOCRINE.

Endocytosis (endo-, -cyto-, -sis) The process by which cells engulf material, which may be liquid (pinocytosis) or solid (phagocytosis). The cytoplasmic membrane folds inwards, carrying the enclosed material into the cell.

Endogenous (endo-, -genous) Arising or developing from within. *See also* EXOGENOUS(1).

Endometritis (endo-, -metr-, -itis) Inflammation of the endometrium.

Endomyocardium (endo-, -myo-, -cardi-) Comprises both the myocardium and endocardium.

Endoneurium (endo-, -neur-) The connective tissue within peripheral nerves that separates individual fibres.

Endoplasmic reticulum (endo-, ret-) A network of membrane-bound channels in the cytoplasm of eukaryotic cells. It is responsible for intracellular transport, and the storage and synthesis of materials.

Endoscopy (endo-, -scopy) Visual examination of hollow organs or cavities of the body (e.g. stomach) using a fibre-optic endoscope, which is also a tool for biopsy.

Endospore (endo-, -spor-) A spore formed within a cell or hypha, by asexual or sexual reproduction. *See also* EXOSPORE(2).

Endothelium (endo-) The inner cellular layer of all body cavities and of the cardiovascular system. *See also* EPITHELIUM.

Endotoxin (endo-, -toxi-) A heat-stable lipopolysaccharide found in bacterial cell walls, especially in those classified as Gram-negative, and which is released after the death of the cell. Endotoxins possess pyrogenic properties. *See also* EXOTOXIN.

Endotracheal (endo-, -trache-) Within or through the lumen of the trachea.

Enophthalmos (en-, -ophthalmo-) Abnormal recession of the eyeball into the orbital cavity.

Enteral feeding (enter-) A method of supplying nutritional support by tube to a patient unable to ingest sufficient quantities of food in the normal way. It may be accomplished via the mouth or nose (nasogastric), or through a fistula (gastric, duodenal, or jejunal). *See also* PARENTERAL FEEDING.

Enteric (enter-) Refers to the small intestine.

Enteritis (enter-, -itis) Inflammation of the mucous membranes of the intestine, and, in particular, the small intestine.

Enteropathogenic (entero-, -patho-, -genic) Capable of producing disease of the intestine.

Enteropathy (entero-, -pathy) Any disease or disorder of the intestine.

Enterotoxin (entero-, -toxi-) A bacterial exotoxin affecting the intestine.

Enuresis (-ur-, -sis) Involuntary urination. *See also* DIURESIS *and* INCONTINENCE.

Enuretic alarm An electrical device that responds to a few drops of urine, employed to evoke a conditioned response in those, especially children, affected by nocturnal enuresis.

Enzootic (en-, -zoo-) Refers to a disease endemic in an animal community.

Enzyme (-zym-) A protein involved in biochemical reactions as a catalyst.

Eosinophilia (-phil-, -ia) An excess of eosinophils in the blood.

Epidemic (epi-) Refers to a disease caused by factors not generally present in an affected region or community, often spreading rapidly, and of high morbidity. *See also* ENDEMIC *and* PANDEMIC.

Epidermoid (epi-, -derm-, -oid) Similar to, or part of, the epidermis.

Epididymectomy (epi-, -didym-, -ectomy) The removal of the epididymis by surgery.

Epididymo-orchitis (epi-, -didymo-, -orch-, -itis) Inflammation involving the epididymis and the testis.

Epigastrium (epi-, -gastr-) The upper middle region of the abdomen.

Epileptiform (-lep-, -form) A condition resembling epilepsy.

Epiphora (epi-) Abnormal overflow of tears.

Epiphysis (epi-) The end of a long bone containing a secondary ossification centre, which lays down spongy bone. It is separated from the diaphysis by a cartilaginous epiphyseal plate, which is replaced by bone in early adulthood, thus preventing further growth.

Epistaxis (epi-) Bleeding from the nose.

Epithelioid (epitheli-, -oid) Similar to epithelium.

Epithelium (epitheli-) The thin cellular layer covering all internal and external surfaces of the body. *See also* ENDOTHELIUM.

Eructation (e-) Belching; the removal of accumulated gases from the stomach through the mouth. *See also* FLATUS.

Erythema marginatum (eryth-) A red patch in which the centre is faded and the margins raised.

Erythrocyte sedimentation rate (erythro-, -cyte) The erythrocyte sedimentation rate (ESR) is the rate of settling of erythrocytes when a known volume of blood is treated with an anticoagulant and allowed to stand under controlled conditions. The ESR varies in many conditions.

Erythrogenic (erythro-, -genic) 1. The production of erythrocytes. 2. The production of erythema.

Erythropoietin (erythro-, -poie-) A hormone secreted by the kidneys (or liver in the foetus), which stimulates erythropoiesis.

ESR ERYTHROCYTE SEDIMENTATION RATE.

Ethmoid bone Forms the supporting structure for the nasal cavities. It is located on the floor of the cranium and between the orbits. *See also* CRIBRIFORM PLATE.

Euthyroid (eu-) Refers to the normal function of the thyroid gland.

Evanescent Passing quickly, vanishing, or unstable.

Exchange transfusion (ex-, trans-, -fus-) Transfusion involving the gradual replacement of blood with that of a donor. Blood is removed from the recipient in small quantities and is replaced by an equal volume transfused simultaneously.

Excision (ex-, -cis-) The removal of tissue or structures by surgery. *See also* RESECTION.

Excrescence (ex-) A growth, usually abnormal, from a surface.

Excretion (ex-) The removal of waste or unwanted material from the body.

Exfoliation (ex-) Peeling in scales or layers.

Exocrine (exo-) Refers to the function of exocrine glands (e.g. sweat glands and the pancreas), which secrete substances via a duct. *See also* ENDOCRINE.

Exogenous (exo-, -genous) 1. Arising or developing from external causes. *See also* ENDOGENOUS. 2. Additions to an outer surface that produce growth.

Exospore (exo-, -spor-) 1. The outer layer of a spore wall. 2. CONIDIUM. *See also* ENDOSPORE.

Exotoxin (exo-, -toxi-) A heat-labile protein secreted by multiplying bacteria, and having effects away from the focus of the infection. Exotoxins are extremely toxic to man. *See also* ENDOTOXIN.

Expectorate (ex-) To remove matter (e.g. mucus and sputum) from the lungs by coughing.

Extensor (ex-, -tens-) A muscle responsible for extending a limb, thereby increasing the angle of the joint. *See also* FLEXOR.

Extracellular fluid (extra-) Fluid found outside cells (e.g. plasma, cerebrospinal fluid, lymph, and interstitial fluid).

Extravasation (extra-, -vas-) The escape of fluid, which may often be blood or blood components, from ducts or vessels, and its accumulation in the surrounding tissues. *See also* EXUDATION *and* TRANSUDATION.

Exudation (ex-) The escape of fluid, which may contain cells or cellular debris, from tissues or capillaries into surrounding tissues. It often occurs in inflammatory reactions. *See also* EXTRAVASATION *and* TRANSUDATION.

——————————— F ———————————

Facultative Refers to the ability to adapt to particular circumstances or perform a function, but which is not obligatory. *See also* OBLIGATE.

Familial Refers to the family, and to disorders that tend to occur more frequently among members of a family.

Fascia Fibrous tissue enclosing and separating groups of muscles and organs.

Fat 1. Adipose tissue. 2. A lipid formed by esterifcation of glycerol and fatty acids. *See also* TRIGLYCERIDE.

Fatigue Weariness and reduced efficiency resulting from exertion. It may range from lassitude to exhaustion. The threshold of fatigue may be lowered in illness. *See also* LASSITUDE, LETHARGY, *and* PROSTRATION.

Fatty acid An acid containing a hydrocarbon chain and a terminal carboxyl group (-COOH). It may be saturated (e.g. stearic acid) or unsaturated (e.g. arachidonic acid). Fatty acids are utilised for fat synthesis (by esterification with glycerol); free fatty acids (FFA) in plasma are metabolised to meet energy requirements.

Fauces The passage from the mouth to the pharynx; the throat.

Febrile Refers to fever; feverish.

Femur The long bone of the thigh.

Fermentation The conversion of complex organic compounds (e.g. carbohydrates) into simpler compounds (e.g. alcohols). Fermentation takes place in anaerobic conditions and in the presence of an enzyme. *See also* CATABOLISM *and* GLYCOLYSIS.

Fertility The capacity for conception.

Fever Raised body temperature above the normal (37°C; 98.6°F). *See also* HYPERPYREXIA, HYPERTHERMIA, *and* HYPOTHERMIA.

FFA Free fatty acid. *See* FATTY ACID.

Fibrinoid (-oid) Similar to fibrin.

Fibrinolytic (-ly-) Refers to the enzymatic dissolution of fibrin.

Fibroid (fibr-, -oid) 1. Formed of, or similar to, fibrous tissue. 2. A leiomyoma. Fibroids is a term used colloquially to denote a leiomyoma occurring in the uterus.

Fibrosis (fibro-, -sis) The abnormal formation of fibrous tissue; the degeneration of a tissue into a fibrous mass.

Fibrous (fibr-, -ous) Composed of fibre.

Fibula The outer, smaller bone in the lower leg. *See also* TIBIA.

Filamentous Thread-like.

Filtration angle The angle at the periphery of the anterior chamber of the eye. It is the principal drainage site for aqueous humour.

Fimbria 1. A border; fringe-like. 2. A fine filamentous appendage of some bacteria, which is shorter than a flagellum.

Fission (fiss-) Splitting into two or more components.

Fistula An abnormal or surgically created channel or communication between two internal organs, or leading from an internal organ to the exterior of the body.

Flaccid In a relaxed and weak state.

Flaccid paralysis (para-) Paralysis with loss of tendon reflexes and reduction of muscle tone. *See also* SPASTIC PARALYSIS.

Flagella, flagellum (flagell-) Fine filamentous structures attached to some cells (e.g. spermatozoa), and used for motility.

Flatulence The accumulation of excessive amounts of air or gas in the gastro-intestinal tract.

Flatus Gas or air in the gastro-intestinal tract, which is expelled from the anus. *See also* ERUCTATION.

Flexor (flex-) A muscle responsible for bending a limb, thereby reducing the angle of a joint. *See also* EXTENSOR.

Floaters Small spots in the field of vision which appear to move, caused by deposits in the vitreous humour of the eye.

Focus The point of concentration or the principal centre of a process.

Foetus An unborn offspring. In man, the term is used during the period from 8 weeks after conception up to birth. *See also* EMBRYO *and* NEONATE.

Follicle A small sac, pouch, or cavity.

Follicular carcinoma (carcin-, -oma) A neoplasm of the thyroid gland that is composed of epithelial follicles without formation of papillae.

Fomites Inanimate objects (e.g. clothing) that can harbour micro-organisms and act as agents of transmission. *See also* RESERVOIR OF INFECTION.

Free fatty acid *See* FATTY ACID.

Fructosaemia (-aemia) The presence of fructose in the blood.

Fructose (-ose) A ketohexose sugar found in honey and sweet fruits.

Fructosuria (-uria) The presence of fructose in the urine.

Fulminant Refers to a disease that occurs suddenly and with great intensity. *See also* INSIDIOUS.

Functional (funct-) Refers to the function of an organ, as opposed to its structure.

Fungating Indicates a fungus-like appearance with marked proliferation.

Furuncular Resembling a furuncle (boil).

Fusiform (-form) Resembling a spindle.

—————————— G ——————————

Gag reflex (re-, -flex) The reflex contraction of muscles in the pharynx resulting in the closure of the glottis, cessation of breathing, and retching or vomiting. It may be caused by touching the back of the pharynx.

Galactokinase (galacto-, -ase) An enzyme produced in the liver, which catalyses the formation of galactose 1-phosphate from galactose and ATP.

Galactorrhoea (galacto-, -rrhoea) 1. Spontaneous secretion of milk after the period of breast feeding is completed. 2. Excessive flow of milk.

Galactose (galact-, -ose) An aldohexose sugar, isomeric with glucose, obtained from lactose, milk sugar, or sugar beet.

Gall bladder The organ used for storing and concentrating bile produced in the liver. When required, bile leaves the gall bladder via the cystic duct.

Gamete (gam-) A reproductive cell (e.g. ovum and spermatozoon).

Gametocyte (gameto-, -cyte) A cell (e.g. oocyte and spermatocyte) that produces gametes.

Gamma radiation (radi-) Radiation of short wavelength emitted from the nucleus of a radioactive substance.

Gammopathy (-pathy) The abnormal proliferation of lymphoid cells that produce immunoglobulins. *See also* MONOCLONAL GAMMOPATHY *and* POLYCLONAL GAMMOPATHY.

Ganglion (ganglio-) 1. A group of neurones outside the central nervous system. 2. The term ganglia refers to specific centres in the brain (e.g. basal ganglia). 3. A fluid-filled enlargement of the sheath of a tendon.

Gangrene Necrosis and putrefaction of tissues as a result of occlusion of their blood supply.

Gastrectomy (gastr-, -ectomy) The complete or partial removal of the stomach by surgery.

Gastric (gastr-) Refers to the stomach.

Gastric acid (gastr-) The generic term for hydrochloric acid in gastric juice.

Gastric glands (gastr-) The glands found in the mucosal membrane lining the stomach, and which secrete gastric juice.

Gastric juice (gastr-) The fluid secreted by the gastric glands containing hydrochloric acid, enzymes, and mucus.

Gastric lavage (gastr-) Lavage performed to remove stomach contents.

General adaptation syndrome The sum of all non-specific responses of the body to prolonged systemic stress.

Genetic (gen-) 1. Refers to birth, reproduction, or origin. 2. Inherited or congenital, as of a disease.

Genetic counselling (gen-) Advice, based on genetic information, given to couples as to the likelihood of passing potentially hereditary anomalies to their children.

Genus A taxonomic category that comprises species of broadly similar characteristics, but which differ in detail. Similar genera belong to the same family.

Germinal cell (germ-) 1. A cell capable of division and differentiation. 2. A cell derived from the epithelial layer lining the seminiferous tubules and involved in spermatogenesis.

Germination (germ-) 1. The developmental process within a fertilised ovum. 2. The developmental beginning of a spore or seed.

Gestation Pregnancy; the period from fertilisation of an ovum to birth.

Gingivae (gingiv-) The gums, consisting of mucous membranes and connective tissue.

Gingival papillae (gingiv-) The portion of the gums between the teeth.

Gingivectomy (gingiv-, -ectomy) The removal of gingival tissue by surgery.

Gland A secretory or excretory cell, or a collection of such cells.

Globus hystericus A subjective sensation of suffocation, often described as a lump in the throat.

Glottis (glott-) The passage between the vocal cords in the pharynx.

Glucose (gluc-, -ose) A monosaccharide hexose utilised as the main source of energy. Excess glucose is converted to glycogen and fat. Glucose is an end-product of carbohydrate metabolism.

Glucose loading (gluc-, -ose) Administration of glucose in sufficient quantities to enable its rate of metabolism to be assessed.

Glucose tolerance (gluc-, -ose) The ability of the body to maintain the plasma-glucose concentration within normal limits after glucose loading.

Glucuronide A metabolite formed by the conjugation of glucuronic acid with a compound (e.g. morphine) to facilitate its elimination.

Glutathione A peptide composed of glutamate, cysteine, and glycine, and which takes part in several redox reactions. It also functions in the transport of amino acids across membranes.

Glycogen (glyco-, -gen) A long-chain polysaccharide polymer of glucose. It is formed from excess glucose and stored as an energy reserve. It is stored mainly in the liver, but is also found in the muscles.

Glycolipid (glyco-, -lip-) A lipid containing a carbohydrate component.

Glycolysis (glyco-, -lysis) The enzymatic conversion of glucose into simpler compounds (lactate and pyruvate) carried out in anaerobic conditions. It results in the storage of energy in the form of adenosine triphosphate (ATP). *See also* CATABOLISM *and* METABOLISM.

Glycoprotein (glyco-) A conjugated compound consisting of a protein and a carbohydrate component.

Glycosaminoglycan (glyco-) A polysaccharide compound which is a component of many mucins. It may be combined with a protein.

Glycosuria (glyco-, -uria) The presence of glucose in the urine.

Goitre   An enlargement of the thyroid gland, which is usually visible as a swelling at the front of the neck.

Goitrogenic (-genic)   Capable of producing a goitre.

Golgi apparatus   A specialised structure within a cell. It is situated near the nucleus and provides the site for synthesis of carbohydrate side-chains of substances (e.g. glycoproteins and mucopolysaccharides). Its functions include the transportation of these synthesised products.

Graft   1. To implant or transplant organs or tissues. 2. The organs or tissues used in the procedure.
See also ALLOGRAFT.

Granulation tissue (gran-)   Newly formed tissue associated with healing of wounds or ulcers. It consists of blood vessels and other cells, and has a red appearance.

Granulocyte (gran-, -cyte)   A granule-containing cell, especially a leucocyte, which contains basophil, eosinophil, and neutrophil granules.

Granuloma (gran-, -oma)   A benign neoplasm composed of granulation tissue.

Gravid (grav-)   Pregnant; containing a developing foetus.

Grommet   A small plastic tube that is inserted through the eardrum to allow air to enter and dry out excessive secretions in the middle ear.

Gustatory   Refers to the sense of taste.

Guthrie test   An investigative test to detect the presence of elevated concentrations of phenylalanine in the blood of neonates.

Gynaecology (gynaeco-, -logy)   The study of disease(s) of the female reproductive system.

Gynaecomastia (gynaeco-, -mast-, -ia)   Excessive development of the mammary glands in the male. They may be functional.

--------------------- H ---------------------

Haemangioblastoma (haem-, -angio-, -blast-, -oma)   A benign neoplasm in the brain consisting of blood-vessel cells or angioblasts.

Haematemesis (haemat-, -sis)   The vomiting of blood.

Haematoma (haemat-, -oma)   A swelling composed of blood, usually clotted, and resulting from a haemorrhage.

Haematuria (haemat-, -uria)   The presence of blood in the urine.

Haemochromatosis (haemo-, -chromato-, -sis)   A chronic inherited disorder of iron metabolism in which excessive amounts of iron are deposited in tissues.

Haemodialysis (haemo-, -dia-, -lysis)   The removal of water, electrolytes, and waste products (e.g. urea and creatinine) from the blood using a special apparatus. Solutes diffuse across a semipermeable membrane (usually made from cellulose) into a dialysate solution. Diffusion of certain substances (e.g. calcium and acetate) also takes place from the dialysate into the blood. *See also* PERITONEAL DIALYSIS.

Haemoglobinuria (-uria)   The presence of haemoglobin in the urine.

Haemolysis (haemo-, -lysis)   The destruction or dissolution of erythrocytes, with the resultant liberation of haemoglobin.

Haemopoiesis (haemo-, -poiesis)   The process of formation and development of blood cells.

Haemoptysis (haemo-)   The coughing up of blood or mucus stained with blood.

Haemorrhage (haemo-, -rrhage)   Bleeding; the escape of blood from blood vessels.

Haemorrhoidectomy (-ectomy)   The removal of haemorrhoids by surgery.

Haemosiderin (haemo-)   An iron-protein complex present in tissues as a storage form of iron and used to form haemoglobin.

Haemostasis (haemo-, -stasis)   1. A process that stops bleeding. It may be physiological or induced. 2. The arrest of blood flow through a vessel or to a particular part of the body.

Half-life   The time required for the concentration of a substance to decline by 50%. The half-life of a drug is the time required for plasma concentrations to decline by 50%, provided that elimination occurs by first-order kinetics. It provides a measure of the rate of drug elimination.

Hallucination   An apparent sensory perception (e.g. auditory, visual, or olfactory) which is not present or is non-existent. *See also* DELUSION.

Hallucinogen (-gen)   A substance that produces hallucinations.

Hamartoma (hamart-, -oma)   A growth of cells and tissue that resembles a neoplasm, and in which normal cells of the organ show an abnormal degree of proliferation and mixture.

Hamstring   Any one of the tendons at the back of the knee.

Heartburn   A burning sensation usually felt behind the sternum, but which may rise to the neck. It is caused by reflux of gastric contents into the oesophagus.

Hemiparesis (hemi-)   Partial paralysis or muscular weakness affecting one side of the body.

Hemiplegia (hemi-, -plegia)   Complete paralysis affecting one side of the body. *See also* DIPLEGIA, PARAPLEGIA, *and* QUADRIPLEGIA.

Hepatic (hepat-)   Refers to the liver.

Hepatic-portal system (hepat-)   The flow of venous blood from the digestive organs to the liver via the hepatic portal vein. After passing through the liver, the blood leaves via the hepatic vein to rejoin the systemic circulation.

Hepatocellular (hepato-)   Refers to, or affecting, liver cells.

Hepatocyte (hepato-, -cyte)   A liver cell.

Hepatolenticular (hepato-)   Refers to the liver in association with the lentiform nucleus (a part of the basal ganglia in the extrapyramidal system).

Hepatoma (hepat-, -oma)   A malignant neoplasm of the liver parenchymal cells.

Hepatomegaly (hepato-, -megaly)   Enlargement of the liver.

Hepatosplenomegaly (hepato-, -spleno-, -megaly) Enlargement of the liver and the spleen.

Hereditary (hered-) Genetically transmitted from parents to offspring. *See also* CONGENITAL.

Hereditary spherocytosis (hered-, sphero-, -cyto-, -sis) A form of haemolytic anaemia, inherited as an autosomal dominant trait, in which the defective cytoplasmic membranes of erythrocytes are lost as the cells pass through the spleen.

Hermaphrodite Having both male and female sex organs.

Hernia The protrusion of part of an organ through an opening in the surrounding structures. *See also* UMBILICAL HERNIA.

Herpetic Refers to, or having the characteristics of, herpesviruses or herpesvirus infections.

Heterotrophic (hetero-, -trophic) A type of nutrition in which complex organic molecules are required as the source of carbon for synthesis of organic compounds. *See also* AUTOTROPHIC.

Heterozygous (hetero-, -zyg-) Possessing different alleles at a given position on a chromosome pair. *See also* HOMOZYGOUS.

Hiatus A break or gap; an opening.

Hindbrain The posterior part of the embryonic brain that develops into the cerebellum, pons, and medulla oblongata. The term may also be applied to these areas in the fully developed brain.

Hippocampus An area of grey matter involved in emotional behaviour and memory.

Hirsute Possessing abundant hair.

Histamine A substance present in most body tissues, especially mast cells, connective tissue, basophils, and platelets. Its actions are mediated through two types of receptors, H_1 and H_2. Stimulation of H_1-receptors produces smooth muscle contraction (e.g. in the intestines and bronchioles), vasodilatation of small blood vessels resulting in hypotension, and an increase in capillary permeability causing oedema. Stimulation of H_2-receptors produces an increase in gastric acid secretion.

Histology (histo-, -logy) The study of tissue anatomy and physiology with respect to cellular structure and microscopical evaluation.

Histoplasmosis (-osis) A fungal infection primarily involving the reticulo-endothelial system, and caused by *Histoplasma capsulatum*.

Homoeostasis (homoeo-, -stasis) The tendency towards stability and equilibrium in the internal environment. This is achieved by dynamic processes and a system of control mechanisms (e.g. negative feedback).

Homogeneous (homo-) Possessing similar or uniform composition.

Homozygous (homo-, -zyg-) Possessing a pair of identical alleles at a given position on a chromosome pair. *See also* HETEROZYGOUS.

Hormone A chemical substance released from one part of the body (usually an endocrine gland) and transported in the bloodstream to another organ where it exerts its action.

Host 1. An animal or plant that harbours a parasitic microorganism. *See also* DEFINITIVE HOST *and* INTERMEDIATE HOST. 2. The recipient of transplanted tissue obtained from a donor.

Hyaline Possessing a glassy translucent appearance.

Hyaline membrane disease A respiratory disease of neonates, characterised by the development of a lining of eosinophilic hyaline material in the terminal respiratory passages.

Hydronephrosis (hydro-, -nephro-, -sis) Distension of the ureter and renal pelvis due to obstruction of the outflow of urine. Atrophy of the kidney may occur.

Hydrops (hydro-) The accumulation of serous fluid in any tissue or body cavity.

Hydrosalpinx (hydro-, -salp-) The accumulation of watery fluid in a Fallopian tube.

Hydrostatic (hydro-, -stat-) Refers to the pressure of a fluid when in a state of equilibrium.

Hydrotherapy (hydro-, -therap-) The treatment of a disorder by immersion in, external application of, or administration of, water.

Hyperactivity (hyper-) An excessive increase in physical activity.

Hyperbaric (hyper-, -bar-) Greater than normal pressure or weight; gases under greater than atmospheric pressure.

Hyperbilirubinaemia (hyper-, -aemia) An excess of bilirubin in the blood. Conjugated hyperbilirubinaemia is an excess in the blood of bilirubin that is combined with glucuronic acid, sulphate, or other substances (i.e. conjugated bilirubin). Unconjugated hyperbilirubinaemia is an excess in the blood of free bilirubin.

Hypercalciuria (hyper-, -calci-, -uria) An excess of calcium in the urine.

Hypercapnia (hyper-) An excess of carbon dioxide in the blood.

Hypercholesterolaemia (hyper-, -aemia) An excess of cholesterol in the blood.

Hyperglycaemia (hyper-, -glyc-, -aemia) An excess of sugar in the blood.

Hyperirritability (hyper-) An excessive responsiveness to slight stimuli.

Hyperkeratosis (hyper-, -kerato-, -sis) Hypertrophy of the epidermal layer of the skin.

Hyperkinesia (hyper-, -kine-, -ia) Excessive activity or motor function. *See also* HYPOKINESIA.

Hyperopia (hyper-, -opia) Long-sightedness, in which the focal point of parallel rays of light is behind the retina, so that the near point is further away than normal.

Hyperoxia (hyper-, -ox-, -ia) An increase in the oxygen concentration in tissues caused by breathing hyberbaric oxygen or air.

Hyperphagia (hyper-, -phagia) Excessive eating.

Hyperphosphataemia (hyper-, -aemia) An excess of phosphates in the blood. *See also* HYPOPHOSPHATAEMIA.

Hyperplasia (hyper-, -plasia) The increase in size of, or part of, an organ, as a result of an increase in the number of cells. *See also* HYPERTROPHY *and* HYPOPLASIA.

Hyperpnoea (hyper-, -pnoea) An abnormal increase in the depth and rate of breathing. *See also* APNOEA, DYSPNOEA, ORTHOPNOEA, *and* TACHYPNOEA.

Hyperpyrexia (hyper-, -pyr-, -ia) A very high body temperature of at least 40.5°C (105°F). *See also* FEVER, HYPERTHERMIA, *and* HYPOTHERMIA.

Hypersensitivity (hyper-, -sens-) An enhanced and exaggerated response to a foreign substance (allergen). It is usually mediated by the immune system. *See also* ALLERGY *and* ATOPY.

Hyperthermia (hyper-, -therm-, -ia) An abnormally high body temperature, particularly one induced therapeutically. *See also* FEVER, HYPERPYREXIA, *and* HYPOTHERMIA.

Hypertonia (hyper-, -ton-, -ia) Enhanced tone of muscles or arteries.

Hypertrophy (hyper-, -trophy) The increase in size of an organ, or part of an organ, as a result of an increase in cell size.
See also ATROPHY *and* HYPERPLASIA.

Hyperuricaemia (hyper-, -uric-, -aemia) An excess of uric acid in the blood.

Hyperventilation (hyper-) 1. Deep breathing which is abnormally prolonged and with increased frequency. 2. An increase in gaseous exchange in the lungs. It causes a fall in the plasma-carbon dioxide concentration.
See also HYPOVENTILATION.

Hyperviscosity (hyper-) Abnormally excessive viscosity.

Hypnotic (hypno-) 1. Produces sleep. 2. Refers to hypnotism.

Hypoalbuminaemia (hypo-, -aemia) An abnormal deficiency of albumin in the blood.

Hypochlorhydria (hypo-, -ia) An abnormal reduction in the secretion of hydrochloric acid in gastric juice.

Hypochondrial Refers to the hypochondrium.

Hypofibrinogenaemia (hypo-, -aemia) An abnormal deficiency of fibrinogen in the blood.

Hypogeusia (hypo-, -ia) Impaired sense of taste.

Hypokinesia (hypo-, -kine-, -ia) An abnormal decrease in activity or motor function. *See also* AKINESIA, BRADYKINESIA, DYSKINESIA, *and* HYPERKINESIA.

Hypophosphataemia (hypo-, -aemia) An abnormal deficiency of phosphates in the blood. *See also* HYPERPHOSPHATAEMIA.

Hypophysectomy (-ectomy) The removal of the pituitary gland by surgery.

Hypoplasia (hypo-, -plasia) Underdevelopment of an organ or part, usually implying fewer than the normal number of cells. It is less severe than aplasia. *See also* AGENESIS, APLASIA, DYSPLASIA, *and* HYPERPLASIA.

Hypoproteinaemia (hypo-, -aemia) An abnormal deficiency of protein in the blood.

Hypotension (hypo-, -tens-) An abnormally low blood pressure.

Hypothermia (hypo-, -therm-, -ia) A body temperature below normal, which is only usually of clinical significance when it falls below 33°C (91°F to 92°F). It may be therapeutically induced to reduce tissue metabolism and oxygen requirement. *See also* FEVER, HYPERPYREXIA, *and* HYPERTHERMIA.

Hypoventilation (hypo-) A reduction in gaseous exchange in the lungs which causes hypercapnia. *See also* HYPERVENTILATION.

Hypovolaemia (hypo-, -aemia) An abnormal decrease in the volume of circulating blood in the body.

Hypoxaemia (hyp-, -ox-, -aemia) A deficiency of oxygen in the blood.

Hypoxidosis (hyp-, -ox-, -sis) An impairment in function of cells caused by a reduction in the supply of oxygen.

Hysterectomy (hyster-, -ectomy) The removal of the uterus by surgery.

Hysterotomy (hystero-, -tomy) 1. Incision of the uterus. 2. CAESAREAN SECTION.

----------- I -----------

Iatrogenic (iatro-, -genic) Produced by doctors; usually applied to adverse conditions produced as a result of treatment by a doctor. Causes may include inappropriate manner, examination, or discussion, and medical or surgical procedures. *See also* NOSOCOMIAL.

Idiopathic (idio-, -path-) 1. Refers to a condition of unknown aetiology. 2. Refers to a primary disease (i.e. one not resulting from another disease).

Idiosyncrasy (idio-) An individual characteristic not shared by others. It includes behaviour, habit, and a response to agents that is peculiar to an individual.

Ileac (ile-) 1. Refers to the ileum. 2. Refers to ileus.

Ileostomy (ileo-, -stomy) A surgical procedure to establish an opening (stoma) from the ileum to the surface of the abdomen. The term may also be applied to the opening itself. *See also* COLOSTOMY *and* UROSTOMY.

Iliac (ili-) Refers to the ilium.

Immunisation A process of increasing a subject's resistance to infection. *See also* ACTIVE IMMUNISATION *and* PASSIVE IMMUNISATION.

Immunocompromise A diminished immune response caused by external factors (e.g. immunosuppressants, radiotherapy, or malignant disease). *See also* IMMUNODEFICIENCY *and* IMMUNOSUPPRESSION.

Immunodeficiency A disorder characterised by the inability to produce an immune response. It may affect any part of the immune system. *See also* IMMUNOCOMPROMISE.

Immunosuppression Inhibition of the immune system by the administration of immunosuppressants (e.g. azathioprine or corticosteroids) to prevent rejection of transplant tissue. It may be selective, and complete or partial. *See also* IMMUNOCOMPROMISE.

Immunosurveillance The concept of a detection and monitoring function of the immune system. It is responsible for recognising neoplastic cells and their destruction by an immune response.

Immunotherapy (-therap-) Therapeutic measures involving active and passive immunisation, stimulation or suppression of the immune system, or establishing the ability to produce an immune response.

Impaction Firmly packed or wedged.

Impotence (im-) The inability to perform sexual intercourse due to the failure to achieve or maintain an erection.

In utero Within the uterus.

In vitro Occurring outside the living body. *See also* IN VIVO.

In vivo Occurring within the living body. *See also* IN VITRO.

Incision (in-, -cis-) The cut produced by a sharp implement during surgery.

Incontinence (in-) Loss of voluntary control of defaecation (faecal or rectal incontinence) or urination (urinary incontinence). *See also* DIURESIS *and* ENURESIS.

Incubate To provide the ideal conditions (e.g. temperature and humidity) for growth and development.

Incubation period The interval of time between exposure to a pathogenic micro-organism and the first appearance of clinical features of the infection.

Indolent (in-) 1. Slow-growing. 2. With little or no pain.

Induration (-dur-) The hardening of a tissue or organ.

Indwelling catheter A catheter that remains in position.

Infant Refers to a child from the neonatal period up to 12 months of age. *See also* NEONATE *and* PREMATURE INFANT.

Infection 1. The invasion of a host by pathogenic, or potentially pathogenic, micro-organisms, and their subsequent multiplication. *See also* INFESTATION. 2. An infectious disease.

Infestation The invasion or habitation of a host by surface-dwelling parasites. *See also* INFECTION(1).

Infiltration (in-) The accumulation within a tissue of a substance not normally present, or in concentrations in excess of the normal.

Infusion (in-, -fus-) 1. The intravenous administration of a fluid, other than blood, for therapeutic purposes. The fluid flows in by gravity. *See also* INJECTION(1) *and* TRANSFUSION. 2. A dilute solution of a vegetable drug prepared by macerating the drug in hot or cold water, and straining.

Inhalation (in-) The inspiration of air or other substances into the lungs.

Injection (in-, -ject-) 1. The parenteral administration of a fluid for therapeutic purposes. The fluid is forced in using a syringe. *See also* INFUSION(1). 2. Congestion of a part.

Innervation (in-) The nerve supply or distribution to an organ or tissue.

Inoculation (in-) The introduction of micro-organisms (or any other antigenic substance) into living tissue or culture media. The process may result in disease, or be used to stimulate an immune response or to study the cultured material.

Inoculum (in-) An agent or substance introduced into tissues by inoculation.

Inotropic Influencing the contractility of muscles, especially the myocardium. There may be a negative influence resulting in reduced contractility, or a positive influence resulting in enhanced contractility.

Insertion (in-) 1. The process of implanting or setting. 2. The site of attachment.

Insidious Refers to a disease that develops or spreads with few signs or symptoms relative to its severity. *See also* FULMINANT.

Interferon A protein produced by most cells in response to viral infection, and which induces the production of anti-viral substances by non-infected cells. Interferons also have complex effects on immunity and cell function; they suppress lymphocyte function, lower the threshold for mast-cell histamine-release, and may have antineoplastic effects.

Interleukin A specific lymphokine that affects antibody production and influences T-cell differentiation and production.

Intermediate host The host in which a parasite undergoes asexual reproduction or is in the larval stage. *See also* DEFINITIVE HOST.

Interstitial (inter-) Refers to the spaces within or between tissues.

Intestinal flora The bacteria that are normal residents of the intestine.

Intolerance (in-) 1. The inability to endure or withstand. *See also* TOLERANCE. 2. An unfavourable response.

Intracranial pressure (intra-, -crani-) The pressure of the cerebrospinal fluid in the subarachnoid space.

Intractable Uncontrollable and unresponsive to remedial measures.

Intraluminal (intra-) Within the lumen of a tubular tissue or organ.

Intrathecal (intra-, -thec-) 1. Within a sheath. 2. Within the subarachnoid space.

Intrinsic factor A glycoprotein secreted by the mucosal cells of the stomach, and which is necessary for the absorption of vitamin B_{12}.

Intubation (in-) Insertion of a tube into a body cavity, especially into the trachea to maintain the airway.

Involution (in-) 1. A reduction in the size of an organ. It may be degenerative, physiological, or follow enlargement. *See also* ATROPHY. 2. Turning towards the inside.

Ion-exchange resin A polymer of high molecular weight, whose component ions are exchanged for other ions of the same charge in the surrounding medium.

Ionising radiation (radi-) High-energy electromagnetic radiation that is capable of producing ionisation (e.g. X-rays and gamma radiation).

Iridectomy (irid-, -ectomy) The removal of part of the iris by surgery.

Irradiation Exposure (which may be therapeutic) to electromagnetic waves. *See also* RADIATION(1).

Isotonic (iso-, -ton-)   1. Applied to different solutions that exert equal osmotic pressure with respect to a particular membrane. 2. Applied to a solution that exerts the same osmotic pressure as serum (e.g. sodium chloride 0.9%).

Isotope (iso-)   A chemical element possessing the same atomic number as another, but having a different atomic mass.

J

Jacksonian epilepsy   Jacksonian epilepsy is characterised by seizures that occur on one side of the body and move systematically from one group of muscles to the next. The cause is a discharging focus in the motor cortex of the brain.

K

Kallidin   A polypeptide and a member of the group of kinins.

Kallikrein-kinin system   The enzymatic cascade system resulting in the formation of the inflammatory mediators, kinins.

Kartagener's syndrome   An inherited pulmonary disorder characterised by immotile cilia, which results in defective mucociliary clearance.

Karyolysis (karyo-, -lysis)   The destuction of a cell nucleus, in which it swells, lyses, and loses its chromatin. *See also* KARYORRHEXIS *and* PYKNOSIS.

Karyorrhexis (karyo-, -rhex-)   Disintegration of the cell nucleus. It results in dispersal of chromatin throughout the cytoplasm in the form of granules which are finally removed from the cell. *See also* KARYOLYSIS *and* PYKNOSIS.

Keratitis (kerat-, -itis)   Inflammation of the cornea.

Keratoconjunctivitis (kerato-, -itis)   Inflammation of the cornea and the conjunctiva.

Keratolysis (kerato-, -lysis)   Separation or loosening of the outermost layer of skin, the stratum corneum.

Keratomalacia (kerato-, -malacia)   Dryness and softening of the cornea caused by severe vitamin A deficiency. Corneal ulceration, night blindness, and complete visual loss may occur.

Kerion   A raised granulomatous lesion associated with tinea infections, and thought to be caused by an immune response. It is inflamed, pustular, and wet and spongy in appearance, and heals in a short time.

Keto acid   An organic acid with a ketone group ($>C=O$) and a carboxyl group ($-COOH$).

Ketoacidosis (keto-, -osis)   Acidosis resulting from the accumulation of ketones in body tissues and fluids.

Ketogenic (keto-, -genic)   Refers to the ability to form ketones.

Ketonuria (keto-, -uria)   The presence of ketones in the urine.

Kinin   A polypeptide (e.g. bradykinin and kallidin) formed in plasma as a result of the action of the enzyme, kallikrein. Kinins have powerful vasodilator properties, increase capillary permeability, cause smooth muscle contraction, and stimulate pain receptors.

Krebs' cycle   The cyclic process of metabolism resulting in the complete oxidation of acetyl-coenzyme A. Carbon chains of carbohydrate, fat, and protein are metabolised to form carbon dioxide, water, and adenosine triphosphate.

Kyphosis (-osis)   Excessive curvature of the spine in the thoracic region; hunchback.

L

Labial (labi-)   Refers to a lip, or, more commonly, the labia that constitute part of the female external genitalia.

Labyrinthectomy (-ectomy)   The removal of the labyrinth of the inner ear by surgery.

Labyrinthine   Refers to the labyrinth of the inner ear.

Lachrymation (lachry-)   Tear production and flow.

Lactation (lact-)   1. Milk secretion. 2. The period of milk secretion after childbirth.

Lactoferrin (lacto-, -ferr-)   An iron-binding protein that possesses antimicrobial activity, and which is found in tissue fluids (e.g. breast milk, saliva, and tears) and neutrophils.

Lactose (lact-, -ose)   A disaccharide found in milk.

Laminectomy (-ectomy)   The removal of the arch of a vertebra by surgery, resulting in exposure of the spinal cord.

Laparotomy (laparo-, -tomy)   An incision through the abdominal wall, but also applied to that in the loin.

Large cell carcinoma (carcin-, -oma)   A malignant neoplasm composed of large anaplastic cells, and originating especially in a bronchus.

Larva   An independent stage in the life-cycle of some organisms, characterised by motility, and in some cases, feeding.

Laryngeal (laryng-)   Refers to the larynx.

Laryngectomy (laryng-, -ectomy)   The removal of the larynx by surgery.

Laryngospasm (laryngo-, -spas-)   Muscle spasm of the larynx, resulting in its closure.

Lassitude   Weakness; tiredness. *See also* FATIGUE, LETHARGY, *and* PROSTRATION.

Latent   Present but not active; dormant.

Lavage   Washing-out or irrigation of an organ.

Laxative   Having the action of softening and promoting the discharge of faeces.

Lentigo (lent-)   A yellowish-brown spot on the skin caused by melanin deposition.

Lesion   A pathological condition (e.g. infection, injury, or malignant disease).

Lethargy   A condition characterised by extreme drowsiness, weakness, and complacency. *See also* FATIGUE, LASSITUDE, *and* PROSTRATION.

Leucocytosis (leuco-, -cyto-, -sis)   An abnormal increase in the number of leucocytes in the blood. *See also* LEUCOPENIA.

Leucopenia (leuco-, -penia) An abnormal deficiency in the number of leucocytes in the blood. *See also* LEUCOCYTOSIS.

Ligation (lig-) The application of a thread-like material (e.g. catgut, wire, cotton, or silk) around a vessel or part, used to constrict it.

Lipid (lip-) A member of a large and diverse group of fat and fat-like organic compounds containing carbon, hydrogen, and oxygen, and characterised as water-insoluble. They are classified as simple lipids (e.g. oils), compound lipids (e.g. phospholipids), or derived lipids (e.g. fatty acids). They act as a source of energy, constituents of cell structure, and serve other metabolic functions.

Lipoprotein (lipo-) A combination of lipid and protein that renders the lipid water-soluble. The group includes low-density lipoproteins that deposit cholesterol in cells, and high-density lipoproteins that remove cholesterol from cells and transport it to the liver for elimination.

Lithotripsy (litho-, -tripsy) A procedure to crush a bladder calculus, with subsequent irrigation and removal of fragments.

Lobectomy (-ectomy) The removal of one or more lobes of an organ (e.g. thyroid gland) by surgery.

Local Confined to a small area; not systemic.

Locomotor (-mot-) Refers to motion, or parts of the body responsible for motion.

Lucid Clear and understandable.

Lung-hilum A depression in the mediastinal surface of each lung at which the bronchus, blood and lymph vessels, and nerve supply enter.

Lymphadenectomy (lymph-, -aden-, -ectomy) The removal of a lymph node by surgery.

Lymphadenopathy (lymph-, -adeno-, -pathy) Any disorder of the lymph nodes.

Lymphoblast (lympho-, -blast) The immature precursor cell of a lymphocyte.

Lymphoreticular (lympho-, -ret-) Refers to the reticulo-endothelial system of the lymph nodes.

Lysis (ly-, -sis) Dissolution or disintegration; decomposition.

Lysosome (lyso-, -some) An organelle enclosed by a double membrane and found in many types of cell. It contains hydrolytic enzymes that have intracellular digestive functions.

Lysozyme (lyso-, -zym-) An enzyme found in various tissue fluids (e.g. saliva and tears) that is capable of breaking down bacterial cell walls.

M

Maceration The softening of tissues caused by soaking.

Macroglossia (macro-, -gloss-, -ia) Enlargement of the tongue.

Maculopapular Characterised by the presence of macules and papules.

Malabsorption (mal-) Defective gastro-intestinal absorption of nutrients.

Malaise A non-specific feeling of illness, uneasiness, or discomfort, often signifying a disturbance of body function.

Malignant 1. A condition that is life-threatening, virulent, or recurrent. 2. Possessing properties of anaplasia, invasive growth, and metastasis. *See also* BENIGN.

Malnutrition (mal-, -nutri-) A disorder of nutrition, which may be caused by an insufficient intake of nutrients, unbalanced diet, or defective utilisation of nutrients.

Mammography (mammo-, -graphy) Examination of the breasts using X-rays.

Manipulation (man-) 1. Treatment using the hands. 2. In physiotherapy, it refers to the movement of a joint beyond its active limit.

Mantoux test A diagnostic test to determine the sensitivity to tuberculin. A positive hypersensitivity reaction indicates the presence of the tubercle bacillus, although the infection may be inactive. It is carried out prior to BCG (Bacillus Calmette-Guérin) vaccination.

Marfan's syndrome An inherited disorder characterised by partial dislocation of the lenses of the eye, abnormally long and thin hands and feet (especially fingers and toes), and cardiovascular abnormalities.

Mastectomy (mast-, -ectomy) The removal of a breast by surgery.

Mastoidectomy (mast-, -ectomy) The removal of the mastoid process or mastoid air cells by surgery.

Mastopathy (masto-, -pathy) A disorder of a breast.

Maxilla The bone that forms the upper jaw.

Meconium The dark green viscous liquid discharged from the bowels of a neonate. It consists of bile, amniotic fluid, and debris.

Mediastinum (medi-) The mass of tissues in the thoracic cavity, excluding the lungs. It extends from the sternum to the vertebral column, and includes the heart, oesophagus, thymus gland, and other structures.

Medulla Refers to the innermost part of a structure. Sometimes called the marrow.

Medulloblastoma (medullo-, -blast-, -oma) A malignant neoplasm of the cerebellum composed of undifferentiated cells resembling the neural tube.

Megaloblast (megalo-, -blast) A large immature nucleated cell, the precursor of an abnormal erythrocyte.

Melaena The passage of dark tarry faeces, which contain occult blood as a result of haemorrhage within the gastro-intestinal tract.

Membrane A thin lining or covering tissue of a surface or cavity, or the dividing tissue of a space or organ.

Membrane depolarisation (de-) 1. Neutralisation of polarity across a membrane. 2. In neurones, the reversal of the resting membrane potential when stimulated; the positive potential of a membrane with respect to the potential outside the cell.

Menarche (men-, -arche) The time when the first menstrual period begins.

Mendelian laws The law of segregation which states that allelic pairs of genes segregate from one another and pass to different gametes; the law of independent assortment which states that genes that are not alleles are distributed to the gametes independently of one another.

Meningo-encephalitis (meningo-, -encephal-, -itis) Inflammation of the brain and the meninges.

Menorrhagia (meno-, -rrhagia) Excessive blood loss during regular but possibly prolonged menstruation. *See also* OLIGOMENORRHOEA.

Mesenteric vein (mes-, -enter-) The vein that receives blood from the mesentery.

Mesentery (mes- -enter-) The portion of the peritoneum that attaches the intestine to the abdominal wall.

Mesothelioma (meso-, -oma) A malignant neoplasm of the mesothelium.

Mesothelium (meso-) The epithelial membrane of the pleura, pericardium, and peritoneum.

Metabolism (meta-) The sum of the chemical processes occurring in an organism, including anabolism and catabolism, and the biodegradation of foreign substances and drugs.

Metacarpal (meta-, -carp-) Refers to the bones of the hand, between the wrist and the fingers.

Metatarsal (meta-, -tars-) Refers to the distal part of the foot between the instep and the toes.

Metatarsophalangeal (meta-, -tarso-, -phalang-) Refers to the metatarsal bones and the phalanges.

Micro-abscess (micro-) A very small localised abscess.

Microcephaly (micro-, -cephal-) An abnormally small head.

Microflora (micro-) Micro-organisms characteristic of a particular part.

Microsomal enzyme (micro-, -zym-) An enzyme associated with microsomes, especially in liver cells.

Miliary Refers to characteristic lesions that are small and resemble millet seeds.

Milk-alkali syndrome A syndrome caused by an excessive intake of milk or absorbable alkali over a prolonged period.

Mineral An inorganic solid of uniform composition found in the crust of the earth.

Miosis (mio-, -sis) Contraction of the pupil of the eye.

Mitochondria (mito-, -chondri-) Double-membraned intracellular organelles located in the cytoplasm, and which are the principal sites of energy production.

Mitosis (mito-, -sis) Cell division that results in two daughter cells of identical genetic composition to the parent cell.

Monoclonal gammopathy (mono-, -pathy) Gammopathy in which there is an increase in a single immunoglobulin clone. *See also* POLYCLONAL GAMMOPATHY.

Mononeuropathy (mono-, -neuro-, -pathy) A disorder affecting one nerve only. *See also* POLYNEUROPATHY.

Morbid 1. Diseased; refers to, or affected by, disease. 2. Refers to mental thoughts that are unhealthy or tend towards abnormality.

Morbidity 1. A morbid condition. 2. The ratio of the number of people within a population suffering from a disease to the number unaffected. *See also* MORTALITY(2).

Morphology (morpho-, -logy) The study of the structure and form of living organisms.

Mortality 1. The mortal quality; destined to die. 2. The death rate; the ratio of the total number of deaths to the total population of a specified group. *See also* MORBIDITY(2).

Motor (mot-) Refers to motion or movement, and its nervous and muscle control.

Mucin (muc-) A glycoprotein or mucopolysaccharide compound, constituting the main component of mucus.

Mucinous (muc-, -ous) Resembling or marked by the production of mucin.

Mucocutaneous (muco-, -cut-) Refers to the mucous membranes and the skin.

Muco-epidermoid (muco-, -epi-, -derm-, -oid) Characterised by epithelial cells and cells that produce mucus.

Mucoid (muc-, -oid) Resembling mucus, or mucin.

Mucolytic (muco-, -ly-) Refers to the thinning, digestion, or dissolution of mucus.

Mucopeptide (muco-) Any glycosylated peptide derived from a glycoprotein.

Mucopurulent (muco-, -pur-) Characterised by the presence of mucus and pus.

Mucosa (muc-) A mucous membrane.

Mucous (muc-, -ous) Refers to mucus; secreting mucus.

Mucous membrane (muco-) A mucus-secreting membrane lining body cavities that open to the external environment (e.g. gastro-intestinal and respiratory tracts).

Mucus (muc-) A viscous secretion of mucous glands and membranes that prevents body cavities from drying out. The main constituent of mucus is mucin.

Muscle tone (ton-) The state of resting tension and contraction of muscle, which maintains form and provides passive resistance to stretch or elongation.

Muscularis mucosa (muc-) The muscle layer of a mucous membrane.

Musculoskeletal Refers to the muscles and the bones.

Mutagenic (-genic) Causing mutation.

Myalgia (my-, -algia) Pain in a muscle or muscles.

Mycosis (myco-, -sis) Any fungal infection.

Myelocyte (myelo-, -cyte) An immature leucocyte formed from a myeloblast, which further develops into a type of granular leucocyte.

Myelogenous (myelo-, -genous) Originating in the bone marrow.

Myeloid (myel-, -oid) 1. Refers to, derived from, or similar to, bone marrow. 2. Refers to the spinal cord. 3. Resembles myelocytes.

Myeloproliferative (myelo-) Refers to, or characterised by, the proliferation of bone marrow or any of the blood cells derived from bone marrow.

Myelosuppression (myelo-) Inhibition of bone-marrow function.

Myoclonus (myo-) Clonus occurring in a particular muscle or group of muscles.

Myopathy (myo-, -pathy) Any muscle disorder.

Myositis (myo-, -itis) Inflammation of voluntary muscles.

Myotomy (myo-, -tomy) Incision or dissection of muscle.

N

Naevocytic (naevo-, -cyt-) Refers to, or composed of, naevus cells.

Naevus (naev-) 1. Any birthmark. 2. A circumscribed, usually hereditary, malformation of the skin and occasionally the oral mucosa. It is caused by hyperplasia of tissue (e.g. blood vessels, epidermis, or connective tissue).

Nail fold The fold of skin around the base and sides of a nail.

Navel UMBILICUS.

Nebuliser A device that converts a drug solution into a fine mist, which can be inhaled into the lungs.

Necrolysis (necro-, -lysis) Exfoliation and separation of tissue caused by necrosis.

Neonatal asphyxia BIRTH ASPHYXIA.

Neonate (neo-) A newborn child; usually refers to the first 30 days of life. *See also* EMBRYO, FOETUS, *and* INFANT.

Nephrectomy (nephr-, -ectomy) The removal of a kidney by surgery.

Nephritis (nephr-, -itis) Inflammation of the kidneys, affecting the glomeruli, tubules, or interstitial tissue.

Nephrogenic (nephro-, -genic) Refers to, originating in, or caused by, the kidneys.

Nerve A cord-like structure consisting of a collection of nerve fibres, which emerge from the spinal cord (nerve root) and innervate body structures (nerve terminal).

Neural tube (neur-) The embryonic central nervous system.

Neuralgia (neur-, -algia) Any disorder of a nerve or nerves causing intermittent, but frequently intense, pain.

Neurilemma (neur-) The outer membrane covering the Schwann cell of a nerve fibre.

Neuritis (neur-, -itis) Inflammation of a nerve or nerves. It may result in pain, numbness, paraesthesia, muscle wasting, and loss of reflexes.

Neurofibromatosis (neuro-, -fibr-, -oma-, -osis) An inherited autosomal dominant disorder characterised by multiple skin neurofibromas and pigmentation.

Neurogenic (neuro-, -genic) Refers to, originating in, or caused by, the nervous system.

Neurology (neuro-, -logy) The study of the nervous system and its diseases.

Neuromuscular (neuro-) Refers to nerves and muscles.

Neuromuscular junction (neuro-, junct-) The site of contact between the axon terminal of a motor neurone and the membrane of a skeletal muscle cell.

Neuromuscular transmission (neuro-, trans-) The transfer of a nerve impulse across a neuromuscular junction to a muscle cell, which is mediated by acetylcholine.

Neurone (neuro-) A nerve cell. It consists of the axon, cell body, and dendritic processes.

Neuronitis (neuro-, -itis) Inflammation and degeneration of neurones.

Neuropathy (neuro-, -pathy) Any disease or disorder of the nervous system.

Neurosecretory (neuro-) Refers to the secretory functions of nerve cells.

Neurosis (neuro-, -sis) A mild personality disorder characterised by emotional disturbances and anxiety, but without distortion of reality. *See also* PSYCHOSIS.

Neurotransmitter (neuro-, -trans-) An endogenous substance that is released from the axon terminal of a presynaptic neurone, and diffuses across the synaptic cleft to bind to a receptor site on the target cell. It may have an excitatory or inhibitory effect. *See also* SYNAPSE.

Neurotropic (neuro-, -tropic) Possessing an affinity for nervous tissue.

Neutropenia (-penia) A deficiency in the number of neutrophils in the blood.

Night blindness Poor vision in dim light, especially at night, although vision in brighter light may be good.

Nissl granules (gran-) Granules found in the cell body of neurones, and composed of endoplasmic reticulum and ribosomes.

Nitrogen balance The state of equilibrium between nitrogen intake and excretion.

NMR *See* NUCLEAR MAGNETIC RESONANCE SCANNING.

Nocturia (-uria) Excessive urination at night.

Nocturnal Refers to activities that occur during the night. *See also* CIRCADIAN RHYTHM *and* DIURNAL.

Node (nod-) A normal or pathological swelling, tissue mass, or a collection of cells.

Normal pressure hydrocephalus (hydro-, -cephal-) A syndrome characterised by the clinical manifestations of hydrocephalus, but without an increase in intracranial pressure. It occurs in adults and may be associated with previous episodes of hydrocephalus. Presenting symptoms include dementia, apraxia, and urinary incontinence.

Normocalcaemia (normo-, -calc-, -aemia) A normal plasma-calcium concentration.

Nosocomial (noso-) Refers to, or originating in, a hospital. *See also* IDIOPATHIC.

Nuclear magnetic resonance scanning Nuclear magnetic resonance (NMR) scanning is a technique in which images are generated by radio-waves directed at right-angles to protons in a magnetic field.

Nucleic acid (nucle-)   A polymeric compound found in a cell nucleus. The two principal nucleic acids are deoxyribonucleic acid (DNA) and ribonucleic acid (RNA).

Nucleoplasm (nucleo-, -plas-)   The protoplasm of a cell located within the nucleus. *See also* CYTOPLASM.

Nucleus (nucle-)   1. The distinct part of a cell that contains genetic information. 2. A collection of neurones in the central nervous system.

Nulliparous (-par-)   Refers to a woman who has never given birth. *See also* PARITY.

Numb   A condition of complete or partial loss of sensation.

Nystagmus   Involuntary oscillation of the eyeball in one or more planes.

———————————— O ————————————

Oat cell   A cell that resembles the shape of oat grains.

Obligate   Refers to the necessity for particular environmental conditions. *See also* FACULTATIVE.

Obstetrics   The medical and surgical management of pregnancy, childbirth, and the puerperium.

Occipital   Refers to the back of the skull or head.

Occipital artery   The artery branching from the carotid artery and located in the occipital region. It supplies the muscles of the neck and scalp, the mastoid process, and the meninges.

Occult   Obscured or concealed.

Occupational therapy (therap-)   Measures designed to promote recovery from illness or surgery, or to stimulate mental processes. It includes work or hobbies, instruction on the efficient use of recovery aids (e.g. walking sticks), and instruction on the performance of daily functions (e.g. bathing).

Ocular (ocul-)   Refers to the eye; ophthalmic.

Oculogyric crisis (oculo-)   A crisis in which there is prolonged fixation of the eyeballs in one position.

Oligodendroglioma (oligo-, -dendro-, -gli-, -oma)   A malignant neoplasm composed of oligodendrocytes.

Oligomenorrhoea (oligo-, -meno-, -rrhoea)   Diminished menstrual flow. *See also* MENORRHAGIA.

Oligospermia (oligo-, -sperm-, -ia)   A deficiency of spermatozoa in the semen.

Oliguria (olig-, -uria)   Diminished urine production in relation to fluid intake. *See also* POLYURIA.

Omentectomy (-ectomy)   The complete or partial removal of the omentum by surgery.

Omentum   The folded double-layer of peritoneum connecting the stomach to another organ.

Oncogenic (onco-, -genic)   Capable of producing a malignant neoplasm.

Oocyst (oo-, -cyst)   The encysted and fertilised stage in the development of protozoa.

Oophoritis (oophor-, -itis)   Inflammation of an ovary.

Opacity   1. Being opaque. 2. An opaque spot.

Ophthalmic (ophthalm-)   OCULAR.

Ophthalmic tonometer (ophthalm-, ton-)   An instrument to measure intra-ocular pressure.

Ophthalmitis (ophthalm-, -itis)   Inflammation of an eye.

Opportunistic infection   Refers to an infection caused by micro-organisms that are not usually pathogenic, but become so under certain conditions (e.g. immunodeficiency).

Optic chiasma   The cross-over point of the optic nerves.

Optic nerve   The sensory nerve from each eye, which transmits impulses to the visual centre in the occipital lobe of the cerebral cortex.

Orchidectomy (orchid-, -ectomy)   The removal of one or both testes by surgery.

Orchitis (orch-, -itis)   Inflammation of one or both of the testes.

Orf   A viral infection that affects sheep, and produces vesiculopustular dermatitis or stomatitis. It may be transmitted to man.

Organelle   Any permanent membrane-bound structure within a cell that is capable of a specific function involving cellular metabolism.

Organic   1. Refers to an organ. 2. Refers to, or arising from, an organism. 3. Chemical compounds that contain carbon.

Organism   An entire living form.

Orifice (or-)   An opening to a hollow organ.

Orthopaedics (ortho-)   The surgical management of bone and joint disorders.

Orthopnoea (ortho-, -pnoea)   Breathlessness that is relieved by assuming a sitting or upright posture. *See also* APNOEA, DYSPNOEA, HYPERPNOEA, *and* TACHYPNOEA.

Osmolality (osmo-)   Refers to osmotic concentration, expressed as moles of solute particles per kilogram of solvent.

Osmosis (osmo-)   The movement of a solvent from a solution of lower concentration to a solution of higher concentration through a semipermeable membrane separating the two solutions.

Osmotic pressure   The force that causes osmosis.

Ossification (oss-)   The process of bone formation through the action of osteoblasts.

Osteitis (oste-, -itis)   Inflammation of bone.

Osteitis fibrosa (oste-, -itis, fibro-)   A bone disorder characterised by the deposition of fibrous tissue in marrow spaces and increased bone turnover. It results in disorganised structure of the bone and causes impaired strength.

Osteochondritis (osteo-, -chondr-, -itis)   Inflammation of bone and cartilage.

Osteoclast-activating factor (osteo-, -clas-)   A lymphokine produced by lymphocytes that activates and facilitates the action of osteoclasts.

Osteodystrophy (osteo-, -dys-, -trophy)   Defective formation of bone.

Osteogenic (osteo-, -genic)   Refers to tissue involved in the growth and repair of bone.

Osteopathy (osteo-, -pathy)   1. Any bone disease. 2. A form of therapy for bone disease involving manipulative techniques.

Osteotomy (osteo-, -tomy)   Incision of a bone.

Otitis (ot-, -itis)   Inflammation of the ear.

Oxidising agent (ox-)   An oxygen-releasing agent that may be used for its disinfectant and deodorising properties.

Oxygen debt   The extra oxygen used in oxidative metabolism to reconvert lactic acid to glucose, and to restore energy stores depleted during exercise or hypoxia.

---------------------- P ----------------------

Pacemaker   1. A device or structure that initiates and establishes action and the rate of a process or function. 2. The sino-atrial node. 3. An artificial pacemaker used to replace the action of an impaired sino-atrial node by the application of electronic impulses.

Palliative   Refers to the reduction in intensity or severity of a disorder or its symptoms, but not resulting in a cure.

Pallor   Paleness.

Palpable   Perceived by touching.

Palpitation   A rapid and forceful heart beat that may be perceived by the patient. The rhythm can be impaired.

Palsy   PARALYSIS.

Pancreatectomy (-ectomy)   The complete or partial removal of the pancreas by surgery.

Pancreatin   An enzyme mixture obtained from the pancreas of animal source, and containing exocrine pancreatic secretions.

Pandemic (pan-)   Refers to an epidemic disease that extends over a very large area.

Pannus   Vascularisation and granulation tissue over a membrane or structure.

Papilla   A general term for any small nipple-shaped elevated structure.

Papillary carcinoma (carcin-, -oma)   A malignant neoplasm with outgrowths of papillae.

Paracentesis (-centesis)   The surgical insertion of a cannula into a cavity to aspirate accumulated fluid.

Paraesthesia (par-, -aesthesi-)   An abnormal sensation (e.g. burning, tingling, and 'pins and needles'). *See also* ACRO-PARAESTHESIA, ANAESTHESIA, *and* DYSAESTHESIA.

Paralysis (para-)   Loss or impairment of motor or sensory function of a part due to a lesion of the nervous system. *See also* FLACCID PARALYSIS, PARESIS, *and* SPASTIC PARALYSIS.

Paranasal (para-, -nas-)   Situated on the side of the nose.

Paraplegia (para-, -plegia)   Paralysis of the legs and lower part of the body. *See also* DIPLEGIA, HEMIPLEGIA, *and* QUADRIPLEGIA.

Parasitology (-logy)   The study of parasites.

Parathyroidectomy (-ectomy)   The removal of one or more of the parathyroid glands by surgery.

Parenchyma   The functional part of an organ, excluding the supporting tissue.

Parenteral (par-, -enter-)   Refers to administration by a route other than by the gastro-intestinal tract. It usually refers to the administration of injectable preparations for a systemic effect.

Parenteral feeding (par-, -enter-)   A method of supplying nutritional support via a peripheral vein, central vein, or an arteriovenous shunt. It is used when the enteral route cannot be utilised. It may be given either as a supplement or as the sole source of dietary provision, in which case it is referred to as total parenteral nutrition (TPN). *See also* ENTERAL FEEDNG.

Paresis   Partial or incomplete paralysis.

Parietal   1. Refers to the wall of a cavity or organ. 2. Refers to the region near the parietal bone of the skull, which constitutes the greater part of the sides and roof.

Parity (par-)   Refers to a woman with respect to her having borne children. *See also* NULLIPAROUS.

Parotid   Situated near the ear.

Parotitis (-itis)   Inflammation of the parotid gland.

Paroxysm   1. Exacerbation or recurrence of a disease, or symptoms of a disease. 2. A spasm.

Partial pressure   The pressure exerted by each of the component gases in a mixture. *See also* TENSION(2).

Parturition (part-)   The process of giving birth; childbirth, labour, or delivery.

Passive immunisation   The injection of immune serum containing the required antibodies to provide immediate, although short-lived, protection from infection. *See also* ACTIVE IMMUNISATION.

Pediculate   Possessing a peduncle.

Peduncle   1. A stalk-like structure. 2. The stalk of a neoplasm attached to normal tissue.

Pelvic cavity   The pelvic cavity contains the urinary bladder, sigmoid colon, rectum, and the reproductive organs.

Pelvic floor   PERINEUM.

Pelvic inflammatory disease   Acute or chronic inflammation of the structures within the pelvic cavity. It especially refers to bacterial infection of the female genital tract.

Pelvis   The lower part of the trunk formed by the two hip bones, the sacrum, and the coccyx.

Pepsin   The proteolytic enzyme found in gastric juice, which catalyses protein hydrolysis. It is formed from its inactive precursor, pepsinogen, by the action of hydrochloric acid.

Peptic   A general term referring to the stomach, digestion, or the action of pepsin and gastric juice.

Perception   The interpretation and conscious awareness of sensory stimuli.

Perfusion (per-, -fus-)   The normal or artificial passage of a liquid through or over an organ or tissue.

Perianal (peri-)   Refers to the area around the anus.

Pericellular (peri-)   Refers to the area around a cell.

Perihepatitis (peri-, -hepat-, -itis)   Inflammation of the peritoneum around the liver and its surrounding tissues.

Perineum (peri-)   The muscular area between the anus and the scrotum in the male, or anus and vulva in the female; the pelvic floor.

Periodontium (peri-, -odont-)   The connective tissue and bone surrounding a tooth.

Periorbital (peri-, -orb-)   Refers to the area around the orbit of the eye.

Periosteum (peri-, -oste-)   The connective tissue covering bones.

Periostitis (-itis)   Inflammation of the periosteum.

Peripheral (peri-)   Refers to a site away from a centre or located on an outer surface or part.

Peripheral vision (peri-)   Vision produced through stimulation of areas away from the macula lutea by light. *See also* CENTRAL VISION.

Periportal (peri-)   Refers to the area around the portal vein.

Peristalsis (peri-, -stal-, -sis)   A wave of contraction that propels the contents of a hollow organ along its length, brought about by the action of longitudinal and circular muscles.

Peritoneal cavity (peritone-, -cav-)   The space between the peritoneum lining the abdominal cavity and covering the abdominal organs.

Peritoneal dialysis (peritone-, -dia-, -lysis)   The removal of water, electrolytes, and waste products (e.g. urea and creatinine) from the blood using the peritoneal membrane as the dialysing membrane. Dialysate solution is introduced into the peritoneal cavity through an indwelling catheter, and subsequently removed after allowing time for substances to be exchanged across the peritoneal membrane. *See also* HAEMODIALYSIS.

Peritoneum (peritone-)   The serous membrane in the abdomen that covers the abdominal organs and lines the abdominal cavity. *See also* MESENTERY *and* PERITONEAL CAVITY.

Peritonsillar (peri-)   Refers to the region around a tonsil.

Peri-ungual (peri-)   Refers to the region around a nail.

Permeable (per-)   Allowing the passage of fluids and substances. *See also* SEMIPERMEABLE.

Pernicious   A severe and life-threatening disorder.

Personality disorder (dis-)   A behaviour disorder characterised by abnormal behaviour, life-style, and social interaction, which is usually firmly fixed and permanent.

pH   An abbreviation that refers to the hydrogen ion (H^+) concentration of a solution. A pH value of 7 represents a neutral solution, a value of less than 7 represents an acidic solution, and a value of greater than 7 represents an alkaline solution.

Phacoanaphylaxis (phaco-)   A hypersensitivity reaction to the protein of the lens of the eye.

Phacolytic (phaco-, -ly-)   Refers to dissolution of the lens of the eye.

Phagocytosis   Endocytosis of solid material.

Phalanges, phalanx (phalang-)   The bones of the fingers and toes.

Pharmacodynamics (pharmaco-, -dynami-)   The study of drug action with respect to molecular structure, mechanisms of action, and the biochemical and physiological action.

Phenon (pheno-)   A term used in some classification systems to denote a group of strains which share similar phenotypic characteristics.

Phenotype (pheno-)   1. The observable characteristics of an organism as determined by both genetic and environmental influences. 2. The expression of a single gene or gene pair.

Phenylalanine   An essential aromatic amino acid.

Phimosis (-sis)   The inability to retract the prepuce over the glans penis due to the constriction of the orifice of the prepuce. It may be acquired or congenital.

Phlyctenule   A small ulcerated nodule, or a vesicle of the cornea or conjunctiva.

Phospholipase (-ase)   Any of the several enzymes that catalyse phospholipid hydrolysis.

Photocoagulation (photo-)   The controlled coagulation of protein using a high intensity beam of light. It is used primarily to destroy neoplastic cells and in eye surgery.

Photophobia (photo-, -phobia)   1. Visual intolerance of normal light levels. 2. A phobic state caused by well-lit places.

Photosynthesis (photo-, -syn-, -sis)   The synthesis of chemicals employing light as a source of energy.

Physiology (physio-, -logy)   The study of the chemical and physical factors involved in the functioning of living organisms and their component parts.

Physiotherapy (physio-, -therap-)   Physical therapy involving the use of exercise, massage, manipulation, and other methods to aid recovery from illness, to improve and alleviate symptoms, and to prevent physical disability.

Phytate   A form of inositol found in plants, particularly the seeds; a salt of phytic acid.

Pigmentation   Coloration.

Pilo-erection (pilo-)   The upright posture of hair.

Pinocytosis   Endocytosis of liquid materials.

Placenta   The organ that connects the foetus with the inner surface of the maternal uterus. It allows the selective exchange of soluble substances between foetal and maternal blood. *See also* TROPHOBLAST.

Plasmapheresis   The separation of blood cells from plasma. The separated cells are mixed with a plasma substitute and transfused back into the bloodstream. The procedure may be used for collecting plasma components or for therapeutic purposes.

Plasmolysis (-lysis)   The dissolution of protoplasm due to water loss by osmotic action.

Pleomorphism (pleo-, -morph-) The ability to exhibit more than one distinct form.

Pneumonitis (pneumon-, -itis) Inflammation of the lungs.

Poison A substance that can cause structural or functional damage to body tissues when administered or applied by any route.

Polyarthritis (poly-, -arthr-, -itis) Arthritis affecting several joints simultaneously.

Polyarticular (poly-, -articul-) Involving many joints.

Polyclonal gammopathy (poly-, -pathy) Gammopathy in which there is an increase in two or more immunoglobulins. *See also* MONOCLONAL GAMMOPATHY.

Polydipsia (poly-, -ia) Excessive thirst.

Polymenorrhoea (poly-, -meno-, -rrhoea) Abnormally frequent menstruation.

Polymyalgia (poly-, -my-, -algia) Myalgia affecting several muscles.

Polyneuropathy (poly-, -neuro-, -pathy) Neuropathy involving several nerves. *See also* MONONEUROPATHY.

Polypharmacy (poly-, -pharmac-) The concurrent administration of several drugs.

Polyposis (-osis) A disorder characterised by the presence of multiple polyps.

Polyuria (poly-, -uria) Excessive urine production. *See also* OLIGURIA.

Porphyrin A molecular structure consisting of four 5-membered heterocyclic rings. It is found naturally as a chelate with metal ions (e.g. haemoglobin or chlorophyll).

Portal 1. Entrance. 2. Refers to the region of the liver where the portal vein and hepatic artery enter, and the hepatic ducts leave.

Portal hypertension (hyper-, -tens-) An abnormally high blood pressure in the hepatic portal vein. The normal pressure is 5 mmHg to 10 mmHg.

Posterior horn (post-) The dorsal portion of grey matter within the spinal cord containing sensory cells. *See also* ANTERIOR HORN.

Postnatal (post-) Refers to the period after birth. *See also* ANTENATAL, POSTPARTUM, *and* PUERPERIUM.

Postpartum (post-, -part-) Refers to the mother in the period immediately after parturition. *See also* POSTNATAL *and* PUERPERIUM.

Postprandial (post-) Refers to the period immediately following a meal.

Postural Refers to posture or position.

Precursor (pre-) That which preceeds a specific form, usually in a less developed inactive form.

Premature infant A premature infant is an infant that is born between the 27th week of gestation and full term, with a low birth-weight.

Prepatellar (pre-) In front of the patella.

Preservative A substance added to a product to prevent decomposition, by killing or inhibiting the growth of micro-organisms or preventing specific chemical reactions (e.g. oxidation).

Pressor Refers to the tendency to increase blood pressure.

Presynaptic (pre-) Situated or occurring before a synapse.

Priapism A persistent and painful erection of the penis attained without sexual stimulation.

Primary First or of most importance.

Procreation The process of producing offspring.

Proctocolectomy (procto-, -col-, -ectomy) The removal of the rectum and colon by surgery.

Prodromal (pro-, -drom-) Refers to the early, often premonitory, symptoms of a disease. *See also* AURA.

Proglottides The segments comprising the body of a cestode.

Prognosis (pro-, -gno-, -sis) A prediction of the course and outcome of a disease.

Progressive (pro-) Advancing, or increasing in severity.

Projectile vomiting The forceful ejection of vomit.

Prolactinoma (-oma) A benign pituitary neoplasm that secretes prolactin.

Prolapse (pro-) Forward or downward displacement; protrusion.

Proliferate Cellular multiplication resulting in growth.

Prolymphocyte (pro-, -lympho-, -cyte) An immature cell in the intermediate stage between a lymphoblast and lymphocyte.

Prone Lying down, facing downwards. *See also* SUPINE.

Prophylaxis The prevention of disease. *See also* CHEMO-PROPHYLAXIS.

Prostacyclin A substance synthesised by vascular endothelial cells that prevents platelet aggregation on normal vascular tissue. It is also a potent vasodilator.

Prostaglandin A lipid derived from unsaturated 20-carbon fatty acids present in most body tissues. The actions of prostaglandins include increasing or reducing blood pressure, bronchoconstriction or bronchodilatation, reducing gastric secretion, altering platelet adhesiveness, altering intestinal and uterine muscle tone, and mediating inflammation.

Prostatectomy (-ectomy) The complete or partial removal of the prostate gland by surgery.

Prosthesis An articial replacement for a limb or body part, which may be functional or for cosmetic purposes.

Prostration Extreme exhaustion. *See also* FATIGUE, LASSITUDE, *and* LETHARGY.

Protease (-ase) PROTEOLYTIC ENZYME.

Protein A member of a large and diverse group of organic compounds containing carbon, hydrogen, oxygen, and nitrogen, and occasionally sulphur and phosphorus. Proteins are composed of amino acids linked by peptide bonds in a specific genetically determined sequence.

Proteinase (-ase) PROTEOLYTIC ENZYME.

Proteinuria (-uria)   The presence of plasma proteins in the urine.

Proteolytic enzyme (-ly-, -zym-)   An enzyme that catalyses the splitting of peptide bonds of proteins by hydrolysis to form smaller polypeptides.

Protoplasm (-plas-)   The main constituent of all animal and plant cells. It is a viscous, translucent, water-based liquid composed mainly of nucleic acids, proteins, fats, carbohydrates, and inorganic salts. *See also* CYTOPLASM *and* NUCLEOPLASM.

Pseudocyst (pseudo-, -cyst)   Resembling a cyst, but without a distinct wall of epithelial cells.

Pseudomembrane (pseudo-)   A false membrane; resembling a membrane but consisting of a thick fibrinous exudate.

Pseudopodium (pseudo-, -pod-)   A temporary protrusion of cytoplasm in amoebic protozoa, formed to facilitate movement and phagocytosis.

Pseudopolyp (pseudo-)   Resembling a polyp, but caused by hypertrophy of the mucous membrane as a result of ulceration.

Pseudopolyposis (pseudo-, -osis)   A disorder characterised by the presence of multiple pseudopolyps.

Psychiatry (psych-)   The study, treatment, and prevention of mental illness.

Psychic (psych-)   Refers to the mind, mental thoughts, and emotions, including conscious and unconscious manifestations.

Psychogenic (psycho-, -genic)   Having a psychic origin.

Psychomotor (psycho-, -mot-)   1. Refers to combined psychic and motor events (e.g. sensory auras and seizures). 2. Refers to the cerebral origin of voluntary movement.

Psychosis (psycho-, -sis)   A general term for a profound psychiatric disorder of organic or psychic aetiology, and characterised by personality disorders, loss of reality, and often delusions or hallucinations. *See also* NEUROSIS.

Psychosomatic (psycho-, -somat-)   Refers to the appearance or exacerbation of physical symptoms as a result of psychic causes.

Psychotherapy (psycho-, -therap-)   The treatment of certain psychiatric disorders by psychological methods. It includes the use of recollection techniques, group therapy, listening and talking to the patient, offering reassurance and encouragement, developing and increasing self-confidence, and other more complex forms of treatment (e.g. hypnosis).

Puberty   The period during which the secondary sexual characteristics develop, the sex organs become active, and the capability for sexual reproduction is attained.

Puerperium   A period of about 6 weeks after parturition, during which time the reproductive organs of the mother return to their pre-pregnancy state. *See also* POSTNATAL *and* POSTPARTUM.

Pulmonary (pulmon-)   Refers to the lungs.

Pulse   1. The rhythmic arterial dilatation produced by ventricular systole. The pulse-rate is the number of pulsations per minute, the normal being between 50 and 100. 2. Rhythmic and recurrent.

Purine   A widely distributed compound occurring as a derivative form in the body. The purines or purine bases (e.g. adenine, guanine, and xanthine) are constituents of caffeine, theophylline, and the nucleic acids.

Purulent (pur-)   Forming, containing, or discharging pus.

Putrefaction   The enzymatic decomposition of animal and plant tissues by micro-organisms. Protein decomposition is characterised by a foul smell resulting from the formation of putrefaction products (e.g. ammonia and hydrogen sulphide).

Pyaemia (py-, -aemia)   The presence of pyogenic micro-organisms in the blood, resulting in the formation of multiple abscesses.

Pyknosis (pykno-, -sis)   A thickening. It refers especially to cellular degeneration in which the cell nucleus condenses to form a homogeneous mass. *See also* KARYOLYSIS *and* KARYORRHEXIS.

Pyoderma (pyo-, -derma)   Any skin disorder characterised by purulent lesions.

Pyosalpinx (pyo-, -salp-)   Accumulation of pus in a Fallopian tube.

Pyramidal cell   A large pyramid-shaped neurone located in the grey matter of the cerebral cortex.

Pyrexia (pyr-)   FEVER.

Pyrimidine   A widely distributed compound occurring as a derivative form in the body. The pyrimidines or pyrimidine bases (e.g. uracil, thymine, and cytosine) are constituents of the nucleic acids.

Pyrogen (pyro-, -gen)   A substance that causes a rise in body temperature.

Pyuria (py-, -uria)   The presence of pus in the urine.

──────────── Q ────────────

Quadriplegia (quadri-, -plegia)   Paralysis of both arms and both legs. *See also* DIPLEGIA, HEMIPLEGIA, *and* PARAPLEGIA.

Quarantine   The detention and isolation of sources of contagious or communicable disease as a routine procedure, or in suspected or definite cases.

──────────── R ────────────

Radiation (radi-)   1. Electromagnetic waves. *See also* IRRADIATION. 2. Spreading from a central point.

Radioactivity (radio-)   The property of emitting radiation.

Radiobiology (radio-, -bio-, -logy)   The study of the effect of radiation on living cells and tissues.

Radiography (radio-, -graphy)   Examination of internal structures using radiation, which is passed through the body onto sensitised photographic film.

Radioisotope (radio-, -iso-, -top-)   A radioactive isotope.

Radiolabel (radio-) A radioactive isotope that is used to replace a stable chemical element in a compound. It is introduced into the body to study the distribution of a compound with the aid of a radiation detecting device.

Radiotherapy (radio-, -therap-) The therapeutic use of ionising radiation.

Rarefaction Reduction in density and mass but not volume.

Rash A skin eruption.

Receptor (-ceptor) 1. A molecular structure on or within a cell that allows the binding of a specific agent to elicit a specific response. 2. A specialised nerve terminal that responds to sensory stimuli. *See also* SYNAPSE.

Recrudescence (re-) The recurrence of symptoms within days or weeks of their subsidence. *See also* RELAPSE.

Rectosigmoid (recto-) Refers to the region at the end of the sigmoid colon and the beginning of the rectum.

Rectovaginal (recto-, -vagin-) Refers to the rectum and the vagina.

Reflex (re-, -flex) The involuntary and rapid response to a stimulus.

Reflux (re-, -flux) Backward flow or regurgitation.

Refractory Resistant to treatment.

Regurgitation (re-) The return or backward flow of contents.

Rehydration (re-, -hydrat-) The administration of fluids to correct dehydration.

Relapse (re-) The recurrence of a disease after apparent cure, usually within weeks or months. *See also* RECRUDESCENCE.

Remission (re-) The subsidence and cessation of disease symptoms; the period of subsidence.

Replacement therapy (therap-) The treatment of deficiency disorders by the administration of natural or synthetic derivatives of the deficient substance.

Resection (-sect-) The complete or partial removal of an organ or structure by surgery. *See also* EXCISION.

Reservoir of infection A host that carries pathogenic micro-organisms, usually without any harmful effects, and serves as a source of infection. Non-living material may also act as a reservoir. *See also* CARRIER(1) *and* FOMITES.

Residual volume The volume of air in the lungs following maximum expiration. *See also* VITAL CAPACITY.

Resistance 1. An opposite force; counteraction. 2. The ability of an organism to remain unaffected by micro-organisms or their toxins. *See also* ANTIMICROBIAL RESISTANCE. 3. In psychotherapy, the conscious and active opposition to prevent unconscious thoughts from emerging.

Respiration (-spirat-) The complete process of gaseous interchange between the tissues and the external environment. It includes ventilation, and gaseous exchange between the lungs and the blood, and between the blood and the cells.

Respirator (-spirat-) 1. An apparatus to prevent the inhalation of harmful environmental substances. 2. An apparatus to provide artificial respiration or assisted ventilation.

Resuscitation (re-) The emergency treatment to restore life in an apparently deceased patient (e.g. using cardiac massage and artificial respiration).

Retch To make an involuntary and ineffectual attempt to vomit.

Reticulin (ret-) The protein from reticular connective tissue.

Reticulo-endothelial system (ret-) A functional system of potent phagocytic cells found throughout the body, and serving as a defence mechanism. The cells include macrophages and are concentrated in the spleen, liver, bone marrow, and lymph nodes.

Retinopathy (-pathy) Any non-inflammatory disease of the retina.

Retrobulbar (retro-) Situated behind the eyeball.

Retrograde (retro-, -grad-) Backwards; in an opposite direction.

Retroperitoneum (retro-, -peritone-) The area behind the peritoneum.

Retrosternal (retro-, -stern-) Situated behind the sternum.

Rheumatism A general term applied to any disorder characterised by inflammation or degeneration of connective tissue, particularly of joints and muscles.

Rhinorrhoea (rhino-, -rrhoea) A profuse discharge of mucus from the nose.

Ribonucleic acid (-nucle-) Ribonucleic acid (RNA) is found in the nucleus and cytoplasm of all living cells, and processes information from DNA for cellular protein synthesis. The molecular structure is similar to DNA except that ribose replaces deoxyribose, and uracil replaces thymine. Three types exist: messenger RNA (mRNA), transfer RNA (tRNA), and ribosomal RNA (rRNA). *See also* DEOXY-RIBONUCLEIC ACID.

Ribosome (-some) A granule composed of ribosomal RNA (rRNA) bound to specific proteins. Ribosomes are found in the cytoplasm of all living cells.

Rigor 1. Rigidity. 2. A chill or shivering fit, with fever and cold skin.

RNA RIBONUCLEIC ACID.

Rosacea An inflammatory skin disorder characterised by extensive facial erythema, often with papules, pustules, and telangiectasia.

Rubefacient (rub-, -facient) Producing erythema.

Rupture 1. A break or tear. 2. HERNIA.

— S —

Sac A pouch or bag-like structure.

Saccular Resembling a sac.

Sacral Refers to, or situated near, the sacrum.

Sacrococcygeal (sacro-) Refers to the region of the sacrum and coccyx.

Saturated fat A fat composed of a fatty acid that contains only single bonds in the carbon chain. It is found in animal products (e.g. meat and milk).

Scan A visual display of body tissues produced by moving a sensing device over the body, or body part, or by a series of observations to produce a complete image.

Schizogony A type of asexual reproduction in which the nucleus undergoes multiple fission, followed by separation of the cytoplasm into discrete masses around each daughter nucleus.

Sclerosis (sclero-, -sis) Hardening, especially of the nervous system due to connective tissue hyperplasia, and also applied to blood vessels. It is usually of chronic inflammatory origin.

Sclerotherapy (sclero-, -therap-) The injection of a sclerosant.

Scotoma An area of diminished vision surrounded by an area of less diminished or normal vision.

Sebaceous (-aceous) Refers to sebum.

Seborrhoea (sebo-, -rrhoea) Excessive sebum secretion from the sebaceous glands.

Secondary 1. Occurring in second place, or as a result of a primary disorder. 2. Often used to denote metastasis.

Secretin A hormone secreted by the intestinal mucosa, whose actions include inhibition of gastric juice secretion, stimulation of pancreatic juice and bile secretion, and stimulation of intestinal juice.

Secretion The production and release of a specific functional substance by a cell or a gland.

Seizure 1. An epileptic attack. *See also* CONVULSION. 2. A sudden occurrence of a disease and its symptoms.

Self-limiting Refers to a disease that follows a definite course, and is restricted in duration as a result of its own characteristics and not by external factors.

Seminal duct Any of the ducts of the male reproductive organs.

Seminoma (-oma) A malignant neoplasm of the testis, arising from germ cells.

Semipermeable (semi-, -per-) Refers to the selective passage of certain molecules. *See also* PERMEABLE.

Semipermeable membrane (semi-, -per-) A membrane that allows the passage of solvent (e.g. water), but not solutes.

Senility A generalised physical and mental dysfunction associated with ageing.

Sensorineural (sens-, -neur-) Refers to a sensory nerve or the sensory mechanism.

Sensory (sens-) Refers to sensations or to sensory nerves.

Sepsis (sep-, -sis) A condition caused by the presence of pathogenic micro-organisms, or their toxins, in the blood or tissues.

Septic (sep-) Refers to sepsis or putrefaction.

Septum (sept-) A dividing structure or partition.

Sero-mucinous (ser-, -muc-) Refers to serum and mucin.

Serotonin Serotonin (5HT, 5-hydroxytryptamine) is a widely distributed compound found in most body tissues and in high concentration in platelets. Its actions include inhibition of gastric juice secretion, stimulation of smooth muscle, and acting as a neurotransmitter in the central nervous system.

Serous (ser-) 1. Refers to or resembling serum. 2. Containing or producing serum.

Serous membrane (ser-) A membrane that covers structures not exposed to the external environment, and which secretes serum.

Serum (ser-) 1. The clear watery portion of body fluids. 2. The clear liquid part of blood, excluding blood cells and clotting factors.

Serum sickness (ser-) A hypersensitivity reaction occurring 7 to 12 days after administration of a foreign serum or some drugs (e.g. penicillin). It is characterised by arthralgia, fever, lymphadenopathy, skin rashes, oedema, and urticaria.

Sexual reproduction Production of offspring by fusion of male and female gametes. *See also* ASEXUAL REPRODUCTION.

Shear Refers to the distortion of an object caused by two oppositely directed parallel forces.

Shunt 1. To divert or bypass. 2. An anastomosis between two vessels, especially blood vessels.

Shy-Drager syndrome A progressive disorder characterised by orthostatic hypotension and symptoms of autonomic nervous system insufficiency. Generalised neurological dysfunctions follow and include parkinsonism, cerebellar ataxia, and paralysis of the extrinsic ocular muscles.

Sialorrhoea (sialo-, -rrhoea) Excessive salivation.

Sibling Brother or sister; having one or both parents in common.

Sigmoidoscopy (-scopy) Examination of the rectum and sigmoid colon using a fibre-optic sigmoidoscope, which is also a tool for biopsy.

Sinus (sinu-) 1. A cavity or channel. 2. A natural cavity within a bone or other tissue, especially the air cavities within the skull communicating with the nostrils. 3. A venous cavity, channel, or receptacle of blood. 4. A fistula or tract permitting the escape of pus from a suppurating cavity.

Sinus rhythm Normal heart rhythm.

Sinusoidal (sinu-, -oid-) Resembling a sinus.

Slough 1. To separate, shed, or cast off. 2. Necrotic tissue separating from living tissue.

Somatic (somat-) 1. Refers to the body. 2. Refers to body structure excluding the viscera.

Somnolence (somn-) Abnormal drowsiness or inclination to sleep.

Sorbitol A hexahydric alcohol and a sweetening agent. It is metabolised to fructose.

Spasm (spas-) A sudden involuntary painful muscle contraction.

Spastic paralysis (spas-, para-) Paralysis with increased tendon reflexes and spasticity of the muscles. It is commonly caused by motor neurone lesions. *See also* FLACCID PARALYSIS.

Spasticity (spas-)   A non-specific condition of increased muscular tone with exaggeration of the reflexes.

Species   A taxonomic category that comprises strains possessing common features. Similar species belong to the same genus.

Sphincter   A circular muscle that constricts and closes an orifice or passage.

Splenectomy (splen-, -ectomy)   The removal of the spleen by surgery.

Sputum   The substance expelled from the respiratory passages by coughing.

Squamous (squam-)   Scaly, or covered in scales.

Stasis   The stoppage or slowing of the flow of a fluid.

Stasis eczema   A chronic inflammatory skin disorder of the lower legs caused by venous insufficiency. It is characterised by brown pigmentation, oedema, and ulceration.

Steatorrhoea (steato-, -rrhoea)   An excessive amount of fat in the faeces.

Stenosis (steno-, -sis)   The narrowing or constriction of a vessel, passage, or duct. *See also* COARCTATION *and* STRICTURE.

Stomatitis (stomat-, -itis)   Inflammation of the oral mucosa. *See also* ANGULAR STOMATITIS.

Stopple   GROMMET.

Strangulated   Tightly constricted and with diminished blood supply.

Strangury   Painful and slow urination caused by spasm of the bladder and urethra. *See also* DYSURIA.

Stress   1. Exerted pressure; force. 2. The total response to adverse stimuli, which elicits homoeostatic mechanisms. The stimuli may be of any origin, and if the compensatory mechanisms are inadequate, they could cause or precipitate disorders. *See also* GENERAL ADAPTATION SYNDROME.

Stricture (strict-)   The closure or abnormal narrowing of a vessel, passage, or duct. *See also* COARCTATION *and* STENOSIS.

Stridor   A harsh and loud breathing sound caused by a constricted airway. *See also* WHEEZE.

Strip   1. To apply pressure along a vessel, using the finger, to move the contents. 2. To remove a large vein by surgery.

Stroke volume   The amount of blood pumped out of a ventricle in each heart beat. *See also* CARDIAC OUTPUT.

Stupor   Almost complete unconsciousness, in which the subject responds only to forceful and vigorous stimuli. *See also* COMA.

Subacromial (sub-, -acro-)   Beneath the acromion, which is the lateral projection of the scapula over the shoulder joint.

Subacute (sub-)   Refers to a disorder with characteristics intermediate between acute and chronic.

Subconjunctival (sub-)   Beneath the conjunctiva.

Subcutaneous (sub-, -cut-)   Beneath the skin.

Sublingual (sub-, -lingu-)   Beneath the tongue.

Submandibular (sub-)   Beneath the bone of the lower jaw.

Submucosa (sub-, -muc-)   The areolar tissue layer beneath a mucous membrane.

Subperiosteal (sub-, -peri-, -oste-)   Beneath the periosteum.

Subphrenic (sub-, -phren-)   Beneath the diaphragm.

Sucrose (-ose)   A disaccharide found in sugar cane, sugar beet, and other plants. It is used as a food and sweetening agent.

Suffocation   Cessation of breathing caused by airway obstruction. *See also* ASPHYXIA.

Superficial (super-)   Refers to, or occurring near, the surface.

Supine   Lying down, facing upwards. *See also* PRONE.

Supportive therapy (therap-)   Measures directed towards maintaining the patient's strength.

Suprapubic (supra-)   Situated above the pubic bone, which is the anterior inferior part of the hip bone.

Supraventricular (supra-, -ventricul-)   Above the ventricles, referring especially to the atria and atrioventricular node.

Surfactant   A substance that reduces the surface tension of fluids.

Suture   A surgical stitch.

Sympathectomy (-ectomy)   The excision or interruption of sympathetic nerves by surgery.

Sympathomimetic   Having an action which mimics that produced by stimulation of sympathetic nerves. *See also* ADRENERGIC.

Symptomatic   1. Refers to a symptom or symptoms. 2. Indicative of a specific disorder. 3. Refers to treatment directed towards alleviating symptoms.

Synapse   The site of functional proximity between neurones, at which transmission of an impulse occurs. *See also* NEUROTRANSMITTER *and* RECEPTOR(2).

Syndrome   A set of distinct and characteristic symptoms that occur together; a symptom complex.

Syrinx   A tube or fistula.

Systemic   Refers to the whole body. *See also* LOCAL.

Systole   The period during which the heart, and especially the ventricles, contract. *See also* DIASTOLE.

Systolic pressure   The maximumum arterial blood pressure, which occurs during ventricular systole. *See also* DIASTOLIC PRESSURE.

T

Tachypnoea (tachy-, -pnoea)   Abnormally rapid breathing. *See also* APNOEA, DYSPNOEA, HYPERPNOEA, *and* ORTHOPNOEA.

Tactile (tact-)   Refers to the sense of touch.

Taxonomy (tax-, -nom-)   The structured classification and naming of organisms.

Temporal (tempor-)   1. Refers to the lateral portion on both sides of the head, in the region of the temple. 2. Refers to time; temporary.

Tenesmus Straining, particularly on defaecation or urination, which may be accompanied by pain.

Tension (tens-) 1. The state and degree of stretch or strain. *See also* ARTERIAL TENSION. 2. The partial pressure of a gas in a fluid (e.g. the pressure of oxygen (PaO_2) or carbon dioxide ($PaCO_2$) in arterial blood).

Teratogenesis (terato-, -gen-, -sis) The production of developmental abnormalities in the foetus.

Teratoma (terat-, -oma) A malignant neoplasm composed of several tissue types, which are usually foreign to the site in which it occurs. Teratomas form most commonly in the ovaries or testes.

Terminal 1. Refers to an end or extremity. 2. Refers to the last stages of a fatal disease.

Tertiary In third place.

Testicular feminisation syndrome A syndrome affecting males and characterised by the development of external secondary female characteristics, but with the testes present. It is thought to be caused by target-organ resistance to testosterone.

Tetany 1. Excessive neuromuscular excitability caused by abnormal calcium metabolism. It is characterised by flexion of the wrists and ankles, muscle twitching, cramp, laryngospasm, and convulsions. 2. Sustained tonic muscle contraction.

Therapeutics (therap-) The branch of medicine that is concerned with the treatment of disease.

Thoracotomy (thoraco-, -tomy) Incision of the chest wall.

Thrombectomy (thromb-, -ectomy) The removal of a thrombus by surgery.

Thromboplastin (thrombo-) A substance that promotes coagulation of blood.

Thymectomy (thym-, -ectomy) The removal of the thymus gland by surgery.

Thymoma (thym-, -oma) A malignant neoplasm consisting of thymic tissue.

Thyroid storm A rare and life-threatening disorder caused by the sudden exacerbation of hyperthyroidism.

Thyroidectomy (-ectomy) The complete or partial removal of the thyroid gland.

Tibia The inner, larger bone in the lower leg. *See also* FIBULA.

Tinnitus A sensation of noises in the ear (e.g. ringing, buzzing, or clicking).

Tolerance Refers to the ability to endure, or become less responsive to, a drug or toxin, especially during a period of continued exposure. *See also* CROSS TOLERANCE *and* INTOLERANCE(1).

Tone (ton-) The state of organs and tissues in which function and firmness is normal. *See also* MUSCLE TONE.

Tonsil A small aggregation of large lymph nodes within a mucous membrane. The pharyngeal tonsil (adenoid) is found in the nasopharynx, the two palatine tonsils are found on the sides of the oropharynx, and the two lingual tonsils are found at the base of the tongue. The term tonsils usually refers to the palatine tonsils.

Tonsillectomy (-ectomy) The removal of one or more tonsils by surgery, usually referring to the palatine tonsils and sometimes also the lingual tonsils.

Topical (top-) Refers to a specific area of a surface.

Total parenteral nutrition *See* PARENTERAL FEEDING.

Toxaemia (tox-, -aemia) 1. The presence of bacterial toxins in the blood. *See also* ENDOTOXIN *and* EXOTOXIN. 2. Metabolic disturbances.

Toxic (toxi-) Refers to a poison or toxin.

Toxicology (toxico-, -logy) The study of the preparation, identification, and action of poisons and toxins, and their antidotes.

Toxigenic (toxi-, -genic) Producing a toxin.

TPN Total parenteral nutrition. *See* PARENTERAL FEEDING.

Trabecula A term for connective tissue that anchors or supports.

Tracheitis (trache-, -itis) Inflammation of the trachea.

Tracheobronchial (tracheo-, -bronch-) Refers to the trachea and bronchi.

Tracheostomy (tracheo-, -stomy) A surgical procedure to establish an opening into the trachea through the neck. The term may also be applied to the opening itself.

Traction (tract-) The application of a longitudinal pulling force to a structure.

Transcription The transfer of genetic information, with reference to the process by which a single strand of DNA serves as a template for the formation of the messenger RNA (mRNA) base sequence. *See also* TRANSLATION.

Transferase (trans-, -ase) An enzyme capable of transferring a chemical entity from one molecule to another, such that the chemical entity does not exist in a free state during the transfer.

Transfusion (trans-, -fus-) The administration of donor blood or blood products (e.g. plasma, serum, or blood substitutes) into the circulatory system. Prior to transfusion of whole blood, selection and cross-matching is carried out. The same blood group is selected and tested by cross-matching with the recipient's serum. Both the recipient and donor blood is tested for atypical antibodies. *See also* EXCHANGE TRANSFUSION *and* INFUSION(1).

Transitional cell A cell of the transitional epithelium, which lines some hollow organs (e.g. bladder). The cells are large and round and are capable of distension. This property prevents rupture and allows the organ to expand.

Transitional epithelium *See* TRANSITIONAL CELL.

Translation The production of a specific protein on the ribosome of a cell, as determined by the base sequence on the messenger RNA (mRNA) molecule. *See also* TRANSCRIPTION.

Transplantation (trans-) A procedure to graft tissues or organs from one part of the body to another, or from one person to another. *See also* ALLOGRAFT.

Transudation (trans-) The outflow of serum or other body fluids through a tissue membrane or surface as a result of inflammation or other causes. The transudate has a low content of protein, cells, and cellular debris. *See also* EXTRAVASATION *and* EXUDATION.

Transurethral (trans-, -urethr-) Refers to a procedure performed through the urethra.

Trauma 1. A physical wound or injury. 2. An emotional shock, especially one having a lasting psychic effect.

Tremor Involuntary shaking or trembling.

Trichotillomania (tricho-, -mania) A compulsive impulse to pull out the hair.

Trigeminal nerve The fifth cranial nerve, the sensory portion of which innervates the face, nasal cavity, mouth, and teeth, while the motor portion innervates the muscles involved in chewing.

Triglyceride (tri-, -glyc-) A fat composed of three molecules of fatty acid esterified with glycerol. It is stored in adipose tissue.

Trimester (tri-) A three-month period of time.

Trophoblast (tropho-, -blast) The cell layer through which a developing foetus receives nourishment from the mother, and which forms part of the placenta.

Trophozoite (tropho-, -zo-) The active and feeding stage in the life-cycle of a protozoal micro-organism.

Tunica A covering.

Turgor Refers to a state of fullness or swelling; normal appearance and fullness.

U

Ulcer An open lesion on an external or internal surface of the body, produced by sloughing of necrotic tissue usually as a result of inflammation.

Ulceration 1. The formation of an ulcer. 2. ULCER.

Ultrasound (ultra-) Sound with a frequency above 20 000 Hz and inaudible to the human ear. Its properties are dependent on the power level used. It may be used for diagnostic purposes using echo reflection techniques, physiotherapy, or to selectively destroy tissues.

Ultraviolet radiation (ultra-, radi-) Radiation emitted from beyond the violet end of the visible spectrum.

Umbilical hernia The protrusion of part of the intestine through the abdominal wall at the umbilicus, but under the skin and subcutaneous tissue.

Umbilicus The navel, marking the attachment site of the umbilical cord, which connected the developing foetus to the placenta.

Unconjugated hyperbilirubinaemia *See* HYPERBILIRUBINAEMIA.

Underwater seal drainage A closed drainage system in which a tube leading from the pleural cavity is immersed in a container of water. This allows air, blood, and fluid to be drained from the pleural cavity, and lung expansion to be maintained.

Ungual Refers to a nail or nails.

Unipolar (uni-) 1. Possessing only one pole or process. 2. At one end of a cell. 3. Used to describe affective disorders characterised by depressive periods only. *See also* BIPOLAR.

Urate A salt of uric acid (e.g. sodium urate).

Ureteric (ureter-) Refers to the ureter.

Urethral (urethr-) Refers to the urethra.

Uricosuric (urico-, -ur-) Refers to the promotion of uric acid excretion.

Urostomy (uro-, -stomy) A surgical procedure to divert the flow of urine from the bladder to an opening (stoma) created on the surface of the abdomen. A length of intestine is isolated, usually from the ileum, and inserted between the ureters and the stoma, thus acting as a drainage channel for urine. The term may also be applied to the opening itself. *See also* COLOSTOMY *and* ILEOSTOMY.

Urothelial (uro-) Refers to the epithelium of the urinary bladder.

Uterine (uter-) Refers to the uterus.

Uterorectal (utero-, -rect-) Refers to the uterus and the rectum, or to a communication between them.

Uvula A pendent fleshy structure, referring especially to the cone-shaped structure within the oropharynx descending from the soft palate.

V

Vaccination 1. The injection or oral administration of a vaccine to induce active immunity. *See also* ACTIVE IMMUNISATION. 2. Historically, the term was applied to inoculation with cowpox virus (vaccinia) to induce immunity to smallpox.

Vaccine A preparation of antigenic material used for active immunisation against specific bacteria or viruses. *See also* ANTISERUM.

Vacuole A cavity formed in the protoplasm of a cell.

Vagotomy (-tomy) The complete or selective interruption of the vagus nerve by surgery.

Vagus nerve The tenth cranial nerve, which consists of motor and sensory fibres. It innervates the muscles of the pharynx, larynx, respiratory system, oesophagus, stomach, small intestine, gall bladder, part of the large intestine, and the heart.

Valvotomy (-tomy) Incision of a valve, especially a heart valve.

Varicose (varic-, -ose) Refers to, or characterised by, a distended and tortuous vein, artery, or lymph vessel.

Vascular (vas-) 1. Refers to blood vessels. 2. Implies a profuse blood supply. *See also* AVASCULAR.

Vasculitis (vas-, -itis) Inflammation of a vessel, especially of a blood or lymph vessel. *See also* ARTERITIS.

Vasoactive (vaso-) Refers to an effect on the tension and internal diameter of blood vessels. *See also* VASOCONSTRICTION, VASODILATATION, *and* VASOMOTOR.

Vasoconstriction (vaso-) A reduction in the diameter of blood vessels, especially the arterioles. *See also* VASODILATATION.

Vasodilatation (vaso-) An increase in the diameter of blood vessels, especially the arterioles. *See also* VASOCONSTRICTION.

Vasodilation VASODILATATION.

Vasomotor (vaso-, -mot-) Refers to the contractility of the muscular walls of the blood vessels. *See also* VASOACTIVE, VASOCONSTRICTION, *and* VASODILATATION.

Vasospasm (vaso-, -spas-) Spasm of blood vessels, resulting in vasoconstriction.

Vector A carrier of an infective agent, which promotes the transfer of infection.

Vegetation 1. Any plant-like or fungus-like growth. 2. A clot attached to a diseased heart valve, and composed of platelets, fibrin, and infecting micro-organisms.

Vegetative 1. Refers to nutrition and growth. 2. Refers to involuntary or unconscious function. 3. Refers to the cellular resting phase, in which the cell is not involved in replication. 4. Refers to asexual reproduction.

Venesection (ven-, -sect-) Incision of a vein.

Ventilation The breathing process resulting in the gaseous exchange between the lungs and the external environment. *See also* HYPERVENTILATION, HYPOVENTILATION, *and* RESPIRATION.

Ventricle A cavity, especially of the brain and heart.

Ventriculo-atrial shunt (ventriculo-, -atri-) An anastomosis created between a cerebral ventricle and a cardiac atrium using a plastic tube, to allow drainage of cerebrospinal fluid.

Ventriculo-peritoneal shunt (ventriculo-, peritone-) An anastomosis created between a cerebral ventricle and the peritoneum using a plastic tube, to allow drainage of cerebrospinal fluid.

Vermiform (vermi-, -form) Resembling the shape of a worm.

Vernal Refers to the spring.

Vesiculation (vesic-) The formation of vesicles.

Vesiculopustular (vesic-) Refers to vesicles and pustules.

Vestigial Refers to the degenerated remnants of a structure which was functional during embryonic or foetal development, or in primeval species.

Villus A small projection or protrusion, especially from a mucous membrane of the small intestine.

Viraemia (-aemia) The presence of viruses in the blood.

Virilisation The development of male secondary sexual characteristics, especially applied to such changes in females.

Viscera (viscer-) The organs within the body cavities, especially those of the abdomen. *See also* SOMATIC(2).

Viscosity The resistance to flow caused by molecular cohesion, commonly applied to liquids as the resistance to shear forces.

Vital capacity (vit-) The total volume of gas expired from the lungs after maximum inspiration and expiration. *See also* RESIDUAL VOLUME.

Vitamin (vit-) An organic compound required by the body in small amounts for metabolism. Vitamins are generally obtained from the diet and are classified as water-soluble (e.g. vitamin C) or fat-soluble (e.g. vitamin D).

Volvulus A knot or twist in the gastro-intestinal tract, resulting in obstruction.

Vomitus 1. The forcible ejection of the contents of the stomach through the mouth. 2. The matter ejected by vomiting.

W

Wheeze A whistling sound made during breathing, especially that associated with asthma or the mechanical obstruction of the trachea or bronchi. *See also* STRIDOR.

X

X-rays Radiation of short wavelength produced by electrons emitted at high speed from a heated cathode and bombarding a heavy metal anode.

Z

Zoonosis (zoo-, -sis) An animal disease capable of being transmitted to humans under natural conditions.

Zygote (zygo-) A term applied to a fertilised ovum (formed by the union of a male and female gamete) before it divides.

COMBINING FORMS, PREFIXES, AND SUFFIXES

Introduction

Many words, including medical terms, are composed from one or more word roots derived from classical Greek and Latin. A knowledge of these word roots may facilitate the comprehension of a wide range of terms, without needing to consult a dictionary.

The following list comprises combining forms, prefixes, and suffixes of some of the most commonly used word roots that make up many of the medical terms used throughout this publication. It is not, however, intended to be a comprehensive etymological list.

A hyphen following a term indicates that the term is used in the prefix position, while a hyphen preceding a term indicates the suffix position. Combining forms may appear in any position within a word, and are identified in this list by hyphens at both ends of the term.

A definition is given under the form that bears the closest resemblance to the actual word root. Some forms which are merely deviations in spelling have been listed, with a cross-reference to the main entry. There may be several combining forms of the same word root, and those most commonly used have been grouped together as one entry, although it should be noted that this list is not exhaustive. If a particular form differs significantly and would appear in the alphabetical listing at a distance from the main entry, it has been listed separately with a cross-reference to the main entry. The reader's attention has been drawn to terms that have the same meaning but are derived from different word roots, by the use of cross-references. In these cases, the definitions have been given under all the terms.

For those terms that have more than one definition, any cross-reference follows on immediately after the definition to which it applies. If the cross-reference applies to all of the stated definitions, it starts on a new line after the last definition.

The reader should consult the glossary for examples of the breakdown of words into combining forms, prefixes, and suffixes, which have, where appropriate, been listed in brackets after the word itself.

---
a
---

a- Without, not. The prefix becomes *an-* before a vowel or *h*.

ab- From, off, away from.

-able Capable of.

ac- *See* ad-.

-aceous Of the nature of, resembling, forming.

-acou- Hear. Alternative spelling, -acu-.

-acro- At an extremity, topmost.

-acu- 1. Needle. 2. *See* -acou-.

ad- To, toward. The prefix becomes *ac-*, *af-*, *ag-*, *ap-*, *as-*, or *at-* before words beginning with *c*, *f*, *g*, *p*, *s*, or *t* respectively.

-aden-, -adeno- Gland.

-adip-, -adipo- Fat. *See also* -lip- *and* -stear-.

-adren-, -adreno- Adrenal gland.

-aemia Of or in the blood. Alternative spelling, -emia.

-aer- Air, gas.

-aesthesi-, -aesthesio- Perception, feeling, sensation. Alternative spellings, -esthesi-, -esthesio-.

af- *See* ad-.

ag- *See* ad-.

-agra Painful seizure.

-alb- White. *See also* -leuc-(1).

-alg-, -algesi-, -algio-, -algo- Pain. *See also* -odyn-.

-algia Painful condition. *See also* -odynia.

-algio- *See* -alg-.

-algo- *See* -alg-.

-all-, -allo- Other, different, abnormal.

-alve- Channel, cavity.

amb-, ambi- On both sides.

-ambly- Dullness, dimness.

-amyl-, -amylo- Starch.

an- 1. *See* a-. 2. *See* ana-.

ana- 1. Up, upward, positive. 2. Back, backward. 3. Excessive, again.
The prefix becomes *an-* before a vowel.

-ancyl-, -ancylo- *See* -ankyl-.

-andr-, -andro- Male, man.

-angi-, -angio- A vessel, usually a blood vessel. *See also* -vas-.

-anis-, -aniso- Unequal, dissimilar, asymmetric.

-ankyl-, -ankylo- Bent, crooked, looped. Alternative spellings, -ancyl-, -ancylo-.

ant-, anti- Against, opposed to.

ante- Before, in front of.

-anthrop-, -anthropo- Human.

anti- *See* ant-.

ap- 1. *See* ad-. 2. *See* apo-.

apo- 1. Detached, separated. 2. Formed from. The prefix becomes *ap-* before a vowel.

-appendic-, -appendico- Appendix.

-arachn-, -arachno- 1. Arachnoid membrane. 2. Spider.

-arch-, -archae-, -arche-, -archi- 1. Original, first, primitive. 2. Leader.

-arter-, -arteri-, -arterio- Artery.

-arthr-, -arthro- Joint. *See also* -articul-.

-articul- Joint. *See also* -arthr-.

as- *See* ad-.

-ase Enzyme. *See also* -zym-.

-asis Condition, state of, process. *See also* -ia, -iasis, -ism, -osis, *and* -sis.

-astro- Star.

at- *See* ad-.

-atel-, -atelo- Incomplete, not perfect.

-atri-, -atrio- Atrium of the heart.

-aur-, -auri- Ear. *See also* -ot-.

aut-, auto- Self, self-induced.

-axi-, -axio- Axis.

azo- Signifies the presence of –N=N– in a molecule.

─────────── b ───────────

-bact-, -bacter-, -bacteri-, -bacterio- Bacteria.

-balan-, -balano- Glans penis or glans clitoridis.

-bar- Weight.

-bas-, -basi-, -basio-, -baso- 1. Base, foundation. 2. Chemical base.

bi- Two. *See also* -dipl- *and* dis-(2).

-bili- Bile. *See also* -chol-.

-bio- Life. *See also* -vit- *and* -zo-.

-blast-, -blasto- Germ, bud, embryonic cell.

-blenn-, -blenno- Mucus. *See also* -muc- *and* -myx-.

-blephar-, -blepharo- Eyelid. *See also* -cili-(2).

-brachi-, -brachio- Arm.

-brachy- Short.

-brady- Slow.

-brom-, -bromo- 1. The presence of bromine. 2. Smell.

-bronch-, -broncho- Bronchus.

-bucc-, -bucco- Cheek.

─────────── c ───────────

-cac-, -caco- Bad, abnormal. *See also* -dys- *and* mal-.

-caec-, -caeco- 1. Blind. 2. Caecum. Alternative spellings, -cec-, -ceco-. *See also* -typhl-.

-calc- 1. Stone. *See also* -lith-. 2. Heel. 3. Calcium. *See also* -calci-.

-calci-, -calco- Calcium or its salts. *See also* -calc-(3).

-canth-, -cantho- The angle of the eye.

-caps- Container.

-carb-, -carba-, -carbo- Charcoal, coal, carbon.

-carcin-, -carcino- Cancer, malignancy.

-card-, -cardi-, -cardio- 1. Heart. 2. The cardiac orifice of the stomach.

-carp- Wrist.

cata- Down, lower, under, against, negative.

-caud- Tail.

-cav- Hollow. *See also* -cel-(2), -cen-(1), *and* -coel-.

-cec-, -ceco- *See* -caec-.

-cel-, -celo- 1. Hernia, swelling, tumour. 2. Cavity, hollow. *See also* -cav- *and* -coel-. 3. Abdomen. *See also* -celi- *and* -ventr-(1).

-cele 1. Tumour, swelling, hernia. 2. Cavity. *See also* -coele.

-celi-, -celio- Abdomen. *See also* -cel-(3) *and* -ventr-(1).

-celo- *See* -cel-.

-cen-, -ceno- 1. Hollow, empty. *See also* -coen-.

-centesis Piercing, puncturing, perforating.

-cephal-, -cephalo- Head.

-ceptor Receiver, taker.

-cerebr-, -cerebro- Brain.

-cervic- Neck. *See also* -trachel-.

-cheil-, -cheilo- Lip. *See also* -labi-.

-chem-, -chemi-, -chemo- Chemical.

-chol-, -chole-, -cholo- Bile. *See also* -bili-.

-choledoch-, -choledocho- Common bile duct.

-cholo- *See* -chol-.

-chondr-, -chondro- Cartilage.

-chondri-, -chondrio- Granule.

-chondro- *See* -chondr-.

-chord-, -chordo- Cord.

-chrom-, -chromo- 1. Chromium. 2. Colour. *See also* -chromat-(2).

-chromat-, -chromato- 1. Chromatin. 2. Colour. *See also* -chrom-(2).

-chromo- *See* -chrom-.

-chron-, -chrono- Time.

-cide Killing, destroying. *See also* -cis-(2).

-cili-, -cilio- 1. Cilia, hair-like. 2. Eyelid. *See also* -blephar-. 3. Some internal structures of the eye.

circa-, circum- Around.

-cis- 1. Cut. *See also* -sect- *and* -tomy. 2. Kill. *See also* -cide.

-clas- Break.

co- *See* con-.

-coel-, -coelo- Cavity, hollow. *See also* -cav- *and* -cel-(2).

-coele Cavity, hollow. *See also* -cele(2).

-coelo- *See* -coel-.

-coen-, -coeno- Common feature, shared. Alternative spellings, -cen-, -ceno-.

-col- 1. Colon. 2. *See* con-.

-colp-, -colpo- Vagina. *See also* -vagin-.

com- *See* con-.

con- With, together. The prefix becomes *co-* before *h* or a vowel; *col-* before *l*; *com-* before *b*, *m*, or *p*; and *cor-* before *r*. *See also* syn-.

contra- Against, opposite.

-copr-, -copro- Faeces.

cor- *See* con-.

-corp-, -corpor- Body. *See also* -somat-.

-cortic-, -cortico- Cortex, rind.

-cost-, -costa- Rib. *See also* -pleur-(3).

-crani-, -cranio- Skull.

-crescent Grow, increase. *See also* -cret-(2).

-cret- 1. Separate, distinguish. 2. Grow, increase. *See also* -crescent.

-cry-, -cryo- Cold.

-crypt-, -crypto- Hidden, concealed.

-cut- Skin. *See also* -derm *and* -derma-.

-cyan-, -cyano- Blue.

-cycl-, -cyclo- 1. Round, circle, cycle. 2. Recurring.

-cyst-, -cysti-, -cysto- Bladder, cyst, sac. *See also* -vesic-.

-cyt-, -cyto- Cell.

-cyte Cell.

-cyto- *See* -cyt-.

---

d

-dacry-, -dacryo- Tears. *See also* -lachry-.

-dactyl-, -dactylo- Finger, toe. *See also* -phalang-.

de- Down, away, removal from.

-deca- Ten.

-dendr-, -dendro- Tree, tree-like structure.

-dent-, -denti-, -dento- Tooth. *See also* -odont-.

-derm Germ layer, skin. *See also* -cut- *and* -derma-.

-derma-, -dermat-, -dermato-, -dermo- Skin. *See also* -cut- *and* -derm.

-desis Binding, fusion.

-dextr-, -dextro- To the right.

di- 1. *See* dia-. 2. *See* dis-.

dia- Across, apart, between, completely, through. The prefix becomes *di-* before words beginning with a vowel.

-didym-, -didymo- Testis. *See also* -orch-.

-dipl-, -diplo- Twice. *See also* bi- *and* dis-(2).

dis- 1. Reversal, separation, apart. 2. Duplication. *See also* bi- *and* -dipl-.
The prefix becomes *di-* before words beginning with a consonant.

-dors-, -dorsi-, -dorso- 1. Back. 2. Back of the body.

-drom-, -dromo- Course, running, conduction.

-dur- Hard. *See also* -scirrh- *and* -scler-(1).

-dynam-, -dynami- Power.

-dys- Bad, difficult, disordered, painful. *See also* -cac- *and* mal-.

---

e

e- Out from, away from, expel. *See also* ex-.

ect-, ecto- Outside, outer, outermost.

-ectasia, -ectasis Dilatation, distension, expansion.

ecto- *See* ect-.

-ectomise, -ectomy Removal of.

-ede- *See* -oede-.

em- *See* en-.

-emia *See* -aemia.

en- Into, on, inside. The prefix becomes *em-* before *b*, *p*, or *ph*.

-encephal-, -encephalo- Brain.

end-, endo- Within, inner.

-enter-, -entero- Intestine.

ep- *See* epi-.

epi- Upon, over, above, in addition, outer. The prefix becomes *ep-* before a vowel.

-epitheli-, -epithelio- Epithelium.

-eryth-, -erythr-, -erythro- Red, redness. *See also* -rub-.

-eso- Within, inside. *See also* intra-.

-esthesi-, -esthesio- *See* -aesthesi-.

-eu- Good, well, easily.

ex- Out of. *See also* e-.

exo- External, outward.

extra- Outside, beyond, in addition to.

─────────────── f ───────────────

-faci- Face.

-facient Make, causing to become.

-febr- Fever. *See also* -pyr- *and* -pyret-.

-ferent Carry.

-ferr-, -ferro- Iron.

-fibr-, -fibro- Fibre.

-fiss- Split.

-flagell- Whip.

-flect- Bend, divert. *See also* -flex-.

-flex- Bend, divert. *See also* -flect-.

-flu- Flow. *See also* -flux-.

-flux- Flow. *See also* -flu-.

-form Shape, resembling. *See also* -oid.

-funct- Perform, serve.

-fund- Pour. *See also* -fus-.

-fus- Pour. *See also* -fund-.

─────────────── g ───────────────

-galact-, -galacto- Milk. *See also* -lact-(1).

-gam-, -gamo- Marriage, sexual union. *See also* -gamet- *and* -zyg-.

-gamet-, -gameto- Refers to a gamete. *See also* -gam-.

-gamo- *See* -gam-.

-gangli-, -ganglio- Swelling.

-gastr-, -gastro- Stomach.

-ge-, -geo- Soil, earth.

-gen-, -geno- 1. Reproduction, producing. *See also* -genic, -genous(2), *and* -gon-(3). 2. Gene. 3. Race.

-genic Producing. *See also* -gen-(1), -genous(2), *and* -gon-(3).

-genit-, -genito- Reproductive organs. *See also* -gon-(2).

-geno- *See* -gen-.

-genous 1. Produced by, arising from. 2. Producing. *See also* -gen-(1), -genic, *and* -gon-(3).

-geo- *See* -ge-.

-ger-, -gero- Old age. *See also* -presby-.

-germ- Bud.

-gero- *See* -ger-.

-gingiv-, -gingivo- Gingivae, gums.

-gli-, -glio- 1. Glue-like. *See also* -glutin-. 2. Neuroglia.

-glomerul-, -glomerulo- Glomeruli of the kidneys.

-gloss-, -glosso- Tongue. *See also* -glott- *and* -lingu-.

-glott- Tongue. *See also* -gloss- *and* -lingu-.

-gluc-, -gluco- Sweet, glucose. *See also* -glyc-(1).

-glutin- Glue. *See also* -gli-(1).

-glyc-, -glyco- 1. Sweet, sugar. *See also* -gluc-. 2. Glycerin. 3. Glycogen.

-gnath-, -gnatho- Jaw.

-gno- Know.

-gon-, -gono- 1. Seed. *See also* -sperm-. 2. Reproductive organs. *See also* -genit-. 3. Reproduction. *See also* -gen-(1), -genic, *and* -genous(2).

-grad- Step, walk.

-gram Recorded, written. *See also* -graph- *and* -graphy.

-gran- Grain.

-graph-, -grapho- Write, record. *See also* -gram *and* -graphy.

-graphy Write, record. *See also* -gram *and* -graph-.

-grav- Heavy.

-gyn-, -gynaeco-, -gyne-, -gyno- Female, woman.

─────────────── h ───────────────

-haem-, -haemat-, -haemato-, -haemo- Blood. Alternative spellings, -hem-, -hemat-, -hemato-, -hemo-. *See also* -sangui-.

-hamart-, -hamarto- Fault.

-hapl-, -haplo- Single, simple. *See also* -mon- *and* uni-.

-hem-, -hemat-, -hemato- *See* -haem-.

-hemi- Half. *See also* -semi-.

-hepat-, -hepato- Liver.

-hept-, -hepta- Seven. *See also* -sept-(1).

-hered- Heir.

-herpet-, -herpeto- 1. Herpes. 2. Reptile.

-heter-, -hetero- Other, different.

-hex-, -hexa- Six.

-hidr-, -hidro- Sweat.

-hist-, -histio-, -histo- Tissue.

-homeo- *See* -homo-.

-homo-, -homoeo- Unchanging, same, steady. Alternative spelling, -homeo-.

-hydr-, -hydro- Water, hydrogen.

hyp-, hypo- Under, beneath, below, deficient, less than normal. *See also* infra- *and* sub-.

hyper- Above, beyond, excessive, over, above normal. *See also* super- *and* ultra-.

-hypn-, -hypno- Sleep. *See also* -somn-.

hypo- *See* hyp-.

-hyster-, -hystero- 1. Uterus. *See also* -metr-(2). 2. Hysteria.

--------------------- i ---------------------

-ia Condition, state. *See also* -asis, -iasis, -ism, -osis, *and* -sis.

-iasis Condition, process, particularly a morbid one. *See also* -asis, -ia, -ism, -osis, *and* -sis.

-iatr-, -iatric-, -iatro- Physician, medicine, medical treatment.

-ichthy-, -ichthyo- Fish.

-idio- Self, one's own.

il- *See* in-.

-ile-, -ileo- Ileum.

-ili-, -ilio- Ilium.

im- *See* in-.

in- 1. In, on. 2. Implies a negative. The prefix becomes *il-* or *ir-* before words beginning with *l* or *r* respectively, and *im-* before words beginning with *b*, *m*, or *p*.

infra- Below, beneath. *See also* hyp- *and* sub-.

inter- Between, among.

intra- Within, on the inside. *See also* -eso-.

ir- *See* in-.

-irid-, -irido- Iris of the eye, iridescent.

-isch-, -ischo- Deficiency, suppression.

-ism Condition, state, action. *See also* -asis, -ia, -iasis, -osis, *and* -sis.

iso- Equal, alike.

-itis Inflammation.

--------------------- j ---------------------

-ject- Throw.

-jejun-, -jejuno- 1. Jejunum. 2. Hunger.

-junct- Join.

--------------------- k ---------------------

-kary-, -karyo- Nucleus.

-kerat-, -kerato- 1. Horn. 2. Cornea.

keto- Signifies the presence of the carbonyl group ($>C=O$) in a molecule.

-kine-, -kinesi-, -kinesio- Motion.

--------------------- l ---------------------

-labi-, -labio- Lip. *See also* -cheil-.

-lachry- Tears. *See also* -dacry-.

-lact-, -lacto- 1. Milk. *See also* -galact-. 2. Lactic acid.

-laev-, -laevo- To the left. Alternative spellings, -lev-, -levo-.

-lal-, -lalo- Speech, talk, babble. *See also* -lexis *and* -pha-.

-lapar-, -laparo- Flank, loins, abdomen.

-laryng-, -laryngo- Larynx.

-later-, -latero- Side.

-legia Reading. *See also* -lexis.

-leio- Smooth.

-lent- Lentil.

-lep- Seize.

-lepsis, -lepsy Seizure.

-leuc-, -leuco- 1. White. *See also* -alb-. 2. Leucocyte. Alternative spellings, -leuk-, -leuko-.

-leuk-, -leuko- *See* -leuc-.

-lev-, -levo- *See* -laev-.

-lexis, -lexy Speech. Often used instead of -legia to denote reading. *See also* -lal- *and* -pha-.

-lig- Bind, tie.

-lingu- Tongue. *See also* -gloss- *and* -glott-.

-lip-, -lipo- Fat. *See also* -adip- *and* -stear-.

-lith-, -litho- Stone, calculus. *See also* -calc-(1).

-logy Study of, science of.

-ly-, -lys-, -lyso- Loose, dissolve.

-lymph-, -lympho- 1. Lymph, lymphatic system, lymphocytes, or lymphoid tissue. 2. Water.

-lys- *See* -ly-.

-lysis Loosening, dissolving.

-lyso- *See* -ly-.

--------------------- m ---------------------

-macr-, -macro- Large. *See also* -mega-(1) *and* -megal-.

mal- Bad, abnormal. *See also* -cac- *and* -dys-.

-malacia Softening.

-mamm-, -mammo- Breast. *See also* -mast-(1).

-man- Hand.

-mania An abnormal preoccupation.

-mast-, -masto- 1. Breast. *See also* -mamm-. 2. Mastoid process.

-medi-, -medio- Middle. *See also* -mes-.

-medullo- Medulla.

-mega- 1. Great, large. *See also* -macro- *and* -megal-. 2. One million or a million times.

-megal-, -megalo- Large. *See also* -macro- *and* -mega-(1).

-megaly Enlarged.

-meio- Less, smaller. Alternative spelling, -mio-.

-melan-, -melano- Black, dark.

-men-, -meno- 1. Month. 2. Menses.

-mening-, -meningo- Membrane, meninges.

-meno- *See* men-.

-mer-, -mero- 1. Part. 2. Thigh.

-mere Part, segment.

-mero- *See* -mer-.

-mes-, -meso- Middle. *See also* -medi-.

meta- 1. After, beyond. 2. Change.

-metr- 1. Measure. 2. Uterus. *See also* -hyster-(1).

-metra-, -metro- *See* -metr-(2).

-micro- 1. Small. 2. One-millionth.

-mio- *See* -meio-.

-mit-, -mito- Thread-like.

-mne-, -mnem-, -mnes- Memory, remember.

-mon-, -mono- Single. *See also* -hapl- *and* uni-.

-morph-, -morpho- Form, shape.

-mot- Move.

-muc-, -muco- Mucus. *See also* -blenn- *and* -myx-.

multi- Many. *See also* poly-.

-my-, -myo- Muscle.

-myc-, -mycet-, -myceto-, -myco- Fungus.

-myel-, -myelo- 1. Bone marrow. 2. Spinal cord. 3. Myelin.

-myo- *See* -my-.

-myring-, -myringo- Tympanic membrane.

-myx-, -myxo- Mucus, slime. *See also* -blenn- *and* -muc-.

---

n

-naev-, -naevo- Mole, naevus. Alternative spellings, -nev-, -nevo-.

-narc-, -narco- Stupor, numbness.

-nas-, -naso- Nose.

-ne-, -neo- New.

-necr-, -necro- Dead.

-neo- *See* -ne-.

-nephr-, -nephro- Kidney. *See also* -ren-.

-neur-, -neuro- Nerve.

-nev-, -nevo- *See* -naev-.

-nod- Knot.

-nom-, -nomo- Law, usage, custom.

non- Implies a negative.

-non-, -nona- Nine.

-norm-, -normo- Usual, normal.

-nos-, -noso- Disease. *See also* -path- *and* -pathy.

-nucl-, -nucle-, -nucleo- Kernel, nucleus.

-nutri- Nourish. *See also* -troph- *and* -trophic.

---

o

-octa- Eight.

-ocul-, -oculo- Eye. *See also* -ophthalm-.

-odont-, -odonto- Tooth. *See also* -dent-.

-odyn-, -odyno- Pain, distress. *See also* -alg-.

-odynia Painful condition. *See also* -algia.

-odyno- *See* -odyn-.

-oede- Swell. Alternative spelling, -ede-.

-oid Having the form of, resembling. *See also* -form.

-ol Denotes an alcoholic or phenolic compound.

-ole-, -oleo- Oil.

-olig-, -oligo- Little, few, scanty. *See also* -pauci-.

-oma Abnormal growth, neoplasm, tumour.

-omphal-, -omphalo- Umbilicus, navel.

-onc-, -onco- Swelling, mass, tumour.

-onych-, -onycho- Nails of fingers or toes.

-oo- Egg, ovum. *See also* -ov-.

-oophor-, -oophoro- Ovary.

-ophthalm-, -ophthalmo- Eye. *See also* -ocul-.

-opia Vision.

-or-, -oro- Mouth. *See also* -stom-.

-orb- 1. Circle, sphere. *See also* -spher-. 2. Eyeball.

-orch-, -orchi-, -orchid-, -orchido-, -orchio- Testis. *See also* -didym-.

-oro- *See* -or-.

-orth-, -ortho- Straight, upright, normal, correct.

-ose 1. Full of. *See also* -ous. 2. Carbohydrate.

-osis Action, condition, process, especially a morbid one. Often used to denote an abnormal increase. *See also* -asis, -ia, -iasis, -ism, *and* -sis.

-osm-, -osmo-   1. Osmosis. 2. Odour.

-oss-   Bone. *See also* -ost-.

-ost-, -oste-, -osteo-   Bone. *See also* -oss-.

-ot-, -oto-   Ear. *See also* -aur-.

-ous   Possessing, full of. *See also* -ose(1).

-ov-, -ovi-, -ovo-   Egg, ovum. *See also* -oo-.

-ox-, -oxy-   1. Oxygen. 2. Pointed. 3. Acid.

--------------------- p ---------------------

-paed-, -paedo-   Child. Alternative spellings, -ped-, -pedo-.

pan-   All, completely, entire.

par-   *See* para-.

-par-   To give birth to; bear. *See also* -part-.

para-   Near, beyond, apart from, beside, abnormal. The prefix becomes par- before a vowel.

-part-   To give birth to; bear. *See also* -par-.

-path-, -patho-   Disease. *See also* -nos- *and* -pathy.

-pathy   Disease. *See also* -nos- *and* -path-.

-pauci-   Few. *See also* -olig-.

-ped-, -pedo-   1. Foot. *See also* -pod-. 2. *See* -paed-.

-pend-   Hang down.

-penia   Deficiency of.

-pent-, -penta-   Five.

-pep-, -peps-, -pept-   Digest.

per-   Through. *See also* trans-.

peri-   Around, about, surrounding.

-peritone-, -peritoneo-   Peritoneum.

-pexy   Fixing, fixation.

-pha-   Speak. *See also* -lal- *and* -lexis.

-phac-, -phaco-   1. The lens of the eye. 2. Freckle, mole. Alternative spellings, -phak-, -phako-.

-phag-, -phago-   Eat, ingest, engulf.

-phagia, -phagy   Eating, swallowing.

-phago-   *See* -phag-.

-phagy   *See* -phagia.

-phak-, -phako-   *See* -phac-.

-phalang-, -phalango-   The bones of the fingers or toes. *See also* -dactyl-.

-pharmac-, -pharmaco-   Drug, medicine.

-pharyng-, -pharyngo-   Pharynx.

-phen-, -pheno-   1. Show, display. 2. Refers to benzene.

-phil, -phile, -philia, -philic   Like, have an affinity for, attraction. *See also* -tropin.

philo-   Affinity for, attraction.

-phleb-, -phlebo-   Vein. *See also* -ven-.

-phobe, -phobia   Abnormal fear of, aversion to.

-phon-, -phono-   Sound.

-phore   Denotes a carrier.

-phot-, -photo-   Light.

-phrag-   Fence in, block.

-phren-, -phreno-   1. Mind. *See also* -psych- *and* -thym-(1). 2. Diaphragm.

-physio-   1. Nature. 2. Physiology. 3. Physical.

-phyt-, -phyto-   Plant.

-phyte   1. Plant. 2. Pathological growth.

-phyto-   *See* -phyt-.

-pil-, -pilo-   Hair. *See also* -trich-.

-plas-   Mould, shape.

-plasia   Development, formation.

-plasty   Moulding, shaping; plastic surgery.

-plegia   Paralysis, stroke.

-pleo-   More.

-pleur-, -pleuro-   1. Pleura. 2. Side. 3. Rib. *See also* -cost-.

-ploid   Refers to the degree of multiplication of chromosome sets.

-pnea   *See* -pnoea.

-pneo-   Breath, blowing, respiration. *See also* -pneuma-(2), -pneumo-(2), -pnoea, -spir-(2), *and* -spirat-.

-pneuma-, -pneumat-, -pneumato-   1. Air, gas. *See also* -pneumo-(1). 2. Breath, respiration. *See also* -pneo-, -pneumo-(2), -pnoea, -spir-(2), *and* -spirat-.

-pneumo-, -pneumon-, -pneumono-   1. Air, gas. *See also* -pneuma-(1). 2. Respiration. *See also* -pneo-, -pneuma-(2), -pnoea, -spir-(2), *and* -spirat-. 3. Lungs. *See also* -pulmo-.

-pnoea   Breathing, respiration. Alternative spelling, -pnea. *See also* -pneo-, -pneuma-(2), -pneumo-(2), -spir-(2), *and* -spirat-.

-pod-, -podo-   Foot. *See also* -ped-.

-poie-   Make.

-poiesis   Formation, production.

poly-   Much, many. *See also* multi-.

post-   After, beyond, behind.

prae-, pre-   Before, in front of. *See also* pro-.

-prax-   Conduct, action.

pre-   *See* prae-.

-presby-, -presbyo-   Old age. *See also* -ger-.

pro-   Before, in front of. *See also* prae-.

-proct-, -procto-   Anus, rectum. *See also* -rect-.

-pseud-, -pseudo-   False, spurious, apparent.

-psych-, -psycho-   Mind. *See also* -phren-(1) *and* -thym-(1).

-ptosis   Falling, sinking down, drooping.

-pulmo-, -pulmon-, -pulmono-   Lungs. *See also* -pneumo-(3).

-pur-   Pus. *See also* -py-.

-py-, -pyo-   Pus. *See also* -pur-.

-pyel-, -pyelo-   Pelvis of the kidney.

-pykn-, -pykno-   Thick, frequent, compact.

-pylor-, -pyloro-   Pylorus.

-pyo-   *See* -py-.

-pyr-, -pyro-   Fire, heat. *See also* -febr- *and* -pyret-.

-pyret-, -pyreto-   Fever. *See also* -febr- *and* -pyr-.

-pyro-   *See* -pyr-.

---

q

quadr-, quadri-   Four.

---

r

-rachi-, -rachio-   Spine.

-radi-, -radio-   Ray, radiation.

re-   Back, again.

-rect-, -recto-   Rectum. *See also* -proct-.

-ren-, -reno-   Kidney. *See also* -nephr-.

-ret-   Net.

retro-   Backwards, back, lying, situated behind.

-rhea, -rrhea   *See* -rhoea.

-rhex-   Burst, break.

-rhin-, -rhino-   Nose.

-rhoea, -rrhoea   Flowing, running. Alternative spellings, -rhea, -rrhea.

-rrhage, -rrhagia   Excessive or unusual flow or discharge.

-rrhea   *See* -rhoea.

-rrhoea   *See* -rhoea.

-rub-, -rubr-   Red. *See also* -eryth-.

---

s

-sacr-, -sacro-   Sacrum.

-salp-, -salping-, -salpingo-   Tube. *See also* -syring-.

-sangui-, -sanguin-   Blood. *See also* -haem-.

-sapr-, -sapro-   Decaying, putrid, rotten.

-sarc-, -sarco-   Flesh, substance of muscles.

-scirrh-, -scirrho-   Hard. *See also* -dur- *and* -scler-(1).

-scler-, -sclero-   1. Hard. *See also* -dur- *and* -scirrh-. 2. Sclera.

-scope   Instrument for examining.

-scopy   Examining.

-seb-, -sebi-, -sebo-   Sebum, sebaceous.

-sect-   Cut. *See also* -cis-(1) *and* -tomy.

-semi-   Half. *See also* -hemi-.

-sens-   Feel, perceive.

-sep-   Decay, rot.

-sept-   1. Seven. *See also* -hept-. 2. Septum, partition.

-ser-   Whey, watery.

-sial-, -sialo-   Saliva, salivary glands.

-sin-, -sinu-   Hollow, fold.

-sis   Condition, state. *See also* -asis, -ia, -iasis, -ism, *and* -osis.

-somat-, -somato-   Body. *See also* -corp-.

-some   Body.

-somn-, -somni-   Sleep. *See also* -hypn-.

-spas-   Pull, draw. *See also* -tract-.

-sperm-, -spermat-, -spermato-, -spermo-   Seed. *See also* -gon-(1).

-spher-, -sphero-   Ball, sphere. *See also* -orb-(1).

-sphygmo-   Pulse.

-spir-, -spiro-   1. Spiral, coil. 2. Breath, breathing. *See also* -pneo-, -pneuma-(2), -pneumo-(2), -pnoea, *and* -spirat-.

-spirat-   Breathe. *See also* -pneo-, -pneuma-(2), -pneumo-(2), -pnoea, *and* -spir-(2).

-spiro-   *See* -spir-.

-splen-, -spleno-   Spleen.

-spondyl-, -spondylo-   Vertebra.

-spor-, -sporo-   Spore.

-squam-, -squamo-   Scale.

-stal-, -stol-   Send.

-stasis   1. Stand still. 2. Slowing, stopping.

-stat   Stationary, fixed.

-stear-, -stearo-, -steat-, -steato-   Fat. *See also* -adip- *and* -lip-.

-steat-, -steato-   *See* -stear-.

-sten-, -steno-   Narrow, contracted.

-ster-   Solid.

-sterco-   Faeces.

-stern-, -sterno-   Sternum.

-stig-   Spot, mark.

-stol-   *See* stal-.

-stom-, -stomat-, -stomato-, -stomo-   Mouth, orifice. *See also* -or-.

-stomy   Making an opening; an artificial opening created surgically.

-strict-   Compress, tighten, cause pain. *See also* -stringent.

-stringent Compress, tighten, cause pain. *See also* -strict-.

sub- Under, near, almost, support. The prefix becomes *suf-* or *sup-* before words beginning with *f* or *p* respectively. *See also* hyp- *and* infra-.

suf- *See* sub-.

sup- *See* sub-.

super- Above, beyond, excess. *See also* hyper-, supra-, *and* ultra-.

supra- Above, over. *See also* super-.

sym- *See* syn-.

syn- With, together, merging, together, joined, alike. The prefix becomes *sym-* before *b*, *m*, or *p*. *See also* con-.

-syndesm-, -syndesmo- Ligament.

-synovi-, -synovio- Synovial membrane.

-syring-, -syringo- Pipe, tube, cavity, fistula. *See also* -salp-.

---

t

-tachy- Rapid, swift.

-tact- Touch.

-tars-, -tarso- 1. Margin of the eyelid. 2. Instep of the foot.

-tax- Arrange, order.

-tempor- 1. Time. 2. Refers to the forehead.

-ten-, -teno-, -tenont- Tendon.

-tens- Stretch. *See also* -ton-(1).

-terat-, -terato- Monster.

-thec- Sheath, case.

-therap- Treatment.

-therm-, -thermo- Heat.

-thorac-, -thoraco- Chest.

-thromb-, -thrombo- Clot, thrombus.

-thym-, -thymo- 1. Mind, soul, emotions. *See also* -phren-(1) *and* -psych-. 2. Thymus gland.

-thyr-, -thyro- Thyroid gland, shield-shaped.

-tomy Cutting; surgical cutting or incision. *See also* -cis-(1) *and* -sect-.

-ton- 1. Stretch, under tension. *See also* -tens-. 2. Tone.

-top-, -topo- Place.

-tors- Twist.

-tox-, -toxi-, -toxico-, -toxo- Poison.

-trache-, -tracheo- Trachea, windpipe.

-trachel-, -trachelo- Neck, constriction. *See also* -cervic-.

-tracheo- *See* trache-.

-tract- Draw, drag. *See also* -spas-.

trans- Across, through, beyond. *See also* per-.

-traumat-, -traumato- Wound.

-tri- Three.

-trich-, -tricho- Hair. *See also* -pil-.

-tripsy Crushed.

-troph-, -tropho- Nutrition. *See also* -nutri-.

-trophic, -trophin, -trophy Nutrition, growth. *See also* -nutri-.

-trophin *See* -trophic.

-tropho- *See* -troph-.

-trophy *See* -trophic.

-tropic Turning towards, influencing.

-tropin Having an affinity for. *See also* -phil.

-typhl-, -typhlo- 1. Blind. 2. Caecum (blind gut). *See also* -caec-.

-tyr-, -tyro- Cheese.

---

u

ultra- Excess, beyond. *See also* hyper- *and* super-.

uni- One. *See also* -hapl- *and* -mon-.

-ur-, -uro-, -uron-, -urono- 1. Urine. *See also* -uria *and* -uric-(1). 2. Urinary tract.

-ureter-, -uretero- Ureter.

-urethr-, -urethro- Urethra.

-uria Of or in the urine. *See also* -ur-(1) *and* -uric-(1).

-uric-, -urico- 1. Urine. *See also* -ur-(1) *and* -uria. 2. Uric acid.

-uro-, -uron-, -urono- *See* -ur-.

-uter-, -utero- Uterus.

---

v

-vagin-, -vagino- Sheath, vagina. *See also* -colp-.

-varic-, -varico- 1. Twisted, swollen. 2. Varicose vein.

-vas-, -vaso- Vessel, duct. *See also* -angi-.

-ven-, -veno- Vein. *See also* -phleb-.

-ventr-, -ventri-, -ventro- 1. Abdomen. *See also* -cel-(3) *and* -celi-. 2. Front of the body.

-ventricul-, -ventriculo- Ventricle of the heart or brain.

-ventro- *See* -ventr-.

-vermi- Worm.

-vers- Turn. *See also* -vert-.

-vert- Turn. *See also* -vers-.

-vertebr-, -vertebro- Vertebra, vertebral column.

-vesic, -vesico- Bladder, blister. *See also* -cyst-.

-viscer-, -viscero- Organ.

-vit- Life. *See also* -bio- *and* -zo-.

—————————— X ——————————

-xanth-, -xantho- Yellow.

-xen-, -xeno- Strange, foreign.

-xer-, -xero- Dry.

-xyl-, -xylo- Wood.

—————————— Z ——————————

-zo-, -zoo- Animal, life. *See also* -bio- *and* -vit-.

-zyg-, -zygo- Union, joining. *See also* -gam-.

-zym-, -zymo- 1. Enzyme. *See also* -ase. 2. Fermentation.

SELECTED BIBLIOGRAPHY AND REFERENCE SOURCES

This section provides a list of books to enable pharmacists to study the background details relevant to the topics covered in this book. It also serves as a guide to further reading and provides reference sources. Details are included under the following classification:

- anatomy and physiology
- geriatrics
- medical dictionaries
- medicine
- microbiology
- paediatrics
- pathology
- pharmacy
- professional and self-help organisations.

Price Bands

A	up to £9.99	Price bands provide an indication
B	£10 to £19.99	of the relative cost of books. They
C	£20 to £29.99	serve as a basis of comparison, and
D	£30 to £39.99	have been checked prior to going to
E	£40 to £49.99	press.
F	over £50	

Anatomy and Physiology

Gray's Anatomy
P L Williams *et al*
37th Edition
Edinburgh, Churchill Livingstone, 1989
Price band: F

Principles of Anatomy and Physiology
G J Tortora and N P Anagnostakos
5th Edition
New York, Harper & Row, 1987
Price band: B

Geriatrics

Practical Geriatric Medicine
A N Exton-Smith and M E Weksler (Eds)
Edinburgh, Churchill Livingstone, 1985
Price band: E

Medical Dictionaries

Black's Medical Dictionary
W A R Thomson
35th Edition
London, Adam & Charles Black, 1987
Price band: B

Concise Medical Dictionary
E A Martin (Ed)
2nd Edition Oxford, Oxford University Press, 1985
Price band: A

Dorland's Illustrated Medical Dictionary
27th Edition
Philadelphia, W B Saunders, 1988
Price band: C

Heinemann Medical Dictionary
B Lennox and M E Lennox
London, William Heinemann, 1986
Price band: B

Stedman's Medical Dictionary
24th Edition
Baltimore, Williams & Wilkins, 1982
Price band: D

Medicine

Cecil Textbook of Medicine
J B Wyngaarden and L H Smith (Eds)
18th Edition
Philadelphia, W B Saunders, 1988
Price band: F

Clinical Medicine
P J Kumar and M L Clark (Eds)
London, Baillière Tindall, 1987
Price band: B

Davidson's Principles and Practice of Medicine
J Macleod, C Edwards, and I Bouchier (Eds)
15th Edition
Edinburgh, Churchill Livingstone, 1988
Price band: B

The Merck Manual of Diagnosis and Therapy
R Berkow (Ed)
15th Edition
Rahway, NJ, Merck Sharp & Dohme Research, 1987
Price band: B

Modern Medicine
A E Read, D W Barrit, and R Langton Hewer (Eds)
3rd Edition
Edinburgh, Churchill Livingstone, 1986
Price band: C

Oxford Handbook of Clinical Medicine
R A Hope and J M Longmore
Oxford, Oxford University Press, 1985
Price band: A

Oxford Handbook of Clinical Specialties
J A B Collier and J M Longmore
2nd Edition
Oxford, Oxford University Press, 1989
Price band: B

Oxford Textbook of Medicine
D J Wetherall, J G G Ledingham, and
    D A Warrell (Eds)
2nd Edition (2 vols)
Oxford, Oxford University Press, 1987
Price band: F

Oxford Textbook of Psychiatry
M Gelder, D Gath, and R Mayou
2nd Edition
Oxford, Oxford University Press, 1989
Price band: C

Parson's Diseases of the Eye
S J H Miller (Reviser)
17th Edition
Edinburgh, Churchill Livingstone, 1984
Price band: C

Roxburgh's Common Skin Diseases
J D Kirby (Reviser)
15th Edition
London, H K Lewis, 1986
Price band: B

Textbook of Dermatology
A J Rook *et al* (Eds)
4th Edition (3 vols)
Oxford, Blackwell Scientific Publications, 1986
Price band: F

Textbook of Medical Treatment
R H Girdwood and J C Petrie
15th Edition
Edinburgh, Churchill Livingstone, 1987
Price band: C

Microbiology

Bergey's Manual of Systematic Bacteriology
Vol I – J G Holt and N R Krieg (Eds)
Vol II – P Sneath
London, Williams & Wilkins, 1984 and 1986
Price band: F

Pharmaceutical Microbiology
W B Hugo and A D Russell
4th Edition
Oxford, Blackwell Scientific Publications, 1987
Price band: C

Topley and Wilson's Principles of Bacteriology,
    Virology, and Immunity
W W C Topley and G S Wilson
7th Edition (4 vols)
London, Edward Arnold, 1983 and 1984
Price band: F

Paediatrics

Essential Paediatrics
D Hull and D I Johnson
2nd Edition
Edinburgh, Churchill Livingstone, 1987
Price band: B

Pediatrics
H M Maurer (Ed)
New York, Churchill Livingstone, 1983
Price band: C

Pathology

Essential Allergy
N Mygind
Oxford, Blackwell Scientific Publications, 1986
Price band: B

Immunology
I Roitt, J Brostoff, and D Male
2nd Edition
Edinburgh, Churchill Livingstone, 1989
Price band: B

Immunology: An Illustrated Outline
D Male
Edinburgh, Churchill Livingstone, 1986
Price band: A

An Introduction to General Pathology
W G Spector
3rd Edition
Edinburgh, Churchill Livingstone, 1989
Price band: A

Muir's Textbook of Pathology
J R Anderson (Ed)
12th Edition
London, Edward Arnold, 1985
Price band: D

Pathology Illustrated
A T Govan, P S Macfarlane, and R Callander
2nd Edition
Edinburgh, Churchill Livingstone, 1986
Price band: B

Processes in Pathology
M J Taussig
3rd Edition
Oxford, Blackwell Scientific Publications, 1984
Price band: B

Pharmacy

British National Formulary
Royal Pharmaceutical Society of Great Britain and the
  British Medical Association
Number 19
London, The Pharmaceutical Press, 1990 (twice yearly)
Price band: A

Drug Abuse: A Guide for Pharmacists
D H Maddock
London, The Pharmaceutical Press, 1987
Price band: A

Handbook of Non-prescription Drugs
American Pharmaceutical Association
8th Edition
Washington, American Pharmaceutical Association,
  1986
Price band: F

Martindale: The Extra Pharmacopoeia
J E F Reynolds (Ed)
29th Edition
London, The Pharmaceutical Press, 1989
Price band: F

Minor Illness or Major Disease?
C Edwards and P Stillman
London, The Pharmaceutical Press, 1982
Price band: A

Patient Care in Community Practice: A Handbook of
  Non-medicinal Health-care
R J Harman
London, The Pharmaceutical Press, 1989
Price band: B

USP DI
Vols IA and IB: Drug Information for the Health Care
  Professional; Vol II: Advice for the Patient
10th Edition
Rockville MD, USP Corporation, 1990
Price band: F

Professional and Self-help Organisations

Directory of British Associations and Associations in
  Ireland
G P Henderson and S P A Henderson
9th Edition
Beckenham, CBD Research, 1988
Price band: F

The Self-help Guide: A Directory of Self-help
  Organisations in the United Kingdom
S Knight and R Gann
London, Chapman and Hall, 1988
Price band: A

INDEX

Items not found in the Index may be located in the Glossary.

Items not found in the Index may be located in the Glossary.

Items not found in the Index may be located in the Glossary.

Items not found in the Index may be located in the Glossary.

Items not found in the Index may be located in the Glossary.

Items not found in the Index may be located in the Glossary.

Items not found in the Index may be located in the Glossary.

Items not found in the Index may be located in the Glossary.

Items not found in the Index may be located in the Glossary.

Items not found in the Index may be located in the Glossary.

Items not found in the Index may be located in the Glossary.

Items not found in the Index may be located in the Glossary.

Items not found in the Index may be located in the Glossary.

Items not found in the Index may be located in the Glossary.

Items not found in the Index may be located in the Glossary.

Items not found in the Index may be located in the Glossary.